THE HISTORY OF
VETERINARY MEDICINE AND THE
ANIMAL–HUMAN RELATIONSHIP

THE HISTORY OF VETERINARY MEDICINE AND THE ANIMAL–HUMAN RELATIONSHIP

Bruce Vivash Jones

BVetSts, MRCVS, DVetMed(Hon)

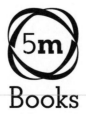

5m
Books

Published by
5M Books Ltd,
Lings, Great Easton,
Essex CM6 2HH, UK,
Tel: +44 (0) 330 1333 580
www.5mbooks.com

A Catalogue record for this book is available from the British Library

ISBN 9781789181180 (hardback)
ISBN 9781789181821 (special binding)
eISBN 9781789181807
DOI 10.52517.9781789181807

Cover graphic: The Uffington White Horse, Oxfordshire – the oldest chalk-cut hill figure in Britain (dated to between 1380 and 550 BCE) – was selected for the cover as a representation of both the long history of the animal–human relationship and of the significance of each to one another.

Book layout by Cheshire Typesetting Ltd, Cuddington, Cheshire
Printed by TJ Books Ltd, Padstow, Cornwall

Dedicated to

those who studied the art and established
the science of veterinary medicine thereby
creating our history

Veterinary medicine is formally one and the same with the better known human medicine, differing simply in the dignity or nobility of the subject

Giovanni Filippo Ingrassia (c.1510–1580)

Animals whom we have made our slaves, we do not like to consider them our equals

Charles Darwin (1809–1882)

Contents

The plates are located between pages 266 and 267

Preface

Early in my veterinary life, when working in the Pathology Department at the Royal Veterinary College London, I was unpacking specimen jars that had been stored for safety at the outbreak of war in 1939. One jar intrigued me; it contained a human heart. It was from Sir Frederick Smith (1857–1929), he had cardiac disease and had requested that his heart be preserved as a teaching aid for students. I investigated and found that he had been a notable veterinarian, soldier, researcher and veterinary historian. I read his books and learned of the history of veterinary medicine; my interest was aroused.

Over the following years I worked in many veterinary capacities around the world, I visited veterinary schools, museums and the site of the original Lyon Veterinary School in France. I began to build a library, joined the British Veterinary History Society, started my own studies, published them and wrote three veterinary historical books, all based around individuals and their lives (one of course devoted to Sir Frederick Smith).

The year 2011 was declared World Veterinary Year with the World Veterinary Association Congress held in Cape Town, South Africa. I was invited to open the Veterinary History Session and spoke on *The Importance of Veterinary History*, reviewing the story from 2000 BC to the 20th century – 4000 years: our history. I emphasised that a knowledge of veterinary history is both important and relevant as it is inseparably allied with progress in social evolution. Judging from the many audience questions I decided it was time for a new examination of the history, from the art to the science.

I realised it was a big subject and would take time, but I wanted to explain the chronology, with the different inputs from the major world civilisations, together with my particular interest, the people who made this history, both good and not-so-good. In 2012 I decided I had better commence writing.

As I was starting at the beginning, about 2000 BC, I thought I should see the two first texts indicating that the veterinary art was known. One, the El-Kahun (or Lahun) veterinary papyrus, is in London at the Petrie Museum of Egyptian Archaeology and the other, the Hammurabi Code with its 282 Laws carved on a magnificent diorite stele is now in the Louvre Museum, so I went to Paris. These two objects made me realise the wisdom of Desiderius Erasmus who wrote in the early 1500s, that to be educated one should read the works of the ancients, and to understand them read them in the original language. As both my hieroglyph and my Akkadian cuneiform competence are somewhat lacking I began to understand the immensity of the project I planned.

Much of my early understanding of the subject derives from two colleagues. One, J.T. Edwards, in the very early days of my career. He was the son-in-law of Sir John McFadyean a pioneering research worker who introduced pathology to the British veterinary profession in the late 1800s. J.T. also had research success, he developed the first attenuated rinderpest cattle vaccine in India in the 1920s, and was very knowledgeable in the classics and history: he was an excellent early mentor. And later when working in the USA I had J.F. Smithcors in my team, Fred was the eminent US veterinary historian and author, and a continual fountain of knowledge. He gave me good guidance on building my veterinary library: the most valuable resource in writing this book.

My purpose is not just to present my interpretation of 4000 years of discovery, but to create a chronology to understand who the people were and what they did. Of previous authors I have found the books by Sir Frederick Smith (England), Emmanuel Leclainche (France), Jean Blancou (France) and D. Karasszon (Hungary) to be valuable guides. In the Introduction I have listed all the names that I could find of previously published veterinary history authors, starting from 1773.

Veterinary history is the core subject and I have expanded the depth of investigation and geographical coverage. I have also endeavoured to identify every species of animal that humans have domesticated, utilised and whose diseases they have encountered. These include mammals, birds, fish and insects (honeybee and silkworm) – all have been domesticated in some form and as a result their diseases have become recognised. For the nine major species my detailed listing of early disease records reveals many problems that have existed, or do still exist, that are seen to be detrimental to welfare.

In writing this book I have come to appreciate and learn from the work of many authors and scholars. Additionally, the help that I particularly value is that of my colleagues who have taken the time to read chapters of the book and advise me on specific points of science, accuracy and selection of illustrations. These, mostly fellow veterinarians, are Anthony Andrews, Clare Boulton, Nancy Burford, Esther Carrigan, Gary Clayton-Jones, John Clewlow, Christophe Deguerce, Dan Fraser, Ronald Roberts, Pierre-Louis Toutain, Mark White and Bradley Viner. I also thank Sarah Hulbert, my commissioning Editor, for her invaluable aid and guidance.

I also have to thank and acknowledge the cooperation and help that I have received from the curators and custodians of the photographs that they have allowed me to use for this book: the Ecole Nationale Vétérinaire d'Alfort, France; History of Medicine Collection, National Library of Medicine, Bethesda, MD; Library and University Collections, University of Edinburgh, Scotland; Royal College of Veterinary Surgeons Historical Collection, London; Royal Veterinary College, London and Veterinary Collections, Medical Sciences Library, Texas A & M University, College Station, Texas.

Unfortunately, in a project taking several years some of my colleagues and friends are no longer here and are greatly missed – Norman Comben and Sherwin Hall for their unique knowledge of the history of our profession, Jean Mann for her attention to detail and help with the Veterinary History Society and Wolfgang Jöchle, a most knowledgeable man and author who enjoyed the classical periods of ancient history.

The difficulty of writing and commenting on the past is our lack of understanding of that environment and social issues of that time. Interpretation and translations can be incorrect, and while I have tried to be impartial I might have ventured into contentious issues in some places. I have tried to follow the admonitory words used by Dr Samuel Johnson, 'Read over your compositions, and where ever you meet with a passage which you think is particularly fine, strike it out and start again.' I hope that I have provided clarity in my writing and have imparted both interest and knowledge. I have to leave it to you to judge, but for any errors of commission and omission which I have made I accept full responsibility and will be grateful for suggestions.

Bruce Vivash Jones

THE HISTORY OF VETERINARY MEDICINE AND THE ANIMAL–HUMAN RELATIONSHIP

Introduction

The purpose of this book is to examine and document the origins of what was initially termed the art, but which has developed into the science, of veterinary medicine. The scope of coverage additionally includes the story of the role that each species has played in its utilisation by, and relationship with, humankind. This indefinite subject, the basis of animal welfare, is now increasingly important to veterinary studies and work. Work that ranges from the management of wildlife to the advanced technologies of modern surgery, now in common use in companion animals. The current veterinary discipline is best described as animal health and welfare.

The development of agriculture, described as the most important innovative change in human history, involved the domestication of animals. This brought into being the need for health care and created welfare considerations. Animals added an essential ingredient to agriculture – they provided economic value, first as meat, and then came the realisation of milk, hides, wool, fats and bones. Later their importance providing traction and transportation, particularly in warfare, was recognised. Animals have also provided unquantifiable value as companions and have significant roles in hunting, sport and prestige.

Early Neolithic humans 'tamed' animals without realising that they were modifying their behaviour. Domesticated animals are essentially social beings; they are kept in herds or groups. This characteristic must have influenced the final selection of the species chosen. The domestication process has four main characteristics: (1) breeding is under human control, (2) the domesticated animal provides a product or service useful to humans, (3) the animal is tame and (4) it has been selectively bred away from its 'wild' progenitor (Mason 1984, pp. vii–viii). These have to be rather broad characteristics. The most important feature of domestication is artificial selection by controlled breeding, but some animals utilised by humans are not controlled (elephants, and not all cats). With certain species breeding has become a very sophisticated science, in particular for poultry and pigs, the providers of the two most widely consumed meats.

The dog was the earliest animal to be domesticated by humans. It appears to have been a mutual process, of providing companionship, a role that has remained a constant feature of human life since it first developed, probably 13,000–15,000 years ago. The dog also acted as a guard and was then found to be of value in herding. This enabled goats and sheep to be captured and controlled. These species naturally live in groups with a leader and a highly developed imprinting characteristic: these traits would have greatly aided the first livestock farmers.

Agriculture started between 7000 and 10,000 years ago with the collection of grain seeds, planting and storing. Livestock began to be domesticated in the Fertile Crescent region of the Middle East from about 8000 BC, and by 6000 BC sheep, goats, pigs and cattle were all involved. Within the next 3000–4000 years agriculture began to be practised in the Indus Valley, China, and South and Mesoamerica.

Humans stopped hunting and began to care for livestock; cattle then also became important for traction, prestige and for sacrificial purposes. Horses were domesticated around 4000 BC, probably in central Eurasia. As animal husbandry developed stock management evolved and the importance of animal health was recognised. The first written evidence of veterinary 'professionals' and veterinary procedures has been dated to around 2000 BC.

We know the species with which humans interact and relate to in various ways, and as a result of this exploitation become in need of veterinary attention. The use of the word 'exploit' in relation to human interaction is probably one that would be contested by some, but animal-human interactions are varied in the extreme by social, religious, ethnic and economic factors as well as the greatest variable: human emotion. For want of a suitable aphorism the title of the book, *Some We Love, Some We Hate, Some We Eat* (Herzog 2010) provides a rather pithy summary of the animal-human relationship.

Veterinary and human medicine are separate endpoints of one discipline and the development of these two branches of medical science will be followed together. Evidence indicates that both evolved at about the same time, had a common root and have shared advances – initially this was mostly with a veterinary adoption or adaptation of learning from its human partner. Later, this has led to knowledge also flowing from animal to human patient. Comparative medicine has a long history and can be traced back to the mythology of Chiron the Centaur and Aesculapius. The collaboration has been frequently broken by human intervention, usually due to religious dogma. There have always been individuals who recognised the value of comparative studies from Aristotle onwards.

From the graphic images that have survived from the Palaeolithic era it is clear that animals have constantly played a significant role in human interpretation of their own lives. The use of these very early images, frequently beautifully executed with significant accuracy, can enable dating, and therefore establish a time frame that gives the basis for creating a record.

One can only produce a reasoned study when there is a written record, which allows for interpretation of the events and beliefs of that time. The cardinal marker in the evolution of writing, following the introduction of hieroglyphs (frequently animal derived) was the development of non-syllabic, non-pictogram characters in Egypt, leading to the creation of the Phoenician alphabet. The use of this by the early Greeks to create the first European language, then expanded by the Roman and Byzantine cultures has enabled writers to place on record almost every aspect of human activity. Finally, the introduction of the printing press to Europe by Johannes Gutenberg around 1445 led to the significant widening of the circulation of information and ideas. The first specific printed veterinary books appeared in the late 1400s and early 1500s, the most important being derived from surviving Roman and Byzantine manuscripts.

Printing enabled and enhanced education, the enlargement of libraries and the establishment of universities. This aided the commencement of training of a specific group of individuals, who were to become known as veterinarians – and the art began to move towards becoming a science. The first school was established at Lyon, France, by Claude Bourgelat in 1761; it was the forerunner of the now global teaching of veterinary medicine and science.

The societal activities of humankind did not arise in only one place. For the purposes of this book three centres of civilisation are studied. The first is Egypt, Mesopotamia and the Aegean (Greece). There were close relationships between these three in trade and cultures, which has developed in Europe into Western civilisation. This has become the dominant global culture for veterinary and human medicine, influenced by the Christian religion.

It is important to also study the other two centres – China and India. These old, sophisticated and highly developed civilisations not only created their own medical science but understood veterinary and human medicine as two parts of one discipline. Again, both were influenced by a spiritual dimension: Confucianism in China and Buddhism in India, each of which affected advances in animal medicine. These cultural centres interacted with other neighbouring communities creating significant spheres of influence. Following the introduction of the Islamic faith in the 7th century AD, a shift in cultural emphasis occurred with the faith becoming dominant across the region from Iberia to Persia and northern India by the 8th century AD. During this period there was intense interest in all branches of science including veterinary medicine, which resulted in the preservation of much Byzantine and Greek knowledge, to which they made contributions, in the Arabic language.

In all of these centres the cultural environment developed with a strong background based in mythology, frequently in conjunction with a belief system – all of these involved animals, as key players in their created semi-spiritual worlds. Out of these imagined environments developed specific concepts as well as a traditional, legendary and, frequently romantic, corpus of folklore beliefs. This is a complex area of study and one that is also plagued by pseudo-scientific ideas: it will be condensed to illustrate major influences, many of which are still detectable.

The format and chapter construction used enables discussion of the major theme by civilisation centre, animal species, and technical and veterinary scientific development. Additionally, individual topics are also discussed on the relationship between animals and humans. Some of these subjects deal with situations where humans involve animals in circumstances that can be seen to act to the disadvantage of animals. For this reason, every effort is made to record the evidence in a dispassionate manner as readers are likely to hold one of two opposing viewpoints.

Warfare provided the prime motive to develop, understand and expand what was to become the veterinary art. When the horse was domesticated, probably starting about 4000 BC it was soon realised that these animals had a greater value when trained to be ridden or to draw vehicles, than to be used as meat. Horses became the principal armament of ancient military forces. This in turn created a need to care for them, feed them well and train them: the record can be traced back about 2500 years to the writings of Xenophon. Horses became more valuable than the foot-soldier and a class of professionals was created who undertook their treatment and care: including treating post-conflict injuries. While veterinary medicine has advanced the cause of equine welfare, in war its longstanding role has been one of aiding a military objective up until the First World War (1914–1918), hopefully the last major conflict in which animals played a significant role. While animal medicine, surgery and welfare would have developed as society advanced, it was warfare that drove its progress.

Dogs have a similar history. While their use in ancient war is possibly exaggerated they did play a significant role as messengers, and still do in guarding. Similarly, they are significant in sport hunting to, it would appear, their enjoyment. This has resulted, over the centuries, in much wounding and injuries, and again canine medicine and surgery advanced to deal with these issues.

Spiritual belief has been, and still is, significant in the animal-human relationship. From very early images animal representation has illustrated not just their value as a food source, but within a wider context. As society has developed, animals have been given mythological god-like roles and also feature in separate religious beliefs and faiths. Almost all beliefs have involved animals in either divination or fables and stories associated with their founder, or by their physical presence. In many religions, if not most at some stage, this has involved sacrifice, frequently with the use of body organs for divination. As religions have evolved, many of these practices have been discarded, but at least two major world religions continue to use ritual slaughter as an important part of their doctrine.

The utilisation of animal products also is affected by religious belief. This is most obvious in the consumption of pig meat, which is eschewed by two major world religions. Another prohibits the eating of bovine meat and another favours vegetarian practice and promotes animal welfare. The impact of these on veterinary medicine is variable. Some may result from early public health concerns; the use of animals in ritual slaughter involves selection of healthy beasts, this may have influenced clinical observation skills.

One area of research into the veterinary past that lags behind its human counterpart is that of the study of the archaeology of animal disease. The resource of graveyards and tombs, together with developing technologies of paleopathology, has enabled the identification of many of the ailments and injuries from which humans suffered in antiquity. Apart from rare graves of pet dogs, diseased animals were either buried in unmarked graves or burned. Animal remains of sacrificial beasts seldom had observable disease problems. However, some recent discoveries indicate an increasing interest in this subject and have helped to add to our knowledge.

In writing this text an effort has been made to place all comment, as far as possible, in the context of the time under discussion: even this is far from infallible as there is no way to truly understand earlier environments, beliefs and cultures in their totality. It is a difficult undertaking and any criticisms of its failure will be accepted.

The end point of this study is the 20th century. Veterinary education commenced in 1762 in France and by 1800 existed in every major European state including, belatedly, Britain in 1791. By the mid-1800s veterinary education was becoming established in the United States, Canada, India, Egypt and Mexico, and by the 1900s was advancing towards a global coverage. With the establishment of veterinary schools, organised research, national disease eradication programmes and, in particular, a profession of specifically trained individuals was created. The art had become the science. The modern era has been well reviewed and discussed elsewhere.

The recording of the history of veterinary medicine has an interesting history in itself. From the beginning there have been individuals working to trace its roots. The earliest printed publications came from France, with the first identified author being P.J. Amoreux at Montpellier, who produced a listing of authors of veterinary related topics up to 1773; followed by C.F. Saboureux de la Bonneterie with *A Translation of old Latin works relating to Agriculture and Veterinary Medicine* (1773) and L. Vitet, Lyon, who wrote *An Analysis of Authors who have written on the Veterinary Art since Vegetius* (1783). Amoreux then elaborated on his earlier work with *An Historical Precis of the Veterinary Art* (1810). All these books were in French, with French authors being prominent as the first writers on veterinary history.

It is not easy to trace early veterinary texts, in particular those in manuscript form. A notable early collector of such works was J.-B. Huzard (1755–1838), Professor at the Alfort Veterinary School and Inspector-General of French Veterinary Schools. He was reputed to have amassed a private library of some 40,000 volumes. While not all of a veterinary nature it did include almost all known printed veterinary works up to 1838 as well as many rare and priceless manuscripts. When the collection was dispersed a significant part was acquired by the Alfort Veterinary School and is held in their library. Fortunately, the collection was catalogued by P. Leblanc and a copy is held in the British Library (BM, No.822, c1). Leblanc also wrote a summary of those items that related to veterinary medicine and animal husbandry. These totalled 5812 works with 1598 directly related to veterinary medicine (up to 1838). At that time by far the majority were by French authors. One category, *Treatises on the Diseases of Different Animals* comprised 216 works, of these 115 were in French and of the remaining 101, just 7 were in English. Huzard's summary was published in English (Leblanc 1848, pp. 214–16).

In 1851 Count G.B. Ercolani, writing in Italian, published the first volume of his *Historico-Analytical Researches on the Writers of Veterinary Science*, with the second volume in 1854. J.C.F. Heusinger, a German national, living in Cassel, France, and writing in French produced *Researches in Comparative Pathology* in 1853, the title is misleading as the text is about historical literature and animal plagues. G.A. Piétremont wrote *The Origins of the Domesticated Horse* (1870) and *Horses in Prehistoric and Historic Times* (1883), both books in French.

The interest in historical veterinary medicine then moved away from France with the *Outline of the History of Veterinary Science for Veterinarians and Students* (1885) by F. Echbaum, Berlin; *History of Cattle Breeding and Medicine in Antiquity* (1886) by Anton Baronski, Vienna, who also wrote *The Training and Taming of Domestic Animals in Prehistoric Times* (1896). A. Postolka, Vienna, contributed *A History of Veterinary Medicine from its beginnings to the Present Times* (1887). All these works being in German.

P. Delprato and L. Barbieri added *The Collection of Works Unedited or Rare* (1867), Vol. XIII in Italian. Part 1 is a consideration of the author Laurence Rusius and Part 2 notes on historical Italian veterinary writers. These were followed by *History of Veterinary Medicine* (in three parts: 1891, 1900 and 1911) by L. Moulé, a particularly good source book in French detailing many early manuscript documents.

Later French authors were M. Laignel-Lavastine with a three-volume *General History of Medicine, Pharmacy, Dentistry and the Veterinary Art* (1936–1939) and A. Senet, *History of Veterinary Medicine* (1953), followed by Emmanuel Leclainche, *An Illustrated History of Veterinary Medicine* (1955), an impressive two-volume production. Authors, writing in Italian include Alessandro Lanfranchi, V*eterinary History* (1935) and Valentino Chiodi, *The History of Veterinary Medicine* (1957). Particular mention must be made of *Danske dyrlaegeinstrumenter gennem 200 ar 1773–1973* (1981) by Gert Espersen, in Danish this is (to the writer's knowledge) the only text available on the history of veterinary surgical instruments and technology; authoritatively written and well-illustrated.

The most valuable English-language book from Continental Europe is *A Concise History of Veterinary Medicine* (1988) by D. Karasszon, Hungary. In recent years there have been several Scandinavian publications discussing their veterinary pioneers Abildgaard and Viborg: and topics such as pig husbandry, all in English.

The first record of veterinary history in English in book form was made by Delabere Blaine as the opening chapter in his *Outlines of the Veterinary Art* (1802). He discussed both the ancient origins as well as the establishment of the London Veterinary College. The *Encyclopaedia Britannica* in the fourth edition, 1806, included a good article on the subject (but under the Farriery title) said to be written by Jeremiah Kirby. Later editions had revised texts by William Dick and George Fleming. The *Short History of the Horse* (1824) by Bracy Clarke includes a section that traces the origins of veterinary literature.

One of the most important contributors to an understanding of veterinary history has been Sir Frederick Smith, who apart from his many papers has left his books, each exceptional and all enhanced by his practical knowledge of veterinary medicine and the profession. *The Early History of Veterinary Literature and its British Development* (1919–1933) in four volumes, remains a valuable and unique resource; *The Veterinary History of the War in South Africa* (1919) gives a first-hand description of the Boer War (1899–1902), characterised by its horrific animal wastage and *The History of the Royal Army Veterinary Corps* (1927) presents a singular history of the introduction and use of veterinarians in warfare. *Ars Veterinaria* (1991) by R.E. Walker is a small unique research based book by a veterinarian who not only made an original translation of the el-Lahun Egyptian papyrus, but comprehensively studied the ancient Greek and Latin veterinary texts. Walker also wrote a valuable appendix on Roman veterinary medicine in *Animals in Roman Life and Art* (1973) by J.M.C. Toynbee.

Another important book, based on original research by Leslie Pugh, is *From Farriery to Veterinary Medicine 1785–1795* (1962) which traces the start of veterinary education in Britain. This is well complemented by *The Royal Veterinary College London: A Bicentenary History, 1791–1990* (1990) by Ernest Cotchin, which documents the establishment and growth of the first British veterinary school. This college can be seen as the fountain-head of English-language veterinary education: spreading to North

America, the Indian subcontinent, South Africa and elsewhere in Africa, Australia and New Zealand. Additionally, a comprehensive study *The British Veterinary Profession: 1791–1948* (1984) was written by Iain Pattison.

American authors have made their contribution, initially with *Veterinary Military History of the United States* (1935) by L.A. Merillat and D.M. Campbell and *A Short History of Veterinary Medicine in America* (1955) by B.W. Bierer, followed by Fred Smithcors *Evolution of the Veterinary Art* (1958), the first English-language narrative account of veterinary medicine from the earliest times to 1850, drawing extensively on the British literature and the derivation of the US veterinary discipline. Smithcors followed this with a more popular presentation, *The Veterinarian in America: 1625–1975* (1975). More recently has been *Veterinary Medicine: An Illustrated History* (1996) by R.H. Dunlop and D.J. Williams, which discusses the subject from ancient to present times.

Early British veterinary publications always showed a curiosity about the origins of veterinary medicine. A short-lived British periodical *The Veterinary Examiner*, in its first December 1832 issue included a lengthy article titled 'The History of Veterinary Medicine', which discussed all the significant Roman, Greek, European and British authors of veterinary subjects. This would appear to be the first British attempt at a history of veterinary literature. The author was probably Bracy Clark, a veterinary surgeon, who was a known scholar (see Appendix 2).

There is available an increasing and invaluable collection of translations of the works of the early Greek, Roman and Byzantine authors. Particularly important is *A Byzantine Encyclopaedia of Horse Medicine* (2007) by Anne McCabe, virtually a translation of the *Hippiatrica*, which can be described as the most important early veterinary book. Equally fascinating is *Pelagonius and Latin Veterinary Terminology in the Roman Empire* (1995) translated by J.N. Adams. Also important is the first historical study to deal with Islamic veterinary medicine, and that of the Mamluk period in particular: *Mamluks and Animals* (2013) by Housni Alkhateeb Shehada. Do not forget the fascinating English translation of the 5th century AD book by Vegetius, *Artis Veterinariae, sive Mulomedicinae*. Published in 1748, not as an historical document, but as an aid to helping the control of the epizootic diseases then prevalent, well over 1000 years after its original publication!

This book is presented in three sections. Part I traces the early development of animal utilisation and veterinary medicine in the Near/Middle East to Greece and then to Western Europe, and the Islamic intervention (Chapters 1–6). Next, East Asia, centred on China and its influence on the neighbouring countries and South Asia with its own culture centred on India and again influencing its neighbours (Chapters 7–8). The American, Australasian and African continents are of interest, all developed their own medical beliefs and practices but apart from Africa had little need of veterinary medicine. Each continent is studied with particular reference to the introduction of European livestock and veterinary medicine as a result of colonial expansion. Veterinary development is studied from its first introduction to the present day. These three chapters (9, 10 and 11) have enabled a full global study to be completed of veterinary medicine and the animal–human relationship.

Part II covers the development of veterinary medicine in Europe from the decline of the Roman Empire through the Middle Ages, the Renaissance and the

Enlightenment to the opening of the first veterinary school and the spread of veterinary education across Europe, then North America, leading to a global veterinary world by the end of the 20th century (Chapters 12–16).

Part III is an historical study of animal utilisation and the animal–human relationship, presented individually for the ten major species and species groups domesticated by humans. Each one includes a detailed chronology of animal disease observations and recognition of causal agents from the ancient records to the modern era (Chapters 17–26).

Throughout the book an effort has been made to reference important ideas, people, and authors and information sources as well as identifying other significant contributors in designated topics, as an aid to further research and study.

Veterinary medicine and animal welfare share a history. The first humans who tried to understand animal diseases were the horsemen and livestock keepers. Our knowledge of their methods and behaviour comes from their early writings: while much of the veterinary activity was probably of little value and frequently harmful the importance of humane animal care was clearly recognised. The most important texts come from the years of the Roman Empire (including the Eastern Empire from 27 BC to AD 1453). There were many writers who are identified in Chapters 1–5: it may help to read the following short biographical notes on these ancient and early authors before starting on the main text, or these pages can be referred to as needed.

Ancient and Early Authors

The preparation of this book has involved the study of as much original source material as could be revealed. It is not until the written (and translatable) word appears that an appreciation of both the knowledge and the reality of the past can be determined and reviewed.

Extant literature indicates an early interest in the discipline of what is now called veterinary medicine. Developing first as a twin or subsidiary to human medicine it then evolved with a separate but related identity. The initial focus varied between cultures, either on the care of economically valuable livestock or for equids used in war. As with its human counterpart the most innovative veterinary ideas developed with the Hellenic culture, taken and used pragmatically by the Romans (to aid their large armies and agricultural economy), continued in the Byzantine Empire, and reincarnated in the Islamic world.

Greek and Roman sources have given us the two primary books of ancient veterinary medicine. Both are compilations, one known as the *Hippiatrica*, by an unknown Byzantine assembler of older writings, and one by a Roman author, Vegetius. These two works are based on essentially the same source material, from Greeks writing in about AD 300–350, but note almost all of the early Greek works have presumptive dates.

Vegetius wrote some one hundred years later and the final versions of the *Hippiatrica* were compiled in the mid-10th century AD. Two other significant Latin veterinary texts have also survived – *Ars Veterinaria* by Pelagonius, 4th or 5th century

AD and *Mulomedicina Chironis* of unknown authorship, written about AD 350–400. Both of these works are mainly derivative. The content of these four books essentially comprise our knowledge of Roman and Byzantine veterinary medicine.

Over many years scholars have tackled the difficult task of translation, challenging because many works are either incomplete or corrupted by scribes or previous translations, and difficult because the subject matter is of a highly specific nature – examples including the names of body parts, symptoms, diseases, plants or insects. Many confusions have arisen from past translations but newer work has helped to resolve some of these. Three recent books, discussed here, are outstanding in providing clarification of the writings comprising the *Hippiatrica* and those of Pelagonius and Herodotus. Other important reference sources up to the early 1900s that have been used are also listed, and identified for their content.

While translation to English conveys the factual content of an original text it does not convey the emphasis given by the original author. Writing and language usage change and the relevance of a technical work presented as poetry (most difficult to translate with accuracy) or an understanding of the original prose-rhythm, much loved by the leading classical authors, is totally lost. Their interpretation of events and emphasis may therefore not be revealed in translation.

The authors and texts listed here are presented in four groupings depending on their veterinary content. An additional group identifies important later reference sources. The believed approximate date of writing is used to rank the entries, but the *Hippiatrica* compilation did not appear until the mid-10th century AD, based on writings from the 2nd and 3rd centuries AD, these were also used by Vegetius in his Latin book of AD 450–500. Both books only became available to Western Europe in the early 1500s, following the introduction of the printing press.

It is recognised that other civilisations have their own veterinary histories. The Chinese were early participants with a structured educational system and the Indian subcontinent developed an original veterinary and animal welfare culture. Additionally, the Islamic Arabic conquerors of large territorial regions in the Middle East, North Africa and Spain became veterinary knowledge seekers, evolving their own systems, but much based on translations of the same early Greek and Byzantine veterinary treatises. These three separate cultural identities and their veterinary histories are discussed later.

Note:* the use of this symbol as a prefix to a name in the following summaries indicates that the individual is themselves discussed in detail elsewhere in these biographical notes.

Veterinary Treatises

Kahun (el-Lahun) Papyrus

This unique hieratic papyrus dating from about 1900 BC, was found in Egypt in 1899 by Flinders Petrie in excavations at Kahun, now Illahun, Fayoum District. An ancient Egyptian style of writing, an abridged form of hieroglyphics, is used on a papyrus of the highest quality, as used for priestly writings in connection with sacred subjects. Only parts have survived: a long narrow strip and six fragments. The latter deal with fish and birds, but it is not possible to determine in what context. The strip has 48 columns of text and 3 horizontal headings. Much of the translation has to be conjecture, but it can be seen to deal with conditions in cattle, and possibly fish and a dog. Translation consulted is by Walker (1964, pp. 198–200).

Praxamus

Praxamus, Greek author described as a student of *Mago of Carthage, lived about 100 BC. He was said to have written on veterinary matters in a typically Greek spirit of originality and observation, and described diarrhoea, indigestion and colic in cattle.

Gargilius Martialis

Quintus Gargilius Martialis (early to mid-3rd century AD), Roman poet and historian. He particularly wrote on gardens, parts of his *De hortis* (*On Gardens*) are extant, as well as two other fragments usually attributed to him. One is on the medicinal value of fruits and the other is *Curae Boum* (*Cures of Cattle*). Opinions on his work are conflicting, ranging from superstitious remedies to veterinary art.

Eumelus

Eumelus, Greek, possibly from one of the Theban cities in ancient Boeotia (part of Voitotia in east-central Greece). Dating from probably the 3rd century AD. He is the earliest author quoted in the *Hippiatrica. It is only due to *Apsyrtus that he is known, who described him as a 'great horse-doctor'. It can be presumed that he practised. The Boeotia region had a militaristic and artistic history and was known in Late Antiquity for horse breeding and racing. His work is quoted by *Varro, *Columella, *Pelagonius and *Anatolius.

Apsyrtus

Apsyrtus, Greek from either Prousa (south of Istanbul) or probably Nicomedia (ancient Greek city in north-west Asia Minor, the metropolis of Roman Bythnia). Apsyrtus lived in the late 3rd to early 4th century AD, a soldier serving under Emperor Constantine, in particular in Scythia along the Danube border. Very little is known about his life, he would appear to have been a senior 'veterinarian' in the imperial cavalry. He wrote a treatise, much of which is used in the *Hippiatrica and forms the foundation text for that compilation; it is the most extensive ancient Greek work on horse medicine that has survived. Apsyrtus is recognised as the most important and original contributor to early veterinary medicine.

Pelagonius

Pelagonius, Roman, possibly born in Illyria (central Balkan region bordering on the Adriatic Sea), wrote *Ars Veterinaria* (*The Veterinary Art*) in Latin, probably during the mid-4th century AD. Little is known of his background; from the work it appears that he concentrated on horses, in particular those participating in racing. This was chariot racing – a particularly dangerous sport for both horse and charioteer.

Injuries and hoof wear were major issues. He copied the letter-writing epistolary style of *Apsyrtus, whom he quotes together with *Columella and others. The writings of Pelagonius have been exhaustively studied (Adams, 1995). This book examines the language of Latin veterinary medicine in a systematic manner; the author has sought to elucidate the anatomical and pathological terminology.

Hippocrates

The author of this treatise, while Greek, is neither the great physician of that name nor is it believed to be the name of the author. The extracts which appear in the *Hippiatrica* are the only work under this name. No reason for the assumed name is given: the author knew his subject, which was horses and mules, not livestock, and is presumed to have practised veterinary medicine. His use of the language is described as 'at the lower end of the literary scale' and the more colloquial style used would indicate that it was written for the layman. The content is similar to other authors included in the *Hippiatrica*.

In the 6th century AD a veterinary book under the name of Ippocras appeared, for a while this was believed to be by Hippocrates but is now recognised to be of Indian origin. This work has a questionable provenance.

Mulomedicina Chironis

This Latin work attributed to Chiron, is believed to have been written about AD 350–400. The origin and authorship has been the subject of much controversy: the author may have been known as Hierocles or Hemerius, or it was a name used to cover the work of several authors; it has one mention in the *Hippiatrica*. References are cited to work by *Apsyrtus, Polycletus, Farnax, Sotio and Hemerius. The text is written in 'rustic' Latin with a coarse use of language and now only exists as a corrupt version. It is however of value as it confirms the state of knowledge of the Byzantine school. There is only one manuscript, Bavarian MS. 243, held in Germany.

Theomnestus

Theomnestus, 4th-century Greek from Nicopolis (capital of the Roman province of Epirus Vetus, on western coast of Greece). Evidence suggests that it was written in AD 313 (but this has been questioned). Theomnestus served in the army of Theodoric, King of the Ostrogoths, either as a veterinarian or as Master of the Horse to the King. He is known to have been a keen horseman who had had a good grounding in medical practice. A significant contributor to the *Hippiatrica* he is the only author to be quoted on grooming and breaking-in. An Arabic translation has provided what appears to be the only complete copy of his treatise (see Chapter 6).

Hierocles

Hierocles, Greek, wrote in the 4th or 5th century AD. A lawyer, he wrote in an elegant manner, following his training in oratory. Some authorities have described him as a plagiarist; although not claiming to be an expert on equine matters, he does describe his own experiences with horses. His work is essentially a paraphrasing of the *Apsyrtus treatise (a custom in antiquity that was neither uncommon nor treated as cheating). He refers to his friend, Bassus (thought to be Cassianus Bassus who compiled the *Geoponika*). Hierocles' writings are one of the major sections of the *Hippiatrica*.

Vegetius

Publius Vegetius Renatus, Roman, believed to have lived between AD 450 and AD 500 in the reign of Emperor Valentinian. A similarly named author, Flavius Vegetius Renatus, wrote on military matters: there is now agreement that they were the same man. Vegetius was a man of letters, had travelled widely and almost certainly had been a soldier in the imperial service. As the mule and horse were essential animals to the Roman army it would be natural for a soldier to have an interest in their health and care.

The writings of Vegetius were lost following the decline of the Roman Empire, until 1528 when a copy was discovered in Hungary by a Count Nuenare. A rather poor translation was made and published in Basel in 1528. It is usually accepted that this was the first printed veterinary work. Since that time many editions have been published in German, French, Italian and English. This has given rise to some confusion: the short Latin title was *Artis Veterinariae, Sive Mulomedicinae*, with the translation of the full title reading, *Books of the Veterinary Art, or Digests of the Art of Curing the Diseases of Mules*. Vegetius was an important author, he not only left a record of the knowledge and practice of veterinary medicine in the later Roman Empire, but he also expressed viewpoints, many based on his own experiences.

Hippiatrica

The *Hippiatrica* is now recognised to be the most valuable veterinary text surviving from the Roman Empire, or specifically from the Greek-speaking culture of the Eastern Empire. Veterinary medicine, both the practice of the art and the evolution of the science, owes its development to the questioning and observant Greeks. That the *Hippiatrica* manuscripts have survived at all is due to its recognition as a work of value. A complex collection of copies and extracts has resulted from the many efforts at transcribing and translating over the centuries. It has value not only in its veterinary medical content, in particular that of Apsyrtus, but also because it preserves a record of veterinary 'science' and practice in the Byzantine Empire. The *Hippiatrica* has been the source of significant study and controversy. Much of this has been clarified by the work of Anne McCabe (2007), which now has to be the source book for detailed examination and study of these early manuscripts.

Medical / Veterinary and Scientific Treatises

Hippocrates

Hippocrates, Greek, born on the island of Cos (Kos) on or before 460 BC and believed to have died about 375 BC at Larissa in Thessaly. He lived in the age of Pericles – Classical Greece. Little is known of his life except that he had learned philosophy, practised medicine and travelled extensively as a physician and teacher; he was consulted by King Perdiccus of Macedon, and Artaxerxes of Persia. Hippocrates was the most famous medical personality of antiquity and is known as the father of human medicine. His dictum 'above all, do no harm' has served as his most valuable contribution to medicine; he rejected superstition in favour of reasoning based on facts, and advocated the study of medicine by the use of careful, namely scientific, research to advance knowledge (Jones 1923).

The best known commentator on Hippocrates is *Galen, who describes a medical leader, but this viewpoint is one which is coloured by his own complex ideas and philosophical theories. Hippocrates made very few veterinary observations, he did value comparative medicine, but appeared to regard animal care as beneath human medicine, this was possibly influenced by early teaching on the soul – possessed by humans but not animals. He left a lasting influence on medicine as a whole, in particular his emphasis on clinical evaluation and problem-oriented diagnosis, record keeping and the rejection of superstitious beliefs, while at the same time having concern for the humane treatment of the patient.

Aristotle

Aristotle (384–322 BC), Greek, born at Stagira in Chalcidice (northern Greece) and died at Chalcis, Euboea. His father, who died when Aristotle was young, was court physician to King Amyntas II of Macedonia. This medical background gave Aristotle an interest in natural history. Initially in 366 BC, he studied under Plato at the Academy at Athens. When Plato died in 347, Aristotle was not asked to take his place and he moved to Mytilene on Lesbos island where his natural history studies, in particular of marine life, fully occupied him. In 342 King Philip II asked him to tutor his son Alexander ('the Great'), he did this for three years, later Alexander became his significant benefactor. In 335 he returned to Athens and started his Lyceum, but had to leave 13 years later due to political problems and handed the Lyceum to his colleague and close friend *Theophrastus. He retired to Chalcis and shortly afterwards died.

Aristotle produced an enormous volume of work on logic, metaphysics, nature, life and mind, ethics, politics and art, much of which is lost. His zoological works, in particular those related to anatomy, physiology, animal welfare and veterinary medicine, have mostly survived.

- *Historia Animalium* (*History of Animals*), ten books: 1–4 a comparative survey of internal organs and external body parts including tissues and fluids, senses and voice; 5–6 reproduction, breeding and embryogenesis; 7–9 feeding differences, habitat, migration, hibernation, social habits, gender differences, veterinary observations, intelligence as well as human reproductive system, pregnancy and obstetrics; 10 discusses the female role in generation.
- *De Paribus Animalium* (*Parts of Animals*), four books in two parts, *De Incessu Animalium* (*On the Progression of Animals*) deals with the material side of living things and the parts of animals used to go from place to place. *De Motu Animalium* (*On the Movement of Animals*) deals with their consequential properties in movement.

- *De Generatione Animalium* (*On the Generation of Animals*), five books, discusses the parts used in reproduction and the reproductive function. This includes the first known discussion of embryology, based on the hen's egg, much of which is still valid.
- *De Anima*, a disorganised work, mainly notes on the philosophy of life and living.

Of these works, all of interest, the most relevant is the *History of Animals* and in particular Book 8: in which Aristotle describes tetanus, scrotal hernia, laminitis, glanders (*melis*), foot-and-mouth disease, bovine pleuro-pneumonia and pulpy kidney disease in sheep. He discusses surgery, umbilical hernia, recto-vaginal fistula, ascites, castration, spaying, the use of cautery to control bleeding, and suturing. Aristotle was, however, incorrect or misled in a few circumstances: he believed in the fatal effects of the bite of the shrew-mouse and also believed the dog could not transmit rabies to humans. The diseases review includes those affecting horses, asses, cattle, sheep, swine, fish, bees, dogs and elephants. Aristotle was an observer, and an avid dissector. He wrote about some 500 species and did dissect 50 of them: among his observations was the finding that the horse did not possess a gall bladder, a fact that was still being overlooked some 1500 years later! He was neither a clinician nor a veterinarian, but was a collector and analyst of knowledge: with anatomy and physiology his main strengths. A remarkable man who can be seen as the first genuine scientist in history and the first contributor to veterinary science. Translations by Peck (1965 and 1970), Balme (1991), Peck and Forster (1961) and Peck (1942).

Theophrastus
Theophrastus of Eresuo, Greek, born on Lesbos island in c.371/370 BC and died c.287/286 BC. A student, associate and successor of *Aristotle, and like his predecessor interested in all parts of knowledge, in particular natural science. Aristotle bequeathed him his library and made him his successor at the Lyceum near Athens, which he headed for 35 years. Theophrastus wrote on several subjects, few of his works survive except for those on botany, where his studies form a parallel to Aristotle's zoological work. These botanical works appear to have survived intact. His collection of observations is regarded as the starting point of Western botanical systematics; he also expressed arguments for vegetarianism based on the affinity between men and animals, in opposition to Aristotle's viewpoints.

Theophrastus left two botanical works: *De Causis Planatarum* (*On the Causes of Plants*) plant physiology, generation, sprouting, flowering, fruiting, climate, cultivation, breeding and diseases; *Inquirere Planatarum* (*Enquiry into Plants*) in nine books, a classification of varieties – trees, plants, shrubs and cereals followed by plant juices and extracts, and in Book 9 the medicinal properties of herbs including specific suggestions for veterinary medications. Translations by Hort (1916 and 1980).

Pliny
Gaius Plinius Secundus (Pliny the Elder) (AD 23–79), Roman, born in Novum Comum in Gallia Cisalpina (northern Italy). Died, as commander of the fleet, at the time of the eruption of Vesuvius, when he went to Pompeii to investigate. Pliny

was high ranking, an accomplished equestrian, much travelled and a prolific author, best known for his 37 book *Naturalis Historia* (*Natural History*). This was planned as an encyclopaedia of all knowledge: animal, vegetable, mineral and human subjects. The entries are a mixture of fact, fable and fiction, in many cases inaccurate, but overall the work is of significant value: he was presenting the available information. At that time Roman medicine barely existed, the adoption of Greek knowledge and influence was still to come: Pliny's advice was to avoid doctors. His medical content should be compared to the more rational approach of *Cornelius Celsus, writing at approximately the same time. Of the veterinary content little original material can be found. Translations by Holland (1601), also French and Greenaway (1986).

Cornelius Celsus
Aulus Cornelius Celsus (c.25 BC–AD c.50) Roman, lived during the reign of Emperor Tiberius, wrote on a wide variety of subjects. Only eight books of *De Medicina* (*On Medicine*) have survived. His influence in Late Antiquity was not significant, possibly because he wrote in Latin and not Greek. The work was later rediscovered, printed and published in 1478: the practical approach and clear layout, for lay readers, as a result of treating his own household (including slaves), caused his work to be highly valued in the Middle Ages.

The eight surviving books include: (1) historical introduction to Greek medicine, dietetics and medical theory as well as stating, 'those who treat cattle and horses, since it is impossible to learn from dumb animals particulars of their complaints, depend only on common characteristics'; (2) prognosis, diagnosis, pathology and therapeutics; (3) treatments for internal ailments, fevers and general diseases; (4) localised diseases; (5) and (6) pharmacology and drug selection; (7) surgery, with good descriptive text including use of spoon of Diocles to extract barbed arrows from the body (a larger version of which was used to extract such arrows from injured horses); (8) skeletal anatomy. The proem in Book 1 provides an excellent survey of the Greek schools of medicine (dogmatic, methodic, empiric) and is recognised as one of the most important ancient sources on this subject. His writings on veterinary medicine are now lost. Their existence is confirmed by *Columella and others, who reference them. Translation by Spencer (1935).

Dioscorides
Pedanius Dioscorides (c.AD 40–90) Greek, of Cilicia (now Turkey), the author of *Materia Medica* (*Materials of Medicine*), a five-book work. This listed herbs, minerals and animal products used in medicine. Dioscorides travelled with Emperor Nero and was possibly a physician in the army; he can also be described as a pharmacologist and botanist. The books list some 700 useful plants and over 1000 drugs. He recorded the effects of these substances on, or in, the body and provided details on preparations and use, including veterinary applications. Dioscorides aimed at accuracy in his descriptions and his records are free from supernatural accounts. His work was used by *Galen, was translated to Arabic and was well regarded in both cultures. Dioscorides' work was much valued in the Middle Ages in Europe, being used for some 1500 years. The last English edition published in 1934.

Galen

Galen of Pergamum (AD 129–c.216) Greek, born in Pergamum (now Bergama, Turkey), well educated in philosophy and rhetoric before he began medical training. Studied in Smyrna, Corinth and for some years in Alexandria before practising in Pergamum in 157, then moving to Rome in 162. He then left, reasons are unclear, before returning in 169 and entering imperial service at the court of Emperor Marcus Aurelius. His reputation as a physician grew. Galen was a polymath: as well as his extensive medical writings he was a highly regarded philosopher with a strong mono-theistic religious belief.

Galen became the leader, in thought and practice, of the medical profession. His medical writing is permeated by his own judgements and, together with the prime sources of information from earlier medical authors, in particular *Hippocrates, there is some difficulty in separating the two inputs. In his own work, of some four hundred medical treatises, of which only 22 have survived, he created a synthesis of Greek medicine embracing theory and practice. This was combined with the knowledge he derived from experimentation, together with his own understanding of humankind and relationships (Johnston and Horsley 2011). He believed in comparative medicine, while *Hippocrates had a low regard for those who looked after animal health, Galen could see positive advantages in cooperation between the two disciplines.

Agricultural Treatises with Veterinary Content

Cato

Marcus Porcius Cato (234–149 BC) Roman, born at Tusculum but mostly lived in the Sabine country, now Umbria, Lazio and Abruzzo. Important Roman statesman and soldier, called Cato the Censor, major personage in Roman political and cultural life. Recognised as the first important writer of Latin prose, his only surviving intact work is *De Agricultura* (*On Agriculture*). It provides sensible, slightly humorous, advice to owners of estates using slave labour, with primary production in wine and olive oil. The work is poorly planned and somewhat disjointed, but gives an interesting insight into Roman domestic life, with economic advice as well as cooking and medical recipes (with a rather over-enthusiastic view of the medicinal properties of cabbage), religious formulae and veterinary advice. The importance of the text was emphasised by *Columella who wrote, 'Cato first taught agriculture to speak Latin' – it was innovative and followed the Greek genre. The background to his treatise is to guide a landowner on how to make money from agriculture. He emphasised the importance of feeding racks for cattle to avoid feed wastage, as well as the provision of clean water and looking to the welfare of livestock. Translation by Hooper and Ash (1935).

Varro

Marcus Terentius Varro (116–27 BC), Roman, born at Reate, in the Sabine country. Varro studied with Aelius (the first important Roman scholar) in Rome and later in Athens. Known for his extensive knowledge: it has been estimated that he completed some 74 works totalling about 620 books. Only two of his works have survived, one of which is *Rerum Rusticarum (On Agriculture)*. Written in 37 BC in a dialogue style, to his wife, Fundania. She had purchased a farm and this was his advice as a practical manual on husbandry. Book 1 agriculture in general; 2 cattle and sheep breeding; 3 other animals including birds and bees. In the books, essentially a compilation, he mentions the names of some 50 Greek agricultural authors. The text is packed with information, and although not as extensive as that of *Columella about 100 years later, the work was highly valued and much read in later years. He emphasised that in all diseases there were three factors to be considered: cause, symptoms and treatment. Great stress is laid on feeding, housing, breeding and care, he noted the low state of Roman veterinary knowledge compared to that in Greece. Translation by Hooper and Ash (1935).

Virgil

Publius Vergilius Maro (70–19 BC), Roman poet, born near Mantua, in Lombardy. His first collection of poems, the *Ecologues*, was completed in 37 BC. He began work on his second major poem, *Georgica (Georgics)* under the advice and guidance of his patron, Maecenas, in the same year and completed it in 29. It attracted the attention of Emperor Caesar Augustus who then encouraged him to write the *Aenid* to celebrate Rome's glory, but Virgil died in 19 BC, before its completion.

The *Georgics* is a didactic poem devoted to farming divided into four books: Book 1 crops; 2 arboriculture; 3 livestock and 4 bees. Of veterinary interest is Book 3, this deals with hygiene and breeding, as well as recognisable diseases and their treatments. The text is of value, Virgil was expressing the views of the time and was not revealing any new knowledge, but the descriptions of symptoms are graphic and informative. Book 4 is devoted to bees, demonstrating the importance of honey in the Roman diet. It also mentions bee diseases and consequences. Translation by Johnson (2009).

Columella

Lucius Junius Moderatus Columella (AD 4–70), Roman, born in Gades (Cadiz), Spain, but moved to Italy where he owned farms near Rome; best known for his work *De Re Rustica (On Agriculture)*. This is the most complete extant work on Roman agriculture. Written AD c.60–65 in 12 books, it presents a systematic approach to farming as a usable manual for owners and managers. The contents are well written: Book 1 introduction, villa plans, slave management; 2 arable farming; 3–5 mostly viticulture and arboriculture; 6–7 animal husbandry; 8–9 poultry, fish, game and bee farming; 10 horticulture (in verse); 11 duties of slave estate manager, farm work calendar; 12 management of female slaves, wine and oil production, food conservation and sale. He defended both the intensive use of slaves as a capital investment, and also the integration of arable and livestock husbandry.

Columella was not only a major landowner, but he took a great interest in every aspect of estate management with a hands-on knowledge of his subject. Further competence is demonstrated by his knowledge and use of the work of Greek, Punic and Roman authors. Emphasis is given to the care, management and hygiene of animals as well as good feeding practices. Some diseases are discussed as well as castration and breeding systems. Sheep are dealt with at length. His description and advice on poultry farming described an organised system that was not excelled until the 20th century. His most important veterinary contribution was the recognition that certain diseases are contagious and that separation of healthy and sick animals is essential, with isolation of the latter. An important and valuable text. Translation by Ash, Forster and Hefner (1941/1968).

Palladius

Palladius Rutilius Taurus Aemilianus (late 4th to early 5th century AD), Roman of high standing, owned properties near Rome, in Sardinia and probably Gaul, the author of the only agricultural treatise to have survived from Late Antiquity. Important because it shows the state of agricultural practice at the end of the Roman Empire and cites sources now lost. Palladius was a practical farmer writing from his own experience. His work *Opus Agriculturae* (*The Work of Farming*) is in 14 books: Book 1 covers various topics related to organising the farm; 2–13 provide a monthly calendar of farm work; 14 deals with veterinary matters. As he makes no mention of slaves (unlike *Columella) he was probably writing for free tenants, and at a time of agricultural recession. The work was an important provider of agricultural information on fruit trees and vineyards to early medieval Europe, but then was neglected. In the 20th century, Book 14, covering veterinary medicine, was discovered (Fitch 2013).

Anatolius

Vindanius Anatolius of Berytus (Beirut, Lebanon) an agricultural writer between first half of 3rd century to early 4th century AD. Essentially a compiler, he produced an almanac covering agriculture and rural life including the care, breeding and medical treatment of animals. Much of the content derives from earlier, now lost manuscripts, in particular that of Diophanes (who used the also lost treatise of *Mago of Carthage) as well as *Democritus, Africanus, Pamphilius, the Quintilii, Tarantinus, Florentius and Apuleius. The works of *Varro and *Columella are quoted. Available evidence indicates that the original text was on an ancient papyrus and then derived from the Arabic translation by a Syriac translation. It was used by Cassius Bassus in his compilation of agricultural knowledge. The veterinary content of *Palladius, in his 5th-century AD compilation, was partly derived from Anatolius. There is little original knowledge content and also some mystical inclusions. Comparisons of content indicate that Mago, Varro, Columella and Anatolius all drew information from a common, now unknown, source.

Geoponika

The *Geoponika* (*Farm Work*) is a collection of agricultural texts and letters made on the instruction of the Byzantine Emperor Constantine VII Porphyrogenitus (AD 913–959). One of the series of anthologies, all written in Greek which included the *Hippiatrica*, that were prepared under his direction; the purpose was to preserve valuable knowledge from over a thousand years of Greek and Latin treatises. The collection is of value as it preserves the names of many agricultural authors of antiquity.

The first full translation into Latin was published at Venice in 1538 and the first translation into English in 1804/5. A recent English translation provides both a much clearer presentation of the content as well as a carefully edited and foot-noted text (Dalby 2011).

Other Texts with Veterinary/Animal Welfare Content

Herodotus
Herodotus (c.480–c.420 BC), born at Halicarnassus (Bodrum, Turkey) then a Greek city under Persian control, died at Thurii in southern Italy. All details of his life are unsure except that he travelled extensively in the Greek world to Asia Minor, Phoenicia, Egypt, North Africa and probably the Black Sea region. His purpose was to meet people and collect information and stories, rather than as a tourist. His narrative is outstanding as a collection of fact, fable and comment: in several places it recounts unlikely stories or he appears to have been gullible, but in other places what was seen as fanciful has been shown by later scientific studies to be correct, some of which are included in this book. The actual date of writing is unknown but it obviously was a life's work. It is the earliest historical narrative (Strassler 2009).

Democritus of Abdera
Democritus of Abdera (470–402 BC), Greek writer on several subjects including agriculture. He has been said to be the first writer on anatomy (unsubstantiated) and also wrote on topics of veterinary medicine, but none have survived. His work is mentioned in *Aristotle's treatise *Historia Animalium* due to his description of a sheep disease, now known as pulpy kidney.

Simon of Athens
Simon of Athens (430 BC), the earliest known Greek writer on the management of horses. No copy of his treatise has survived but earlier authorities have used the names *The Veterinary Art* and *The Inspection of Horses,* which are believed to be the same work; he probably wrote on horse hygiene and management more than disease. *Pliny said that Simon was the first to write about equitation. Simon's views complement those on stable hygiene laid down by *Xenophon and demonstrate how truly advanced ancient Greece was in these matters. Simon was believed to belong to the Eleusinian Order: one of the laws of this secret society was to treat animals kindly.

Xenophon
Xenophon (c.430–354 BC) son of Gryllus, Greek born in Erchia, Athens. Studied under Socrates and at one point, in a complex mercenary career served as a general, is remembered as a philosopher, historian and soldier. Xenophon wrote three works of animal interest, *Hipparchikos* (*The Cavalry Commander*) deals with the management and improvement of the Athenian cavalry. A military treatise which asserts that no art should be practised more than warfare, adding that gymnastics are frivolous! *Peri Hippikon* (*On Horsemanship*) is generally recognised that as a work written over 2300

years ago, its observations and humanity are just as applicable today. The work is the oldest surviving text on horses, but Xenophon acknowledges the prior writing by Simon of Athens. In *Cynegeticus* (*On Hunting with Hounds*) Xenophon writes on dogs and their selection and training – he discusses the hare, deer, boar and wild cats, but does not approve of fox-hunting. Dog care is stressed. Translations by Morgan (2006) and Phillips and Willcock (1999, pp. 33–89).

Mago

Mago of Carthage, reputed to have been a general in the Carthaginian army, wrote, in about 300 BC, a work on agriculture in 28 books, including veterinary advice. In 146 BC Carthage was totally destroyed at the end of the Third Punic War (149–146 BC); the Roman Senate, however, ordered that Mago's work be saved and translated to Latin. No copy now exists.

Diodorus

Diodorus Siculus (c.90–c.30 BC) Greek, of Agyrium, Sicily. The author of the *Bibliotheca Historica* (*Library of History*). The work was planned on a large scale, of 42 books, of which 40 were completed. He travelled widely and lived in Alexandria and Rome. He enjoyed recording interesting and unusual happenings and places: some of which are used in this book.

Grattius

Grattius 'Faliscus' (63 BC–AD 14) Roman, an Augustan poet with one extant work, the *Cynegeticon Liber*, in about 540 hexameters. Dealing with hunting and management of dogs, it overviews, in some 300 lines, dog breeds and breeding, management and ailments. A favourable mention is given to British dogs for 'their courage, speed and resource', as well as commenting on their 'unattractive form and appearance'.

Arrian

Lucius Flavius Arrianus (AD c.86–160), Greek, born in Bithynia, studied with Epicetus, later became friend of Emperor Hadrian, who awarded him senatorial rank. He followed the style of Xenophon and his *Cynegeticus* is modelled on Xenophon's treatise. He also includes a delightful account of his favourite bitch, *Horme* (*Impulse*) (Phillips and Willcock 1999, pp. 90–127).

Aelian

Claudius Aelianus (AD c.170–235) Roman, born in Praeneste (Palestrina) Italy; author and teacher of rhetoric, fluent in Attic Greek. His works (many of which are lost) are valuable because of the quotations from other, now lost works. Aelian writings include a varied and interesting collection of traditions and facts accepted in his Roman world. The two main extant works are *Varia Historia* (*Various Histories*), a collection of anecdotes and short biographies and *De Natura Animalium* (translated as *On Animals, On the Characteristics of Animals* or *On the Nature of Animals*). This major work comprises brief stories of natural history covering virtually all the then known species of animals, sea life and birds. Some are allegorical, some amazing, some bizarre, and many correct. An overall impression of expressing the reality of divine providence in the animal kingdom, with lessons for humankind is produced. The work throws a light on the Roman mind and attitudes: it created a pattern that was later followed in the medieval bestiaries and medical treatises. It is interesting to peruse the facts and fables, natural medicines used by animals and much about bees. Translation by Scholfield (1958).

Oppian
Oppian (late 2nd century AD) Greek, of Cilicia (now Turkey), poet. His most well-known surviving work is the *Halieutica*, a remarkable five book hexameter text dealing with the sea, fishing and the life forms found there. Another work, the *Cynegetica*, is also a hexameter poem in four books related to hunting and use of dogs. The text discusses dogs, giving favourable mention to a British breed called *agassei* which could be a progenitor of the current terrier breeds: originally attributed to Oppian, there now appears to be agreement that it is by another Greek hand.

Nemesianus
Marcus Aurelius Olympius Nemesianus (late 3rd century AD), Roman, a resident of Carthage. Little of his work has survived, but there are 325 lines of his *Cynegetica*, an incomplete poem about hunting, which discusses dog training, diseases and breeds. It is obvious from the text that Britain had replaced Gaul to become a major source of hunting dogs. While well composed and written Nemesianus added little new knowledge. This was probably the last work on hunting written under the empire.

Early Notable Authors and Other Recommended Books

Following the end of the Roman and Byzantine Empires there was a dearth of original writers on veterinary and human medicine in Western Europe. Gradually translations of the ancient manuscripts appeared and were widely read and accepted. As medieval culture evolved its written expression was based mainly in work from the religious houses, with an increasing interest in what was termed 'natural history'. This category expanded to include many other topics. At the same time monasteries – the main centres of medical care, were developing herb gardens as a medication source, creating a separate literary culture (herbals). Knowledge advanced, printing became available and many books appeared. Nine of these authors are listed below, all have either a direct veterinary/animal interest or a medical influence.

Magnus
Albert Magnus (c.1200–1280) German theologian, scientist and philosopher. Worked on zoology, physiology and alchemy. Author of *De Animalibus (On Natural History)*, in the book is incorporated a chapter, *De Falconibus (On Birds)* including remedies for sick and wounded falcons.

Bombastus von Hohenheim

Philippus Aureolus Theophrastrus Bombastus von Hohenheim (1493–1541) Swiss German, better known as **Paracelsus**. An enigmatic, but brilliant philosopher, physician, alchemist, botanist and astrologist: he moved away from ancient texts and introduced a new dynamism to the study and practice of medicine. His original thoughts eventually led to asepsis; he presented a pre-germ theory that diseases were entities in themselves rather than states of being. He developed the discipline of toxicology ('the dose makes the poison'), produced laudanum and prescribed it widely.

Gesner

Conrad Gesner (1516–1565) Swiss naturalist and important investigator into plants and animal life. Major work was *Historiae Animalium* (1551–1558) a five-volume, 4500-page work, now regarded as the beginning of modern zoology (initially banned by the pope). The work bridges the ancient and modern science of zoology; Gesner tried to give an accurate description of animals.

Vesalius

Andreas Vesalius (1514–1564) Belgian, professor at Padua University, Italy where he produced his masterwork (with Johannes Oporinus) *De humani corporis fabrica* (*On the fabric of the human body*) in 1543. His objective was to understand human anatomy and disprove many of Galen's errors. Although not the first human anatomy work it was the best, influencing Carlo Ruini's *Anatomia del Cavallo* 1598.

Caius

John Caius (1510–1573) English physician, studied at Padua under Vesalius, a pioneer naturalist, zoologist and author. In contact with Conrad Gesner with a view to contributing to his work. Published the first British book on dogs, *Of English Dogges: Their Diversities, their Names, their Natures, and the Properties*, 1576. The co-founder of Gonville and Caius College, Cambridge and may have designed the caduceus.

Harvey

William Harvey (1578–1657) English physician, had worked with Fabricius at Padua; notable for his work *Exercitatio Anatomica de Motu Cordis et Sanguinis in Animalibus* (*An Anatomical Disquisition Concerning the Motion of the Heart and Blood in Animals*) published in 1628, at Frankfurt Book Fair. While taking some time to be accepted this remarkable piece of work explained the action of the heart and circulation of the blood. His other important work was *Excercitations de Generatione Animalium* (*On Animal Generation*) published in 1651, noted for his dictum, 'omne vivum ex ovo' (all life comes from the egg). Thought to be the first definitive statement against the spontaneous generation belief.

Browne

Sir Thomas Browne (1605–1682) English physician and polymath. Studied at Montpellier, Padua and Leiden and travelled widely in Europe. Important author, of particular relevance is *Pseudodoxia Epidemica or Enquiries into very many Received Tenets, and commonly Presumed Truths*, published in 1646, where he tried to disprove many zoo-logical and medical fallacies, including the equine gall bladder myth. Very inventive with language and was the first to use the word 'veterinarian'.

Pennant

Thomas Pennant (1726–1798) English naturalist with, for his time, a great curiosity about life forms. He investigated animals, fish and birds, producing good descrip-tions as well as including interesting comments on husbandry and other practices. His most important book was *British Zoology* (1766–1767) in four volumes, also wrote *The History of Quadrupeds, Arctic Zoology* and *Indian Zoology*.

Darwin

Erasmus Darwin (1731–1802) English physician and natural philosopher, wrote sev-eral books and had profound thoughts on many subjects. One of his quotations is 'A fool you know is a man who has never tried an experiment in his life.' His views on evolution foreshadowed those of J.-B. Lamarck – he was the grandfather of Charles Darwin. Most relevant book is *Zoonomia* (1794–1796), this was a system of pathology, mostly based on human disease but also including valuable animal observations.

During this period there was an increasing output of both medical and veterinary books. Three that were to have a great influence on the developing medical and vet-erinary discipline were the works of Galen (from the Roman era) published in Latin in 1490, the *Hippocratic Corpus* (from the earlier Greek time) published in Latin in 1528 and *The Canon of Medicine* by Avicenna, in Latin translation from Arabic which became the standard medical text in many medieval universities and remained in use up to 1650.

It has been thought that the first printed veterinary book was the Vegetius text, published at Basel in 1528, followed by the *Hippiatrica* published in Paris in 1530. This overlooks the earlier work by J. Ruffus, published in Venice in 1492. L. Moulé, the leading early French veterinary historian also records printed books by three authors of the 14th and 15th centuries, published in 1486, 1494 and 1495. These works have not been seen. Those books of direct importance in veterinary medicine are discussed individually in the main text.

A work of particular English veterinary interest is *A Dictionary of Veterinary Medicine* 1805, by Thomas Boardman. This review of diseases and treatments in use in the late 18th and early 19th centuries in Britain covers all major species including the dog and cat. A valuable source on early disease outbreaks on a semi-global basis is *Animal Plagues* Vols 1 (1871) and 2 (1882) by George Fleming, a listing of epizootic disease outbreaks in animals, birds and aquatic life. Volume 1 covers 1490 BC to AD 1800 and Volume 2 1800–1844. Fleming probably used another source, said to be French, to gain such a comprehensive coverage of literature citations.

An interesting, and literary, source are the medieval bestiary books. These were written for, and usually by, monks to serve as an aid to meditation. The bestiaries are a bridge between the ancient works and the just developing natural philosophy concepts, and natural history as a study. The books are profusely illustrated with beautiful illustrations, almost always in brilliant colours and embellished with gold. They are of interest specifically for the illustrations of the animals and birds, and also for the text (much of an allegorical nature) related to each species: this reveals items of contemporary knowledge. The text that has been consulted is the *Liber Bestarium* (MS Bodley 764), written in the 13th century and held in the Bodleian Library in Oxford; it contains 135 images of animals, birds, reptiles and fish, both real and imaginary.

Other important reference sources that have been consulted are *The Oxford Encyclopaedia of Ancient Greece and Rome* (Gagarin 2010) and *The Oxford Classical Dictionary* (Hornblower and Spawforth 2003). Invaluable guides to the history and development of domesticated animals have been *A History of Domesticated Animals* (Zeuner 1963), *Evolution of Domesticated Animals* (Mason 1984), *Cattle: A Handbook to the Breeds of the World* (Porter 2007) and *Domesticated Animals from Early Times* (Clutton-Brock 1981).

An interesting and useful introduction to both ancient and European veterinary literature is the 1891 book, *The History of Roman Literature* (Teuffel and Schwabe 2010) which reviews both Vegetius and his work. Additionally, *The Early History of Veterinary Literature* (Smith 1976) provides a good overview, principally related to the early English-language literature.

References

Adams, J.N. (1995) *Pelagonius and Latin Veterinary Terminology in the Roman Empire.* Leiden: E J Brill

Ash, H.B., Forster, E.S. and Hefner, E.H. (1941/1968) *Columella on Agriculture*, Loeb Classical Library 361, 407, 408. London: Harvard University Press

Balme, D.M. (1991) *Historia Animalium*, Books 7–10 (translation) Loeb Classical Library 439. London: Harvard University Press

Clutton-Brock, J. (1981) *Domesticated Animals from the Earliest Times.* London: British Museum/Heinemann

Dalby, A. (2011) *Geoponika: Farm Work.* Totnes: Prospect Books

Fitch, J.G. (2013) *Palladius: The Work of Farming.* Totnes: Prospect Books

French, R. and Greenaway, F. (Eds.) (1986) *Science in the Early Roman Empire: Pliny the Elder, his Sources and Influence.* London: Croom Helm

Gagarin, M. (Ed.) (2010) *The Oxford Encyclopaedia of Ancient Greece and Rome*, Vols 1–7. Oxford: Oxford University Press

Herzog, H. (2010) *Some We Love, Some We Hate, Some We Eat.* New York: HarperCollins

Holland, P. (1963) *Pliny's Natural History* (1601 translation). London: Centaur Press

Hooper, W.D. and Ash, H.B. (1935) *Cato and Varro on Agriculture*, Loeb Classical Library 238. London: Harvard University Press

Hornblower, S. and Spawforth A. (Eds.) (2003) *The Oxford Classical Dictionary*, 3rd edn. Oxford: Oxford University Press

Hort, A.F. (1916, 1980) *Theophrastus Enquiry into Plants*, Books 1–5 (1916) and Books 6–9 (1980) Loeb Classical Library 70 and 79. London: Harvard University Press

Johnson, I. and Horsley, G.H.R. (2011) *Galen: Method of Medicine*, Books 1–4 Loeb Classical Library 516. London: Harvard University Press

Johnston, K. (2009) *The Georgics: A Poem of the Land*. London: Penguin Classics

Jones, W.H.S. (1923) *Hippocrates*, Vol. 1 (translation) Loeb Classical Library 147. London: Harvard University Press

Leblanc, M. (1848) Enumeration of Works Relating to Veterinary Medicine Published up to the Year 1838. *The Veterinarian*

Mason, I.L. (1984) *Evolution of Domesticated Animals*. London: Longman

Mattern, S.P. (2013) *The Prince of Medicine: Galen in the Roman Empire*. Oxford: Oxford University Press

McCabe, A. (2007) *A Byzantine Encyclopaedia of Horse Medicine*. Oxford: Oxford University Press

Morgan, M.H. (2006) *On Horsemanship*. London: Dover Publications

Peck, A.L. (1942) *De Generatione Animalium*, Books 1–5 (translation) Loeb Classical Library 366. London: Harvard University Press

Peck, A.L. (1965) *Historia Animalium*, Books 1–3 (translation) Loeb Classical Library 437. London: Harvard University Press

Peck, A.L. (1970) *Historia Animalium*, Books 4–6 (translation) Loeb Classical Library 438. London: Harvard University Press

Peck, A.L. and Forster, E.S. (1961) *De Partibus Animalium*, Loeb Classical Library 323. London: Harvard University Press

Phillips, A.A. and Willcock, M.M. (1999) *On Hunting*. Warminster: Aris & Phillips

Porter, V. (2007) *Cattle: A Handbook to the Breeds of the World*. London: Christopher Helm

Scholfield, A.F. (1958) *Aelian on Animals*, Loeb Classical Library 446, 448, 449. London: Harvard University Press

Shehada, H.A. (2013) *Mamluks and Animals*. Leiden: Brill

Singer, C. (1956) *Galen on Anatomical Procedures*. Oxford: Oxford University Press

Smith, F. (1976) *The Early History of Veterinary Literature*, Vols 1–4 (reprint 1912–1918 edition). London: J.A. Allen

Spencer, W.G. (1935) *Celsus on Medicine*, Loeb Classical Library 292. London: Harvard University Press

Strassler, R.B. (Ed.) (2009) *Herodotus: The Histories*. New York: Anchor Books

Teuffel, W.S. (2010) *Teuffels's History of Roman Literature Rev. and Enl. By L. Schwabe*. London: General Books

Walker, R.E. (1964) The Veterinary Papyrus of Kahun. *Veterinary Record* **76**

Zeuner, F.E. (1963) *A History of Domesticated Animals*. New York: Harper & Row

PART I

The Veterinary Art Evolves

CHAPTER I

Egypt, Mesopotamia, The Levant and Persia

In tracing the history of veterinary medicine one is confounded by the mists of antiquity, with only the beliefs, presumptions and folk memories of the time before the written word develops. We know practically nothing about the diseases, relationships and practices of prehistoric humans and their animals. Paleopathology does present some knowledge of human disease conditions, but very little of animal ailments, they are seldom interred in known graves.

When hieroglyphic and cuneiform writings were translated and transcribed they provided the first authentic insight into the ancient civilisations and the peoples who used them. Although they had no understanding of the causes of disease and very rarely any reliable treatments the picture is of societies that had some purpose and organisation. They created their own knowledge resource and had constructed a system of laws by which they were governed.

When these cultural developments evolved, an over-riding factor is seen to be a religion, and with that religion a structure of priests. This class of individuals, because of their claimed understanding and relationship with the gods, created controlling factors that both held the populations in thrall and obligated them to the priestly class. Then, as now, a chief concern of the people was sickness, in themselves, their families and their animals. While the religions who came to their aid were dominated by ritual, it is obvious that they had acquired a level of knowledge and an early understanding of certain aspects of disease. Some of this was sensible and logical, however it was also offered with magic, incantations and invariably ritual animal sacrifice, as a means of expelling the demons believed to be causing the sickness, and as an act of propitiation to the gods.

Without knowing the causes of disease, the concept developed, probably by the priesthoods, that sickness was related to genies, devils and demons who had to be overcome. In ancient times almost all disease and phenomena: floods, lightning, thunder, earthquakes, drought, were believed to have a supernatural origin. If medications and treatment failed, the last resort was spells and incantations to please and placate the gods – and the priests took it to be their task to protect people and animals. It is not easy to fully understand such cultures.

The time and place of the origins of veterinary practice is unknown. It dates from the domestication of animals and the human realisation of the value of this relationship in economic and companionship terms, which can only be understood from a knowledge of how civilisations developed. It is universally agreed that Western civilisation evolved from the Fertile Crescent, 'the land between two rivers' – the Euphrates and Tigris (in modern Iraq). In fact, archaeological studies have revealed that there was a broad cultural evolutionary trend from Egypt in North Africa to modern-day Palestine, Syria, Iraq, western Iran, southern Turkey and with connections to other civilisations in the Indus Valley and possibly China.

Our knowledge of the origins of veterinary medicine is derived from the limited evidence surviving from around 2000 BC. From these fragments a picture of veterinary medicine's development can be traced. The technology of writing developed slowly in disparate and diverse ways. The pre-alphabetic texts are found in three main systems:

- hieroglyphic (pictogram) – Egyptian, on papyrus and wall paintings
- cuneiform (syllabic) – Assyrian, Persian, Phoenician, others, on clay tablets
- symbols (ideogram) – Etruscan, Cretan, others, on plates, coins and wall paintings.

The Egyptian pictograms became highly developed, eventually into a form of cursive script, enabled by the use of the paper-like papyrus, but nonetheless an essentially fragile medium and therefore much of the work has been lost. Cuneiform texts, made by cut reed imprints on moist clay tablets, have survived well and especially when the tablets were baked, which makes them almost indestructible. Some civilisations used symbolic ideograms that have resisted translation, but other images, in the forms of wall paintings and sculptures, indicate that these cultures had an active interest in and use of animals and birds.

The two centres that have left early translatable texts were very different civilisations. In both Egypt and Mesopotamia, at approximately the same time, there are records of veterinary medicine procedures and of recognised specialists working in this field.

Egypt

Egypt provided the first known written document of veterinary medicine; because it is written on papyrus it has only survived in fragments. These were discovered in 1889 by Flinders Petrie in the Fayyum district. The first English translation was by F.L. Griffith in 1898, with a definitive assessment and interpretation being made by Walker (1964, pp. 198–200).

The text, commonly known as the Kahun papyrus, was discovered with other, mostly administrative, papyri and a medical gynaecological treatise (of significant interest in ancient Egypt because of the young age at which many women had their first child). The veterinary papyrus is tentatively dated 1900–1800 BC. As a point of accuracy: Flinders Petrie misunderstood the spelling of the location 'el-Lahun' and expressed it as 'Kahun'. Egyptologists now recognise the correct designation as – the veterinary papyrus of el-Lahun (Driesch 2001, pp. 105–106).

The text is written in cursive hieroglyphics, where the characters are read from left to right and which was the religious manner of presentation, and not in the more common hieratic script. The papyrus was of very good quality, which indicates that it was an important document. All that remains is some six miniscule pieces with a main fragment about 58.5 cm in length and 14.5 cm in width of 48 columns of text. It is seen to be composed according to a plan, with discernible headings – Title, Symptoms, Notice ('what must be read for it', i.e., treatment), Treatment, Prognosis, Development, New examination and New symptoms, Supplementary treatment. There was a system of case reporting, exactly the same as that used in describing human ailments: Egyptian veterinary and human medicine were one discipline.

The first case described is of a bull with 'nest of the worm' then, after a portion of lost text, 'If, after he stretches out *ith*', an unknown word but may mean some kind of noise made by the ox. 'I must insert my hand into the rectum. A bowl of water is at my side. The man's hand comes [on the bull] to caress his dorsal spine'– presumably an assistant pressing on the bull's back. This part of the text is written in red (to give special emphasis, but not explained why) and goes on to explain that the operator, 'must take out the clots, the matter, and the mucus from the rectum' washing his hand after each removal. A possible diagnosis of severe necrotic gastroenteritis has been suggested. A notable record because the case is the first recorded example of manual evacuation of the rectum in an attempt to treat a bovine abdominal ailment.

The second case covers instructions for a bull suffering from having the *nft*, this is a word used for the wind, breath or blowing –a respiratory condition or caused by the wind as the source of the disease. 'If I see a bull suffering from *nftw* [respiratory symptom] his eyes run; his temples are heavy; his gums are red and he has swellings on the neck . . . he must be laid on his side and splashed with water . . . his eyes, his flanks and his limbs should be rubbed with *hns* or *ssw* [unknown plant juices, extracts or oils] . . .', the next piece of the text is missing 'he must be carried out of the water . . . and rubbed with *hns* or *kádt* [unknown plants] . . . he will be bled on the nose and the tail. You must say "he has been bled" and then he will come through it or he will die'. Diagnostic suggestions have been bovine gangrenous coryza, malignant catharral fever, or rinderpest. The rest of the papyrus describes livestock afflicted with buccal and ocular lesions and suffering from profound depression. The fragments include possible mentions of fish and birds.

Study of wall paintings and funerary models indicate that the Egyptians were skilful stockhandlers, they had knowledge of obstetrics and feeding. Illustrations show cattle without horns, as it is believed that there were no hornless breeds in ancient Egypt, possibly they understood a dehorning technique. Depictions of draught oxen show that castration was practised, but no details of the procedures used have survived. The case above, in a bull, describes a 'nest of worms': it is unclear what this means, but the inevitable high stocking rate in the Nile Valley would suggest a parasitism problem.

In the Egyptian assemblage of gods, the healing knowledge was held by the Ibis-headed Thot (who also protected the arts of writing and eloquence). Thot passed the secrets of healing to the Egyptian priesthood and they were used by Imhotep, a priest of Ra, who became the court physician to Pharaoh Djoser, c.2700 BC. Many years later Imhotep was also celebrated as the god of healing (Karasszon 1988, pp. 38–39). In the complex stories of the gods it was Thot who healed the child Horus of an illness, who was then blinded by Set resulting in the Eye of Horus (*udjat*). This hieroglyph became the symbol of protection against disease as well as having healing power, and can also mean 'to make or do' or 'one who does'. The mathematical dimensions of the eye were used to determine the proportions of ingredients in preparing medications. The symbolism of the Horus eye survived for centuries in the 'Rx' pharmaceutical cipher for 'take thou' at the commencement of a prescription, for either veterinary or human use.

Healing and related knowledge in ancient Egypt was incorporated into religious texts, and it appears that priests became medical professionals for humans and animals. The extant literature is limited, for veterinary medicine only the el-Lahun/Kahun papyrus, but for human medicine there is the classical Ebers papyrus. While this dates from 2660 BC to 2160 BC, the copy found originates from about 1650 BC to 1552 BC. Another nine medical papyri have been found in various stages of completeness and readability. The 110-page Ebers papyrus covers many conditions and treatments, including magical spells. The content indicates that Egyptian medicine considered excrements and corrupt materials were capable of penetrating the veins, and therefore bleeding was essential to remove these. The word *metous* was used to describe the arteries, veins and nerves, these were thought to be the points of access for blood, medications and sickness. According to interpretation both the air and secretions, such as saliva, sperm, urine and faeces, were carried to their destinations by various *metous*, including four which connected the liver to the rectum where they carried the faecal matter. Walker (1991, pp. 10–11) has suggested that the Hebrew practices show an analogy with those of the Egyptians by rejecting as food the hind quarters of slaughtered animals, possibly connected with the idea that this body part contained the *metous* that carried excrements, urine and sperm.

Of the other papyri the most important is the Edwin Smith papyrus, dated c.1600–1500 BC, the only surviving Egyptian surgical text, believed to be based on an earlier (3000–2500 BC) papyrus. It covers trauma surgery and also demonstrates that Egyptian medical professionals knew the major internal organs and recognised that the blood vessels were linked to the heart, but did not understand the circulation of the blood. The pulse was recognised, cautery was used, fractures were immobilised and treated, enemas were applied and many salves formulated. Both the sensible application of hygiene and preventive medicine precautions were described.

Laxatives played an important role in medications with an apparent belief that faeces might be related to, or were part of, the cause of disease. Bleeding was important, bleeding from the nose in cattle might be associated with a belief that it was curative for conditions of the head. Bleeding by cutting the throat (exsanguination) was seen as a procedure to allow undesirable materials to be drained from the body, this concept may be the origin of the ritual slaughter practices of some religions today.

There are comparisons to be made in the words and descriptions used in the human and veterinary texts. The word *dgmy* (translated as 'without words') was observed in the el-Lahun/Kahun papyrus referring to a prostrate bull, and the same expression is found in the Edwin Smith papyrus in describing a wounded man with a penetrating head injury – also explaining that he is 'silent in sadness', 'does not speak', 'after something has penetrated into the inside'. In another human case the patient is described as *dgm* or 'someone having received a blow from something coming from the outside', there is also veterinary use of the word. A final note is more explicit – 'the breathing of an external god or death'. It must be appreciated that the Egyptian language used very elaborate means of expression, making precise translation difficult.

From the quality of the papyrus and the priestly script used it is argued that veterinary medicine was of an equal status to that of the human art. The tomb inscriptions of the priest-physicians of Sekhmet state 'The author of the inscription Aha-Nekht. I was a priest of Sekhmet, mighty and skilful in my art, I placed my hand on the patient and I understood [his disease], I was skilful in examining with my hands, I knew about cattle . . .' (Anthes 1928, pp. 33–35, cited by Walker). Medicine was an art that was applied to both humans and animals.

From these papyri was given an insight in to how medicine was organised. Rather than schools of medicine, temples had 'houses of life', which provided quarters for expert copyists who transcribed the ancient medical writings, which went back well over 1000 years. This was necessary as the writing systems were continually evolving to a more cursive form, reserved for the religious documents of the priestly class (Sournia 1992, pp. 42–56).

Priest/physicians, including surgeons, passed their expertise to the members of their family or caste. They were an elite part of the hierarchy of civil servants that worked throughout the country: they had official titles indicating their status, and also assistants of differing grades. No fees were charged, their payment was in food and clothing: some were classed as doctor-priests and some as doctor-magicians. Herodotus (Strassler 2009, pp. 150, 152), following his visit to Egypt, wrote that all doctors were specialists; this was probably correct in the major cities but unlikely throughout the country. Specialisation was well developed with gynaecological, eye, and abdominal problems being the most prominent. He also noted the Egyptian belief that disease was related to ingestion of food and that for three days every month many people went through a ritual of enemas and induced vomiting, to clear their body systems.

Egyptian medicine began with very good practices and systems, however, over the following centuries it stagnated. With medical (and presumably veterinary) practice restricted to the same families and castes, being included as a part of religion and ritual, and being based in texts written many hundreds of years earlier, there was little opportunity for progress. It is interesting to note that when one pharaoh was seriously ill, help was requested from Assyria. The examination procedures that were followed (as listed earlier) by both human and veterinary practitioners were well based and sound but prescribing treatments was essentially empirical, and heavily influenced by magic and incantations to Amon-Re, Isis, or other gods. Unfortunately, the Egyptians created a system that combined logic and magic; they did, however, appreciate good hygiene procedures and laid down medical principles that are still utilised such as regular washing with clean water.

While the existence of 'veterinarians' in ancient Egypt is not proven, what is known is that a priestly caste recognised animal disease, used diagnostic methods and procedures, and instituted treatments. Funerary paintings also indicate that the priests were used to assess the value and health of sacrificial animals and the butchery of the resulting carcases: this indicates a meat inspection role. A parallel can be drawn with Mosaic Law, including the strict texts on ritual slaughter and the inspection of meat – possibly an effect of Egyptian influence on the Jews while they were held in captivity, and remembered after leaving Egypt (Walker 1991, p. 12).

While specific information on veterinary medicine is confined to the one surviving papyrus, a picture of veterinary procedures can be developed from a study of other papyri and wall paintings. Reviewing these Karasszon (1988, pp. 41–45) lists the eight classes of priests. One of these, the *pastophoros*, a separate order dating from the Third Dynasty (c.2686–c.2613 BC), dealt with the designated holy animals and birds: they cared for them, used their behaviour patterns for prophecy and carried their gods in processions. They were experts in the diseases of the animals they cared for, and were said to cure the ailing animal gods when needed. Pastophores were divided into specialist groups for differing types and species of holy animals and birds. They were also the priestly group who examined the meat of slaughtered animals, banning the consumption of meat they considered 'objectionable' – including saltwater fish and pork.

It has been deduced from non-medical papyri that pastophore priests held secret books in which diseases and remedies were described (possibly the el-Lahun/Kahun papyrus was one of these). They were also responsible for the examination of animals before sacrifice, conduct of sacrifice and examination of viscera: they must have acquired some knowledge, now unknown. Pastophores, like other priests, were required to make a vow to keep their knowledge secret. Breaking of the oath was punishable by death – by drinking a decoction of the seed of the apricot-tree devoted to Muth (from which the Latin *mutus* and *mors*, death, are derived). Muth was the god of silence.

Mention has to be made of the 'plagues' identified in the Bible Old Testament, Exodus 7:8. The fifth plague in the time of Moses, which affected cattle, from its description was most probably carbuncular anthrax. The observation that the cattle of the Egyptians, which grazed the lowland pastures of the Nile Delta, were badly affected, whereas those of the Israelites were largely unaffected is possibly significant. The probable reason being that the Israelites were forced to graze the poorer higher land, lying farther from the delta. River basins subject to annual flooding have a reputation for being favourable for the recurrence and spread of anthrax (Smithcors 1958, p. 30).

Mesopotamia

The agricultural prosperity of the 'Fertile Crescent' was the basis of the Mesopotamian civilisation that developed as the evolving cities and empires struggled against each other, each building their own culture. They created innovative agriculture cultivating a wide range of crops and raising domesticated goats, pigs, cattle and sheep (Bourke 2008, pp. 58–59). The first true Mesopotamian urban culture was the Sumerian, whose people developed writing, dating from c.3500 BC. Other city states formed, were absorbed into empires until a dominant autocracy was created by Hammurabi of the First Babylonian dynasty; Semitic in origin it absorbed the earlier well developed Sumerian civilisation. Later his empire was subjugated by the Assyrians, until Babylon was absorbed into the Persian Empire in 539 BC (Saggs 2003, pp. 161–174, 234–249).

Animal produce was a significant part of the diet, based on milk from sheep and goats, also from cattle. Owing to the high temperatures milk was mostly processed to yoghurt, butter, ghee or cheese. A 3rd millennium frieze depicts milk production and milk food preparation: farmers had learned that by showing the cow her calf, milk 'let-down' was triggered, the system was well developed. Most other animal protein came from fish, but sheep meat and sometimes beef was eaten at festivals (mostly from sacrificial animals). There was no taboo on pig meat, large herds were present. Dead asses were fed to dogs. Meat was preserved by salting or desiccation.

Details of Mesopotamian medicine are not readily available as the clay tablet cuneiform texts were limited in their scope being initially introduced for record keeping and then mathematics: writing was more of a shorthand. Medicine began to be studied as evident in their early laws.

The most significant feature of Mesopotamian civilisation was the establishment of a concept of justice headed by the king. The earliest known laws were those of Ur-Nammu, first king of the Ur Dynasty (c.2700 BC), but little of their content has survived. The next legal code was the *Law of Lipit-Ishtar* (c.1950 BC), only fragments have survived, but these include laws 34–37 grouped as 'Fines for damage to a hired ox': of these, law 35 states 'If a man has hired an ox and damaged its eye, he shall pay half its price.' One of the first recognitions of health issues.

Both of these legal codes were written in cuneiform in the Sumerian language and were followed by the *Laws of Eshnunna*, in Akkadian. Dating is unconfirmed but probably two to three hundred years before the next (Hammurabi) legal code. The forty-eight section Eshnunna code, was found on just two clay tablets; most relevant are laws 53–58: 'Responsibility for damage caused by an ox, dog or collapsing wall.' Law 54 states:

If an ox is one that gores and the authorities have notified the owner, but his ox is not kept under control and it gores a man and causes his death, then the owner shall pay two-thirds of a mina of silver.

The expression of a fine in silver seldom resulted in such payment; it was used as a standard by which goods of a similar value would be paid. This law is very similar to the later Hammurabi law 251 also fixing a fine in silver, and is echoed in the Bible, Exodus 21:29, where both ox and man are sentenced to death.

The other Eshnunna laws (55 and 56) relating to damage done by a dog have been interpreted as referring to a rabid animal: if so it would be a very early mention of rabies. If not, it does indicate that dogs were a regular part of society and had to be kept under control. The owners of uncontrolled dogs were subject to a heavy fine, if they had not heeded a warning and a subsequent bite resulted in a human death.

The establishment of the empire by Hammurabi (c.1800–1750 BC) was significant in the history of the Mesopotamia region. He considerably expanded the territory under his control and established his legal code, built on earlier laws. The *Laws of Hammurabi*, dated c.1800 BC, illustrate their debt to previous proclamations, however, they are more extensive and better ordered and presented. Arranged in more than 260 sections they are engraved in cuneiform text on a diorite stele found at Susa, now Iran, in 1902. A carving at the top shows Hammurabi receiving the laws from Shamash, the god of justice. The stele is preserved in the Louvre collection in Paris.

The laws are prefaced by a prologue praising Hammurabi and include an epilogue that establishes their authority, and calls on succeeding rulers to also follow these precepts (these broad principles were observed for the next 1000 years). The laws established a moral code for society: all major human interactions and financial dealings are comprehensively covered. Of relevance is the category 'Professional fees and responsibilities', this includes laws 215–225 dealing with 'fees payable to surgeons of men and surgeons of animals; penalties in the event of failure'. The relevant 'veterinary' laws are as follows.

224 If a doctor of animals performs a major operation on an ox or ass and cures it, the owner of the ox or ass shall give to the doctor one-sixth of a shekel of silver as his fee. [Translations vary, another reads six shekels as the fee. A shekel was a silver coin weighing 16.8 g]

225 If he performed a major operation on an ox or ass and has caused its death, he shall give to the owner one-fourth of its value.

Also of interest are two groups of 'Agriculture' laws with a veterinary relationship.

241–9 Distraint, hire, death and injury of oxen.
245 Anyone who has killed a hired ox by maltreatment or beating shall give the owner another ox.

246 Anyone who has broken a bone of a hired ox shall give the owner another ox.

247 Anyone who has put out the eye(s) of a hired ox shall recompense the owner by paying half of the ox's price.

248 Anyone who has broken the horn(s), has cut off the tail or has hurt the mouth of a hired ox shall recompense the owner by paying half of the ox's price.

249 If a hired ox has died due to an accident, the hirer, if he has sworn to his innocence, remains unpunished.

250–2 Responsibility for damage by a goring ox.
250 If an ox walking on the street tosses and kills someone the resulting point of law should not serve as basis for legal claim.

251 If the owner of a vicious ox has been told about the bad nature of the

animal, does not wrap the ox's horns and does not hold the ox, and the ox kills someone, the owner shall pay ½ mina (308 g silver).

252   The owner of an ox that has killed a slave shall pay ⅓ mina (206 g silver).

263   Responsibility for damage to animals

263   Anyone that has ruined a beast or sheep entrusted to his care should recompense the owner with a beast for each beast and a sheep for each sheep.

For the medical practitioner the penalties were more severe: 'If a surgeon has made a deep incision in a man with a bronze instrument and caused the man to die ... they shall cut off his hand.' It is not known how often such a penalty was enforced, but it must have ensured great care was taken in surgery. Fees were also based on the social class of the patient, for a similar procedure on a slave two shekels were due; for a free man, five shekels; for an aristocrat or priest, ten shekels. Veterinary fees were significantly lower. Penalties for deliberately wounding or harming working animals were severe; the act was classed as criminal.

At this time much attention was given to divination, to determine a disease's cause and for a hoped-for prognosis. An important divination practice was hieromancy, the examination of the internal organs of a freshly slaughtered animal, particularly a sheep's liver. This was conducted by a *baru*, or divination priest, who would try to determine the supernatural force or spirit that was causing the disease. The liver would be examined for any slight variations in appearance. These were then interpreted according to their location – many clay models of sheep livers, presumably made for instruction, have been excavated, carefully marked in squares with symbols. It was a highly developed practice, and used for many purposes, 'For the King of Babylon standeth at the parting of the ways ... to use divinations ... he looketh at the liver' (Ezekiel 21:21).

Unfortunately for veterinary history, only animals in good condition were selected for slaughter, as a result the diviners would rarely have experienced diseased livers or other organs, which could have suggested an explanation for any abnormal external condition. The cost of giving over an animal for slaughter for divination was beyond the means of many of the people, and less costly divination methods were used, such as bird flight, smoke signs or oil drops on water.

Babylonian medicine developed similar, but not identical methods to those in Egypt. A series of 'prescription texts', from the Third Ur Dynasty (just before 2000 BC) have been found (unfortunately incomplete) which note symptoms and a list of medications with preparation instructions. These were mostly oral with some administered by breathing a vapour into the nostrils, or even by sucking into the nostrils (possibly for onward transmission to the palate and alimentary tract). Poultices, potions and bathing with hot infusions were all listed.

There was no advanced knowledge of surgery and very little of anatomy. It was believed that the bodily organs were the seats of the differing parts of human behaviour – the heart was thought to be the source of creative intelligence and the ears that of understanding. Medical practice involved checking the pulse and while it was recognised that blood moved in the veins there did not appear to be any knowledge of the circulation. Procedures such as lancing abscesses and bleeding to remove 'corruption' were mentioned, as are eye diseases (no doubt due to the sandy, dusty environment). Fracture treatment with splints was practised. It is reasonable to assume that all the above was known to the animal healers as well and were used with animals.

The great medical deficiency was the lack of a basic understanding of disease causation. Believing that sickness was due to demonic possession various apotropaic devices were used to avert evil influences or ill-luck. Amulets of various types were worn, and also placed on horned animals, as a protection. Religion played the major role in both protection and diagnosis: the principal god worshipped was Marduk, the son of Ea, the god of magic. Much prognosis was by divination in particular by liver examination, looking for omens. Animals offered to the gods as propitiation were slaughtered on special altars or on the temple roof. The throat was cut by a *nash patri* or sword bearer and the meat was frequently distributed to the priests and onlookers. Ritual sacrificial slaughter was a common practice – for example, to seal a treaty of peace between former enemies a donkey foal was killed.

Healers of humans and of animals had been recognised from very early days in Mesopotamia. From inscriptions in the ancient Sumerian/Akkadian texts (c.2500 BC) the words *asuanshe* and *azagulia* have been found which have been translated as a 'cattle healer'. These individuals were also associated with mystical practices to remove demons. The developing art of veterinary medicine was evolving with a mixture of early medicine and surgery and with the priest and divination.

Of interest is a cylinder seal found in the Sumerian tomb of King Ur-Ningursu, from the Second Dynasty of Lagash (c.2200–2100 BC). The cuneiform inscription reads:

O God Edinmugi, Vizier of the God Gir
who helps pregnant animals give birth
Urlugalidenna the doctor is your servant.

Accompanying the text are drawings of what have been described as gynaecological instruments and equipment, together with an image of Urlugalidenna. This would appear to be the first known named veterinarian. The cylinder seal is in the collection with the Hammurabi stele in the Louvre Museum, Paris.

By the time of Hammurabi the word *Asos* or *Azu* was in use, translated as 'healer' or 'doctor', and linked to either human or animal practitioners. It would indicate that veterinary work was performed by a recognised class of individuals. The groups of medically related workers were strongly hierarchical with physicians the most highly rated followed by surgeons, next veterinary surgeons, and then midwives, wet nurses and exorcists. From extant sources it can be determined that these individuals had a pragmatic and more realistic approach to health, and understood contagion (but probably not why) (Woolf 2005, p. 105). The level of veterinary knowledge is not known but tablets dated between 1000 and 645 BC from the Chaldean Empire (later absorbed into Babylonia) show an efficient livestock management system indicating an understanding of animal management and some healing practices.

Animals featured in the practices of priest-exorcists (*ashipu*), which involved omens, incantations and much ritual to move the evil spirit named as responsible for a disease symptom from a patient to an animal. Usually a goat kid, dressed in the patient's clothes, was placed in the patient's bed for the night. In the morning the exorcist would remove the kid and cut its throat, thus eliminating the cause of the disease. This 'scapegoat' practice was widely used across the Near and Middle East, including being adopted by the early Hebrews. There is no record of the success rate of this procedure, but it was one that survived in England to the 18th century – a dog was used to sleep with the patient to receive the evil spirit, but was allowed to live for another day.

Medical practice in Babylonia developed in a slow and limited way but gradually acquired skills: it has to be presumed that some of the applicable ones would have been followed by the veterinary practitioners. Human life expectancy was short – malaria, smallpox, eye, alimentary tract and sexually transmitted diseases were widespread. Maternal and infant mortality was high. There was little famine as water levels were generally high and harvests were maintained. Disease was endured as a punishment for a sin. The guardian spirits were also believed to cause harm and they were named after the specific organs they attacked, and could be used to make a diagnosis.

The medical culture that arose in Mesopotamia, eventually concentrating in Babylonia, was based on a belief that disease was a supernatural effect of demons, was diagnosed by omens and was treated according to observable symptoms. Treatment by physicians, surgeons or veterinarians was dominated by incantations, magic and religious rites. Malaria, epilepsy and strokes were all identified in the clinical state, resulting in the patient undergoing a vigorous enquiry to identify the sin that had been committed (Saggs 2003, p. 379). It was known how to reduce fractures, remove foreign bodies, amputate limbs, treat cataracts and use a urethral sound to ease stricture. Medication was mostly of plant-origin, with some minerals and animal organs. Cassia, myrtle, belladonna, willow, asafoetida, salt (cleanser) and saltpetre (astringent) were all used. Preparations included infusions, decoctions, salves, embrocations, ointments, enemas and suppositories. It was recorded that oral herbal mixtures could be taken in either beer or milk to improve palatability.

Veterinary surgery was restricted to castration, and the treatment of wounds and fractures. There was little mention of the animal plagues in the cuneiform texts, but these would have been present. Sheep, goats and oxen were the important livestock, plus pigs. Dogs were companions and guards. The onager and the ass (donkey) were kept before the introduction of the horse. A pedigree chart dated to the Chaldean Empire almost certainly depicts onagers, probably in the proto-Elamic era; indicating both stallions and mares, it is highly suggestive of a selective breeding programme (Jöchle 2006, pp. 119–124).

Hammurabi on his death, was followed by his son King Samsuiluna, who in his correspondence not only mentions horses, which had arrived in numbers with the invading nations, but also mentions a bovine veterinarian, Abil-ilisu, in a legal document (Schäffer 1999, pp. 252–254). The Hammurabi Empire fell to the Kassites in 1530 BC and they in turn to the Assyrians: both were Semitic peoples who regarded disease as a supernatural occurrence. Medicine made little progress. Finally, in 539 BC the Babylonian Empire was conquered by the Persians. A closing note – the Mesopotamian civilisation created a sanctuary for the god, Marduk. It was named *Babilim*, in Greek, Babylon.

The Horse Comes to Mesopotamia

Use of the equine animal has been important in human civilisation for both transport and pleasure, but in particular for warfare. Initially the only equid found native in Mesopotamia was the onager (also called hemione or half-ass); they are depicted in the Royal Cemetery of Ur in Chaldea (c.2500 BC) drawing chariots. Other depictions indicate that they were quite widely used by Sumerians in the 3rd millennium BC for pulling wagons and for riding, and were also probably bred (Zeuner 1963, pp. 367–373). The horse did not enter the Mesopotamia region until about 1900 BC, following domestication on the Eurasia steppe. Initial arrival appears to have been from Anatolia (southern Turkey) and the Zagros Mountain region (spanning Iran, northern Iraq and southern Turkey). Images are seen in figurative depictions, from about 1700 BC. That the horse was not named in the Hammurabi Laws would suggest at that time it was not an animal of importance (Zeuner 1963, pp. 317–319).

Visual evidence from Assyrian bas-reliefs show King Assurbanipal (r.668–c.627 BC), a keen hunter, used the horse extensively in his famed lion hunts. His palaces had both stables and breeding facilities. Excavations at Nimrud, the ancient Assyrian city (Iraq), revealed a 7th-century BC cuneiform tablet fragment detailing equine veterinary medication, listing plants and instructions for preparation to anoint the abdomen of a horse with 'cutting abdominal ache', probably a colic remedy. From the mode of presentation, this could have been part of a veterinary almanac (Donaghy 2010).

At some date the ass had also reached Mesopotamia; as they are an African species they would have been a benefit of trade between Egypt and the Levant. It appears that the horse from the north and the ass from the south arrived in the Middle East at about the same time. Possibly the two species met during the Hittite period (c.1680 BC). The ass is first mentioned in the Bible, Genesis 12:16, when the Egyptian pharaoh presented some to Abraham together with other livestock. As a result, cross breeding with the horse began and the mule was produced; it is known that crosses had been made with onagers, but these were unsatisfactory. The ideal animal was found to be the hybrid from breeding a male ass with a female horse – interestingly this is an infertile animal (although some fertile ones have been claimed).

The mule is a valuable equine, highly prized for strength and endurance, good heat tolerance and an ideal haulage and transport animal. The horse is more agile and better used for cavalry and chariot warfare. The ass, while being very useful, is generally despised and mainly used as a beast of burden: the meat is only rarely eaten. Its greatest contribution to mankind has been as the progenitor of the mule. A cross between a male horse and female donkey will produce a hinny, but these are rare (Zeuner 1963, pp. 380–383). The Bible, Genesis 36:24, states that the Edomites and Husites combined the two species and invented mule breeding at Mount Seir, Petra. However, this only appears in the Authorised Version, other translations produce 'hot springs' in place of mules. The Authorised Version may not be an authoritative source for equine history.

The Hittites

Early 20th-century excavations in Anatolia revealed the Hittite Empire – previously it was believed that the Hittites were simply one of the tribes that the Israelites found when they entered Palestine, as listed in the Old Testament, Genesis 15:19–21.

Excavations at Tel-el Amarna and Boghazköy (Turkey) have revealed over 10,000 clay tablets, from which an indication of the scope and longevity of their civilisation can be obtained. This lasted until they were overcome by the Mushki (Phrygians) in about 1200 BC. An (incomplete) Hittite code of laws indicates that animals were important, with sections related to yoking the ox, horse, mule and ass. The pig, plough-oxen and bees also feature. Sheep, goat and cattle meat was eaten, but not pigs or equines. There is no mention of a veterinary (or a medical) class. The rise of Hittite power was partly due to their development of a fast light horse chariot with two spoked wheels, unlike the previous slow onager drawn chariots with solid wheels. It became a potent weapon of war, and was immediately copied by all neighbouring countries.

In the Boghazköy excavations a comprehensive four tablet treatise on the training and acclimatisation of horses for chariot warfare was found. This instruction document was the key to using horses effectively. Written by an author in Mitanni, a neighbouring state, mainly in Syria, south of Hittite lands. Known as the Kikkuli Text (dated c.1360 BC) it contained specialist horse knowledge: probably the earliest known on equine management. Of particular interest are the words used to describe various tactical procedures in warfare: they are similar to Sanskrit (the ancient north Indian Aryan tongue). Other texts indicate that the rulers of Mitanni worshipped Indo-Aryan deities with Indian sounding names and that the rulers used this Aryan language. The finding is one of the earliest records of the relationship between Mesopotamia and Indian civilisations, and an indication of their equine expertise (Gurney 2003, pp. 102, 120).

The Levant: Phoenicia and Israel

The Levant is an area of the eastern Mediterranean. Its importance is its coastline, with the core areas falling in the lands of Syria/Palestine and running from a northern border with Anatolia (southern Turkey) and extending south through current Syria, Lebanon, Israel, the Palestinian lands to the Egyptian Sinai border. The territory has been a key factor in the distribution of knowledge, as well as the probable base from which early pre-alphabetic veterinary and human medicine made contact with the developing Hellenic medical culture centred on the Aegean Sea. The initial reason for these contacts was the trade between Egypt and the Lebanon: Byblos (Lebanon) became a major port. The Egyptians with their constant building works needed Levantine wood, the big cedar trees on the hills and slopes of Mount Lebanon. Egypt's need for the Levantine cedar wood was a major factor in the development of trade between Egypt and elsewhere in the Mediterranean, as well as providing a through conduit eastwards to Babylon. Not only trade but knowledge flowed.

There were many disparate tribes of people in this much fought over region. The history is incomplete because of a dark age (1200–900 BC) and a dearth of relevant cuneiform texts. The information that is available is based on Hittite texts from the north and their invasion, together with Egyptian papyri detailing correspondence with the local kings, and later from the Bible, Old Testament writings. Specific cultures evolved in three locations: Hittites in the north, in the centre various city states (the most active founded by the Phoenicians), and Canaan in the south with the Semitic tribes – Ammonite, Moabite, Edomite, Philistine and the Hebrews, who were first mentioned to be present in Canaan in 1210 BC. Gradually the Hebrews became the dominant tribe with a significant rise in power under King Solomon (960–920 BC).

The Phoenician cities, in particular Tyre and Sidon in the mid-Levant, became dominant, reaching their greatest prominence about 1000 BC. They rapidly built their trading empire across the Mediterranean. Metals became important and the Tyrian maritime economy was able to supply Solomon with the bronze and wood he required to build his temple, aided by an earlier treaty signed with Tyre by his father King David. Phoenicia grew in strength as a collection of city states spread around the Mediterranean.

Animals were of low importance in the Levant, the little agricultural land was mainly devoted to vines, olives and cereals; some sheep, but mostly goats were raised on the poorer soils of the hills. Fish provided the staple protein food. As early as 1600 BC Tyre developed the cultivation of *Murex* shellfish (sea snails) and extraction of the famed purple dye, then known as Tyrian Blue: it became a significant high price export for the clothes of royalty. Phoenician coins frequently portrayed the murex shell, as well as dolphins, equine heads and a bull/lion combat. Generally, food staples were in short supply, imports were necessary including wool for cloth production. Animal sacrifice was common with offerings of blood or a burned sacrifice: lambs or sheep were usually used. While pigs were in the countryside they were not allowed to be used for sacrifice and eating their meat was taboo (Markoe 2005, pp. 2, 48, 110, 114, 158). Of perhaps greatest importance, the Phoenicians developed the use of alphabetic writing, driven by its use recording their trading activities. It became the progenitor of the Greek alphabet and of European languages.

One of the more important early centres was Ugarit (now Ras Shamrah, Syria), a coastal city established before the Phoenicians arrived. Excavations have revealed clay tablets dealing with veterinary procedures, dated about 1500–1300 BC. The inscriptions deal with equine treatment, the tablets were badly damaged and the naming of the disease conditions is unclear, but nasal application is indicated for each one. The medications are of plant-origin: figs, fruits, flour and herbs are listed. The text is the first known description of the equine nasal route of application; while incomplete it demonstrates veterinary knowledge (possibly Canaanite) (Schäeffer 1939, pp. 49, 56). Translation has suggested that the first condition listed is commonly known as 'roaring' (laryngeal hemiplegia), but it is probable that the translation is incorrect, or poorly expressed. Other conditions identified include difficulties with urination and defaecation, putrid discharge (site of discharge not named) and pain – this is probably associated with colic, a not infrequent equine problem. Other ailments are listed; one of these describes 'itching', a symptom of equine mange, a common horse problem (Cohen and Sivan 1983).

Eventually the Phoenician cities were absorbed into the Persian Empire, who were anxious to keep the Mediterranean trading links open. Their city states established around the coast were absorbed by the expanding Greek colonies and then the Roman Empire. One stood alone, the city established at Carthage (Tunisia): it made a final break in the 6th century BC from its Phoenician roots and gradually developed their own language and society – Punic (discussed in Chapter 3).

The land that became Biblical Israel in the south of Canaan was home to other Semitic tribes; it is believed that under their influence the Hebrews abandoned nomadic life and moved to agriculture and an urban civilisation. Their establishment under the guidance of Moses, resulted in laws and cultural practices that continue to affect the Western world. While in Mesopotamia (Babylon) and in the Nile Valley (Egypt) the Hebrews adopted characteristics of those cultures into their own evolving culture. These characteristics, transmitted through the text of the Bible, became a part of the Christian religion. If Christianity had not developed from Judaism it is most probable that the Israelites would today only be recognised as an interesting early tribe in Palestine, of little importance. While there is scant evidence that the Hebrew culture made any significant contribution to veterinary medicine *per se,* the structure of their society and the Mosaic strict legal code has had a profound effect on medical, and veterinary practice.

One has to be cautious in the use of the Bible as an historical source, as there is a scarcity of independent sources that make clear-cut references to the Hebrews, Israel or particular biblical events from the estimated period that the Old Testament covers – the 2nd millennium BC. Where the biblical text is of value, is to get a better understanding of the ancient cultural practices and civilisation. However, as biblical writings, over many centuries, have undergone both differing translations and editorial revisions, caution has to be exercised in utilising the content. There is much confusion in both dates and placings in the biblical text compared with the archaeological record, which leads to disagreement between religious scholars and historians. The Merneptah Stele (c.1208 BC) is often held to indicate the appearance of the Israelite people in Palestine. Housed in Cairo it is the earliest written reference to Israel and the only documentation from Egyptian sources.

Of veterinary and medical interest are two important features of Judaism, the Laws of Moses and the hygienic measures introduced into this early culture. The significant point about Mosaic Law is that it appears to carry many of the features of the earlier legal codes of the Babylonian kingdoms and of Ugarit. The difference is that the Mesopotamian codes were all given by the kings to their god for approval. The Law of Moses came from god to humanity: the emphasis was radically changed.

The major impact of Mosaic Law was that the concept of disease as a punishment for sin was made a reality for the Jews. This was a Babylonian Semitic concept that the Jews adopted; it appeared in the Bible Old Testament and has affected the Western world for many centuries, both animals and humans. Since an affliction was punishment for a sin and only those worthy of a cure were healed, the early Jews had little need for physicians – and no physicians names are in these early records. Veterinary medicine had little opportunity to develop.

The early Hebrew scribes recognised that some plagues affected both humans and animals: 'for that which befalleth the sons of man befalleth beasts . . . so that a man has no pre-eminence above the beast' (Eccles. 3:19); divine displeasure was also considered to be the cause of animal plagues, 'Behold, the hand of the Lord is upon thy cattle which is in the field . . . there shall be a very grevious murrain' (Exodus 9:3). The biblical stories (1 Samuel 5:6) tell that the Philistines defeated the Israelites in battle and captured the Ark, after which God afflicted them with 'emrods'. No satisfactory translation of this word has been made but it is believed these were the same as the tumours and boils also recorded, possibly the bubos of bubonic plague. Another reference, when the Ark was returned, is 'so you must make images of your tumours and images of your mice that ravage the land' (1 Samuel 6:5). Together, and accounting for translation difficulties (mice? rats) this could be a description of bubonic plague, a zoonotic disease.

An important aspect of Mosaic Law was the introduction of a sanitary code that promoted both personal and community cleanliness, and hygiene. This demonstrates a recognition of disease contagion and the need for isolation. The rites of purification as described in Leviticus (for a disease translated, probably incorrectly, as leprosy), illustrate their control measures. First, recognising the disease as punishment for a sin its amelioration was by a priest taking two live birds, killing one and freeing the other to which the disease had hopefully been transferred, then using the blood of the fresh killed bird to sprinkle over the patient for seven days, who was then isolated for seven days. The house of the patient was cleansed with blood and running water, and a sin offering of the sacrifice of two lambs, or two pigeons if the patient was poor. There was a mixture of logic and magic – logical to have isolation and cleanliness, but not to believe in the properties of the number seven or the transference of disease to another being. However, both ideas continued in Western belief for centuries. Note also the belief in the vital properties of blood, a feature that has survived in Jewish, Christian and Islamic religions.

Other Mosaic injunctions that involved animals have lasted within the Jewish and Moslem faiths. A principle one is the prohibition against eating pork, shellfish and certain other foods: it is quite possible that there was a recognition of the risk of parasite transfer behind these, but this is unproven and also demonstrated over the centuries to be unnecessary. An injunction on pork and saltwater fish consumption had already existed in Egypt among other Middle East communities, before the Hebrews made it a prime requirement of their faith.

Moses banned cruelty to animals and imposed penalties for those involved, and also for animal theft, and decreed compensation to the owners for damage to their oxen (as in the Hammurabi Laws). Religious slaughter was an important ritual:

conducted by priests who performed the killing (*shechita*) and judged *bedikah*, the ritual inspection of the meat to ascertain its fitness for consumption. The latter was determined by exsanguination, examination of the lungs (seen to be the most important organ) and the banning of the consumption of certain visceral organs. The hygienic approach was almost certainly inherited from the period of Egyptian captivity. There was a prohibition on eating blood (Deuteronomy 12:23), or the meat of animals dead from natural causes (but such meat could be given to strangers or sold to 'aliens'). Only fresh meat was eaten; the head, feet, kidneys, guts, fatty tissue and non-exsanguinated meat were all forbidden. As previously noted the rejection of the meat from the hindquarters of the animal, now said to be due to the difficulty of removing the blood vessels from these regions, may well be following the practice of the early Egyptians.

Obviously from the inspection of slaughtered animals a body of comparative medical knowledge must have been acquired. It is recorded that pulmonary tuberculosis, kidney abscess, cirrhosis and other liver conditions were all recognised. As time passed, priests became 'health officers', and a group of 'physicians' developed who also looked at alleviating disease conditions. But for a long time, the belief dictated that disease was to be ameliorated by animal sacrifice, prayer, exorcism of demons and self-chastisement. Fevers, rabies and some animal parasites were also recognised, but a religious explanation was given. Also, the 'scapegoat' was used, a much earlier tradition of transplantative curing, probably taken from Egyptian practice.

Finally, it is described in the Bible how Aaron became high priest and his 'sons', the Levites, chose the animals for slaughter, first judging their health and suitability and then performing the sacrifices. Male calves, lambs, goat kids, and doves/pigeons were selected, all had to be devoid of any obvious infirmity: described as blindness, crippled, injured, ulcerous, scabby and itching; the subject also had to possess normal external genitalia. Slaughter for either sacrifice or for consumption was conducted with a specific detailed ritual: this involving the slaughterer, the knife, the procedure and the butchering of the carcase.

The above review illustrates how Judaism and the Mosaic Law preserves cultural practices that the Hebrews had encountered in their Mesopotamia, Egypt and Canaan travels. While many were simply ritual, some were also sensible and practical. Both categories of behaviour became enshrined in the early Jewish *Pentateuch* to later become part of the Bible's Old Testament and thus enshrined into Christian practice. The Hebrews provided a conduit for ancient Near and Middle Eastern beliefs to be transferred to Europe, and these influenced veterinary and human medicine.

Persia

The Persian Empire reached its peak under the Achaemenid kings, starting with Cyrus the Great (560–530 BC) and ending when Darius III (336–330 BC) was defeated by Alexander the Great (356–323 BC). The empire grew from the later Assyrian Kingdom, first assimilating the Medes, followed by Lydia, Babylonia and

Egypt. It was the 'Empire of the Horse', they absorbed the Median horse culture and became skilful in using the animal in war – the horse also became their sacrificial animal (Cook 2002, pp. 154, 160).

Like other developing Middle East cultures, they copied many of their rituals and habits from others: an important Persian ritual was animal sacrifice, initially from Babylonian/Assyrian culture and later following the Greek pattern. The location was an elevated position, preferably on a hill or mountain top. The main sacrificial animal was the horse, but cattle, goats and sheep were also used. Following preparation by the priest, wine would be poured on the altar and secret words sung before the killing. The meat was then cooked and portions placed on herbage, preferably clover. A magus priest was also needed to chant a *theogany*, probably a hymn about the gods. Herodotus wrote that the Persians would wreath the animal with myrtle and then kill with a blessing of prayers.

The Persian religion was a fire cult based on the wisdom of Zarathustra (Zoroaster): his place of birth and dates are unclear, probably about 1500–1000 BC. The religion was conducted by the magi priests based on the laws of *Avesta*, the Zoroastrian holy book. The religion was dualist, contrary to the Babylonian belief which was monistic (a doctrine that there is only one supreme being). The two beings were Ahura Mazda, the wise spirit and Angra Mainyu, the evil genius: the latter was said to have 99,999 specific disease demons. Another religious cult, Mithraism, has been said to have its basis in Mithra or Mitra, a belief from Indo-Persia. It was widespread in the Roman Empire, the actual practices have remained secret, except that it required the killing of a bull (tauroctony). It is now believed that there is probably no relationship to Zoroastrianism or Persia.

The priests of the religious cult were the *magi*, these people were possibly Medes. They were responsible for the care of the holy fire, and functioned as the clergy: they also had the habit of killing with their own hands undomesticated creatures – birds, snakes and others, including ants (Cook 2002, p. 229).

The dog was proclaimed as the sacred animal of Zoroaster. The presence of a dog was believed to aid warding off evil spirits and demons, a dog would be taken to a dying person for them to confess their sins. The *Avesta* gives advice on animal healing and care, with particular reference to dogs. It was also recorded that if a dog refused its medication it was lawful to bind him and open his mouth with a stick (Smithcors 1958, p. 41).

Persian medicine embodied many characteristics of other civilisations and there is a possible relationship to Sanskrit medical texts. One characteristic which it shared with the Jews was a great emphasis on personal and communal hygiene. Herodotus (Strassler 2009, pp. 72, 74) wrote that the Persians were especially concerned with fire and with purity. Neither was allowed to be defiled; therefore it was forbidden to wash in rivers, and privacy was required for all bodily functions. Medicine was essentially a magico-religious practice. Health depended on Ahura Mazda and medicine was in the hands of the priest-physicians. A professional code was laid down in the *Vendidad*, a collection of texts within the *Avesta*. This detailed many topics, in particular hygiene, disease and spells for its prevention, and praise and care of the sacred animals – the dog, bull, otter and *Sraosha* bird. Also listed are training requirements, fees and penalties for malpractice (Margotta 1996, p. 15). Those priests who acted in a medical/surgical capacity had to perform three successful operations (unspecified) upon 'worshippers of evil spirits' before they could be considered qualified. If a patient died after an operation it was regarded as homicide. Fees were levelled according to status – a priest would offer a blessing, and gifts of varying value were provided by others according to their rank. Firdausi (cited by Margotta), writing of Persian doctors and surgeons about AD 1000 said that they were proficient and mentions caesarean section. The priests also acted in a veterinary capacity. They worked for a fixed fee, payment being in kind based on the species being treated: sheep were bottom of the list with the fee being 'the price of a good meal' (Smithcors 1958, p. 41). There is evidence to suggest that at this time some animal diseases were recognised – rinderpest, anthrax and equine colic in particular.

The magi disease control measures were by ritual ceremonials. The emphasis in the religion and medical/veterinary teaching was (as in Babylon) that disease was a manifestation of evil spirits. This affected all dealings with the sick or dead, humans or animals. The religious doctrine of 'impurity' formed the basis for practice; as a result, post-mortem examination was taboo and special rites were required for all who handled corpses. Rather than contaminate the earth, final rites for humans and dogs were for the bodies to be placed in the open for birds (vultures) to consume the carcase, bones were then collected and placed in ossuaries. In later years the Parsee Towers of Silence were used for initial corpse placement. The dog had every protection. In the *Avesta* it was written that a man who beat a dog would have his soul leave his body after terrible torture, and as a result in the 'other world' no dead soul would give him friendship. Ancient Persian literature (*The Spirit of Wisdom*) includes the Prayer of the Moribund, 'I regret my sins . . . I have committed . . . to my beasts; I beat and insulted them, and I allowed them to thirst and killed them unjustly.'

A final Persian note, the divination practice of *hippomanteia* could be used when a decision had to be made on selection of a person from a group of contenders. The story is that in 521 BC it was necessary to choose the next king and it was agreed that the man whose horse would be the first to neigh at sunrise would be chosen. Darius was selected – because he had a clever groom who found a mare in season and rubbed his hands in her urine. At dawn he stimulated the charger of his master, and so Darius' charger was the first to neigh, and he became king. Most likely an apocryphal story, but they were a people who really understood horses and knew their behaviour.

The Near and Middle East Civilisations

It is not possible to understand the actuality of human and animal life in the Middle East 4000 years ago. The attitudes, thought processes and beliefs that moulded the culture of the people and their relationships with animals are only partly understood; from their written texts we can produce a synthesis of ancient life, but it is not necessarily accurate. Study does show that very early in civilisation society soon falls into an ordered system produced by those who provide leadership. This leadership is invariably related to religion, which forms a mutually supportive channel to reach the perceived gods. The gods are seen as the ultimate controllers who possess the power to both protect health and well-being, or create disease and catastrophe. The priesthood mediate this relationship. From the earliest times people have concerns about health – their own, their families and their animals. Health care becomes placed under religious edict and supervision.

The evolution of the Hebrew tribe is particularly interesting, they spent periods of time in both Babylon and Egypt, adopted beliefs that appear in their laws and religion which were then written in the Bible and the Christian religion, producing a lasting impact on Western civilisation: most important was the belief that disease was a punishment for sin, it stifled any real effort to study disease until the onset of the Renaissance.

This first chapter of the veterinary and animal–human relationship history ends in the last centuries of the 1st millennium BC. We know that a form of what we now call veterinary medicine existed 4000 years ago, and almost certainly was recognised many years earlier. There was a recognition of the need for disease control, some therapies have evolved and a gradual appreciation of hygiene was developing. These ideas were carried along trade routes and to the Levant where a growing Mediterranean trade was expanding, first to the Aegean islands where the Hellenic culture arose. The Roman nation started to expand outside of Italy. Carthage was becoming a major trade centre. Europe was becoming significant and seeking medical and veterinary advances.

References

Anthes, R. (1928) *Felseninschriften von Hatnub, Untersuch. Z. Gesch. U. Altertum Aeg.* IX Leipzig

Bourke, S. (Ed.) (2008) *The Middle East.* Lane Cove: Global Book Publishing

Cohen, C. and Sivan, D. (1983) *The Ugaritic Hippiatric Texts: A Critical Edition.* London: American Oriental

Cook, J.M. (2002) *The Persians.* London: Folio

Donaghy, T. (2010) The Origins of Equine Medicine. *Veterinary History* 15 No.3: 232

Driesch, A. (2001) Is there a Veterinary Papyrus of Kahun? *Historia Medicinae Veterinariae* 26: 3–4

Gurney, O.R. (2003) *The Hittites.* London: Folio

Jöchle, W. (2006) The Horse in Ancient Near East: Facts and Fancies. *Veterinary History* 13 No.2

Karasszon, D. (1988) *A Concise History of Veterinary Medicine.* Budapest: Akadémiai Kiadó

Margotta, R. (1996) *History of Medicine.* London: Hamlyn

Markoe, G.E. (2005) *The Phoenicians.* London: Folio

Saggs, H.W.F. (2003) *The Babylonians.* London: Folio

Schäeffer, C.F.A. (1939) *Ugaritica I-III; Ras Shamra Mission,* Nos II, V, VIII. Paris

Schäffer, J. (1999) Abil-ilisu-Ein, Rinderarzt in Babylonien, um 1739 v. Chr. *Dtsch. tierärztl. Wschr.* 106 (6)

Smithcors, J.F. (1958) *Evolution of the Veterinary Art.* London: Balliére, Tindall & Cox

Sournia, J.-C. (1992) *The Illustrated History of Medicine.* London: Harold Starke

Strassler, R.B. (Ed.) (2009) *Herodotus: The Histories.* New York: Anchor Books

Walker, R.E. (1964) The Veterinary Papyrus of Kahun. *Vet. Rec.* 76

Walker, R.E. (1991) *Ars Veterinaria.* Kenilworth: Schering-Plough

Woolf, G. (2005) *Ancient Civilisations.* London: Duncan Baird

Zeuner, F.E. (1963) *A History of Domesticated Animals.* London: Hutchinson

CHAPTER 2

Greek (Aegean and Hellenic) Culture

While Greece is recognised as the second centre of Western civilisation, the details of the very early years of settlement on the coast and islands of the Aegean Sea are unclear. The region was populated by immigrants arriving from Asia Minor, the Levant and through the Balkans. As these early peoples of the Aegean and its coasts, with their mix of cultures and knowledge grew together, they called themselves Hellenes and their country Hellas. The term Greece dates from the completion of their Roman subjugation following the Battle of Actium in 31 BC and the annexation of the remaining territory by Emperor Augustus in 22 BC.

It is important to understand the background to the Greek achievements, but it is best to summarise much of this: the so-called Golden Age of their culture all happened in a period of some 200 years, mostly based around the 5th century BC. This explosion of brilliance and talent was centred on Athens with a population of just 20,000–30,000 free male citizens: it provided the basis of European culture and civilisation.

From the Aegean Islands and Coasts to One Country

The history of Greece can be dated to about 2600 BC when the Minoan culture developed in Crete; the first significant European civilisation. Consolidation and the eventual creation of a common Hellenic entity was slow and based on war and conquest. Later the Minoans were subjugated by the Mycenaeans, who in turn were invaded by the Dorians. There were continuing struggles until the 8th century BC. Gradually a social/economic structure evolved as a series of *polis* or city states emerged mostly around the coastline. These self-governing independent communities, with a primary loyalty from their citizens, grew in strength and formed the basis of Greek civilisation. An important unifying factor was the development of an alphabet from the Phoenician script, producing the early Greek alphabet and language. The urban structure was dictated by the topography. On the mainland there were small coastal areas of plain with mountains behind, those on the Aegean coast, with no mountain shield, built walls to defend their cities. The mainland states created a central citadel (the *acro-polis*) for protection in an emergency (Parker 1997, pp. 66,74). The economies were based on agriculture: cereals, with grassland for sheep, goats and some cattle; the sheep were managed with transhumance, often a cause of friction between neighbours. An understanding of animal husbandry developed and probably an early need for veterinary care.

As coastal communities, ships were essential and trading became increasingly important, focusing on metals, marble and woollen goods. This was followed by the establishment of *coloniae* around more distant Mediterranean coasts. Unlike 19th-century colonies, the local populations were seldom involved, although slaves were important throughout the Hellenic communities. Colony growth and exploitation was important, until it came to face increasing opposition from the growing Carthaginian and Roman empires. In the 7th and 6th centuries BC there were increasing trade and cultural transference with the East – Egypt, Phoenicia, Mesopotamia and India: gradually the Hellenic culture was formed. The 5th century BC was seriously disturbed by the 27-year Peloponnesian war between Sparta and Athens (431–404 BC), but this did not appear to affect the great flowering of Athens.

In the 4th century BC Plato and Aristotle developed a new method of thinking which produced their great metaphysical ideas on the nature of being, truth and knowledge, which have had such a profound effect on European civilisation. They urged the restoration of the early age of the *polis*, as a means of unifying the city states, this failed, and Philip of Macedon defeated the city states at the battle of Chaeronea (338 BC), which initiated the start of unification of the Hellenistic world. Alexander the Great (356–323 BC), who had been tutored by Aristotle, transformed this world with his invasion of the Persian Empire in 334 BC, opening up the resources of the Middle East. This enabled a great expansion of trade to India and even to China, and increased wealth. Trading links across the Mediterranean grew, largely based in metals, marble, luxury products (pots, sculpture) and agricultural produce – in particular woollen goods, based on sheep farming. After Alexander, the Asian territories split to form three independent states, each with a continuing Greek influence. This created a *cosmopolis* – a civilised Hellenised world with Athens as the cultural centre. The new city of Alexandria in Egypt grew and the Museion became the international centre of higher learning and the arts. This reached a peak in the 3rd century BC with far reaching advances in astronomy, mathematics, geography and other sciences, but in particular medicine.

By 185 BC the power of Rome was growing and in 150 BC the first Roman governor, and soldiers, were in place on the east coast of the Adriatic. Finally, following the Battle of Actium (31 BC) Rome took control of the remains of Alexander's Empire. However, while the structure of the Hellenic world was subsumed and broken, its intellectual and metaphysical legacy had by now infiltrated the Roman mind and culture. This period produced great advances for medicine, both human and veterinary, led by Hippocrates (460–375 BC), Aristotle (384–322 BC), Theophrastus (370–287 BC), and the early schools of medicine culminating in the Alexandrian centre of knowledge. Advances that laid the basis for modern medicine and were responsible for directly influencing European human and veterinary practice for many centuries.

The Minoans and the Mycenaeans

The first major European civilisation developed in Crete. This **Minoan** culture (named after the legendary King Minos) flourished between 2600–1100 BC. By about 1600 BC it appears to have been overrun by the Mycenaeans, from the Greek mainland, whose culture was later destroyed by the Dorians from the north, around 1100 BC.

In ancient history, civilisation by definition, means a literate society. This is a necessity because a civilised society is complex and cannot function without records. The Minoan culture left these, initially in ideograms and hieroglyphs then evolving into a script termed Linear A, inscribed on clay tablets, as yet undeciphered. This was followed by Linear B, which has been de-coded as early Greek. From these records and extensive excavations both on Crete and the mainland, a picture of this early culture has been created. They contributed a literature content, an extraordinary variety of pottery, frescos and palaces, and an economic input in wool and cloth production. Animals were important in their cultural achievements, their economy and their religious rituals. Their absorption into the Mycenaean Age marks the beginning of what is termed 'The Greek Miracle' (Taylor and Chadwick 2004, pp. 15–16).

There is little detail available on Minoan religion, except for the remains of many shrines. In all of these sites fired clay votive models of bulls, sheep, goats, pigs, dogs and birds as well as human body parts have been found. These were offered to the gods, possibly with prayers for healing and for protection of livestock (the basis of the economy). The names and nature of the actual gods are unclear and the religion appears to be associated with the natural world. As Greek mythology developed Crete was seen as the birthplace of Zeus and associated with other gods so these early shrines may have been highly significant. Sacrifice played an important part in Minoan culture. Excavated remains indicate that this involved oxen, pigs, goats and, from bones found at ceremonial sites, also human subjects. The bull was important and is shown in wall paintings, often trussed on an altar with the blood being collected from neck incisions. Named for the wall paintings, excavations at Knossos have revealed The House of the Sacrificial Oxen.

Public interest in early Crete is largely due to oxen. The well-known Knossos wall frescos illustrate the ritual sport of bull jumping, which would appear to have been practised by both men and women. While it must have been highly dangerous, the athletic prowess shown is probably somewhat exaggerated. In the same context is the myth of the Minotaur, the half man-half bull monster in the Labyrinth: the story is possibly the most potent symbol of Greek mythology. It reveals the dark side of man's nature with the sense of unrevealed menace and power. While possibly a harsh judgement, the Minoan culture appears to have been both cruel and bloodthirsty. The palaces while extensive were also austere. The use of animals for both sport and sacrifice does not indicate high welfare standards.

Minoan economics was founded on animals: the island offers an ideal terrain for sheep and goats, they provided meat, milk, cheese, hides and wool. The latter product enabled the development of an extensive cloth industry, creating a valuable exportable product. Cattle were also important as a source of meat, milk and hides but in particular as draught animals; total numbers would appear to have been small compared to the extensive sheep population. While the cattle stock was small it appears that large bulls were produced, probably by careful selection and feeding. Pigs were also kept, and dogs as guards, pets and for hunting. Deer, hares, partridge, quail, dove and *agrimi* (wild goat) were all hunted; feral pigs were hunted for their tusks. Asses were not introduced to Crete until the Middle Bronze Age (c.1700 BC) and were soon the recognised beasts of burden. Horses appeared in the Late Bronze Age (c.1600 BC), but remained rare. Cats may have been present, from Egypt. Beekeeping was valued as a source of a sweetening agent.

The human diet was rich in meat, cereals, pulses and various herbs are mentioned. Jewellery and ornamental art frequently illustrate dogs, monkeys, birds, bees, and in particular the *agrimi*, this wild goat had large, attractive horns. There are no records of either disease or medication for either animals or humans. Possibly the island location provided an effective quarantine against the major plagues.

Minoan independence ended with the arrival of the **Mycenaeans** from about 1450 BC. There were extensive earthquakes and destruction about this time, and either internal warfare or conquest by the Mycenaeans occurred, giving them full control by 1300 BC. The Mycenaeans were a war-geared society, with massive walled cities and a fleet of warships. The written evidence of their culture is limited to a few hundred clay tablets (compared to the 3000–4000 Minoan tablets). These were written in Linear B script (early Greek). The limited records of the Mycenaean world are supplemented by archaeological evidence, plus the writings of Homer, much of which is based in the Peloponnesus in the Late Bronze Age.

There is little information extant on Mycenaean religion. Shrines and offerings have been excavated. Most of the classical gods were recognised and some others – Zeus, Hera, Poseidon, Hermes, Athena, Artemis – but it is not clear who was the principal deity. It appears that the belief was based in a coalescence of the Olympian celestial deities and those from the underworld, such as Demeter. Offerings were made of olive oil, unguents and ritual sacrifice of animals: the meat was then eaten.

Agriculture was well organised and based in wheat, barley, olive oil and wool. When Crete was absorbed by the Mycenaeans their wool and cloth industry made this sector the major source of wealth, both local sales and through exports. The main livestock were sheep, goats and cattle. Pigs were fattened. Dogs were used for hunting (mainly deer). While the ox population was small it is notable that these draught animals were treated with affection, and named – Blondie, Dapple, Darkie, Winey and Whitefoot are listed in the records. Oxen may have been used as an early means of barter, or for their hides; copper ingots, in ox hide shape have been found, possibly an early currency. Shepherds, goatherds and ox drivers are mentioned on the excavated tablets, as well as 'yokes', possibly drivers of a yoke of oxen. Equines appear to have been rare, horses are only noted with chariots, and asses only appear once. Saddlers were an important craft with much leather work from ox, sheep, goat, pig and deer hides. Human diet was based on cereals (bread and porridge) with spices, cheese, fruit (mainly figs) together with honey, and wine. The collection and use of herbs and spices was important to both flavour foods and to perfume unguents: these were significant for various purposes for both sexes as well as votive gifts. A mixture of oils and spices, in particular coriander, appears to have been a favourite.

While not specifically mentioned it is highly probable that herbs and spices formed part of therapeutics as both a treatment and preventive. Translation of the surviving tablets has not revealed any mention of disease or health in connection to either animals or humans, similar to the Minoan texts that have been deciphered. As both communities were relatively isolated, at a time when populations were small, it is possible that they had a degree of protection from the human, and animal, plagues that were experienced elsewhere in the ancient world. In the Mycenaean tablets there is mention of a physician (or is translated as such), but no details were given.

With the end of the Mycenaean culture (c.1200–1100 BC), when seemingly it was overrun from the north by the Dorians, following the story of Greek evolution becomes difficult. This period is termed the Dark Age of Greece. For reasons that remain unclear kingdoms vanished, cultures were seriously damaged, the population numbers fell dramatically, central organisational control collapsed and the survivors descended into poverty. Linear B writings ceased and no Greek records exist. Egyptian records describe a 'conspiracy' of foreign countries that all at once were on the move and at war. Some scholars have called the attackers the 'Land and Sea Peoples', but they do not seem to have been a unified force (Thomas 2010, pp. 341–343). Possibly the region was affected by volcanic activity or other natural disasters. It was not a totally negative period. The survivors transformed the Mycenaean inheritance to provide the basis for the creation of the city-states, the appearance of the earliest literature and important cultural developments.

The Rise of Classical Greece

The 8th century BC saw a renaissance with a 200-year period of expansion of *coloniae* around the Mediterranean islands and coasts. In the following two centuries new cultural influences, ideas, behaviours and products, arrived with the increasing trade with Egypt, Syria, Mesopotamia and India. The 5th century BC produced the great flowering of Greek culture, founded and centred on Athens, with the development of philosophy, theatre, drama, sculpture and pottery, and buildings such as the Parthenon.

Names such as Socrates and Herodotus are still widely known as they represent the development of both thought and the investigative, questioning mind. By the 4th century BC Plato and Aristotle had produced their great metaphysical thoughts and ideas on the nature of being, truth and knowledge, which have had such a profound effect on European civilisation and led to the study of life. The descriptive word 'philosophy' initially embraced all intellectual studies, but was essentially a love of wisdom, a discipline that sought truth through reasoning and not empiricism. This then gradually resolved into more precise groupings with 'natural philosophy', embracing astronomy, physics and biology. And out of the latter arose the discipline of medicine.

The Gods of Greece and Veterinary Medicine

It is important to understand the ancient foundations of the Greek culture – the myths of origin. Every culture is based on such myths, but in the Greek case these were particularly strong, providing a unifying factor for the disparate peoples of the Aegean community and resulting in a pantheon of gods that wielded great influence on almost every early Hellenic endeavour. The early peoples depended on the land: they were hunters, shepherds and animal breeders (doubly important as animal sacrifice was an essential religious ritual), they needed gods to protect their farming and their animal husbandry – and they represented them in animal form.

Zeus the all-powerful, head of the pantheon, which included many gods who possessed the power of healing and the power to bring about disease when angered. They could also assume human form and behave like men. Apollo was the master of the creative arts: he could heal but he could also decimate those who gave him displeasure (his arrows, in Homer's story, were the ones which spread the plague when the Greek army was encamped before Troy).

These mythical entities might have had some origin in actual people, in particular Chiron the immortal, the most famous wise and learned centaur who taught medicine and practised surgery on Mount Pelion, Thessaly, in northern Greece. In the mythology Chiron was the son of Cronos the Titan and Philyra the Oceanid. According to the myth he raised and taught Asclepius (Aesculapius in Latin) the son of Apollo and Coronis, who was taken to Chiron on the death of his mother. He also mentored Achilles of Troy, Jason and Peleus the Argonauts, and many others.

Medically, Asclepius was his most important pupil, becoming the god of medicine. Chiron taught him how to treat the sick 'by words, herbs and the knife'. In mythology he had five daughters – each of whom had a medical attribute including Hygeia who taught people how to lead healthy lives (hygiene) and Panacea 'who heals all' – and was the originator of medicines. Two of his three sons were mentioned by Homer – Machaon a gifted surgeon and Polidarius who devoted himself to medicine.

These figures evolved to the Cult of Asclepius and the founding of many temples and healing centres around the Mediterranean. The resident priests or *asclepiads* offered a particular type of religious medicine by calling on the inspiration and benevolence of Asclepius; they instituted and planned various ceremonies of worship. Much of the treatment provided was by the use of baths, diet, light, air and exercise – customs still followed in today's spas. These early developments pointed to a relatively sophisticated approach towards health and healing.

The narrative now moves from mythology to actuality. There is a measure of agreement by historians that it is highly probable that many mythical figures of the late Mycenaean period were historic characters. It is useful to explore what is known, or can be substantiated, about Chiron and Asclepius. Both were historic personalities to Homer when he wrote the *Iliad*, they date to the pre-Homeric period and possibly lived in the 13th century BC, belonging to the tribe of centaurs. In old Greek the word *kentaur* meant 'hunter on horseback of the wild oxen'. The myth of the half horse-half man monster developed much later in the 7th and 6th centuries

BC. The mythical (but possibly not) King Ixion of Thessalia promised rewards to those who eradicated the wild oxen that were devastating his fields. Legend has it that this was achieved by the Kentaurs (on horseback), who became wealthy as a result. There could be historic fact behind the legend (Hausmann and Jöchle 2003, p. 78).

Georges (1879), cited by Hausmann and Jöchle, called the centaurs a tribe who excelled as huntsmen on horseback. Edelstein and Edelstein (1945) presented numerous pieces of evidence that Asclepius, a prince of Trikke, was actually a student of Chiron. Since then, what is claimed to be the first Asclepius treatment centre, built by Prince Asclepius, has been uncovered at Trikkala (the current name). According to further investigations by Hausmann (1982, p. 393, 1984, p. 24), Chiron was the leader of a tribe that invaded northern Greece on horseback, probably from Thracio. At this time, while horses were known in Greece they were used as draught animals, Chiron appears to have arrived at about the same time that horses with riders are first recorded in the Mycenaean records, about 1300 BC.

It is postulated that Chiron bought with him knowledge from the earlier Indo-Germanic and Asiatic traditions and combined these medical approaches to injuries and diseases in humans and animals (Hausmann and Jöchle 2003, p. 78). Mythological and other sources agree that he used a cave as the centre for his school and that his pupils included princes and others from the neighbouring kingdoms. As these were the only people who had the money, motivation and liberty to study – they needed to be healthy to stay in power, and because livestock represented their wealth the loss of a bull, or a cow, was a serious problem. Schwabe (1978) describes Chiron as the educator and warden of the sons of leading Greek families.

Following Chiron two branches of medicine appeared. One, the Chironids, remained mostly in the region of the Pelion Mountains, in Demetrias, a town founded in 294 BC. Their descendants worked in this local region as healers of animals and humans for at least 1000 years according to Hausmann (multiple sources identified in Hausmann and Jöchle 2003, p. 78). The other branch followed the teachings of Asclepius, initially working from caves, as Chiron, but soon moving to specially equipped buildings, which became known as sanctuaries. The Asclepian teaching and health spas spread across the Greek world and later the Roman. In the last two centuries BC and the first two AD the appellation *Asclepiades* was used by these healers. They established a medical tradition based on hygiene, simplicity of treatment, and the use of water and steam baths. The most famous of these *asclepia* was built at Epidauros, with other leading ones at Cnidos and Cos, which in turn later developed into schools of medicine with their own systems. This traditional medicine lived alongside the newer medical philosophy that was being developed by men such as Hippocrates (460–370 BC) who, in his formative years living on Cos, was influenced by this much older tradition.

Chiron has remained a mythical character but is upheld as a symbol of medicine in its many branches. The half man-half horse legend has been popular with veterinary associations, in particular those with a British relationship. The Chiron figure is used on the monograms or heraldic devices of the Royal College of Veterinary Surgeons, British Veterinary Association, Royal Army Veterinary Corps, Australian

Veterinary Association and others. The figure used is depicted as holding a torch, caduceus or a branch. Only one organisation appears to show the correct representation of the historic Chiron the Centaur of medical fame. He was set apart from other centaurs in mythology who had a bloodthirsty, libidinous reputation. In the traditional Greek representations of Chiron (as seen on much ancient pottery) he is shown with human front legs, rather than equine, usually wearing clothes, frequently with a branch over his shoulder, and sometimes with dead hares he has just caught hanging from it. The branch is traditionally from a lime tree, which has significance: when Chiron was born his mother Philyra was so horrified to see her son that the gods pitied her and allowed her to change to a lime tree. From earliest times lime blossom was seen as a remedy and strips of the bark were used for divination. Chiron was portrayed as a wise and gentle teacher of his art. This correct illustration is used as an emblem by the British Veterinary History Society.

Additionally, there is a fascinating discovery and claim related to Chiron. Investigations based on local folklore have led to the finding of what is claimed to be Chiron's original cave. This is detailed by Hausmann and Jöchle (2003, pp. 82–84). Situated in the lower Pelion Mountains, close to the village of Miliés (or Miléae), in the deep cut wooded Peletronic valley is a typical cave dwelling. A bedplate has been carved out of the rock, located close to a mountain stream with 'crystal clear water and very close to an age-old path . . . which (leads) down to the shore' all as described in the legend. At the time of publication there had been no excavation at the site, this requires Greek government consent. A related story is of interest. Greek mythology tells the story of Melampus, described either as a local king or a famous shepherd, the first mortal who, like Chiron, healed animals and people. Another version says Melampus was a pupil of Chiron. An annual Spring Festival is held in Volos (in the Pelion foothills), which is said to date back to the time of Melampus. Several other local festivals also involve the memory of Chiron and his pupils. All obvious mythology, but maybe with an historic nucleus.

The Natural Philosophers

In ancient Greece medicine was not a separate discipline but was seen as a part of a complex of various types of knowledge. As a group these subjects formed the core of philosophical debate, and in particular in the pronouncements of the 'natural philosophers'. Thinking was deemed to be the sole basis of the act or experience of knowing or acquiring knowledge, the idea of experimentation did not arise. The arrival of competing and rival beliefs in the 6th century BC from Phoenicia, Mesopotamia and Egypt, to join the already significant input from Crete and other cultures in the Hellenic region, created a unique mix of concepts. The Ionian philosophers debated the origin of the world around them. One of the earliest causes of discussion was the nature of the 'primary matter' – was it water, air or some unknowable element? Possibly Athens is overemphasised as the centre of this unique intellectual awakening. These thoughts inspired thinkers in the Greek settlements in Ionia (Asia Minor), in Sicily, Cyrene and southern Italy.

It is an over simplification of an involved and complex picture to state that Pythagoras invented philosophy or that Hippocrates originated medicine: their predecessors left no records. There were many individuals who played a part in this sudden burgeoning development of ideas. Some 14 Hellenic Schools evolved each with their own philosophical discipline. Socrates (c.470–399 BC) became the great teacher in Athens, an enigmatic figure who left no writings, but taught Plato (c.428–348 BC). Then there were many schools of thought – Sophism, Cynicism, Cyrenaicism and others, until Plato dominated the field and elaborated the ideas with the theory of forms (to be regenerated in the 3rd century AD as Neoplatonism – a religious and mystical philosophy). The other leaders were Plato's student, Aristotle, who in turn tutored Theophrastus. Socrates, Plato and Aristotle are recognised to have laid the basis of Western science and philosophy.

A Medical Discipline Evolves

The development of medical thought came from a unique group, philosopher-scientists: one of the first was Thales of Miletus (c.624–c.546 BC) an astronomer and mathematician who travelled in the Mediterranean region, Egypt and Babylon, returning with a variety of ideas. He used a single method of analysis and attempted to prove that 'all life springs from water'. A most significant contributor was Pythagoras (c.582–c.497 BC) of Samos: he established a philosophical school at Croton, Southern Italy, following his travels, including Egypt and Chaldea (Babylonia), spending time with the local priests and religious leaders. He appears to have been the first to use the word 'philosophy', meaning love of wisdom. Best known for mathematics he pondered the universe and with his disciples developed the belief of the universality of 'the four elements – earth, air, fire and water'. One concept he adopted was that of the immortality of the soul and after death its rebirth in other animals: this derives from the mythological Orpheus who purified souls in the underworld before releasing them in another animal form. This one abstract belief was to have far reaching consequences for hundreds of years. Pythagoras forbade the eating of flesh, the shedding of blood and banned surgical procedures since such intervention might interfere with the soul.

Also located at Croton was the medical school of Alcmaeon (6th century BC), who studied the origins of the human embryo and was possibly the first to dissect animal bodies. He described arteries and veins, the optic nerve, the Eustachian tube and the brain, which he recognised as the centre of thought and intelligence, and stated that the soul was the source of life. He discounted astrology as being related to good health, which he founded on the equilibrium and balance of properties – wet/dry, hot/cold, bitter/sweet. This developed to the concept of the balance of the four humours, taken further by Hippocrates, and developed by Aristotle and Galen to last for centuries as a foundation block of biological science.

Other early thinkers of note included Heraclitus of Ephesus (active c.550 BC) who pondered the place of man in the cosmos and had the idea that all living phenomena are influenced by a form of fire. Zeno of Elea (c.5th century BC) developed the 'paradox principle' in philosophical reasoning, and its consequences for the study of nature. The Pythagorean influence reached Empedocles (c.500–430 BC) of Agrigentum and Acragus in Sicily. He was a philosopher-scientist who believed in the transmigration of the soul between species and wrote his thoughts as poetry; he valued experimentation and had an interest in medicine. He wrote three treatises on 'Nature' and a medical discourse. Regrettably Acragus was attacked and destroyed by the Carthaginians about 400 BC and most of the work of Empedocles was lost. It is known that he recognised the heart as the centre of circulation, was said to have drained a swamp to control malaria and advanced the theory of the four elements – earth, water, air and fire. This linked to the four humours of the body concept.

There were many individuals whose philosophical ideas led them to medicine. Democritus of Abdera in Thrace (c.460–c.370 BC) is known for his atomic theory of the universe. He would appear to have been a diligent biologist and performed dissections, and while his work has only survived in fragments and quotations, he obviously studied anatomy, physiology and pathology. Aristotle quotes him for his animal dissections and for his observations on clostridial enterotoxaemia, or pulpy kidney in sheep. Aristotle had also noted that the sheep kidney was enveloped in a thick coating of fat and that this could not be penetrated by either moisture or by the wind (a term used to describe various influencing factors), 'Therefore when pernicious influences are contained in the kidney and cannot escape they provoke a putridity which spreads to the heart via the aorta' (Peck 1965, p. 217). He adds 'the sheep die because their kidneys are completely surrounded by suet. This condition is provoked by overeating, as occurs in Leontini in Sicily. One understands why the sheep are made to go out late in the evening so that they will eat less.' The proposal that the animals should have their habits altered is probably one of the first animal disease prevention recommendations (Walker 1991, pp. 14–15). Study of another fragment of his work relates to the structure of horns of cattle with comparisons between horned and hornless animals. His work was cited by Roman agricultural authors in the 4th century AD.

Diogenes of Appollonaria (c.428 BC) on the Black Sea coast, presented a thesis that the basic body must be air as it pervades everything and supports life and intelligence. Of his major work, *On Nature*, only fragments survive, but Aristotle wrote that he left a detailed account of blood channels. Diogenes also considered vision and the senses and how they interpret nature. At Cnidus (modern-day Turkey), Euryphon (probably early 5th century BC) led a school devoted to rational medicine: he demanded facts and based his teaching on animal dissection and post-mortem examinations and was the author of several works, now lost. Members of the Cnidian school became known as empiricists: their beliefs and teaching resembled those of Alcmaeon. Another member of the Cnidian school, Philiston of Syracuse (early 4th century BC) wrote an advanced and significant dissertation, *Of the Heart*, which demonstrated that he had dissected the human heart and major vessels. It was purely anatomical without discussion of disease problems. He also taught medicine to Eudoxas, a mathematician and philosopher.

Hippocrates

The medical school on the island of Cos became the most famous: this was led by Hippocrates (c.460–c.377 BC). While he left very little of his own writings his teachings were widely adopted and became the basis of the Alexandrian School. Hippocrates' importance lies in his move away from mysticism and the suggestion that there was any divine intervention in either the cause or the treatment of disease. He devised a medical system based on ethics, observation, clarity, recording case histories and rational treatment. He urged that research be based on a knowledge and examination of previous discoveries and caused others to sift through the earlier medical writings to extract what was seen to be both useful and interesting. This was combined with his main teaching – clinical observation using all the senses. Hippocrates created the concept of medical scientific enquiry. He relied on natural faculties, with his admonition *primum non nocere* ('above all, do no harm').

While developing a masterly system Hippocrates had no knowledge of anatomy and physiology, as human dissection was banned at that time. He did value comparative studies and wrote about zoonoses, such as rabies, and observed hydatid cysts in a goat brain, but he did not consider that human and veterinary practice had much in common. When discussing luxation of the hip in humans he mentions the same condition in cattle, adding, 'if I may be allowed to make such an observation while treating a medical subject'! In retrospect this was a failing: Hippocrates followed the teachings of Plato concerning the existence of the soul in humankind only, this apparently precluded him from taking an active interest in animal disease.

Hippocrates was a man of his time – his methods of treatment of fractures and wounds would be deemed sensible today, but many of his other methods would not. He used bloodletting, cauterisation, purgatives and emetics, but did lay down lifestyle and dietary rules. He condemned magicians and healers and emphasised that a doctor must understand the human self. One of his most important dictums was that personal experience was of prime importance, yet this was forgotten for centuries. Finally, and most significanly, he emphasised the need to question the patient and to look, touch and palpate, and only then make a diagnosis, consider a prognosis and determine a treatment.

The Hippocratic method was pragmatism, he rejected the Pythagorean theory of the so-called magic geometry and believed that examination of the patient, assisted by his knowledge and experience was the correct way to proceed in medicine. Hippocrates would sometimes use contradictory procedures: treating diarrhoea with vomiting, or cold patients with heat, but always emphasised that this was in an effort to improve knowledge. The writings of Hippocrates were collected soon after his death but then became mixed with other treatises, as a result establishing exactly what Hippocrates wrote, apart from in the case of a few works, is difficult. Later the collection was named the *Corpus Hippocraticum*, it is believed, by a group in Alexandria, when their studies in the medical sciences were being developed.

At the time that Hippocrates was working, magicians and diviners were also active, in particular at the *asclepeions*. The priests would interpret the patients' dreams and miraculous cures were claimed, votive gifts presented with some evidence that psychosomatic and mental problems were helped (Sournia 1992, p. 78). There is little doubt that the regimen of water springs and baths were important. There were clearly two forms of medical practice at that time. One by those following and trained in Hippocratic methods, the other by those performing of religious rituals. There was no real medical system. Doctors were few in number, some travelled and were paid by rich merchants and politicians. Some were also known to have worked for town councils and cared for the poor, slaves and victims of epidemics or earthquakes (Sournia 1992, p. 79). During the period between the death of Hippocrates and the founding of the Alexandrian School, Greek medicine relapsed and the advances were few.

Diocles and Praxagorus

One important contributor to medical knowledge was Diocles of Carystus (4th century BC), a town on the island of Euboea. Little is known of his life, but he lived at about the same time as Aristotle. Also known as Diocles Medicus he had a reputation as a philosopher and physician and was an important representative of the Dogmatic school. He wrote in Attic Greek, while most other similar texts were in Ionian Greek. None of his writings have survived intact and he is only known from surviving fragments and many quotations by other writers. Pliny stated that he was second only to Hippocrates in his knowledge and ability.

Diocles' most famous work was on animal anatomy, based on his own dissections. This is said to have been the first anatomical treatise and he was the first to use the word anatomy; he insisted that the nerves were the 'channels of sensation'. Other works were on dietetics, a major interest, and also on physiology, embryology and medical botany (he is believed to have compiled a herbal manual). It is clear Diocles worked to reorganise Greek medicine on both theoretical and practical lines. His name is remembered by his invention of the Dioclean *cyanthiscus* (the spoon of Diocles), invaluable as a safe way to extract arrows and foreign bodies from wounds in humans and animals.

Mention must be made of Praxagoras of Cos (c.340 BC). Very little known of his life and none of his writings have survived. He was well quoted by his contemporaries, and by Galen (AD c.130–200). He is now believed to have been one of the most important medical thinkers and researchers during the period between Hippocrates and the start of the Alexandrian School. Praxagoras distinguished between arteries and veins, but saw the arteries as air tubes for the *pneuma* (the life force) and the veins as the vessels to carry the blood: together he believed that these two created the body's heat. He recognised the pulse and thought it was of value in diagnosis. Praxagoras had his own variation of humoral theory and recognised eleven humours; he considered digestion to be a form of putrefaction, a belief that persisted until the 19th century. His important link in the chain of medical evolution was that he taught Herophilus (c.335–c.280 BC), who was later to be a significant member of the Alexandrian School.

Plato and Aristotle

The most important person in the development of philosophy was Plato, a Dogmatist (their opinions were forcibly asserted as if unchallengeable) and while not a medical man he analysed the human sciences in his dialogues. Plato was important because he separated the idea of a god for humans from animals, and therefore deprived animals of a soul: this concept was to affect the animal-human relationship for centuries. He acknowledged that four elements made up the human body, but attributed a major role in its functioning to *pneuma*, the concept of air and fire which formed the 'breath of life' and led to the movement of the bodily organs and their functioning. This idea was revived by the 'pneumanists' in the 17th century AD as the word became more broadly translated as the 'soul'. Plato's importance is emphasised by his being the core figure of the trio: Socrates who trained Plato, who trained Aristotle.

Aristotle was raised in a medical household, his father was court physician to Philip I of Macedon. He moved to Athens to study under Plato at his Academy. Plato regarded him highly, however on his death, Aristotle was not appointed as his successor. As a result, he moved to Mytilene on the island of Lesbos and fully involved himself in the study of natural history, in particular marine biology. Here he met Theophrastus who became his pupil and successor.

In 342 BC Philip II of Macedon invited him to return to the mainland to act as tutor to his son Alexandros, later Alexander the Great, who was greatly influenced by his three-year tutelage and later became Aristotle's greatest benefactor. Pliny wrote that he made available to Aristotle 800 talents of silver (26.2 kg), as well as providing him with hundreds of men, who collected plants and animals for his research. Additionally, Alexander sent him animals and plants discovered during his conquest of the Eastern territories. Following to his nephew being involved in a plot and being executed, Aristotle became disgraced on Lesbos and returned to Athens. Here he started the Lyceum, his own philosophical (Peripatetic) school, was joined by Theophrastus and worked for 13 years producing an impressive corpus of work, now mostly lost. He was not happy in his location, being situated outside Athens town, as he was regarded as a stranger. After the death of Alexander, he was accused of violating the gods because he had erected an altar for his late wife. To avoid execution he moved to Chalcis, and shortly afterwards died. He left both his Lyceum and his library to Theophrastus.

While Aristotle is important in his own right he is particularly important for veterinary medicine. His work as a 'natural-scientist' produced the first classification of the animal kingdom. Zoology was one of his major interests with treatises including *Parts of Animals*, *The Gait of Animals* and *Generation of Animals*. These included his many original observations, such as the movement of the limbs: those of the horse were diagonal whereas in the camel they were lateral. He recorded the absence of the gall bladder in the horse, noted the ages up to which horses and mares were capable of procreation and described how teeth could be used to indicate age. He observed the influence of castration on the growth of the deer's antlers, that a camel could go for four days without water and that cattle preferred clear drinking water to muddy. His carefully observed and recorded stages of incubation and maturation of the chicken embryo remain as valid now as when first written. His studies on reproduction and inheritance heralded the beginning of genetics.

Aristotle's masterwork in his biological series was *Historia Animalium* (*The Story of Animals*). In this he gives detailed information on some five hundred species, of which he dissected about fifty. His reports are of importance as he began to formalise the disciplines of anatomy and physiology, he laid the groundwork for later studies and he used the observations of others to extend his descriptions. There are errors (possibly of transcription), most notably his teaching that the heart has three cavities: he believed that the heart was the seat of intelligence. A detailed explanation of these segments of Aristotle's work has been given by Karasszon (1988, pp. 74–77). In Book VII of *Historia Animalium* Aristotle deals with his concept of pathology and disease causation following the Hippocratic doctrine of the four humours (based on the four qualities, four elements and four moistures – blood, phlegm, yellow bile and black bile).

Disease is discussed in horses, ass, cattle, sheep, pigs and dogs, as well as fish, bees and elephants. The equids receive a major part of the coverage: he recorded that horses at pasture are generally healthy except for foot problems, and describes the loss of their hoofs followed by regrowth, but the possible cause is not explained. He stated that stabled animals are much more prone to disease with *ileus,* being cited with the symptom of abdominal pain; as castration was suggested as a remedy it is probable that this was strangulated scrotal hernia, not uncommon in uncastrated horses. Tetanus is described with recognisable symptoms. Another syndrome termed *melis* in the ass, with blood-stained nostril discharge and lung symptoms is almost certainly glanders. Laminitis is described and a syndrome called heartache is probably broken wind. Bladder displacement and blistered prepuce are all described. Aristotle believed in the bite of the shrew-mouse and its poisonous effect with boils and death: most likely this condition was due to anthrax, with sudden death in a believed healthy animal. The shrew-mouse fallacy was widely believed up to the 18th century AD. A very detailed examination of Aristotle's equine disease records has been provided by Donaghy (2010, pp. 234–236).

Cattle were stated to suffer from two epidemic diseases, *podagra*, the foot sickness, and *craurus*. From his descriptions the former was probably foot-and-mouth disease and the latter contagious bovine pleuro-pneumonia (he describes fever and when opened the lungs were 'disintegrated'). Castration of calves is described by cutting off the end of the scrotum but not stating how the testicles were removed. The incision was stopped with hair, to allow for suppuration.

Aristotle described three diseases of pigs – *branchos* and two *crauras*. The first showed swellings of the throat, jaw and foot and elsewhere, which rapidly decay and result in death: probably due to anthrax or possibly foot-and-mouth disease. The other two appear to be fever related, one with diarrhoea: possibly swine fever. He recognised so-called measly pork with encysted larvae in the tongue and correctly stated that this does not exist in suckling piglets, mention is also made of acorns as a cause of abortion in the sow and of pig skin diseases. Ovariotomy was practised and he describes the operation as being undertaken after a two-day fast, the animal hung up by the hind legs and the ovaries removed by an incision in front of the pubes (groin) and the wound stitched. He wrote that similar procedures are undertaken in the camel and cockerels.

Dogs were said to suffer from three diseases: *lyssa* (rabies), which produced a lethal madness and was spread by the bite (but he stated that man is the only animal that is not affected if bitten); *quinsy*, a throat related condition, usually fatal; *podagra*, a painful, gouty, foot condition. Aristotle also recorded that elephants suffered from tympanitis, with flatulence and diarrhoea being listed as the most frequent symptoms. Diseases of both bees and fish are also described. A range of surgical procedures are mentioned apart from castration and ovariotomy; treatment of damaged tendons in the horse, surgery for the correction of topical conditions, as well as the use of cauterisation, swabs and sutures. No indications of success rates or side-effects are given.

This major treatise by Aristotle was a remarkable text, due to his own contributions as well as his collection of other relevant information. It shows that at this very early date a significant amount of veterinary knowledge had been acquired. His work became a primary source for future investigators of animal diseases. There were many writers on Greek agriculture, while they were known to and quoted by the Romans, their works are now lost: these would have indicated the practical application of the Aristotelian knowledge; the Roman author, Varro (116–27 BC), reveals this. Later in the Roman Empire, in the terminal Byzantine period, the Greek superiority in veterinary knowledge was again recognised.

Theophrastus, has to be remembered for his veterinary contribution. As first a student of, and later successor to, Aristotle he was not only a philosopher but a keen biologist. He wrote two books on plants. *Historia Plantarum (Enquiry into Plants)* includes a section identifying those plants of value in the treatment of animal diseases. Theophrastus is remembered as the first person to create a systemisation of plants which is seen as providing the basis for modern botanical systematics.

Greek Veterinary Practice

Karasszon (1988, pp. 70–71) observed that while Hippocrates did not practise animal healing, he did exert a significant influence on contemporaneous veterinary medicine with his humoral-pathological concepts, teachings on patient examination and his rational empiric medication proposals. His followers opened *zooiatreions* where sick animals were treated according to his methods. Castration, bleeding, cauterisation and trepanation were all performed with the animals constrained in a holding device (*mechanê*). The Hippocratian *crasis* doctrine of the four humours was used, with animals being described as sanguine, phlegmatic, choleric and melancholic. These practices were encouraged by the increased interest in horse, and chariot, racing and the development of cavalry units in the armies.

There is no literature that describes early Greek veterinary practice as an occupation, nonetheless, from the establishment of stadia for horse and chariot racing and zoological collections it follows that there must have been some level of veterinary care. In the earliest extant Roman work on agriculture, Varro lists more than 50

Greek authors who had written on agriculture, livestock and health problems. The majority of these are now lost but the content cited demonstrates that Greek veterinary practitioners were using Hippocratic procedures.

It is known that there were *hippiatroi* or 'horse doctors'. Their existence is confirmed by the excavation of gravestone monuments with figures holding gelding irons and knives. One, dedicated to Eutychos a horse doctor, is in the Athens Archaeological Museum; another similar inscription naming Metrodorus as a horse doctor of Lamia (Thessaly) who treated horses without charge, has been dated to c.130 BC (Fischer 1988, pp. 191–192). Fischer also reported on an Egyptian papyrus dated 257 BC, then under Greek influence, with reference to a man as a *hippiatrikon*, which possibly indicates that these equine practitioners were present in the 3rd century BC.

Praxamus (c.100 BC) described as a student of Mago of Carthage, but whose work now appears to be lost, described diarrhoea, indigestion and colic in cattle. Hecker (*History of Medicine*, 1829, cited in Smith, 1976, vol. I, p, 12) noted that he wrote in a typically Greek spirit of originality and observation. Another early writer whose work is now lost was Epicharmus of Syracuse (5th century BC), a poet who wrote on animal healing, quoted in Columella's treatise.

Simon of Athens and Xenophon

Simon of Athens (5th century BC) wrote a treatise that has only survived in fragments and quotations from other writers. A member of the Eleusinian Order he dedicated an equine sculpture cast in bronze, erected at the temple of the Order in Athens. It was said that his own exploits were recorded in relief on the pedestal (Xenophon 2014, pp. 13–19). One of the three laws of the order was to treat animals with kindness, the rituals of the order were secret and are unknown. It has been suggested that Simon wrote two works: *The Veterinary Art* and *The Inspection of Horses* but it is probable that there was only one treatise. Simon did not discuss specifically veterinary matters but concentrated on hygiene, selection and management. A 12th century AD manuscript (No.25l, old No.13, Library Emmanuel College, Cambridge) includes work believed to be Simon's. In translation this deals with selection of horses in significant detail, revealing that Simon not only knew his subject but described it with a clarity that is equally applicable today (Smith 1976, pp. 7–8).

Xenophon (430–354 BC) was a student of Socrates – a philosopher, historian and soldier. He was a general, and while an Athenian he usually sided with Sparta in the wars. He wrote in Attic Greek including two books on horses and one on dogs. *Hipparchikos* (*The Cavalry Commander*) deals with cavalry management. His more important text was *Peri Hippikon* (*The Art of Horsemanship*); it demonstrates that the Greeks had a clear understanding of the selection, management, training and hygienic care of horses. The outstanding characteristic of his treatise is the emphasis on humanity, he impresses on his readers what he called his first and best precept, 'Never act with anger towards a horse', a rule unfortunately that was ignored by generations of farriers and others. Xenophon does not deal with disease (apart from a reference to what is termed rheumatism and his admonitions on hoof care). The most important veterinary interest is in Chapter IV. This deals with stable cleanliness and care of the feet. It is emphasised that owners should closely supervise feeding to prevent other horses robbing the food, and give attention to the stable floor. He was, correctly, concerned that maximum care must be given to the foot, dirty stables that allow urine to collect result in problems. Xenophon understood management and hygiene. This was before horseshoes: he stated that a moist and smooth floor will ruin the best feet and that the floor must be of cobblestones and each to be about the width of a horse's foot, to ensure that the feet would be dry and the sole exposed to circulating air. Xenophon's principles were, 'for his mouth you must take as much care to make it soft as you take to make his hoofs hard'. While Xenophon did not write about disease in the horse he observed that, 'his master shall very often have an eye on the animal . . . because you can easily tell when the horse refuses his feed'. He noted, 'In the horse, as in the man, all diseases are easier to cure at the start than after they have become chronic and have been wrongly diagnosed' (Xenophon 2014, pp. 27–29).

Cynegeticus (*A Treatise on Hunting with Hounds*) by Xenophon, has only survived in a poor state in later transcribed manuscripts. It was probably an early work, about 391 BC, but it is seen as 'a vivid and personal account of hunting as practised in his day' (Phillips and Willcock 1999, pp. 25–26). He was a great advocate of hunting and urged young men not to despise it, 'for from these pursuits they would be well prepared for war and for other activities'. Two types of hunting dogs, castorian and vulpine, are described, the former was said to be purebred and the latter a dog/fox-cross, but the two breeds (believed terrier type) had become interbred. Canine defects (mostly of appearance) are listed in detail as conformation was felt to be most important. The greater part of the treatise concerns these dogs and hare hunting. Next he deals with fawn and deer hunts and using Indian dogs (but with no description) and finally wild boar hunts, seen as the most dangerous for dogs and hunters. Here the hunter is advised to use Indian, Cretan, Locrian and Laconian hounds as well as nets, javelins, boar-spears and traps. Xenophon makes no mention of canine diseases but gives very specific instructions for mating, care in pregnancy, feeding of the puppies and training them, on the leash, from eight months of age. Every dog was named and presumably responded to these, he lists 45 names as suggestions. And all short 'so that it will be easy to call them'. In the *Cynegeticus* the dogs are purely an aid to hunting, there is no suggestion of them being companions or pets. However, it is almost certain that the dog-handlers would have developed close relationships.

The Alexandrian School

Following Alexander the Great's death in 323 BC his empire was broken up between his warring generals. Egypt came under the control of General Ptolemy, later to become King Ptolemy I *soter* (saviour) and founder of the Ptolemaic Dynasty, which was to last for almost 300 years, until conquered by Rome under Julius Caesar. Ptolemy produced a sound economic basis for the country. He moved the capital to Alexandria (founded by Alexander the Great) and built an impressive city and harbour. Part of his legacy to the city was the Pharos, the massive lighthouse remembered as one of the seven wonders of the ancient world, and famously he constructed the Museion, a scientific centre.

The Museion was an enormous building housing laboratories, an astronomical observatory, reading rooms and a dining area as well as the library, which allegedly grew in size to hold 700,000 scrolls. It became the centre of Hellenistic culture attracting men of literature and science from all over the Mediterranean region: both Euclid and Archimedes spent time there. It was, however, essentially a Greek city and not Egyptian. Ptolemy tried to introduce a new religion with a new god, Serapis, but its acceptance by the Egyptian people was limited. Serapis was an animal incorporation of Osiris and was worshipped as Apis, a black bull, with divine signs. Later Serapis worship was united with the Isis cult and spread across all Greece and into the Roman Empire. This belief was strongly animal related, as was the horse cult centred on the enormous Poseidon temple built by the sea at Alexandria. The animal–human relationship and bond was a major feature of Hellenic/Egyptian life.

The Alexandrian School was generously financed by the Ptolemies and existed for some 800 years (300 BC to AD 500) with the first three centuries being seen as the 'golden age'. Alexandria was the centre of the civilised Hellenic world for both higher learning and the arts. Far reaching advances were made in all sectors of science, and in medicine some fundamental discoveries were made. Previous religious constraints on human dissection and experimentation were removed. First by the availability of human corpses, when the rulers allowed the still warm bodies of executed prisoners to be made available, and then vivisection was also conducted. Tertullian, one of the early Christian writers, passed harsh judgement on vivisectors, although his observations do not appear to have survived in print. The first comparisons between human and animal dissections were made; Alexandria was where not only comparative anatomy began but also the detailed study of human anatomy. Physiology also made advances, aided by vivisection studies.

These liberal policies opened the way for two practical physicians to advance knowledge: Herophilus of Chalcedon (c.335–280 BC) and Erasistratus of Ceos (c.304–250 BC): 'they were given criminals from prison by the kings and dissected them alive: while they were still breathing they observed parts which nature had formerly concealed, and examined their position, colour, shape, size, arrangement, hardness, softness, smoothness, connection . . . Nor is it cruel, as most people allege, by causing pain to guilty men – and only a few at that – to seek out remedies for innocent people of every age' (Barnes 1989, pp. 377–379). Celsus in *De Medicina* wrote that Herophilus dissected 600 live prisoners.

Herophilus studied the brain and described the cerebral ventricles, the meninges and the various sinuses of the dura; he differentiated nerves and tendons, traced several nerves and was the first to describe the eye and optic nerve. He also demonstrated that both veins and arteries contain and transport blood, but the arteries also held 'pneuma'. He studied the pulse and constructed a water chronometer device to measure the exact pulse rate. He was the first to describe the structure and function of the duodenum, which he also named. Erasistratus provided the first detailed examination of the trachea, oesophagus and the structure of the throat. He described how the entrance to the larynx and trachea was covered by the epiglottis and how this structure enabled both swallowing and breathing (Karasszon 1988, p. 83). He also studied the nervous system, recognised the brain as the seat of intellect and determined that the nerves had either a motor or a sensory function. Both men made enormous contributions to anatomy and physiology and began to recognise pathology as a discipline. They endeavoured to move medicine in a rational direction. They both emphasised the importance of exactness, thorough examination and scientific observation.

These men also had to counter the long Greek association of medicine with philosophy. Eristratus' pathology was based on the idea of overfilling, which in his mind was the cause of all disease, and on the concept that nature abhors a vacuum. He was said by his followers to have associated with the Peripatetic philosophers. Herophilus was also much exercised by the notion of causation, he cast doubt on all causes by many powerful arguments, and came to a sceptical conclusion, 'whether or not there are causes is by nature undiscoverable, but in opinion I am made hot and cold and am filled by food and drink' (Barnes 1989, p. 378). He was the first in a long line of medical sceptics which culminated in Sextus Empiricus, the 2nd century AD physician and Pyrrhonist. This school of thought advised that we should suspend judgement about virtually all beliefs and that we should neither believe nor deny. These ideas have influenced philosophers up to the present day. The sceptics followed the principle that everything should be tried, as medicine has a sole aim – healing the patient.

During a period of some 400 years when the Empirical School dominated medicine, great advances were made in *materia medica* and surgery: opium was introduced from the East into Greek therapeutics, as was the use of sulphur to treat skin conditions. Herbals were written, and poisonous plants and snakes listed. Surgical advances included treatment of hernia and fistula, lithotripsy to crush bladder calculi, and cataract removal. However, coprotherapy utilising both faeces and many animal parts was also supported by the Empirics, a practice which harmed medical advances for both humans and animals.

The decline of Alexandria as a medical centre followed attacks by religious heretics and vandals and finally capture by the Arabic tribes. Eventually the library was consumed by fire, said to be in AD 642 (having previously been damaged, or destroyed by fire and then rebuilt, in both 48 BC and AD 272 as a result of Roman military activity).

The Hellenistic Culture and Greece

The mix of beliefs and peoples who populated the islands of the Aegean Sea and its coasts created a culture that, for some still unexplained reason, broke out of and away from the religiously dominated systems of the Nile Valley and the Near and Middle East, to establish a new approach to the world. In almost every field of human endeavour – the humanities (philosophy, literature, the arts) and the sciences (natural and physical phenomena), the results are still to be seen in surviving architecture and arts, and remembered in the written word.

A discipline of 'natural philosophy' evolved. This was part of the overall search for meaning – of life, the world and the universe. One of the first philosophers was Thales of Miletus, who used a single method of analysis to attempt to prove that all life springs from water. And so, living beings were studied. For veterinary medicine, as a part of the total medical discipline, the developments and discoveries that arose from this creative period were not only the most important in the developing story of medicine, but would remain so for the next 1000 years.

Veterinary medicine had already developed to recognise a systematic approach (Egypt), to understand cleanliness and hygiene (Babylon and Egypt), and to utilise isolation (Mesopotamia). Some remedies, of varying effectiveness, had been discovered. There was a recognition of the benefits of animal welfare, but mainly for economic rather than humane reasons (with the possible exception of Zoroastrian beliefs in Persia). A veterinary profession did not exist, nor veterinary practice as now understood.

The name of Hippocrates is remembered as *the* leader in Greek medicine. He worked to train his students to study not only earlier medical work, but above all to study the patient, with clinical observation using all the senses. He established the concept of scientific enquiry and devised a system of ethics, observation, clarity, recording case histories and rational treatment and his notable admonition, 'above all, do no harm'. Hippocrates valued comparative medicine but did not study animal disease. His precepts and concepts, however, did pass into the methods and behaviour of the Greek *hippiatroi* or horse doctors. Not yet a profession but recognised specialists in animal disease problems.

Important veterinary observations were also made and Aristotle, one of the most remarkable men of ancient Greece, wrote of his studies and dissections of animals. He can truly be called the first veterinary scientist: he was not a clinician; he was an observer and recorder. Many diseases are described in his writings, some with great accuracy, for all species of livestock, and some exotic animals. Not only was his work notable, but while it was read by his contemporaries, and by the Romans and Byzantines – it was then neglected for centuries. Aristotle provided the basis for veterinary anatomy, physiology and pathology.

There was the beginning of a veterinary structure in ancient Greece, based on practical medicine and humane behaviour. Knowledge had grown, but it was the Romans who took the Greek texts and exploited their expertise. They recognised the Greek contribution and bemoaned the fact that Rome had not developed good veterinary practices. These were, however, to happen much later in the Eastern Byzantine Roman Empire, with Greek veterinary expertise again leading the way.

References

Barnes, J. (1989) Hellenistic Philosophy and Science, in *Greece and the Hellenistic World* (Ed.) Boardman, J., Griffin, J. and Murray, O. Oxford: Oxford University Press

Donaghy, T. (2010) The Origins of Equine Medicine. *Vet. Hist.* **15**

Edelstein, E.J. and Edelstein, L. (1945) *Asclepius: A Collection and Interpretation of the Testimony*. Baltimore, MD: John Hopkins Press

Fischer, K.D. (1988) Ancient Veterinary Medicine: A Survey of Greek and Latin Sources and Some Recent Scholarship. *Medizinhistor. Jnl.* **16**

Georges, K.E. (1879) *Ausführliches Lateinisch-Deutsches Wörtebuch in vier Bänden*. Leipzig: Hahn'sche Verlag

Hausmann, W. (1982) Chironica Ars. Antike Autoren ueber Cheiron. *Dtsch. Tierarztl. Wochenschr.* **89**

Hausmann, W. (1984) Cheiron. Eine weitere Sammlung und Auslegung von Zeugnissen. *Dtsch. Tierarztl. Wochenschr.* **91**

Hausmann, W. and Jöchle, W. (2003) The Discovery of Chiron's Cave. *Veterinary History* **12** No.1

Karasszon, D. (1988) *A Concise History of Veterinary Medicine*. Budapest: Akadémiai Kiadó

Parker, G. (Ed.) (1997) *Atlas of World History*, 4th edn. London: BCA

Peck, A.L. (1965) *Historia Animalium*, Books 1–3 (translation) Loeb Classical Library 437. London: Harvard University Press

Phillips, A.A. and Willcock, M.M. (1999) *Xenophon and Arrian on Hunting*. Warminster: Aris and Phillips

Schwabe, C.W. (1978) *Cattle, Priests and Progress in Medicine*. Minneapolis, MN: Minnesota University Press

Smith, F. (1976) *The Early History of Veterinary Literature*, Vol. 1. London: J.A. Allen

Sournia, J.-C. (1992) *The Illustrated History of Medicine*. London: Harold Starke

Taylor, W. and Chadwick, J. (2004) *The Mycenaeans*. London: Folio

Thomas, C.G. (2010) The Dark Age in *The Oxford Encyclopedia of Ancient Greece and Rome* Ed. Gagarin, M. New York: Oxford University Press

Walker, R.E. (1991) *Ars Veterinaria*. Kenilworth: Schering-Plough

Xenophon (2014) *The Art of Horsemanship*, (Trans. Morgan, M.H). Mineola: Dover Publications

CHAPTER 3

Carthage

Carthage occupies a very minor place in the history of veterinary medicine, but it deserves a significant mention due solely to the writings of one man: Mago of Carthage.

As Rome increased its power and conquered more lands it realised that being situated in the near centre of the Mediterranean Basin meant that it had to have complete control of the sea. Greece was subjugated first and then Carthage, who controlled the western Mediterranean with its fleet and network of bases and territories. This gave the Romans total control of the sea and over extensive additional lands in North Africa and the Iberian Peninsula. To achieve this dominance a substantial navy was created.

As discussed in more detail in Chapter 1, the Phoenician people living on the Levantine coast became traders and developed extensive links around the Mediterranean. One of their major cities, Tyre, established a settlement, probably in the 8th century BC, on the coast of modern-day Tunisia. Using the local language, they chose the name *Kart-hadasht* (New City). Later it was renamed *Carthago* by the Romans.

The city, applying its parent Phoenician expertise in maritime trade, came to dominate the western Mediterranean in the 5th century BC. This was based not only on their trading, but also on the huge agricultural surpluses they began to produce. They had created a cornerstone agrarian-based economy. Diodurus Siculus (c.90–30 BC), the historian, wrote of the luxuriant and well pastured land with cattle, sheep and horses, together with wheat production and olive and vine cultivation. The Carthaginians soon developed their own culture, artworks, architectural style and Punic, a Phoenician-related language.

With their fleet the Carthaginians blocked further expansion of the Greek *coloniae*, and enjoyed enormous growth in the 2nd century BC. They had, however, reached their peak and now came up against the increasing power of Rome, whose main strength was in their army; Carthage was a naval power and so Rome built ships.

The confrontation resulted in the three Punic Wars. The Second Punic War (BC 218–201) ended with the Roman army, commanded by Scipio, defeating Hannibal and the Carthaginian army at Zama in 202 BC. The power of Carthage was broken and they struggled to pay the heavy war indemnity imposed by the peace treaty. After a few years of peace Rome believed that Carthage was planning a resurgence, with a revival of its fortunes. Cato the Elder urged the Senate to destroy Carthage 'once and for all'. They had troops at the nearby city of Utica and issued a final ultimatum in 149 BC – 'abandon Carthage and settle inland', which resulted in the Third Punic War (149–146 BC). The city was razed in the spring of 146 BC.

For many centuries the rulers of Carthage were descendants of General Mago, known as the Magonids. One of this family, known as **Mago of Carthage** became famous for his agricultural knowledge and treatise. Described as a retired army general, probably correct due to his family connections, his life dates are unclear but he is believed to have been active at the end of the 4th century BC (Lancel 2012, p. 235).

The Mago treatise was probably written in the 4th–3rd century BC, but possibly later, it comprised 28 books. From the surviving citations, almost all from the Roman writers Varro, Columella, Pliny the Elder and Gargilius Martialis, an idea of the content can be deduced. Opening sections covered basic practical agricultural economics and then the cultivation of vines, olive and fruit trees, various plant varieties, grains, milling procedures and wine. Livestock sections included the selection of, and cattle breeding, diseases of cattle and veterinary procedures (including castration), mules and horses, sheep and poultry and general livestock management, including bees. Mago, of Phoenician origin, would probably have known the Canaan veterinary knowledge revealed in the Ugarit cuneiform tablets (Chapter 1) which indicated equine disease diagnostic features and therapies. This was possibly also a link back to Mesopotamia and their early veterinary knowledge.

Mago's work became widely known in the Mediterranean region and valued for its content. When Rome decided that Carthage had to be eliminated, the Senate ordered the total destruction of the city, with the unique exception of Mago's writings. By Decree 18 of the Senate the treatise was to be translated from the Punic into Latin. This translation was made by Decimus Junius Silanus, at the expense of the Senate, after the destruction in 146 BC. Later a translation into Greek was made by Cassius Dionysius in 88 BC. An abridged Greek version of the text, in six volumes, was also made by Diophanes of Nicaea in the 1st century AD: it was from this version that extracts were selected to be placed in the 9–10th-century AD Byzantine *Hippiatrica* (all these datings are imprecise).

It is obvious that Mago had accumulated and recorded significant advances in agriculture, he was the intellectual heart of the Carthaginian agricultural success. Rome, pragmatic as usual, in particular wanted his experience of cattle breeding, and so the knowledge of Carthage passed into their hands. Columella, who used more quotations from Mago's work than any other surviving agricultural authors' texts, called him 'the father of agronomy' – the agricultural prosperity of the Carthage lands had confirmed this.

Except for Mago's treatise the great library at Carthage on papyrus and leather scrolls was partly burned and partly given to local Numidian rulers. This was not only a significant loss but a great irony as the Phoenicians were the people responsible for transmitting the alphabet (from which Latin and Greek were derived) to the West. With the total occupation of Greece, Rome achieved European supremacy and absorbed the knowledge of both Carthage and the Hellenic world. While they respected and valued the Hellenic culture, they made every effort to eliminate that of Carthage – except for Mago's treatise.

Reference

Lancel, S. (2012) *Carthage, A History*. London: Folio

CHAPTER 4

The Roman Empire

The Roman story begins in the 7th and 6th centuries BC with a group of villages on and around the Palatine Hill. The people, mainly shepherds, were dominated by the Etruscans, who had settled in the region to the north. They were wealthy traders who between 625 and 600 BC established themselves as the overlords of Rome. Etruscan rule introduced the Romans to an artistically brilliant eastern Mediterranean influenced culture, that also contributed good masonry and metalwork skills. The Etruscans were probably the source of an alphabet, which enabled the development of the Latin language (the Etruscan tongue has never been translated). Etruscans were interested in animals, in particular horses and cattle: as demonstrated from the wall illustrations in their, still remaining above and below ground, tombs.

In about 509 BC the Romans overthrew the last Etruscan king, Tarquin the Proud, to establish an independent Roman republic. Expansion began gradually, first gaining mastery over the central Italian Latins by conquest or alliance, and by granting Roman citizenship: a confederacy was established, linked by roads. It was an agricultural economy. France and the Iberian peninsula were conquered, Carthage defeated, Greece and the north African territories assimilated. Following a continual series of conquests, the empire reached its peak in AD 117.

Animals Within the Roman Economy

The Roman world thrived because, apart from their military skill, they were exceptional builders and lawmakers. They created an effective society (slave-based) linked by a superb road system enabling swift communications. Agriculture was the basis of the economy, with wheat and olive oil the main products, but livestock production increased with population growth. With 90% of the people living in the country, and with agricultural labour based on slaves, all sectors of farming became of significance. Oxen were valued for transport of goods. Equines were important: mules were the work animals, in particular for the extensive army wagon trains, but horses were the status animals for the wealthy classes and later for the cavalry, when they learned from their opponents how to use them in warfare. Dairy cattle, sheep, goats, pigs and poultry all became significant to meet the food needs of the increasing urban populations.

As the empire matured the dog and talking birds became popular companions, the cat was regarded as a useful mouse catcher. There was extensive shipment and trade in wild animals from all parts of the empire, for the bloodthirsty spectacles in the many amphitheatres. Some were shipped to Rome from as far afield as India: these were paid for by the emperor or by wealthy public sponsors.

Before the problems of corruption and overpopulation most free people lived quite well with both fish and pork being popular staples. A wide variety of poultry, wildfowl and other birds were consumed as were eggs, cheese, varieties of bread and olive oil. In the later days of the empire, as wealth grew, so did an appetite for exotic and extravagant foods. Recipes for these dishes can be read in the only surviving Roman cookbook by Apicius. There are many records of the varieties of gluttony: the Emperor Vitellius fed his guests on the brains of pheasants and peacocks, and at a dinner party (at Trimalchio's feast described by Petronius) in Nero's time, a huge wild roast pig was carried to the guests with palm leaf baskets hanging from its tusks holding varieties of dates, and pastry piglets around the body, which was cut open to release live birds. Greed reached possibly the greatest extremes ever.

Most people ate frugally – a breakfast of bread and fruit followed by *prandium*, a light lunch about noon with the main meal, *cena*, taken at the workday's end, at sunset. The poor depended on *puls*, a porridge of ground wheat mixed with water maybe with an egg, cheese or honey if available. Slaves were fed on bread together with any cheap foodstuffs available including the remains of any *garum*, the fish sauce widely eaten by the more affluent classes. In Rome, the poorest citizens depended on a free issue of wheat, at the peak of the empire this was said to be 200,000 people each month, requiring constant replenishment of supplies. In the later days of the empire provision of food for the growing population became a problem in Rome and other major cities.

The Art of Medicine in Ancient Rome

Medical, both human and veterinary, practices in the early Roman world had evolved from a mixture of folklore, magic and religious rituals, including animal sacrifice. The basis of the medical art was belief in the supernatural. Roman medicine derived from the Etruscans, whose origin is unclear, but many aspects of their Etruscan culture can be traced back to the Levant and the Middle East.

Medical practice in Etruria was based on the ancient art of divination. The first Etruscan diviners used augury. The augers made their predictions based on a variety of observations, by first marking the four cardinal points with *lituus* (an unclear procedure) and then on the flight, cries and behaviour of birds. This was a particularly ancient art and the augers were of high social standing. The other group of diviners were the haruspices who made predictions based on the study of the viscera of sacrificial animals. The chief organ used was the liver, it is believed that the word *haruspex* (soothsayer) comes from the Chaldean *har* meaning liver, confirming its Mesopotamian origins (Margotta 1996, p. 33).

These two groups of divination oracles with their temples became absorbed into the early Roman culture. Etruscan priests served as both doctors and veterinarians. The success of their efforts is not known but Theophrastus wrote in his *History of Plants* that 'Aeschylus in his elegies says Etruria is a land rich in remedies and that the Etruscan race make medicine.' The Etruscans were a significant influence in their understanding of public health and clean water. The construction in Rome of the *cloaca maxima* or great drain, a sewer still in existence, took place under the 6th century BC rule of Tarquinius Priscus. They were also responsible for the first aqueduct, finally completed in 312 BC.

There were few medical or veterinary professionals for the greater part of early Roman history. The work of treatment and cure was, in major households, assigned to a trusted slave. For the rest of the population religious shrines and family folklore provided the prescriptions for hoped-for cures. Over time freed slaves who had shown some proficiency opened shops – this provided an opportunity for Greek slaves in particular, who were able to introduce and exploit the more rational procedures from their homeland.

The first Greek doctor in Rome is said to have been Archagathus, in 219 BC. A more forceful influence was created by Asclepiades who arrived in Rome in 91 BC: he was successful in attracting clients from among the local high society – but also drew criticism, particularly from Cato the Elder for being a person of a vanquished nation treating noble Roman citizens. Asclepiades, who probably adopted his name because of its ancient healing predecessor, was an Epicurean and introduced the Methodist school of medicine (from Alexandria). He recognised the *pneuma* as the source of life. The reasons for his success were probably that he prescribed diets and medications that pleased his patients, and his surgical skills were competent: he followed a Latin rule of *cito, tuto et jacunde* (quickly, safely and agreeably). Following his death many Greek doctors moved to Rome and at least 14 adopted the same name, claiming to be his pupils (Sournia 1992, p. 85).

Of the many doctors, few achieved distinction except Soranus of Ephesus, who arrived about AD 100, he was not only well educated, but also wrote a treatise on human generation and dystokia, as well as advice on paediatrics. It was not until Galen (AD 130–210) arrived in Rome from Greece in the early AD 160s that some science and rational medicine was achieved – and his influence reigned supreme in Europe for 15 centuries after his death.

Roman Veterinary Authors

The haruspice diviners were the first 'professionals' to provide advice on treatments for animal disease. Later their art was influenced by similar methods in Greece, using the same sacrificial organs. The practice and development of veterinary medicine in the Roman Empire can be traced by the written record. The few treatises that have survived are mostly compilations of earlier works, but as attribution was given we know that there was extensive literature available from Greece on agriculture, including veterinary. Many names are quoted but their work is lost, however, a small number of the extant papers do present a picture of the husbandry methods, diseases and the treatments. The work of each of these authors is reviewed in the Introduction.

Marcus Portius Cato (234–149 BC) Cato the Elder, also known as Cato the Censor, a Roman senator known for his opposition to what he saw as the 'Hellenisation' of Roman culture. In advice to his son he wrote 'They [the Greek physicians] have sworn to kill all barbarians with their drugs, and they call us barbarians. Remember that I forbid all physicians for you'. He served in the army, was appointed *censor* in 184 BC and tried to preserve Rome's customs against outside influences. Like most men of his class he had large estates and showed a particular interest in agriculture. Only one of his written works has survived, *De Agri Cultura* (On Agriculture) written about 160 BC, the earliest Roman agricultural and veterinary text. It provides a picture of the state of ancient Roman agriculture and their veterinary methods.

Remembering Cato's violent antipathy to Greek medicine, it does appear that some of his recipes emanate from that source. His own medical philosophy, which he tried to impose on Rome's citizens, is carried through to his advice for animal care. He had a favourite nostrum based on cabbage and praised its universal value in every form – raw or cooked, as a food or a broth – both internally and externally. To quote, 'It aids digestion wonderfully. It benefits the bowels, and the urine [of one who eats cabbage] is a universal remedy'; crushed leaves put on 'all wounds and tumours . . . will cure all these sores . . . it will purge wounds full of pus and cancers . . .'.

The more specific veterinary remedies recommended by Cato show a lack of rationality with much of the advice almost pure folklore. A complex herbal mixture for administration to working cattle, who were the basis of farm transport, also included 'three live coals and three pints of wine', and when administered the attendant should hold himself upright, be fasting at the time and feed the medication from a wooden dish. The use of burning coals, the wooden dish, fasting and standing upright by the attendant are all founded in very ancient beliefs. Pig dung plasters were recommended for snake bite in cattle; for sickness in a working oxen, 'give it at once one raw hen's egg. See that it is swallowed whole'. More practical, the advice to coat the feet of working oxen with tar had some reasoning, 'smear the bottom of the hoof with liquid pitch before you drive them anywhere on the road'. There was a recognition of sheep scab and external parasites, both use of salves and washing were recommended.

Cato did have some understanding of both preventive medicine and animal welfare, 'nothing pays better than to treat your work oxen well', and stressed the value of clear, clean water for livestock. His emphasis demonstrated the importance of cattle as draught animals. Cato described agriculture with a slave population as the primary source of labour; he was the typical pragmatic Roman. He wrote 'An owner should be a seller . . . let him sell the old work oxen, blemished cattle, blemished sheep . . . old wagon, worn-out tools, the aged or diseased slave and everything else that he does not need'. These were attitudes for which he was criticised, but were commonplace. Many farms were small, under 200 acres, had few oxen and most labour was by slaves (but he does recommend flattering the ox driver, 'so that they will more cheerfully care for the oxen'). Wheat, vines and olive trees were major crops, sheep for wool was the main livestock profit area. Cato mentions pigs but not as an important species and poultry had not yet developed as a sector.

Marcus Terentius Varro (116–27 BC) is remembered as one of the most learned and scholarly Romans, he served the state, becoming a *praetor*, fought in the army and was a prolific writer. Of some 74 works in an estimated 620 books, most of which are only known by title, only one has survived in its entirety: *Rerum rusticarum libre tres* (*Three Books on Agriculture*), written in 37 BC, his 80th year, as a manual for Fundania, his wife who had just acquired a farm. It is a sensible guide and an exposition of the agriculture of its time. The text covers many aspects of agriculture from crops, vines, fruits to fish and bees as well as livestock including poultry. He quotes extensively from Greek authors and Mago the Carthaginian, and understood the economic contribution of agriculture. The value of the book was shown by its readership in Europe for many hundreds of years post-Roman Empire.

There had been an advance in perception of disease, Varro recognised contagion as a factor in epidemic disease and attributed the cause to minute invisible animalculae. He suggested that these may come with the wind from miasmatic areas, such as swamps, to peopled regions. Not only was this an anticipation of the germ theory of disease, but the concept of a disease-bearing miasma rising from the ground persisted into the early 1800s. He was unable to proffer specific measures for epidemic prevention but did recommend closing windows and doors when the winds blew from unhealthy locations, and recommended only having small groups of animals rather than large herds – 'Because a pestilence quickly takes possession of a large herd and sweeps it to destruction.' He was perceptive in disease causation stating that when establishing a home or farm, 'precautions must be taken against swampy places . . . because as they dry, swamps breed certain animalculae which cannot be seen . . . and which we breathe . . . into the body where they cause grave maladies.' Yet it was several generations before the Pontine marshes were drained and Rome was freed from malaria.

Varro read the Greek literature extensively and recognised that equine medicine was as complex as human so that 'on this account in Greece the veterinarians are most frequently named *hippiatroi* or horse doctors'. He saw the need for both a trained veterinarian to undertake complex procedures, and for a good stock manager, in particular for sheep, to perform what he saw as two levels of healing work. He understood that veterinary (like human) medical action required a study of the cause, and then of the symptoms and finally the treatment for each disease. Varro believed the common causes of disease in cattle were overwork, excesses of heat or cold or lack of exercise; he was concerned by what he termed 'fever' – gasping breath, open mouth and a hot body. The treatment was to cool the animal with water, rub with oil and wine, and to cover with a blanket. If this did not cure, then bleeding from the head was suggested. There was always a practical pragmatic Roman approach. One reason for his two levels of veterinary care was that if all the care was in the hands of a medically trained slave 'the death of such a single such skilled slave wipes out the entire profit of a farm'!

Varro knew the Romans started as a race of shepherds and 'penalties to this day are assessed in terms of cattle or sheep according to the ancient custom'. He stressed the value of cattle, 'our word for money *pecunia* comes from *pecus*, cattle, which is the foundation of all wealth . . .'. Killing an ox was a capital crime in ancient Rome, slaughter was only allowed when they were no longer fit for work. Castration was undertaken at two years old, 'as they recover with difficulty if the operation is performed sooner, while if it is done later they are apt to be stubborn and useless'. Neither cattle nor sheep were considered as meat animals, Varro assumed that every farmer would have pigs and poultry for this provision. He noted that the Latin word for a pig, *sus*, is derived from the Greek meaning 'to offer as a sacrifice'.

The veterinary practices discussed by Varro are a minor part of his writing but illustrate the major problems then encountered in livestock farming. He states that the medications should be written down by the overseer of the stock and carried with him. Advice is given on cattle husbandry, in the summer they should be protected from flies, the floors of housing should be paved, able to drain and all dung cleared away. Pregnant sows should be individually housed and poultry examined for mites. Bees are given special mention (honey was the only sweetener) and their diseases recognised, 'Bees contract a malady of the bowels from their first spring pasture . . . and can be cured by giving a urine drink.' Sheep had to be watched for scab and those affected not sheared, wounds from shearing should be anointed with liquid tar.

Warranties of health were expected at the sale and purchase of livestock, including dogs, except for goats, 'no sane man ever guarantees that goats are without malady, for the fact is that they are forever in a fever': this could have been brucellosis. Many medications are proposed, but few would have had any significant effect. If the husbandry, housing, feeding and water supply measures proposed by Varro were all followed they would have significantly reduced disease incidence. His agricultural treatise both described Roman farming and contained early concepts of microbiology and epidemiology. Varro demonstrated a significant knowledge of agriculture; he was one of 20 men chosen by Gaius Julius Caesar in 59 BC to produce a great agrarian scheme for the resettlement of Capua and Campania.

Publius Vergilius Maro (70–19 BC), more commonly Virgil, was one of the most famous Latin poets. His second major work, *Georgica* (*The Georgics: A Poem of the Land*), a title derived from ancient Greek, etymologically meaning 'to work the earth'. Virgil began the poem in 37 BC, under the urging of Maecenas his patron, completing it in 29 BC. A part of this work, a manual of agriculture in verse, is in praise of animal breeding and healing. In Book 3 he deals with animals, mainly with hygiene – in horses, cattle and sheep. He took current local knowledge and clothed it 'in language of unparalleled beauty, which has secured their preservation'. His verses give us the most vivid description of the animal plagues in ancient times: these are particularly illuminating.

The work should be read with caution as there is no evidence that Virgil was either a stock-keeper or had any practical involvement in farming. He was presenting a poetic celebration of the land and including a picture of livestock husbandry and disease problems faced by the Roman farmer in 29 BC. His descriptions are enlightening, for sheep scab and its treatment, 'the shepherds drench the whole flock in sweet streams . . . or they besmear their bodies after shearing with bitter lees of oil . . . and black bitumen . . . the distemper is nourished and lives by being covered'.

Virgil described *Oestrus ovis* infestation, severe footrot needing surgical intervention and use of the cautery. He also described how ignoring the signs of what was an infectious disease without using ruthless methods of control would leave 'old grazings empty up to the far horizon'.

A severe malady of the horse is described, in true poetic gory detail (it was probably anthrax), for which the only remedy was wine. The disease also affected cattle, 'the bull too, smoking under the oppressive shere, drops down, and vomits out of his mouth blood mingled with foam, and fetches his last groans'. A plague, possibly rinderpest, in the province of Noricum (present-day Austria) is described. It was a severe epizootic and the air was heavy with the odour of dead animals with birds and fish also affected, and even sacrificial animals died before the ceremony, 'and delivered over to death all the race of cattle'. Pigs are mentioned as suffering from severe coughing and having symptoms of what would appear to be anthrax infection. 'Pale Tisophone, sent from the stygian glooms to light, rages . . . drives before her diseases and dismay . . . by droves and flocks she deals destruction, and in the very stalls heaps up carcasses . . .'. Of all the diseases described anthrax is most clearly indicated, he writes of the danger of the fleece and hides, to humans handling them with 'fiery pustules and filthy sweat overspreading his noisesome body'. A disease of sheep, possibly liver fluke infestation is noted with listlessness, wasting and dropsy, and when used for sacrificing the knife is hardly marked with blood.

Grattius Faliscus (c.63 BC–AD 14) was a Roman poet in the Age of Augustus; only one extant work, *Cynegeticon Liber*, of 541 hexameter lines exists. This was found in a manuscript in about AD 800, only one copy of this now exists in a later manuscript of the early 16th century, included with a copy of *Cynegetica* by Nemesianus. The text covers hunting methods, types of game, selection of horses, dogs and their management and care (this last section in verses 150–430). Twenty-two different breeds of dogs are listed, of which only one was of Italian origin. Five breeds were of outstanding merit including one called the 'Britain' and adding it was worthwhile to take the long journey to these 'utmost shores' – the breed would appear to have been a formidable mastiff-type.

Diseases are discussed, mange and skin conditions were the most serious problems and many medications were tried, including taking mangy hounds to sulphurous pools on the slopes of Mount Etna. Coughs, foot disease and lameness were also problems. Surgery to lance and drain abscesses and to repair disembowelment injuries from boar hunts are mentioned including an 'antiseptic' procedure before the intestines were returned to the abdomen, they were cleansed and then washed in the 'urine of the enemy who had dealt the blow'. Grattius recognised rabies as a major scourge and quotes the removal of the 'worm in the tongue' as a sure preventive, a procedure dating back to Aristotle. There was well developed canine care with disease recognition, some small advances in medications and significant developments in surgery, while primitive, possibly in advance of human practice.

Aulus Cornelius Celsus (c.25 BC–AD 50) was a prolific author in the time of Emperor Tiberius. His only surviving work is *De Medicina*, believed to be part of a much larger treatise. He also wrote on veterinary medicine, this work is lost but known from the many quotations from it, in particular by Columella. Celsus was well educated and his work, which covers diagnosis, pharmacy and surgery, is the best source of Roman medical knowledge. He was not just a compiler, he displayed original thought. He differed from Hippocrates in several ways, and saw that methods used in veterinary work might have a place in human practice. He drew attention to the importance of objective as well as subjective signs of disease, and is remembered today in the dermatology field. Celsus discussed in detail how to stop bleeding and how to clean wounds to prevent complications. He stated four cardinal signs of inflammation *rubor, calor, dolor, tumor*: redness, heat, pain and swelling. The treatment of broken bones by reduction, immobilisation, splinting, bandaging and fixation by wax and resin pastes is detailed in a workmanlike manner (Margotta 1996, p. 35).

Rabies in the human is described. Eye problems, common in both humans and animals in the dry sandy regions around the Mediterranean, are discussed in detail. Particular emphasis is given to examination of the head; much value was associated with various cranial procedures, in particular cautery of the scalp to cure 'the sacred disease' (epilepsy). These procedures were also used on animals. Many surgical procedures are explained, recognised by the Roman instruments that have been excavated – forceps, scalpels, hooks, sounds, probes, tongs, lithotomes and trephines are discussed – and a modified Diocles spoon, a V-shaped iron instrument to open wounds and remove arrowheads. All of these have equal application in veterinary work and account for the many mentions of the Celsus text.

Celsus was probably not a medical man by training, but his medical text is an excellent exposition of how medicine should be practised, written before the establishment of a sound medical structure in the Roman world and while belief in folklore and supernatural influences held sway. He advocated a logical and complete approach to a patient, together with an emphasis on the physician understanding the position of the bodily organs. His medicine was based on three practical strategies: diet, medications and surgery. Of these he emphasised surgery, as this demonstrated some action being taken.

The Celsus manuscript was discovered in AD 1426 and issued in print in AD 1428. It was the first printed medical text. The loss of the veterinary treatise has to be regarded as a tragedy for the animals of the Middle Ages, when a sensible and practical approach to medicine was much needed in the veterinary field. Celsus has to be also remembered as an early believer in the One Medicine approach.

Lucius Junius Moderatus Columella (AD 4–70) was born in Gades (Cadiz, Portugal) the old Punic colony, Columella was a Roman citizen. He served in the army, achieving the rank of *tribune* in Syria. Returning to Italy he owned extensive estates in Latium. He was well educated, knowledgeable and wrote well using the Latin language in a rich and erudite manner, described as 'stylish prose'. His period of life is confirmed by his mentioning that Marcus Varro was a contemporary of his grandfather, and also that he lived at the same time as Cornelius Celsus, Seneca and Pliny the Elder, by whom he is quoted. He lived outside Rome on a farm, which he called *Ceretanum*, possibly located at Caere in Etruria (Boyd Ash 1941, pp. xiv–xv). Of his several books, only *De Re Rustica* (translated as *On Rural Affairs, On Agriculture* or *On Husbandry*) has survived. Written about AD 60–65 it does not appear to have been widely read in the later Roman years, and was only known from fragments until the complete manuscript was discovered in monastery libraries between 1414 and 1418. It was later realised that this was the most complete surviving treatise on Roman agriculture.

The work is arranged in 12 books, of which numbers 6–9 deal with livestock breeding and rearing covering oxen, horses, mules, sheep, goats, pigs, dogs, poultry, bees and fishponds. Veterinary procedures are discussed in Book 7 and bees and their care in Book 9. Columella understood farming, the many aspects of practical husbandry and knowing how to run a profitable business. He obviously had experience of managing livestock. He emphasised hygiene and suggested that any *villicus* (agriculturalist) should have experience in medicine, should inspect his animals daily and have an infirmary in which to place sick animals. He stressed that sick and pregnant animals should be isolated. There was a recognition of the importance of endemic disease and he advocated keeping livestock in small groups to prevent epizootic diseases getting a hold. During his discussion of animal health issues, he quotes many authorities including Celsus and he gives much praise to Mago, and his Punic work, 'the father of agronomy, inasmuch as his 28 memorable volumes were translated into the Latin tongue by senatorial decree' (see Chapter 3).

In an analysis of the Columella treatise Walker (1991, p. 26) identifies the close similarity between the description of a specific disease of cattle, to that found in the Egyptian el-Lahun papyrus (c.1900 BC); the same signs are listed and presented in a similar style. Walker posits that the knowledge, of certain diseases, had been passed down through the generations and cultures and that this was particularly noticeable in sheep and cattle maladies, such as malignant catarrhal fever, rinderpest and diseases of the feet and mouth. As this knowledge was transmitted, so were many customs and superstitions.

Columella described many diseases, he understood contagion, recognised parasitism, knew surgical procedures, such as castration, and believed in good husbandry practices for hygiene, housing and correct feeding. He was a confident practitioner of surgery. He copied Greek practice in the use of embryotomy in sheep to save the life of the ewe. Bleeding was frequently recommended, either by venesection or by cuts to the palate. He used astringents on wounds and the cautery on suppuration. His 12 agricultural books display both an organised system, as well as an authority conveyed by his practical advice, accompanied by his critical use of Greek, Punic and Roman authors. His citations of Virgil, together with Book 10 on horticulture written in hexameter verse, all gave his work additional credibility among well-educated Roman landowners. For centuries his writings were thought to be unsurpassable, and possibly limited the expression of new ideas (Karasszon 1988, p. 97).

Gaius Plinius Secundus (AD 23–79), commonly Pliny 'the Elder' to distinguish him from his nephew, was a prominent Roman. He had an international and a diverse career: held an equestrian command, was active in legal practice and through a series of senior positions earned a reputation for integrity. He was a member of council for both Emperors Vespasian and Titus, and was given command of the Misenum Fleet based in the Bay of Naples. He was a prolific author on many subjects but is particularly remembered for his 37 book *Naturalis Historia* (*Natural History*) a monumental encyclopaedia of information that he claimed included

20,000 important facts derived from 2000 books. His work is particularly important as Pliny not only usually notes his sources by name, but it provides almost the only compilation of information on the Roman world that has survived in the original. Study indicates that our knowledge of ancient agriculture, medicine, metallurgy and the great artists of that time would be diminished if the work had been lost like so many others.

While Pliny sometimes presents a garbled summary of his information, overall the work is a superb overview and reflects the mood of Roman society and the way that it lived. As it is a mixture of fact and fable it has to be read with care. The observations on veterinary medicine are mainly a compilation from Aristotle, Varro and Columella. However, in many of his sources, in particular Cato, Mago, Celsus, Virgil and Dioscorides he barely mentions their contributions to veterinary medicine. The most reliable veterinary content is from Columella in discussing animal health and hygiene. Pliny also includes a miscellany of dubious observations such as, the ass is unable to endure cold and hates water and the ox is the only animal that walks backwards in feeding. For rabies prevention in the dog docking the tail is recommended, and the use of hair of the dog as a treatment for a bite from a rabid dog is advocated.

Pliny, reflecting the beliefs of the time, elaborated on magic and superstitions as well as discussing contemporary medicine, both human and veterinary. Of the many remedies that he lists he reflects then current views, to utilise some quite bizarre and disgusting medications – dried camel brain, camel urine, hyena eye, lion fat, fresh blood and crocodile dung. The book and its varied content was much valued when it was first printed in 1469, its importance indicated by this being soon after the Bible, and before the works of Celsus. For many years Pliny was the knowledge source that challenged those trying to advance medical and veterinary medicine.

Pliny was in command of the Misenum Fleet based on the opposite side of the Bay of Naples when Vesuvius erupted on 24 August AD 79. Following his natural curiosity and duty he led a detachment across the bay to offer help. Landing at Stabiae he died following inhalation of the volcanic fumes. His nephew (Pliny the Younger) wrote that his uncle read all the time, even in the baths and while eating. A quite remarkable man.

Pedanius Dioscorides (AD c.40–90) a Greek physician, pharmacologist and botanist was born in Anazarbus, Cicilia (Turkey). Enrolling in the Roman army as a surgeon he travelled extensively. During this period, he collected herbs, plants and every claimed medication from the regions he visited. In about AD 64–77 he produced five books under the title *De Materia Medica* (*On Medicinal Materials*, with a subtitle *On the Preparation, Properties and Testing of Medicines*). The work remained in print for centuries, with the last English-language edition being published in 1934. It was said to have been used by Galen and remained the standard text for both medical and veterinary reference until the Renaissance, forming the core of European pharmacopoeias up to the 19th century. Avicenna (AD 980–1037), renowned for *The Canon of Medicine*, a medical encyclopaedia, based his medication writings on the Dioscorides text.

The work is presented in five books: 1 Herbs, ointments and oils; 2 Animal food products, honey, milk, wheat and so on; 3 and 4 Plants and roots; 5 Wines and medications from mineral sources (including lead acetate, copper sulphate and calcium hydroxide). There was an appendix on poisons, including arsenic and mercury with antidotes. Over 600 plants are listed. There is evidence that Dioscorides tested suggested medications; as well as listing treatments he discussed the disease management in certain cases. He also examined the earlier texts and included information from Cratenas, Andreas of Carystos and Theophrastus (who had listed plants for veterinary medication). He provided the first mention of opium as an anaesthetic. To obtain accuracy Dioscorides used distillation to refine his medicines: his apparatus was composed of a retort and a helmet held close.

Dioscorides makes frequent reference to dogs. He specifically included the milk of the bitch in a comparison of differences between the milks of the domesticated animals. Of importance was his writing on rabies where the dog is clearly identified as the vector of the disease. He discusses the disease and rabid dogs, and lists what were considered to be sovereign remedies. His commentary indicates that hydrophobia was widespread and well recognised as a serious issue. Particular attention was paid to treating the bite: he had realised that poison had been injected into the flesh and regarded large bite wounds as less dangerous, as they would have copious haemorrhage and recommended that smaller wounds be opened up to allow for more effective flushing out of any injected poison (Merlen 1971, p. 79).

Dioscorides achieved a unique reputation, his work became the prime source of information on medicines, widely read for 1500 years. The text was never lost and was used in Latin in the medieval times, and in Arabic in the Islamic world. Its influence can be seen in the Anglo-Saxon leech books. The finest original manuscript in existence was created in about AD 515 in Constantinople and passed to the Holy Roman Emperor in Vienna. Known as the *Vienna Dioscorides*, it is termed the Juliana Anicia Codex. In the later Byzantine period – 4th to 15th centuries – it was used as the original for copies in Greek and in Arabic (see Chapter 5). It is now entered on the UNESCO Memory of the World Programme.

Lucius Flavius Arrianus Xenophon (AD c.86–160), commonly Arrian of Nicomedia (present-day Izmit), was Greek but a Roman citizen. While his dates and early life are unclear he became a leading Greco-Roman. Initially studying philosophy under Epicetus he served in the military in many locations, was appointed *consul* and became a friend of Emperor Hadrian, who appointed him to the Senate and then governor of Cappadocia. Arrian was an historian and a respected author, Xenophon was his hero on whom he modelled his writing and to some degree his life. Of his several books, only two have survived in full. One is his *Cynegeticus* (*Hunting Man* or *On Hunting*). It is an interesting work because 'you can walk the streets of Athens and talk to a real Roman gentleman about a subject on which he is both knowledgeable and enthusiastic' (Phillips and Willcock 1999, pp. 90, 167).

The importance of the book is in the great detail given to the selection, care and management of the dogs (hounds). He stressed bitches should not be bred until three years old and not after seven; that mating must take place in seclusion, and that the male should have 60 days rest before being used again. The recommended diet was of a farinaceous food – bread, dried and moistened with water. When hunting, hounds were given lumps of salted suet for energy, and then after fed the bowels of the deer or other animal hunted (termed *praemia* or *curée*). This diet does not appear to be good nutritionally and may have accounted for the frequently mentioned skin diseases. Puppies were given liver broth and raw eggs, as were 'sickly' dogs. Great care was taken after the hunt to rub down the dogs and put them on dry bedding. A daily routine of four runs was advocated, with constant care by kennel boys.

The serious disease problems noted were mange and other skin and ear problems (ringworm, fleas, lice and fly maggots are recorded). A suggestion to control spread of the skin diseases was that the kennel boys should sleep between the dogs. Merlen (1971, pp. 67–72) observed that this idea had some sense, reducing the contact between dogs was helpful as canine parasites – fleas, lice and so on, only have a short lifespan on humans. Unwell dogs had gravy from fat meats added to their meal or roasted ox liver grated over food.

Animal sacrifice also played a role in the activities of the professional hunter. A sacrifice to Artemis, goddess of the hunt, was recommended for good hounds and also after a successful hunt. A collection box was sometimes used for an annual Artemis sacrifice – a sheep, goat or calf; after the offering the carcase was fed to the hounds.

Claudius Galenus or Aelius Galenus (AD c.129–c.216), commonly known as Galen of Pergamum (Bergama, Turkey), was educated in philosophy and rhetoric before beginning medical training in Smyrna, Corinth and for some years in Alexandria, before practising in Pergamum in AD 157, and then moving to Rome in AD 162. Galen then left, for unclear reasons, before returning in AD 169 and entering imperial service at the court of Emperor Marcus Aurelius. Galen's reputation as a physician grew and his public demonstrations of dissection of animals, most frequently pigs and Barbary apes, were popular. As a result of treating gladiators he developed expertise in wound treatment. Galen was a polymath: as well as his extensive medical writings he was highly regarded as a philosopher with his heroes being Plato, Hippocrates and Aristotle. He also had a strong monotheistic religious belief.

Galen became the leader, in both thought and practice, of the Roman medical profession. He had a strong personality and was thought to be conceited, cruel and vindictive. His medical writing is permeated by his own judgements combined with the prime sources of information from earlier medical authors, in particular Hippocrates; there is difficulty in separating the two inputs. He incorporated the ancient Greek theory of the four humours as well as his own theory of four temperaments into his understanding of medicine. In his work, of some 400 medical treatises, of which only 22 have survived in full, he created a synthesis of Greek medicine embracing theory and practice, and he inaugurated therapeutic scepticism. Galen combined this with the knowledge that he derived from experimentation, together with his own understanding of humankind and relationships. Galen's diagnostic supremacy was based on his acute powers of observation and experience.

He was particularly important because he summarised and systematised all medical knowledge from ancient times. Anatomy and physiology were his most productive research areas, but as his anatomical knowledge was based on animal dissection, particularly of monkeys, this sometimes led to errors when transposed to the human body (Singer 1956). Owing to the religious prohibition on human dissection his observations remained unchallenged until the rebirth of anatomical studies in the Renaissance.

Galen believed in the value of comparative medicine and his animal dissections were most detailed, he studied the brain, cranial nerves and the eye and showed that severing the recurrent laryngeal branch of the vagus nerve in a pig prevented the vocal cords functioning. Among his many investigations he produced cardiac arrest in animals by cutting the nerves to the heart, this dispelled the ancient misconception that nerves came from the heart rather than the brain. He understood the role of the spinal nerves and came close to understanding blood circulation. In his physiology the fundamental principle of life was the *pneuma*, which entered the body by the trachea. This had three forms – 'animal spirit' in the brain; 'vital spirit', which controlled the heart, blood flow and body temperature; and 'natural spirit' based in the liver and was the centre of nutrition and metabolism.

While Hippocrates had a low regard for those who looked after animal health, Galen could see the positive advantages in cooperation between the two evolving disciplines; among other proposals he suggested examining an animal for health before its products (milk) were given to humans. In *De Anatomicis Administrationibus* he refers to specific individuals who undertook animal healing (Johnston and Horsley 2011).

Galen had a reputation for his prescriptions: these were complex mixtures usually containing opium. Many of his treatments were derived from the concept of *contraria contrariis*, the theory of opposites. As well as medications he was an advocate of physiotherapy, but regarded surgery with disdain, after treating gladiators and injured slaves. He recommended the interpretation of dreams by doctors and the use of medical astrology. At the same time Rome was introducing public health – sewers, public latrines, clean water, other health care measures and early hospitals (Sournia 1992, p. 92).

Galen did not gather a group of scholars to follow in his footsteps and after his death his works remained unused in Europe until the 13th century, when they were translated from Arabic copies. His death marked an end to serious anatomical and physiological research. The first printed copy of his works, together with the *Corpus Hippocratica* represented the medical achievements of antiquity. His ideas then became the most important input into Western medical thought and practice (Mattern 2013). When his work was rediscovered it was valued and accepted by the new societies and cultures of the time, because his belief in one god was acceptable to Christians, Jews and Moslems. His authority and his mistakes, which created perpetual errors, went unchallenged for almost 1500 years, but as a physician, observer and experimenter he was remarkable and his contribution deserves to be remembered (Margotta 1996, p. 43).

Claudius Aelianus (AD c.170–c.230), commonly Aelian, a Roman, born at Praeneste (Palestrina) in Italy was an author and teacher of rhetoric. Fluent in Attic Greek he was known as 'honey-tongued', he devoted himself to the Greek authors, and their ways. In one of his surviving treatises, *De Natura Animalium* (*On the Nature of Animals*) he describes the characteristics of each species. These are a series of brief natural history stories describing almost all the then known (and believed) species of animals, aquatic life and birds. He presents an 'attitude' towards each species, this reflected the then views and influenced later concepts and welfare approaches.

There was no veterinary content but the work is important, as a tentative early step into zoology classification. The text was much valued and utilised by later Christian writers because it created an impression of expressing the reality of divine providence in the animal kingdom, with lessons for humankind. The approach was later used in the monastic medieval bestiaries and medical treatises. The species descriptions range from the allegorical to the bizarre (the mythical Basilisk is included) but many are correct; natural medicines used by animals and fables are all included.

Oppian (2nd century AD) of Anazarbus, was a Greco-Roman poet. A series of didactic poems in hexameter verse have been attributed to him: *Cynegetica* on hunting; *Ixeutica* on catching birds and *Halieutica* on fishing. There is now a belief that the first was composed by another Oppian and the second by Dionysus.

The *Halieutica*, dedicated to Emperor Marcus Aurelius, is a remarkable five books of 3500 lines of text dealing with the sea, fishing and the aquatic life forms. There is an encyclopaedic listing of aquatic creatures and fishing, together with several comments on fish health and some on specific copepod parasitic infestations, even drawing an observant comparison with gadfly (*Hypoderma* spp.) attacks on cattle. The *Cynegetica* is a shorter poem relating to hunting with dogs. Written about 50 years after Arrian's work it is dedicated to the Emperor Caracalla. Oppian mentions 22 breeds of hounds including 12 not listed by any other author, but all were from countries visited by Caracalla. There is little of veterinary interest but there is an account of a small dog 'called the Agasseus which the painted Picts in Britain reared', the breed was praised for fierceness and hunting skills (Merlen 1971, pp. 58–59). The observation demonstrates both the availability of information, and interests, in the widespread Roman Empire.

Vindanius Anatolius (c.3rd to 4th century AD) of Berytus (Beirut, Lebanon), was an agricultural writer and compiler. His best known work was a farming almanac that included information on the care, breeding, treatment and healing of animals. While Varro and Columella are quoted the majority of the content derives from early, now lost, books in particular that of Diophanes (who had used the also lost treatise of Mago) as well as Democritus, Africanus, Pamphilius and others. There is little original knowledge included but the almanac represents a useful summary of the state of animal health at that time. The changing climate of Roman attitudes is illustrated by the inclusion of the Democritus cure for 'erysipelas' in sheep – bury a live animal at the entrance to the sheep fold and then drive the flock through the gateway. This appalling mystical remedy survived in Europe until the 18th century. Both Cassius Bassus (*Geoponika*) and Palladius used the text for their books.

Quintus Gargilius Martialis (early to mid-3rd century AD), a Roman poet and historian. Of the many works believed to be his, few have survived. He particularly wrote on horticulture and gardens, and parts of his *De Hortis* (*On Gardens*) are extant. Of other fragments usually attributed to him, one is on the medicinal value of fruits and the other is titled *Curae Boum* (*Cures of Cattle*). From this limited evidence it is difficult to judge the importance of Gargilius. Columella quotes him, and Teuffel and Schwabe (1891, cited in Smith 1976, vol. 1, p. 13) remarked on his knowledge of agriculture and medical botany, adding that he was well read and 'exhibited intelligent physiological views'. An early 20th-century edition of *Encyclopaedia Britannica* refers to him as a writer on the veterinary art and on agriculture. Other commentators regard him as unimportant and his writings as a collection of superstitious remedies.

Eumelus (c.3rd century AD), only known by quoted extracts that follow the pattern of the Antique agricultural tradition; he is one of seven authors from that period who are quoted in the *Hippiatrica* compilation. Their roots can be traced back, through Hellenic agricultural texts with derivation from Mago of Carthage. Eumelus, who wrote on both horses and cattle, is probably the earliest of the authors quoted. Recent study (McCabe 2007, pp. 98–121) of the content of the *Hippiatrica* has shown the extent of the Eumelus writings, his sources and how later authors have utilised him as their source; in particular Apsyrtus, Theomnestus, Hierocles and *Mulomedicina Chironis*.

There is no known background detail for Eumelus. He can only be dated in relation to Apsyrtus, who referred to him as 'the great horse doctor'. He wrote in Greek and was called a Theban, but this only indicates the region of his residence, possibly near Boeotia, which had a reputation for horse breeding, racing and hunting. From the content of his work it is obvious that he was both well read and also practised veterinary medicine. Eumelus valued the earlier writings of Varro, Columella, Cassius Dionyius, Anatolius and Julius Africanus. The valuable and fascinating comparison of the extracts by McCabe of the writings of the various authors on similar topics shows how veterinary knowledge moved between Latin and Greek manuscripts to reach a larger readership.

The Eumelus texts discuss wounds, eye conditions, cough, digestive ailments and parasites; sometimes these entries just list the symptoms seen, and rarely the believed cause, others are simply a heading or a prescription. Bloodletting and wound treatments are identified. In the medication recipes is one using silphium root, the famed herb harvested in Cyrene, the Greco-Roman province (Libya). It was widely used in medicine, and even depicted on Cyrene coins. The plant apparently died out and what it actually was is unknown. The Eumelus recipe required bean-sized pieces of root in honey and warm water to be given as a drench. In recipes where a broth was required made from a chicken or a puppy, it is noted that in his copy Eumelus always omitted the puppy. His remedies generally reflected the theory of the humours.

The Eumelus writings also reflect the movement in the later Roman Empire towards a revival of superstitious beliefs. Examples are seen in the recommendation that an animal's own blood or faeces be used in treatment. Bleeding was regularly advocated and faeces were commonly applied to wounds to stop bleeding. The left nostril was regarded as being 'weaker' than the right and was frequently recommended to be used for administering medications. The person administering medication was often told to be fasting: to treat corneal scars the operator was to use his fasting saliva, and after chewing salt to then spit into the affected eye. For a horse with boils, before they fill with pus the 'veterinarian' was told to seize the boil with three fingers while saying 'I defeat you.' Amulets were advocated: a whole dock plant in a cloth bag hung around the neck was a supposed cure for respiratory symptoms. Many of the remedies were harmless, but useless, folklore.

Marcus Aurelius Olympius Nemesianus (late 3rd century AD), a poet and resident of Carthage. Little of his work has survived, except for 325 lines of his hexameter verse *Cynegetica*, an incomplete didactic hunting poem written about AD 282–284. He explains the procedures of breeding, rearing and training dogs and details the advantages of having differing breeds, 'from Sparta, Molossia and Britannia, Pannonia, Spain, Libya and Tuscany'. It is obvious that Britain had replaced Gaul as a major source of hunting dogs, 'the fleetest hounds, the best in the world for the chase'. While well composed and written with much coverage of hunting methods, there is little of specific veterinary note. The poem is of interest as it is the last known work on hunting written under the empire. The theme of 'the battles of the countryside' can be traced from Xenophon, Arrian and Oppian writing in Greek, to Grattius and Nemesianus in Latin. They are the primary information sources on dogs in the ancient world. The earliest extant *Cynegetica* manuscript is dated at AD 825; it was first printed in Venice in 1534.

Apsyrtus (3–4th century AD) was a Greek Roman citizen, possibly from Prousa (south of Istanbul) or Nicomedia (ancient Greek city, which under the Roman Empire was the metropolis of Bythnia). Emperor Constantine lived there for six years prior to AD 330 when he decided on Byzantius for his new capital. The early life of Apsyrtus is not well documented, his place of origin is based on a biographical entry in the *Souda*. More recent study suggests that he was a native of Clazomenae (McCabe 2007, p. 129) and had early medical training there and possibly also in Alexandria. This is unconfirmed, as is the suggestion by Björck (1944, p. 4) that Apsyrtus should be dated as between AD 150–250, this date, however, would not fit with other authors who wrote in his time. McCabe observed that he does not have a Christian name but one found more often in mythology in the imperial period.

As a soldier he campaigned in the legions under Emperor Constantine on the River Danube, in particular in Scythia (a territory ranging over Eastern Europe and Central Asia). He met with the Sarmatians, a nomadic tribe living in the hills around the Black Sea, and studied their equine practices. He would appear to have been a senior 'veterinarian' in the imperial cavalry. In that time, he wrote a treatise, much of which is used in the *Hippiatrica* (See Chapter 5) and forms the foundation text for that compilation; it was the most extensive work on horse medicine in ancient Greek, that has survived. He was knowledgeable in the early Greek agricultural and medical authors, he utilised these and added his own views on earlier studies together with his own work and observations.

The Apsyrtus text is the most important principle source of information used in the *Hippiatrica*. While the various versions of the book vary, Apsyrtus represents about one-third of the content, and much of the quotations from other authors are based on his writings. His approach to equine veterinary practice, using both ancient tradition and his experience, with that of Theomnestus, demonstrates the advances they made. Apsyrtus wrote well in an epistolary manner, it is not known if these were genuine letters and answers, but it was a not uncommon literary practice of the time. The work is in four categories: letters on diagnosis, cause of illness and treatment;

essays on classification, mostly on serious diseases such as glanders, colic and also hoof care; formulae for medications; and finally magical cures. In differing versions of the *Hippiatrica* his quotations list 21 spells (of which nine were for glanders). He also suggests the use of amulets as a means of disease prevention. These were the practises of the time, commonly used in agriculture, with horses in particular and generally in healing.

In his writings Apsyrtus demonstrates that he was a practical healer of animals and recognised many ailments. He showed experience of management, feeding and treatment of injuries (in particular those resulting from warfare). He identifies four presentations of *malleus* – articular, moist, subcutaneous and dry, but does not list signs or symptoms for most of these. Smith (1976, p. 46), experienced in equine disease, suggested that the moist form could be glanders, the subcutaneous form farcy and the dry form anthrax. Other descriptions suggest farcy of the limbs, and strangles. The use of the word *malleus* for such a variety of problems appears confusing until one realises that the term implies that the animals had been 'knocked down' as if hit by a hammer: it was a generic term for all sudden onset or epizootic diseases.

He describes diseases of the small intestine and advocated manual removal of faeces as a routine procedure in intestinal disorders. Rupture of the intestine is described, as is ruptured kidney – both recognised to be fatal. Scabies is discussed but not mentioned as being contagious. Laminitis is termed 'barley disease', understanding the digestive origin of the problem. Eye conditions are described with treatment. Tetanus is well described with treading on a nail and puncturing the foot as a cause. Treatment was by placing the horse in a bath of hot sand, or in the dung heap. Castration is described in detail: securing the scrotum and contents, exposing the testes by incision, placing a ligature on the vascular cord, cutting through the wall dividing the two sacs and dividing the cremasteric cord by a very hot iron. The wounds were packed with wool soaked in oil and pitch and removed on the third day. The subject was fasted on the day and kept on a reduced diet for a few days.

Human medicine was used as a source for advice on healing limb fractures, below the knee were considered curable with splints and bandages for 40 days; fractures above the knee were deemed untreatable. Sections also deal with plants and poisoning, insects, reptiles and the shrew-mouse bite (possibly cases of anthrax). There are many 'cures', grouped as drenches, ointments, poultices and emollients. Apsyrtus states that he has tested each one, but writes little on signs and symptoms of disease. Bleeding was used but in moderation, generally his treatment methods avoided stress. He quotes Eumelus as well as Aristotle, Simon, Xenophon and Mago. He describes Mago as the best for diseases of cattle and their remedies.

Apsyrtus becomes significant when the history of cavalry in the Roman army is examined. For a long time, horses were not used as an effective fighting unit, while their opponents understood their use in war. In the time of Constantine, the Romans began to use their equine force effectively; this meant that veterinary knowledge and care became an essential part of the army structure. Apsyrtus is recognised as the most important and original contributor to early veterinary medicine.

Pelagonius (4th–5th century AD), Roman, possibly born in Illyria (central Balkans bordering the Adriatic Sea), wrote *Ars Veterinaria* (*The Veterinary Art*) in Latin, probably during the mid-4th century AD. Little is known of his background. He copied the letter-writing epistolary style of Apsyrtus, whom he quotes together with Columella and others. His writing is equine oriented, in particular related to racing. In Roman times this was mostly chariot racing – a particularly dangerous sport for both horse and charioteer. Injuries and hoof wear were major issues. Magic and magical practices, amulets and the binding of objects to the patient to provide protection and many questionable curative procedures are suggested. One of his treatments (cited by Smith 1976, p. 35) for 'pestilential fever' (?anthrax) was the ashes of a swan buried alive, and another for treatment of equine ophthalmia included swallows' nests. Pelagonius was a great believer in bleeding as a part of treatments.

Vegetius admired his treatise, but scholars who have examined his work state it to be of little value. The range of diagnostic features and treatments discussed are not highly regarded. It was, however, the first Latin book on horse diseases, later translated into Greek and included in the *Hippiatrica*, alongside the writings of Apsyrtus, which Pelagonius had used as his source. The work was first published in Florence from an old codex. The writings of Pelagonius have been exhaustively studied by J.N. Adams (1995). This valuable book examines the language of Latin veterinary medicine in a systematic manner. The author has sought to elucidate the anatomical and pathological terminology used in these treatises, providing a significant aid to further studies.

Hippocrates (possibly 4th century AD), Greek author of an unknown treatise, which survives only through extracts, some 120, which appear in the *Hippiatrica*. They are the only known work under this name, while it is certain this is not the great physician of the same name, it is commonly believed to be a nom de plume and no reason for the assumed anonymity is given. The author, of the Byzantine school, knew his subject, which was horses and mules, and is presumed to have practised veterinary medicine. His use of language, written in the first person, is described as 'at the lower end of the literary scale' (McCabe 2007, p. 244) this more colloquial style would indicate that it was written for the layman. The contents are similar to the other authors included in the *Hippiatrica*. While no sources are named the writing is in the Cassius Dionysius–Mago tradition, but drawn from Eumelus, Pelagonius, Apsyrtus and others. Problems related to the hoof (*podagra*), the eye and the digestive tract represent the main content. An interesting inclusion is the description of the use of ant mandibles to suture wounds and incisions. Rarely are disease causes given, bleeding is recommended and reference made to humoral theory.

A veterinary treatise attributed to *Ipocras Indicus* appeared in about the 6th century AD, translated from the Arabic to Latin it shows a relationship to Greek texts but not to the Hippocrates cited in the *Hippiatrica*. The name of a veterinary Hippocrates is found in two ancient Greek codices held in Paris (Smith 1976, p. 34). One is described as being by Sostratus and Hippocrates, the other by Osandrus and Hippocrates. Sostratus and Osandrus are not known as Byzantine writers. The name Sostratus has been given to a probably fictional brother of Hippocrates of Cos, said to be an equine healer.

Theomnestus (4th century AD) was Greek, of Roman citizenship. His background is unclear, his treatise suggests that he was from Nicopolis, but there were several towns of this name. He was based for some time at Carnuntum in Pannonia (mainly current Hungary, Austria and Croatia). Theomnestus has been variously described as a veterinarian in the army of Theodoric, King of the Ostrogoths, or Master of the Horse to the King, and as a friend of the Roman Co-Emperor Licinius: all of these statements have been questioned.

He is recognised as one of the seven Late Antique authors, based in the Mago-Greek agricultural tradition, to be quoted in the *Hippiatrica*. Theomnestus was not only a veterinarian but was a keen horseman, he wrote well and knew medical theory, possibly having had a medical education. His treatise is of particular interest because he both quotes from previous sources, in particular Apsyrtus, and cites his own experiences including two case histories, which are unique in antique veterinary literature: these confirm his career in the army. His treatise is notable compared to the others quoted in the *Hippiatrica* in that there is no mention of magic, spells or incantations. This may be due to the Edicts of Emperor Constantius II against sooth-sayers and magicians, which influenced the use of such practices. Theomnestus was obviously both a keen and active horseman, his instructions for breaking, grooming and management follow the pattern of the early writings of Simon and Xenophon in both discussing the points of the horse and selection together with emphasis on care of the foot. Much of this was written about his own horses – unlike other *Hippiatrica* authors but following Simon and Xenophon. His advice was aimed at the amateur as well as the professional horseman who rode horses and horse doctor who cared for them.

The veterinary context is well presented and lists the main disease issues and discusses glanders. He tried to define a disease and showed that he understood anatomy. The case histories are written with good descriptions. The first details a crossing of the Alps in such bad weather that the soldiers froze to death in the saddle and the horses developed 'tense' bodies which froze if they stopped moving. He termed the condition *tetanos* and obviously regarded some as tetanus and treated them accordingly; his tetanus remedy required 31 ingredients, but he added that his own horse, which was affected, recovered after being kept warm. The other case history is also drawn from this march: one of the soldiers had been giving his horse salt in large quantities at regular intervals. The symptoms are described, as well as his palliative care, which enabled the horse to recover, he wrote that the king was so pleased with the result that he rode the horse himself. Theomnestus was the fourth most frequently quoted author in the *Hippiatrica* compilation.

An additional link to the veterinary past is that although Theomnestus had written a treatise, it is only quoted in parts in the *Hippiatrica* and this in turn has come down in history in various interpretations in differing manuscripts. In the late 9th century AD a learned Arabic translation by Ibn Akhi Hizam appeared, titled *Kitab al-Baytara* (*Book of Horse Medicine*) and is attributed to Theomnestus. The work has been care-fully studied (McCabe 2007, pp. 182–191), and compared to the extracts used in the several *Hippiatrica* recensions. It is not known if this is a translation of the original treatise, or a carefully created compilation of the extracts and fragments of quota-tions used elsewhere. It does, however, provide documentary evidence of the influ-ence that the Greek authors had on the development of Arab veterinary medicine.

Chiron (c.4th century AD) was the supposed author of a Latin work, *Mulomedicina Chironis*, believed to have been written about AD 350–400. Its origin and authorship has been the subject of much controversy. The author may have been known as Hierocles or Hemerius, or the name was used to cover the work of several authors; it has one mention in the *Hippiatrica*. The text includes references to work by Apsyrtus, Polycletus, Farnax, Sotio and Hemerius. The original manuscript, which is long lost (but known to have existed because Vegetius quotes it extensively), was found as a 15th-century AD copy. This was discovered in 1885 in the collection of the Royal Bavarian Academy of Science: MS. 243.

Written in 'rustic' Latin with what has been described as a coarse use of language, it now only exists as a corrupt version, but is of value in describing the state of Roman knowledge in the 4th century. The text is essentially a compilation with Apsyrtus extensively quoted, and recognised as 'the master' of veterinary medicine. Study of the quoted extracts suggest (McCabe 2007, p. 11) that it may have its origins in a much earlier Greek work on equine medicine which had originally used the centaurs' name. It also shows that a Latin translation of the Apsyrtus work was made before the *Mulomedicina* compilation.

In ten books, based on body systems, there is a detailed description of procedures and diagnostic methods, with the usual confusion seen by the widespread use of the word *malleus* to indicate more than one disease. A range of curative treatments is also presented. There is emphasis on advising prophylactic and preventive measures including isolation, fumigation and the burial of dead stock. Book 1 opens with a detailed description of bleeding (*depletura*), described as the treatment of choice as it is the most powerful procedure the veterinarian has available. The reasoning is that indigestible foods produce corruption in the blood (which has to be removed with fasting or a controlled diet at the same time). Bleeding is recommended as a seasonal procedure in the spring, to remove polluted blood that has accumulated during the winter. The procedure is explained in detail as well as explaining the use of the *sagitta*, a phlebotomy instrument. Book 2 is a compilation of extracts from Apsyrtus, Sotio and Farnax. Chiron's chapters follow the pattern of Emperor Diocletian's Edict of about AD 302 in which, as a part of measures to control inflation he lays down price controls on a whole variety of goods and services, including certain veterinary procedures (Walker 1991, p. 20). Book 3 covers fevers and the differential diagnosis of different types of colic by rectal examination. There is also a most detailed section on *Purgio capitis*: the head is regarded as being of the greatest importance and it is discussed in relationship to rabies, heart pain, frenzy, turning in circles and tumours. A most complex procedure is described, involving bleeding the patients, medication with herbs and oils (to purge) and the application of mustard poultices and cauteries to the head. The procedure is named in Diocletian's Edict. Book 5 includes a detailed description of rectal prolapse and its treatment by submucosal resection; a procedure that then became unknown for centuries. The treatment of uterine prolapse in the mare using an inflated bladder to aid recovery is also described. Book 7 is devoted to castration of the horse.

This rather puzzling treatise is worthy of more attention. It has been noted that while its teaching falls short of that of Apsyrtus it is an advanced veterinary text for its time. The references to Polycletus, Farnax and Sotio are three authors whose names are not known elsewhere. The work was used as a primary source by Vegetius.

Publius Vegetius Renatus (AD c.450–500), commonly Vegetius, was a Roman, believed to have lived in the reign of Emperor Valentinian. A book, *Epitoma rei Militaris* on military matters by Flavius Vegetius Renatus is believed to be by the same person. Vegetius was a man of letters and wrote in excellent Latin, he had travelled widely, almost certainly as a soldier in the imperial service. He was typical of the class of well-educated Romans, in several places while quoting other authors he is critical of their use of Latin. As the mule and horse were essential animals to the Roman army it would be natural for a military author to have an active interest in the maintenance of equid health and operational capacity. Vegetius was fond of animals, in particular horses, was interested in veterinary science and wanted to see its status raised in Italy to that it held in Greece. The writings of Vegetius were lost following the decline of the Roman Empire, until in 1528 a copy was discovered in Hungary by a Count Nuenare. He had a rather poor translation made, dedicated to King Ferdinand of Hungary and Bohemia, and published in Basel in 1528. Since that time many editions have appeared in German, French, Italian and English. This has given rise to some confusion: the short Latin title was *Artis Veterinariae, Sive Mulomedicinae,* with the translation of the full title reading, *Books of the Veterinary Art, or Digests of the Art of Curing the Diseases of Mules.* Each translator appears to have given their own version of title and content. The original Latin title was correct: Vegetius was presenting a compilation of knowledge mostly related to mules, these were the valuable animals (more costly than horses) widely used in the Roman army.

Later J.M. Gesner made an accurate translation, said to be assisted by Morgagni the famous anatomist, published in 1735: his title (in Latin) was *Four Books of the Veterinary Art, or Art of Curing the Diseases of Mules.* An English translation was titled, *Of the DISTEMPERS OF HORSES and of the ART OF CURING them as also of the Diseases of OXEN and of the Remedies proper for them* (all capital letters as printed text). A subtitle was included, 'Of the best method to preserve them in health and restore them when sick, and to prevent the spreading and Communication of Infectious Distempers according to the Practice of the ancient Romans'.

The author of the English translation is unknown, except for the words on the title page that the person was 'the Author of the Translation of Columella'. The translator's preface includes '. . . Columella wrote of best methods of breeding and managing horses and other sorts of cattle, [and] has given an account of many of the diseases . . .', reflecting his previous translation. Printed in 1748 by A. Millar in the Strand, London, it was obviously intended to contribute to understanding the cattle plague (rinderpest) problem, 'to see if it would help to produce any answers to the cattle murrain that was sweeping the country'. This was possibly the prime reason to produce the English translation at that time.

Vegetius was an important author, he left a record of the knowledge and practice of veterinary medicine in the later Roman Empire and he expressed viewpoints, many based on his own experiences. He was concerned at the state of veterinary practice and took it upon himself to collect the opinions of authors and those who practised the veterinary art, together with human physicians. His primary objective was to produce a book that would prevent veterinary medicine falling into decay. Study of his text indicates that his primary sources were Columella, Chiron (including his Apsyrtus sections) and Pelagonius. The latter work was probably only written shortly before Vegetius; of this when commenting on the eloquence of the other authors 'Pelagonius did not have it, but Columella abounded in it.'

In his introductory words Vegetius deplores the lack of veterinary education and training in the Roman world. He states that a trained person who undertakes the medical care of animals should be regarded by the public in a similar manner as that accorded to those who practise human medicine. Vegetius was worried about the standing of veterinary practitioners, 'the Profession which undertook the curing of the Distempers of Cattle, seemed to be attended with less Honour and Dignity, therefore it has been practised by men of less Figure and Character, and they who have taught, and written of it have been men of very little eloquence'. In the practical Roman way, he sees the need for a profession that can save the army and the state, as well as agriculture, the heavy losses that were being incurred by animal disease. In a further comment, comparing those who cared for animals with a physician, he wrote 'the curing of slaves is not considered a mean or vulgar thing, and they are often sold at a lower price than horses or mules'!

Vegetius offered sound sensible advice on stock management to mitigate the effects of disease, in the Roman era outbreaks of plagues of epizootic disease were the greatest threat to the livestock industry. To paraphrase his words – whenever any infectious disease showed, there should be an immediate change of pasture and cattle should be moved to a remote place (the belief was that a change of air was of great benefit). Sick cattle should be separated from the sound and all communication be prevented between the two groups. Cattle should never be put into places where the sick had been kept, which included stables, stalls, cribs, ponds, wells and the ground on which they had laid. It was stated that dead animals should be buried deep in the ground and cattle kept away from the burial area. All very sound and reliable advice – however, he did not advise slaughtering sick animals (understanding contagion but not infection), but said that they should be kept and given medication, hoping that they would live.

The English translation is presented as four books. Book 1 deals with the signs of sickness of different diseases; the *maul* or *malleus* is said to be most dangerous, in its three manifestations – wet, dry or farciminosus (possibly glanders); other ailments discussed are scabies, possibly epizootic lymphangitis, seven types of fever, arthritis, colic, tetanus and gut helminths. All are related to equines. Procedures listed are bleeding, use of the cautery and drenches. Isolation of sick animals is emphasised. Book 2 is mostly equine and deals with diseases of the head. These are specifically discussed as vertigo, frenzy and cardiac disease including medications and surgery; also discussed are problems with the eyes, lips and teeth. Book 3 covers cattle diseases, specifically, cattle pestilences and recognising specific diseases such as rinderpest, foot-and-mouth disease, tetanus and tuberculosis. Emphasis is given to methods to prevent disease spreading. Also discussed are worms in wounds (maggots); kidneys, urine, testicles; other diseases of the horse, poisonous plants and bites from snakes, spiders, shrew-mice, scorpions and mad dogs. In Book 4 the English translation omits the first four chapters, as it was felt to be full of errors (such as stating the bovine head has only two bones), the rest discusses ageing of horses, specific drenches, medicines, ointments and malagma (a dressing to be applied for softening a hard part). The work of Gargilius Martialis is quoted. Above all Vegetius, while not able to list many cures (by today's standards), could recognise and diagnose many diseases, as listed above. He emphasised good management, feeding and care. While equines were the primary interest, cattle also feature.

The point was made that animals cannot talk, therefore the veterinary task was much harder than that of the physician. Emphasis was given to care and compassion in treatment, it was stressed that animals should be looked at every day. Among other observations, Vegetius wrote that 'frequently medicines were sold for profit and not to cure'. The book contains much sound and sensible advice. One quotation applies just as well today: 'that which contributes principally to the benefit of horses and mules (and all animals) is the Love and Diligence of their owner, or of him who has the charge of them committed to him, or even the keeper himself who feeds them'. The Vegetius text is important, not just as a book in its own right, but also because there was no significant advance in veterinary knowledge between the date of his work and its availability in print (1528) – almost 1000 years.

Hierocles (c.4th–5th century AD) was a Greek and by profession a lawyer or jurist. Very little else is known of his background, he was highly educated, wrote well and elegantly, a result of his training in professional oratory. He was obviously very fond of horses and appears to be knowledgeable in both equine care and veterinary medicine. Whether he actually practised is debatable, he uses the phrase 'our traditional art', which has led to the belief that he is writing from experience, although he does not state that.

His writings are based on those of Apsyrtus, whom he acknowledges, he also quotes from other authors, most of whose work is now lost. His treatise was in two books which others have tried to reconstruct (McCabe 2007, p. 284), the extracts included in the *Hippiatrica* have caused his name to be remembered. As a major contributor to that compilation he is also recognised as one of the seven Antique agricultural authors. He implies he was a friend of Cassianus Bassus who compiled the *Geoponika* (but this produces a confusion in dating). Hierocles' work, from the way that it is written and phrased appears to be directed more at the educated layman rather than a professional horse doctor. An extensive study has been made by McCabe (2007, pp. 208–44).

Hierocles presents the most detailed veterinary treatise after Apsyrtus. He emphasised the need for a proper diagnosis based on the signs and symptoms shown, and noted that as human doctors can ask questions veterinarians must take time and care in their examination. Like Apsyrtus he believed in manually unloading the contents of the rectum and terminal colon in treating intestinal disorders. Both the selection of horses and the need for hygiene procedures are discussed. Fever (*malis*) is a major topic being seen in four forms; the disease (recognised as glanders) is seen as the most dangerous. Emphasis is given to conditions of the eye and treatment of cysts; he was a believer in bleeding patients, differing from Apsyrtus who did not approve of heavy bleeding, in particular in weak, sick animals. The treatise includes a list of drugs used: refreshing drinks, purgatives, enemas and barley gruel were an important part of his medication advice, together with the extensive use of vinegar as a wound and skin dressing. Magic spells are also proposed. A Latin translation of Hierocles has been preserved in nine manuscripts, translated by Bartholomew of Messina for King Manfred of Sicily, in the 12th century renaissance (McCabe 2007, p. 239).

Palladius Rutilius Taurus Aemilianus (4th or 5th century AD) from the form of his name was a Roman of high standing, but otherwise little is known of him apart from his own statement that he owned farms on Sardinia and near to Rome. His treatise *Opus Agriculturae* (*The Work of Farming*) was probably written about AD 370. While the work contains little new knowledge, it is mainly a compilation of other authors observations, it is of importance because it presents a picture of agricultural practice at the end of the Western Roman Empire. It is the last of such books, in a series dating from the 2nd century BC treatise by Cato, to survive. While principally concerned with arboriculture and vineyards the whole farming sector is covered in sequence based on calendar months, including a book of veterinary medicine. This was only discovered in 1925 and is available in a new translation (Fitch 2013).

The veterinary book opens with the recommendation to care for the farm workers, feed them well, provide adequate liquid refreshment and protect them against 'creatures with spines or poison'. The organisation of the text, by species, is prefaced by a listing of the plants and fruit products in medications of various types (chemical, animal and seeds) used for livestock treatment. In general, the advice is based on Columella. While there is much common sense and good advice it also includes many practices that are unchanged from 500 years previously, in particular the utilisation of bleeding as part of treatment and the inclusion of magic spells. The work shows a stagnation and decline in veterinary practice. Cattle with 'pain in the stomach and intestines' are said to be 'calmed by the sight of a duck or swimming birds'. This treatment was said to work with even greater success with mules and horses.

Palladius' work was recognised in the 6th century AD, but then vanished until rediscovered in 1418 and used as an agricultural reference source through the Middle Ages up to the Renaissance. An English translation appeared about 1442. When printed books became available some 20 editions appeared between 1472–1543: Palladius was a major influence on European medieval agriculture.

Roman Medicine

As the Roman Empire expanded and the wealth of the ruling classes grew the interest in medicine increased. The early folklore and temple rituals were replaced by practitioners of the superior knowledge acquired from Greece. In the late Republic Greco-Roman medicine became important and the title of *medicae* was adopted. Julius Caesar recognised the value of these immigrants and granted Roman citizenship to all medical practitioners resident in Rome, as an inducement to stay and to tempt others to follow (Cruse 2004, p. 195). Caesar also granted them certain tax exemptions: medical professionals had become valued.

Roman medicine made advances, the writings of Celsus and the work by Dioscorides in creating a pharmacopoeia were important, but the over-riding influence and dominant figure was Galen. He was in Rome when it was successful, wealthy and expanding; his written works drew together the medical theories and practices of the Greek and ancient world. His medicine was based in the Hippocratic formula of preventive measures such as diet and exercise. Herbal medicine was becoming standardised, surgical expertise evolved, public health advanced hygiene with public baths, clean water supply and sewage disposal. There was, however, no formal medical education or medical profession structure. Medical individuals could be highly regarded and were used by wealthy patrons, but much family medicine was conducted at home with temple medicine still playing a significant role.

Following Galen's death there began a long decline in Roman medical science; it was part of the decline of the empire, which was reflected in widespread corruption, poverty, oppression of minorities and civil strife. There was little time for rational thought with an increasing onslaught of plagues and pestilences. The doctors could not help and people turned to religion and magic. Christianity was spreading as a belief and it included a mystical element – it offered brotherhood and charity to all. The Jesus miracles were praised, bodily ills can only be cured with divine aid was the message. Medications were rejected in favour of holy oil, prayers and the laying on of hands. The Christian religion built on this and grew, they did shelter the sick, which eventually lead to hospitals, but the church viewed the care of the sick as a moral obligation incumbent on its members – not doctors, and so superstition grew (Margotta 1996, p. 44).

Roman Veterinary Medicine

Veterinary medicine in the Roman world was not treated as a sister vocation to human practice. Those working in the veterinary field were frequently regarded as of a low status. The most important early contributors to veterinary knowledge were Varro, Columella and Chiron, with their basic knowledge, as in human medicine, derived from the Greek. They were followed by the most important book on Roman veterinary practice, written by Vegetius. His book was a good distillation of veterinary knowledge in the later Roman Empire and a statement on the poor state of their veterinary medicine – no clearly defined 'professionals' and the treatment of the subject as being inferior to human medicine. Those who practised it were seen as low status, and in Roman society this was important.

There is considerable confusion over the names used to describe those who undertook veterinary work. In surviving literature, the earliest mention is in the Varro treatise where he recognises a *medicus* to be called in when an intelligent herdsman was unable to deal with a problem. Varro also noted that the knowledge was derived from a Mago-Greek source, and it was known that the Greeks also had recognised individuals as horse doctors, which in Latin became *equarius medicus*. Both Columella and the Latin translation of Chiron use the term *veterinarii* but Vegetius refers to such individuals as *mulomedicus*. This latter term is also used in the Diocletian *Edict* and also in the Theodosian *Code*. Vegetius was referring to private individuals as was Diocletian but Theodosius refers to *mulomedici* who were hereditary public slaves. The term *veterinarius* was a recognised title in the military, particularly used with the *immunes* (those soldiers with identified skills who were exempted from general duties).

Walker (2013, pp. 304, 313–314) has identified the veterinary titles that have appeared in eight known inscriptions – *mulomedicus* (3), *medicus veterinarius* (2), *medicus iuementarius* (1), *medicus pecuarius* (1) and *medicus equarius et venator* (1). He also points out that the word *veterinarium*, translated as 'veterinary hospital' is probably incorrect and that it actually refers to the picket lines of the many baggage animals or *veterinae*, which were located in the centre of the Roman camp, to avoid pandemonium in the event of an attack. This wide range of titles indicates the lack of any clear definition of the veterinary specialist in Roman society and would reflect the poor state of veterinary medicine. Individuals would have had a place and status in the military, but in the wider world had to depend on personal expertise and reputation.

The demands for veterinary practice were based in the extensive animal related interests of the Roman economy in separate distinct categories.

Equine

Equine work was the best developed and most highly regarded: mules were essential to the army for the baggage train and all manner of haulage work, horses were initially status symbols and subject to great care. Breeding was well developed and horses were sent to Rome from all parts of the empire. In the later empire the horse cult was important, epitomised by Emperor Caligula (AD 37–41) with his favourite horse Icinatus, to which he erected a temple and planned to elevate him to rank of consul, but his death supervened. Nero (AD 54–58) not only robed his racehorses in extravagant togas, but appointed his favourites to high posts and paid them high salaries. Hadrian (AD 117–138), an enthusiastic hunter, erected a magnificent tomb for his horse Boristhenes, and Commodus (AD 180–192) had the hoofs of his horse Pertinax, gilded. Such exaggerated worship of horses was also seen later in Arab behaviour (Karasszon 1988, p. 105).

Livestock

Livestock veterinary work was mostly undertaken by the farmers. The big landed estates were the primary producers of livestock and had herdsmen (usually slaves) who had competence in dealing with most ailments, if there was a particular problem a veterinary specialist could be called upon. The level of on-farm practice was probably adequate for many procedures. An interesting light on such practice is seen in *The Golden Ass*, the only Latin novel to have survived in its entirety, written by Lucius Apuleius Madaurensis (AD 125–170), it is an irreverent and amusing story of a man transformed into a donkey, for his misdemeanours. He was threatened with castration, and then heard a neighbouring farmer say 'and then home to fetch my gelding irons . . . I undertake to return him to you as gentle a beast as any wether in my flock' (Graves 1950, p. 179). That such surgery was commonplace indicates the level of knowledge, and ability of an ordinary, average farmer.

Even with the advances that had been made, the lack of basic knowledge of the aetiology of disease and of the mechanism of medications led to problems in diagnosis and treatment: there were many erroneous concepts related to farm livestock health and disease. In this environment, as advances slowed, fallacious doctrines were accepted, together with an increasing reliance on spells and incantations.

Army Veterinary Service

An army veterinary service must have existed, but there is little information available. With such a dependence on mules for transport, horses for officers and the cavalry there was an obvious need. Both Apsyrtus and Theomnestus were in military service, while neither described the rank they held, from the context it would appear to have been quite senior. Walker (1991, p. 332) cites an inscription to one Gaius Anfidius, described as a *hippiatros* (horse doctor) who served in Egypt as a military veterinarian. As noted the interpretation of the word *veterinarium* is probably more accurately read as the park for the pack animals (*veterinae*). Presumably this was the place where the *veterinarii* were located: these people were classified as *immune*. Exactly how these were ranked related to the *mulomedicus*, or perhaps the titles were interchangeable over time, remains unclear. They would have needed some facilities to undertake the care of the animals and these were presumably close to the place where the mules and horses were kept, but not as a hospital.

Government Veterinary Service

A government veterinary service was included in the imperial *cursus* system, the key link in the maintenance of the empire. The administrative centres were joined by major roads which enabled rapid movement of messages, officials and government transportation. Along these routes were sited rest houses for travellers, and care and exchange of mounts and draught animals. Included in the personnel were grooms and staff to repair vehicles, and *mulomedici* who provided veterinary care. As there could be significant numbers of equids and cattle at these relay stations health care was important. It appears that these *mulomedici* were usually trained slaves.

Roman Veterinary Practices

These are difficult to describe with accuracy, the procedures and medications are known but exactly who used them, and what their official position or status was, as already outlined, is unclear. Those providing veterinary service for the army and imperial cursus worked almost wholly with equids, plus some cattle used in transportation. On farms, and the bulk of agriculture was on large estates with veterinary work the responsibility of herdsmen. These were men of some knowledge and were stated to carry notebooks on diseases, care, and recipes for medications. Final responsibility would be with the estate owner or manager who had to ensure that the herdsman (usually a slave) was competent and who would decide if a specialist was required – indicating veterinarians in general practice, but details are few. There was no formalised veterinary education, and probably recognition for their expertise only in a limited area or region.

In all texts dating back to Varro and Columella certain basic principles were advocated: hygiene, cleanliness, good housing, well cared for flooring, fresh water, quality feed, careful attention to all stock, every day checking and isolation of sick animals. Breeding was seen to be of fundamental importance (in particular for horses), together with good husbandry. The basic precept was – attend to health to avoid sickness. Roman authors were always conscious of the need for good animal welfare, it is not known how many Roman farmers really adhered to this advice, which is just as sound today.

Equine Medicine

Equine medicine was not only the best developed practice but was clearly defined by the Diocletion Edict listing the five major procedures:

- *Depletura* (bleeding) – the most common, to remove corrupted blood due to indigestion and tiredness, based on the humoral balance and well described by Vegetius.
- *Purgationes capitis* (purging the head) – the head was seen as the centre of sight, hearing, taste and smell ability, and therefore controlled the whole body. Mostly treated by bleeding from specified sites to remove corrupted blood from around the brain. An important procedure, defined by Chiron.
- *Purgationes* (general purging) – bleeding from specific sites to remove corrupted blood, in particular, from the brain. Great care was emphasised, at the same time oral purging medications were used to remove undigested food.
- *Tonsurae* (clipping) – the procedure to keep the horse 'looking good' was regarded as being important for both the horse and the rider. This was obviously intended for riding horses, which were the most valuable and socially well regarded animals. Several fashions were described.
- *Aptaturae pedis* (foot care) – the advice was to always check hoofs after work, keep clean, trimming was important. Many hoof salves were recommended (incorporating tar, fat, oils). The use of the *soleae ferreae*, hipposandals, as a means to protect a dressing on the foot, was obviously quite widespread; a modified form was also used for cattle (Walker 2013, p. 324).

Bovine Medicine

The basic rules for breeding cattle and rearing calves were identified by Varro and Columella. The emphasis was on draught animals, there was little bovine milk production on an agricultural basis. Castration was undertaken by the herdsmen. While mature cattle were slaughtered as a food item it was of minor importance, but veal was commonly eaten and often formed a part of the soldiers' diet; other stock would be specifically fed and raised for sale for sacrifice.

The majority of medications proposed for cattle ailments were derived from the initial writings of Columella, who acknowledged a debt to the Greek and Mago treatises. Walker (2013, pp. 326–327) studied the available cattle disease treatment literature from the Egyptian c.1900 BC Flinders Petrie papyrus and has traced a theme suggesting that little new knowledge was accumulated over the centuries, but also emphasised the good early powers of observation. The major diseases discussed by Columella are difficult to interpret, the epizootic plagues were termed varieties of *malleus* and obviously included rinderpest, bovine pleuro-pneumonia and foot-and-mouth disease. The medications were applied to treat symptoms, not causes; the formulae were mainly herb or plant based (some would have had activity, based on modern knowledge of active principles).

Draught oxen, whose main uses were for transport and ploughing, received particular care because of their value to the farm. Apart from fractures the main problems were injuries to the feet and bruising, and oedema following faulty neck yokes or accidents. Rest was seen as important; many accidents arose because the oxen were over-worked and tired. Foot injuries were treated with dressings of oils, grease and pitch, frequently with a covering of wool and the use of the *soleae ferreae* (the iron hipposandal). This allowed the whole foot or one hoof to be protected while the wound, or incision to drain pus, commenced healing. A foot boot made from plaited straw or basket work is also mentioned. Columella advised that cattle, sheep and goats with similar ailments should all be treated using the same procedures and with similar medications.

Ovine and Caprine Medicine

Emphasis was given to breeding and using sound stock. Sheep, and ewes in particular, were considered animals that needed particular care in management and required constant surveillance. Embryotomy, following the Greek procedure to remove a retained foetus to save the ewe's life was employed. The knife was very similar to those used in current practice. The main cause of sheep ailments was considered to be the weather – either bright sunshine or cold winters. The methods described to control diseases now termed pulpy kidney and braxy, show they knew how to control the problem without understanding the cause. The main sheep crop was wool, and skin diseases were well recognised; plant-based medications were used that would have had some anti-parasitic effect. Foot rot was described, as were disease symptoms that would indicate that infestations with liver fluke and gut helminths were common. It was, however, stressed that good husbandry, hygiene, nutrition and management would keep a flock healthy and resistant to severe disease problems – except for epizootic plagues, where it was advised to immediately split the flock into isolated groups.

Porcine Medicine

Swine were popular as a meat source (sucking pigs and porkers) and also as a fat source, used for many applications. The description of diseases by Columella is confused but foot-and-mouth disease and anthrax can be recognised. Several skin problems were seen. Bleeding was a frequent first treatment and various herbal medications were used. It was recommended that if disease appears in a group of pigs the best solution was to slaughter and butcher them all for sale. The human health hazard would have been significant.

Canine Medicine

Dogs were particularly important for hunting, the literature emphasises their role in a sport that was considered to be a manly art, and an important part of an educated Roman's life. As with other species much stress was placed on the selection of breed and their breeding and rearing. All sources indicated that weak puppies should be destroyed, and careful attention paid to their nutrition. Meat, bones and barley bread were the main components of the diet. Guard dogs in training were never allowed to eat the meat of the stock or flock they were to guard. Of the early authors Varro appears to have been the most welfare aware, for both the bitch and her puppies. He also recommended that one should not purchase a sheep dog from a butcher as it would be found to be lazy and have a liking for fresh meat, he was always practical.

Diseases of dogs were not well categorised. Skin problems, mange, fleas and ticks were all known and recognition was given to the anti-parasitic activity of sulphur. Several varieties of foot disease (*podagra*) are noted; rabies (*lyssa*) and its transmission risk was known but some symptoms listed indicate a confusion with canine distemper. More common ailments such as coughs, diarrhoea, constipation and so on, would appear to have been treated with the same medications used for livestock.

Avian Medicine

As the Roman world matured, poultry of all types – chickens, ducks, geese, guinea fowl, pigeons and a variety of wild birds were all intensively reared for both meat and egg production. The methods were well described by Columella. Diseases were recognised, in particular a syndrome of oral/nasal/ocular signs termed 'pip': a word that probably covered several ailments. Plant-based medications were used, ectoparasites were obviously a problem but overall the systems appear to have been profitable and not greatly influenced by disease. Emphasis was given to good husbandry, hygiene, cleanliness and fresh water and feed supply. The availability of slave labour would have enabled an adequate labour force.

Castration appears to have been the major surgical intervention, and was utilised for horses, cattle, pigs, sheep and poultry. Applied to such a variety of species must have created a significant level of expertise. The importance of this procedure is demonstrated by the carving of gelding irons seen on the gravestones of some horse doctors. As identified in the review of Roman veterinary authors work, the methods of treatment for fractures and accidental injuries followed those used in human practice.

The Story of Roman Veterinary Medicine Ends

Veterinary practice in the Roman world was defined by two factors – first, the original knowledge, cited by Varro and expanded by Columella, derived from Greek and Carthaginian sources. Second, the veterinary vocation had a low status. As the empire grew in size and power it became status conscious: the medical man was well regarded, but not his veterinary counterpart. There was no formal training and the people employed in veterinary medicine had a variety of titles.

Roman veterinary knowledge is found in four Latin works, the *Mulomedicina Chironis*, and those by *Pelagonius*, *Vegetius* and *Palladius*: these are all essentially compilations. The most significant book was that by Vegetius, much based on the Chiron book, which in turn utilised the Apsyrtus knowledge. There is little information that describes the everyday work of practice and in particular the surgical techniques used. There are indications that veterinary surgery had reached a significant level of proficiency, Walker (2013, p. 332) has discussed this. The advance of medicine, both human and animal, in the later years was slowed because time was taken up with intricate and involved theories of medicine, and in particular the doctrine of *Methodos* (methodism) which tried to explain the symptoms of a disease by concepts that were based in an ignorance of the structures and working of the body. Such debate, while of a philosophical interest, did little to progress medicine. The veterinary art in the Roman world could have developed towards becoming a science, but it stagnated, unlike the developments in the Greek-speaking eastern half of the empire. The hallmark of Roman veterinary medicine was the concentration given to examination of the patient to produce an analysis of the visible signs of illness. The procedures and medications used for treatment were consistent with the knowledge of the time. The measures used to combat the animal plagues were more thoroughly grounded with a more efficient approach than those used in contemporary human medicine (Bodson 2003, pp. 1592–1593).

Those who led the veterinary fraternity expressed genuine concern about welfare and expressed a sympathy for the animals in their care; it also has to be remembered that there were shocking examples of cruelty accepted in the believed interests of efficiency or disease prevention. While overall it was recognised that good welfare and care contributed to a profitable business the Romans were above all pragmatic as far as livestock were concerned. They did, however, demonstrate an affectionate, frequently excessive, relationship to certain individual horses and dogs.

The Roman Empire became too large and extensive to administer efficiently. Diocletion tried to bring a measure of control by dividing the empire into four regions, each with its own emperor (the Tetrachy) about AD 293. After more problems and internal strife Theodosius (the last emperor to rule the whole empire) divided it into Western and Eastern Empires in AD 395. The Western Empire was unable to control the internal problems and halt the invaders, it succumbed in AD 476 and finally ended in AD 493. Initially the new rulers tried to preserve many of the features of Roman life, but gradually these disappeared. The story of veterinary medicine now moves to the East in what was to become the Byzantine Empire, but claiming the continuity of its Roman origins.

References

Adams, J.N. (1995) *Pelagonius and Latin Veterinary Terminology in the Roman Empire.* Leiden: Brill

Björck, G. (1944) Apsyrtus, Julius Africanus, et l'hippiatrique grecque. *Uppsala Universitets Arsskrift* **4**

Bodson, L. (2003) *The Oxford Classical Dictionary* (Ed. Hornblower, S. and Spawforth, A.). Oxford: Oxford University Press

Boyd Ash, H. (1941) *Columella on Agriculture: I-IV.* Cambridge, MA: Harvard University Press

Cruse, A. (2004) *Roman Medicine.* Stroud: Tempus

Fitch, J.G. (2013) *Palladius: The Work of Farming.* Totnes: Prospect

Graves, R. (1950) *Apuleius: The Golden Ass.* London: Penguin

Johnston, I. and Horsley, G.H.R. (2011) *Galen: Method of Medicine*, Books 1–4 Loeb Classical Library 516. Cambridge, MA :Harvard University Press

Karasszon, D. (1988) *A Concise History of Veterinary Medicine.* Budapest: Akadémiai Kiadó

Margotta, R. (1996) *History of Medicine.* London: Hamlyn

Mattern, S.P. (2013) *The Prince of Medicine: Galen in the Roman Empire.* Oxford: Oxford University Press

McCabe, A. (2007) *A Byzantine Encyclopaedia of Horse Medicine* Oxford: Oxford University Press

Merlen, R.H.A. (1971) *De Canibus: Dog and Hound in Antiquity* London: J.A. Allen

Phillips, A.A., Willcock, M.M. (1999) *Xenophon and Arrian on Hunting with Hounds* Warminster: Aris and Phillips

Singer, C. (1956) *Galen on Anatomical Procedures* Oxford: Oxford University Press

Smith, F. (1976) *The Early History of Veterinary Literature.* London: Allen

Sournia, J.-C. (1992) *The Illustrated History of Medicine.* London: Starke

Walker, R.E. (1991) *Ars Veterinaria.* Kenilworth: Schering-Plough

Walker, R.E. (2013) Appendix Roman Veterinary Medicine, in (Ed.) Toynbee, J.M.C *Animals in Roman Life and Art.* Barnsley: Pen & Sword Books

CHAPTER 5

The Eastern Roman Empire (Byzantine)

Byzas, ruler of the Greek city of Megara, in about 660 BC, established a colonia on a triangular peninsular on the west (European) side of the Bosphorus. It was a key trade position on the maritime route between the Black and the Aegean seas, and controlled a land route between Europe and Asia. With the sea on three sides it was easily defended and the Golden Horn Bay on the north side provided a natural harbour. The settlement grew and prospered by farming the fertile Thracian hinterland, to become a large grain producer, and the surrounding seas yield good fish harvests. The local Bythnians were reduced to Byzantine serfs.

Over the centuries the town was a target of seizure by the Persians and by Greek groups. When the Romans appeared in the 2nd century BC the Byzantines sided with them, until civil disputes disrupted the alliance. The civil unrest was put down by Septimus Severus in AD 196 who partly destroyed the walls and old town before building a circus, hippodrome and kynegesion (hunting theatre) and other structures. In 324 Constantine defeated his rival Licinius and with his new-found Christian belief began to restructure the Roman Empire. He refounded Byzantium as a new city.

Constantinople Founded

Constantine wanted a city that would demonstrate his imperial power. The buildings were sited partly around the Severan forum and his new palace was attached to the circus with his imperial box. He built the Church of the Holy Wisdom (which later became the site for the Hagia Sophia) and embellished the city with art from both Rome and gifted from all around the empire. It is not clear if he had intended the city to be the Christian capital of Europe, Constantine clearly saw the city as a celebration of himself, rather than as a rival to Rome: it was dedicated in 330 and renamed Constantinople. Constantius II succeeded his father in 337 and in 340 created a senate in Constantinople on an equal footing to that in Rome. In the 4th century the Roman Empire was becoming ungovernable and suffered from civil strife, corruption and barbarian invasions: various subdivisions were attempted (the Tetrarchy) until Theodosius redivided the empire into East and West in 395.

The Eastern Roman Empire Established

The Latin west gradually lost contact with the Greek east. Then in 410 Rome fell. The Western Empire, then based in Ravenna, ended in 476 when Odovacar deposed Romulus Augustus, the last western emperor, and was elected King of the Germanic tribes that had invaded Italy. In 493 Theodoric, a Goth, overthrew Odovacar, established the Ostrogoths and was recognised by the Byzantine emperor, who gave him official status. Theodoric adopted Roman ways and his regime mimicked Roman practices. Over a long period, the West slowly restructured under local rulers in Britain, France, Spain, North Africa and in Germanic and Slav regions. The Roman concept of empire was durable and in many areas of Europe there was little change, life carried on as before.

The Eastern Empire was to survive for a further 1000 years, during which time it was almost continually at war with invaders on the outside, and struggled with civil strife and religious controversies from within. However, the city itself grew, mainly due to the efforts of Theodosius II (r.408–450) who built the massive protective walls, and Justinian (r.527–565), responsible for the Church of Hagia Sophia and many other buildings.

A further threat developed in the Arab world, invigorated by the Islamic religion; Arabic peoples swept across North Africa, into Europe, across Anatolia and attacked Constantinople in 693. Finally, the empire was reduced to Greece and part of Asia Minor, with mercenary armies, little wealth and no orderly succession of emperors – they simply deposed each other. From the 5th century Christianity was the only unifying force, but itself was split by heresies and schisms. In 1054 the Eastern Church broke with Rome to become the Greek Orthodox Church: the two parts of empire were finally separated.

Byzantine Medicine and Culture

While Byzantium failed in many respects it had a brilliant culture – it was the centre of eastern Mediterranean trade and had access to the riches of Asia. Its architects, artists and monks were highly regarded and travelled to the West to both work and educate. Constantinople became the depository of ancient knowledge. There were some original medical contributions, but it acted mostly as repository of previously existing knowledge (Sournia 1992, pp. 98–99).

Medicine continued to be practised across the empire after the fall of Rome. Doctors and veterinarians continued to practise in the West, but the professions began to falter. Plagues and epidemics ravaged Europe: there were many undiagnosed diseases described as 'plague', but they all had a common factor of a high death rate. Medical progress stalled, and when doctors were unable to help, the people turned to magic, incantations, temple sacrifices and increasingly to the church. All they could offer was prayers and sympathy, but it was a helping hand. Gradually, over quite a long period, pilgrim rest houses became hospices and laid the ground for hospitals.

There is no reliable evidence of how veterinary practice fared, but in the worsening situation of epizootic diseases and a growing belief in the power of both 'magic' and the church, it also declined.

In the East, medicine did not collapse in the same way, there was still a flow of medical and veterinary literature in letters, almanacs and treatises, and several notable medical authors are recognised. These authors both mentioned and fostered the traditional ancient writers. The words of Hippocrates, Dioscorides and Galen lived on in the works of Orbasius (325–403), Paulus of Aegina (died c.690), Alexander of Tralles (6th century) and others. The Byzantine world grew in cultural superiority while Western Europe sank into intellectual obscurity.

Orbasius of Pergamum was a tutor to the Emperor Julian (r.331–336). He later joined the imperial court and started on a monumental medical encyclopaedia in 70 volumes. The work was more Hellenic than Galenic and included works by Archimedes, Dioscorides and Antyllus (a surgeon of the 3rd century). The final encyclopaedia, only parts of which have survived, was written on a scale greater than the Corpus Hippocraticum and Galen's treatises. He did not produce just a simple compilation of earlier authors, but commented on their work and demonstrated how Byzantine medicine had turned away from all the disputing medical schools, which had become a feature of Roman medicine (Sournia 1992, pp. 100–101).

Alexander of Tralles (c.526–c.605) travelled widely, then settled in Constantinople, and later died in Rome. He is remembered as one of the leading ancient physicians and his writing is recognised as being very original, he was not a compiler. His main work was titled *Twelve Books of Medicine*, this was well regarded as he attempted to describe all known diseases, and catalogue them. Based on his personal experience he also stressed the importance of examining patients and making a diagnosis, but he also recommended the use of charms and amulets. His only other extant work is *De Lumbricis* (*On Worms*), now seen as the first parasitology treatise.

The influence of the church, a major force in the Byzantine culture, initially did not appear to affect the work of medicine. Cosmas and Daimian, martyred under Diocletian, had become the patron saints of surgeons. Society was becoming Christianised and the churches created valetudinaria, a similar concept to the hospice; gradually almost all monasteries and convents created 'hospitals'. The church then began to play an increasingly significant role in medical life and in treatment, supported by their teaching, such as Jesus healing the blind man and the raising of Lazarus. People turned away from those still active Hellenic *asclepeions*, looking instead to the church to keep themselves healthy. However, the civil authorities were well aware of potential human disease issues and sound public health measures were introduced, based in hygiene and clean water.

Human medicine gradually declined as the most knowledgeable men, aware of the constant pressure from the Turks and other invaders, emigrated to the West with their books and the didactic treatises of Hippocrates, Dioscorides, Oribasius and Paul of Aegina, these formed the basis of medical education in Europe. Following the fall of the city in 1453, the manuscripts were taken by the Islamic conquerors and translated into Arabic making a fundamental contribution to the development of their medical and veterinary sciences.

Byzantine Veterinary Medicine

The value of veterinary medicine was always better appreciated in the Eastern Roman Empire, it followed from the recognition of the *hippiatroi* (horse doctors) and because of the traditional Hellenic skills in agriculture (linked to the writings of Mago). Following the break with Rome the importance of cavalry became emphasised. The equine fighting tactics of the invading tribes of Avars, Slavs and Persians were copied and the Roman cavalry was reorganised on the models of the Avars and Turkish invaders. A strong cavalry needed good veterinary support; this allowed for original thought and expertise to be transmitted among the military.

Agriculture was well developed and important to Byzantium, as there was less cultivable land than in the West. Horse breeding became a major enterprise, not just for the military, but to support the, also essential, sport of chariot racing to entertain the public. The popularity of the sport was such that when two conflicting political factions developed in the city they took their names, the Blues and the Greens, from two of the four colours worn by the charioteers. Clashes eventually led to a civil war with significant loss of life.

For veterinary medicine the great importance of the Byzantine period was that Constantinople became the depositary and guardian of the intellectual activity of ancient Greece and Rome, it became the trustee of the best knowledge. Later between the 12th to 15th centuries this knowledge passed into the West, assisting the growth of the Renaissance.

There was considerable literary activity in the 4th and 5th centuries, as seen by the work of Apsyrtus, Hippocrates, Theomnestus and Hierocles, all written in Greek (the work of these authors is discussed in the Introduction). Following this period there appears to have been a gradual decline, or any work that was written has not survived.

In the 10th century, under the influence of Emperor Constantine VII (913–959) who had the designation Porphyrogenitus (born in the purple), there was a revival in interest in Greek science. Constantine, who was well read and both an author and scholar, created a learned circle for the writing of history. He encouraged activity in literature and the arts, a revival which lapsed on his death. Two of the sciences in which he was interested were the veterinary art and agriculture, and he employed authors to collect every fragment of information that had been written on these subjects and to compile them as treatises. As the original writers had been dead for some 400 years it follows that much information must have been lost. Constantine realised that if action was not taken quickly much more would vanish. The texts and fragments in both Greek and Latin were collected and arranged under the names *Hippiatrica* (veterinary) and *Geoponika* (agricultural). Both were remarkable works, saving the knowledge of the later Roman Empire. Vegetius had described the state of the art in the Western Empire and the *Hippiatrica* achieves the same for the later Eastern. Note that *Hippiatrica* is usually spelt in Latin translation, but *Geoponika* in the Greek form.

The *Hippiatrica*

A difficulty in both translation and interpretation of the *Hippiatrica* content is that since the final compilation in Byzantium there has been much copying and revision. This has resulted in five recensions (or revisions), now held as 22 manuscripts (25 copies in all) dating from the 10th to the 16th century (McCabe 2007). The term *Corpus Hippiatricum Graecorum* is also used, this refers to the group of translations and copies that have been found. Recent studies indicate that the 10th-century work is possibly an update of a previous compilation from the 5th/6th centuries, no longer extant, rather than a first attempt to gather together information that would otherwise be lost.

The history of the travels of the original Greek manuscript(s) from Byzantium is complex and in detail poorly understood. Two main channels developed. As the Eastern Empire declined and collapsed, many documents were taken to Western Europe, mostly deposited in monasteries, as the then chief centres of learning. Those remaining in Byzantium were taken by the Turkish conquerors and translated to Arabic (some by way of Syriac translators). Many of these Arabic translations survived and in the later Middle Ages were translated back into Latin. It is unavoidable that with changes in both language and script, and with double translation, various forms of corruption have crept in over the years – parts lost, no longer understandable, deleted or added to. Recently these have been the subject of significant scholarly research which has provided much clarification of the texts and the authorship, but there is still much that needs further exploration.

Attention to the existence of the work now known as the *Hippiatrica* was due to the French king Francis I (1494–1547). He was an avid patron of the arts (he persuaded Leonardo da Vinci to move to France, bringing the *Mona Lisa* painting with him). Francis started the standardisation of the French language, worked to improve the royal library and had agents looking for rare manuscripts: among these were the Byzantine texts on equine medicine. His advisors suggested that a translation would aid the lack of veterinary knowledge in France and also help improve the French cavalry. Jean de la Ruellius was appointed as the translator. He was a learned man in both Latin and Greek, had studied medicine and had already translated the work of many ancient medical authors including Hippocrates, Galen, Celsus and Dioscorides. He was helped in the translation by Peter Ruellius, believed to be his brother. The dedication to the king is dated 1528 and publication was in 1530. A Greek version by Simon Grynaeus of a similar, but not identical text, was published in Basel in 1537.

What is both interesting and frustrating is that neither Ruellius nor Grynaeus reveal the identity of the manuscripts that they were working from. While scholars of the classics have preferred the Grynaeus translation, it is the Ruellius version that has been preferred for its veterinary content. A third version, in French, was produced by Dr J. Massé in 1563 under the (translated) title of *Veterinary Art* or the *Grand Marshal*: Massé recorded that he had used both Latin and Greek sources. There were also three translations published in Italy in 1543, 1548 and 1559.

The valuable and scholarly book by Anne McCabe (2007), based on one of the 22 known manuscripts, has provided an excellent exposition of the work. The manuscript chosen is held in France and is known as the 'M recension: Parisinus gr. 2322', dated to the 10th century. The M recension is written on a fine parchment in a plain hand. After passing through many hands it was acquired in 1603 for the Royal French Collection under Henri IV. It is believed that Ruellius used Parisinus gr. 2245, dated to the late 15th century; this is in the B recension, one of the three recensions that represent the complete compilation, or encyclopaedia. The other principal manuscript is the D recension, with the RV and E manuscript copies making the five principal versions.

There is no simple or single discussion about the contents of the *Hippiatrica*. No copies of the manuscripts agree, probably due to the multitude of copiers and scribes who worked on the compilations in Greek and Arabic/Syriac. The contents of the texts are essentially a record of veterinary medicine in Byzantium. It is full of cures, which dominate, and descriptions of symptoms and diagnostic conclusions. The manuscripts include many names, some 150 are mentioned, but most do not feature as quoted authors.

The main authors and the number of excerpts of their writings which are used are listed in the following table (based on McCabe). While there are some 1223 excerpts of the original writings included in the M recension compilation, the number and length of those included have a great variation. The two best explored versions of the book show, in the table, a wide difference in selections. Such variations exist between all the recensions making it somewhat difficult to understand the content. It depends on which copy you read.

It is not the number of excerpts that count but the total volume of text: Apsyrtus holds by far the largest amount of content, with Hierocles, Theomnestus and

Table 5.1

Author	McCabe (M recension) Parisinus 2322	Ruellius (acc. Massé) Parisinus 2245
Apsyrtus	372	121
Heirocles	114	107
Pelagonius	369	48
Hippocrates	124	36
Eumelus	77	31
Theomnestus	72	31
Anatolius	15	10
Tiberius	–	10
Didimus	–	5
Archedemus	–	3
Himerius	–	1
and others (1 each)	(80)	
Total	1223	Not given

Pelagonius comprising the major part of the remainder (but these are all very much based on the Apsyrtus text). The principal sources were seven Late Antique veterinary texts: the works of Eumelus, Apsyrtus, Theomnestus, Hierocles, and Hippocrates together with a Greek translation of the Pelagonius treatise and the equine chapter of the Anatolius agricultural manual (as discussed in the Introduction).

That the *Hippiatrica* manuscripts have survived at all is due to its recognition as a work of value. It has value not only in its veterinary medical content, and in particular that of Apsyrtus, but also because it preserves a record of veterinary 'science' and practice in the Byzantine Empire. Apsyrtus is notable because he had written the most extensive early Greek treatise on horse medicine, which has survived, in part, in the extracts used in the compilation.

While primarily a manual of the Greek practice in the care, management, diseases and ailments of the horse it is a vast work of reference that was originally presented (but somewhat disorganised by later copyists) as each author's discussion of a health problem and its treatment, together with a listing of the medications and recipes that were recommended. A wide range of prescriptions, massages, Roman bath treatments and the use of incantations and magic are described.

The *Hippiatrica* is particularly valuable as it presents the original author contributions in their own language, providing a unique source of information on the formative years of the specialised veterinary art, reflecting also the role of the horse, and its care, in Roman life. The compilation is remarkable both for its expression of the advanced state of Greek veterinary medicine and equine care, and following translation and publication in 1530, for its influence on veterinary knowledge and education in Western Europe at a time when there was revival in learning.

The *Geoponika*

The *Geoponika* (*Farm Work*) is a collection of agricultural texts and letters presented as a compilation, made on the instruction of the Byzantine Emperor Constantine VII Porphyrogenitus (AD 913–959). This is one of the series of anthologies, all written in Greek, that were prepared under his direction. An illuminating picture of agricultural practice through the writings of Greek and Roman authors in the late classical period, is presented. As the individual authors of the ancient texts are named, the collection is of particular value, preserving the names of many agricultural authors of antiquity. An ancestor work was a shorter compilation of agricultural knowledge made by Cassianus Bassus in the 6th century AD which has survived by being translated into Arabic.

The *Geoponika* comprises 20 books each divided into chapters, this was at the instruction of Constantine who wished the information to be presented in an orderly manner. The name of the compiler is not known. Books 1–14 are solely devoted to crops, vines and fruit (a good picture of agricultural practice); Book 15 deals with honey, bees and diseases; Book 16 horses and breeding; Book 17 cattle and breeding, Book 18 sheep and goats and breeding; Book 19 dogs, hares, deer and swine;

Book 20 fish. The veterinary content is quite minimal and based on sources cited in veterinary treatises: the aim was to acquaint the farmer with more important problems rather than to provide a medication manual. The works of some 12 veterinary and animal health care authors are quoted, including Apsyrtus, Theomnestus, Pelagonius and Xenophon.

There is much superstition and use of magic and incantations cited, together with sound advice and sensible procedures, which demonstrates the diversity of agricultural and veterinary practice at the time. While produced at the same time as the *Hippiatrica* the veterinary content is of a totally different quality, as shown by this quotation, 'All the diseases of animals are almost unknown, for how is a person to understand them, or of whom can he inform himself of the internal diseases of animals? If you pour into his nostrils powdered silphicum [possibly asafoetida] with genuine black wine, you will cure every unknown disease.' This different standard of knowledge adds credence to the belief that the *Hippiatrica* was in fact an updating of an earlier compilation work, now no longer extant.

The first full translation into Latin was published at Venice in 1538 and the first translation into English in 1804/5 (Owen). A recent translation into English (Dalby, 2011) provides a much clearer presentation of the content as well as a carefully edited, and foot-noted, text.

The *Orneosophion* and the *Hieracosophion*

Two other compilation works of interest were produced during the later Byzantine period, in the 13th century. Both were treatises on falconry but they did not appear to have been a significant influence in medieval Europe. The *Orneosophion* (*The Wisdom of Training Birds*) mostly discusses methods of training falcons. The *Hieracosophion* (*The Wisdom of Treating Falcons*) while based in hunting procedures and training also has veterinary content.

The latter book was probably prepared by Demetrios Papagomenos, court physician to Emperor Michel Palaeologus (1201–1283). The Crusader armies had attacked and occupied Constantinople in 1204 but the Byzantines regained control, under Palaeologus in 1260, in what was now only the shell of the empire. The text is said to be of interest (Karasszon 1988, p. 118) as it covers the selection, management, care and diseases of falcons. The practice of falconry had become popular with royal households and nobles across Europe. The content is discussed in Chapter 24 which covers all avian species and their diseases.

The Ottoman occupation of Constantinople in 1453 ended the Roman Empire. While Byzantium was a late flowering of, essentially Greek veterinary knowledge, it made a valuable contribution to the progression of European veterinary development towards the Renaissance.

References

Dalby, A. (2011) *Geoponika: Farm Work.* Totnes: Prospect Books

Karasszon, D. (1988) *A Concise History of Veterinary Medicine.* Budapest: Akadémiai Kiadó

McCabe, A. (2007) *A Byzantine Encyclopaedia of Horse Medicine.* Oxford: Oxford University Press

Owen, T. (1804/5) *Geoponika: Agricultural Pursuits.* Published privately in two volumes

Sournia, J.-C. (1992) *The Illustrated History of Medicine.* London: Starke

CHAPTER 6

Islamic Veterinary and Human Medicine Develops

The disintegration of the Roman Empire left Europe in a chaotic situation: the Balkans and Anatolia region remained as the Byzantine Empire while Central and Western Europe became backward and unstable. The Roman Church was growing in influence. The new cultural and political force was Arab Islamism which had conquered and stabilised most of the Middle East, North Africa and Spain. The Islamic influence in the veterinary story is important. The early Arab tribes had little veterinary knowledge, but they valued horses and held them in high esteem. When, as conquerors, they realised the value of the Greek veterinary treatises held by Byzantium and had translations made, they ensured this knowledge was never lost.

Little is recorded of Arab culture and life before the introduction of the Islamic belief. Arabia was a bleak, arid land on the edge of the Roman (Byzantine) and Sasanian (Persian) empires. It was populated by a mixture of tribal nomadic and oasis dwelling people, mostly traders or reliant on trade. There was no dominant religion and many gods, with idols, were worshipped. It had evolved as a somewhat fatalistic society with a strong belief in astrology, and astral magic played a significant role in the resolution of many problems including that of animal and human health. They were aware of other cultures. Some 6th-century Arabic manuscripts have survived, one is a translation from Latin of an agricultural treatise, but with little veterinary content: it reveals their interest in obtaining knowledge. Eight Arabic manuscripts from the 7th-century are known (Smith 1976, p. 58).

The horse was the most important animal and the Arabs developed an amazing horse cult, which became particularly important under Islam, providing the cavalry that enabled rapid conquest of other lands. The camel was also important – they bred them, used them for transport, ate them, made butter and cheese from their milk, used their hides for leather, hair for cloth, carpets and blankets. Both pigs and dogs were traditionally regarded as unclean (*kelb*), except for the greyhound, which was regarded as a noble animal, and like the horse a good friend to an Arab man. The Arab greyhound (*sloughil*) and the Persian greyhound (*saluki*) were used for hunting, they were highly esteemed – at night they were given blankets and talismans to ward off evil demons. A well-bred dog could cost as much as a good saddle camel. Equally important were falcons, used for hunting, and also symbolising wealth and power (see Chapter 24): summarised in their proverb 'A good falcon, a fast greyhound or a noble horse is more precious than twenty women.'

The Islamic Era

Early in the 7th century AD a religious movement began in Mecca when the Prophet Muhammad began to call men and women to moral reform and submission to the will of God, as expressed in the divine messages revealed to him, and later recorded in a book, the *Qur'an* or Koran. The Islamic era is dated from 622, when Muhammad had to flee Mecca to Medina, as there was initial opposition to his views. Before long he returned to Mecca with followers, termed companions, who shared his views; he cleared the city of idols and statues and Islam became the religion of the Arab peoples.

Muhammad preached a powerful message confirming the monotheistic teachings of Abraham, Moses and Jesus, the earlier prophets. This belief created in the Arab people an energy which, driven by horses, carried the new religion to the world, using the proselytising influence of the sword and spear. The advance was rapid, the first caliphs captured Syria in 637, Egypt in 639, Persia in 640 and the southern Mediterranean coastal region by 674, the same year that an Arab fleet laid an unsuccessful siege to Constantinople. Within the next 50 years, parts of northern India, central Asia and Spain were added, but incursion into Europe was stopped in 732 at Tours, France. One reason for the easy victories, achieved with such speed, appears to have been that the conquered lands were parts of other empires in decline, the local peoples were inclined to change one ruler for a new one, who might be better. During the first 250 years after Muhammad's flight from Mecca a vigorous Arab Islamic culture developed.

The Muslim Empire under the ruling Umayyad Caliphate moved the capital from Mecca to Damascus in 661. In 749 they were overthrown by the Abbasid dynasty, who moved the capital to Baghdad – and began the most glorious age in Islam's history, lasting for five centuries. By the 10th century rival caliphates were established in Spain and Egypt, but the social and cultural community survived. The Arabic language was used throughout and Jewish, Christian and other religious groups remained, as a part of the cultural advances.

Islam Discovers Science

The roots of Arab science can be traced to the Nestorian scholars. Nestorius of Antioch, Patriarch of Constantinople, provoked the anger of the church in Rome by announcing Christ's duality – separating his humanity from his divinity. This was a declared heresy and he was imprisoned, eventually dying in Upper Egypt in 451. The Syrian followers of Nestorius were exiled and found shelter in the Sasanian Empire (Persia) at the school founded by Shapor I at Jundishapur (Gundeshapur), in modern-day Iran. It became home to the Nestorians and they were able to exploit their educational and missionary strengths. As a group the theologians took artisans, physicians and scribes with them and established a flourishing medical school and hospital. This was to be an important factor in the development of Arabic medicine:

the medical advisor to the Prophet Muhammad, Al-Harith ibn Kalada, had studied at Jundishapur. This created a confidence in Greek medicine, which resulted in Muslims accepting and agreeing with the medical activities of the faithless 'scientists'.

Following their conquests, the ruling Arabs, with their all-important Islamic belief, appear to have had little problem with those of their new peoples who remained faithless, provided they paid their *jizya* tax, a poll-tax required of non-Muslims. They soon found that the Jewish communities had expertise in medicine and that some Christians understood the Greek texts, of which they were aware. The Nestorian Syrian monasteries had translated much of Greek work (medical and other texts) to Syriac and their libraries had become the depositories of the records and achievements of the Roman Empire. Both the Persians and the Arabs wanted copies. At first their interests were broad – philosophy, astronomy, mathematics, chemistry and medicine were all sought. They had no ethnic prejudice and took up education with great enthusiasm.

From the late 8th to 12th centuries in Mesopotomia, Egypt, Sicily, Spain and elsewhere Muslim scholars were active: libraries were created, books written, schools established and public lectures presented in the mosques. The translators were mostly Nestorians, whose first language was Syriac, but who could understand Greek; they were chiefly responsible for transferring this knowledge to the Arabs. The translation work was initially intensive, with the encouragement of the Abbasid Caliphate. The essential part of their work was to expand the Arabic language in both vocabulary and idiom to make it a medium in which these new concepts of science and philosophy could be expressed in a precise manner (Hourani 2010, p. 87). A major role was played by the most famous translator of the time, Hunayn ibn Ishaq (808–73), also called Johannitus, and his colleague Thabit ibn Qurra. Ibn Ishaq was also an important medical author who contributed many sensible observations, such as emphasising that medicine is divided into two parts – theoretical and practical. Virtually all of Greek culture was translated, with the most interest expressed in philosophy (Aristotle, Plato and some neoplatonic works); medicine (human and veterinary); the exact sciences (mathematics and astronomy) and occult sciences (astrology, alchemy and magic). The boundaries of science were indistinct.

Since these translations from Greek were the origin of Arabic science, it initially continued to develop following the Greek tradition. Mixed with the Greek translations were some from Persia and India, the latter providing numerals (now termed Arabic) which aided mathematical studies. While there was enthusiastic curiosity and a search for knowledge for its own sake, there was also a very practical purpose, driven by a need for medical help for both the human population and also for their much valued horses. The new medical knowledge was easily accepted by the conservative Islamic society: doctors were highly respected individuals. Baghdad, as the capital of the Abbasid Dynasty, grew to be a great cultural centre. Under the rule of al-Mansur (r.754–775) every available foreign book was translated into Arabic. Al-Mansur is of interest as he represented another strand of Arab belief – he favoured astrologers, and used them to help him choose the site for Baghdad (Maxwell-Stuart 2010, p. 87).

Al-Mansur was a leader in creating the Islamic intellectual tradition. It was recorded that he had a chronic indigestion problem, which was only cured after he was treated by Gurgis ibn Buhtisa, a Nestorian Christian physician. He then had him live in Baghdad where he appears to have been the first to start the translation of the Greek works, and is credited with being the founder of the first medical school and hospital there. Early Arab scientists began by explaining the content of the Koran in a manner that showed there was no conflict with scientific studies. Then began the monumental task of translation of almost every manuscript that they could find in Greek, Syriac, Hebrew and Sanskrit. A succession of caliphs supported this effort.

An important feature of this period was the construction of the *Bayt al-Hikma* (*The House of Wisdom*), said to have been commissioned by Caliph Abdallah al-Mamun, son of legendary Caliph Harun al-Rashid, who reigned from 813 until the time of his death in 833. The building was constructed in the 8th century and played an important role in the translation movement: it was possibly originally the library of al-Mansur that then became a public academy. It was destroyed, together with most of its collection, in the 1258 siege of Baghdad by the Mongols. One factor that helped the Arabic transfer of information was their acquisition, in the late 750s, from China, of the method of making paper from linen and hemp. By 795 there was a factory in Baghdad producing various qualities of paper: at this time Europe still relied on vellum (animal skins).

Islam, Astrology, the Occult and Science

Arab culture before Islam tended to embrace superstitions and magic elements. Astrology was generally accepted and astrologers were both much used and well regarded for making important decisions. It had become a fantasy mixture of spirits, magic and superstition with elements of Babylonian, Indian and Persian cultures. This dream world was inhabited by the *rukh* (roc) bird, magic steeds and legendary beings who healed, or were endowed with other powers. It would appear that the Prophet accepted the existence of *jinn* (spirits). Usually they were good spirits and devotees of Islam, but other types were malignant and evil carriers of disease. These were all part of a complex belief system – the good lived on earth, in water or in air, and the bad in wells, ruins or filthy marketplaces. One spirit was known as Azazel, a fallen angel who appears in the traditions of Islam, Judaism and Biblical Christianity. It is said that Allah's favourites were the saints (*vali, marabut*), and *hakim*, the wise physicians who could ward off bewitching and the 'evil eye', as they knew *baraqq*, the blessing of healing power. The Koran speaks of *djennet* (Eden) and *djehennem* (hell), and angels and devils (Karasszon 1988, pp. 119–120).

These beliefs, existing in the Arab imagination, blended well with Islam. They already attributed their wonderful horses to a mare who had been inseminated with sperm from the famous horses bred by Suleiman al-Hakim (Solomon the Wise), King of Israel and Judea. By this they attributed the power of Islam to the Arab horses which 'were swift, stout, enduring and at the same time, wantless'. The Prophet's miraculous winged part-horse animal, al Buraaq, who took the Prophet from Mecca to Damascus and back one night, had supernatural talents and was surrounded by legends (Karasszon 1988, p. 116). The well-known stories of the *Arabian Nights* feature magic horses, and poets who wrote in praise of them.

In Mesopotamia, the early belief system was related to the stars and the heavens: this developed into, what has been termed, the first science – astrology. It spread to the Arab regions and was widely used when important decisions had to be made. Astrology with magic and folklore remedies were a part of everyday Arab health care before Islam, and continued after Muhammad's proclamation. When al-Mansur decided to create Baghdad as his capital he decided on a circular city, following Euclidian geometric principals, and much astrological consultation (Lyons 2009, p. 55). There was a rapid acceptance of a blend of Muslim belief, astrological divination and Greek science: a pragmatic resolution of the science versus religion debate. The decision was made that astral magical powers were ultimately derived from God and conveyed via rays by angels and spirits, and these were the entities with whom humans made contact. As a result, no conflict of interests or beliefs was recognised.

Human and Veterinary Medicine in the Islamic World

Islamic medicine was unlike the medical practice of the later Roman and Byzantine Empires. The Western concept had become based in superstition, divine causation and exorcism, and stultified. The Arab approach progressively developed clinical training and an understanding of surgery, pharmacology and epidemiology. The important difference between European and Islamic medicine was the Christian Church. This had taken the position of European moral authority, but was based on a theology which viewed illness as a divine punishment. Arabs developed a more Galenic approach and looked to balance the humours and to try to find a cause, but they also consulted the stars before bleeding or undertaking surgery. The Christian belief at that time regarded animals as being without a soul – they were brute creatures: this was bad for animal welfare and care. The Muslim community held the horse, in particular, in high regard and encouraged veterinary medicine for most species. When the Crusader invasions to capture Jerusalem began in 1099, the Arab society was shocked by their lack of hygiene and sanitation procedures (Lyons 2009, p. 20). Muslims practised ritual ablutions before prayers, five times a day; their religion provided a positive health/hygiene input.

There was a system of organised research in the Islamic world, following an understanding of developments in other cultures. A body of Arabic science developed, including philosophy, mathematics, astronomy, medicine (human and veterinary) and optics. It was referred to as *falsafa*, which meant 'natural philosophy' or a complete system of knowledge (Lyons 2009, p. 65). Medical schools were established in many places: Baghdad, Cairo, Cordoba and Damascus were the leading centres and in Cairo and Cordoba significant veterinary schools were sited. A relationship grew with the Salerno school in Italy, the first western medical teaching establishment: Muslim knowledge was read and absorbed into European medicine.

Islamic Medical Authors

As the Islamic world evolved, two principal centres of medicine developed, in the Eastern Caliphate led by Rhazes and Avicenna, both Persian, and later in the Western Caliphate with its capital in Cordoba (Spain) led by Averroes, Maimonides and Albucasis. Apart from these leaders there were many other contributors. These are listed chronologically below, partly derived from Al-Khalili (2010, p. 272).

Jabir ibn Hayyan (c.720–815), known as Geber the Alchemist in Western Europe, laid the basis for chemical science. Made significant advances in practical chemistry and is known as the inventor of the *al-ambiq* (alembic or retort), used for distillation. He is said to have been the first chemist to study both faeces and blood.

Al-Jahith (c.776–869) a leader in biological sciences rather than medicine. His main work, *Kitab al-Haywan* (*Book of Animals*) is a broad discussion with some early concepts on evolution, an indication of the Arab animal interest.

Ali ibn Sahl (c.838–870) was a physician and Jewish convert to Islam, tutor to Rhazes. His major work (c.850) *Firdaws al-Hikma* (*The Paradise of Wisdom*) is mainly devoted to medicine (including embryology), based on Greek and Hindu sources.

Ibn Zakariyya al-Razi (865–932), also known as *Rhazes*, was a Persian who studied medicine in Baghdad and lived in Tehran and Baghdad. Renowned as the greatest Islamic clinician of his lifetime and into the Middle Ages; was a noted scholar in mathematics, astronomy, religion and medicine. Of his writings 237 works have survived with over half devoted to medicine. His most important treatise was a monograph on smallpox and measles *Kitab al-Judari wal-Hasbq* (*The Book of Pestilences*): it included excellent descriptions as well as the first, defined treatment regimens (while it is quite clear that he is discussing smallpox there has been some controversy about the second disease – chickenpox or measles). His other important work was *Kitab al-Hawi*, known in the West as *Liber Continens*, an encyclopaedia of medical practice and treatment. Translated to Latin in 1279 and printed in 1486 it was an important medical book in Europe for centuries. He produced the *Kitab al-Jani al-Kabir* (*The Great Medical Compendium*) also called the *Liber Medicinalis ad almansoren*, essentially a compilation of Greek, Byzantine and Persian texts. Rhazes was responsible for the management of several hospitals and was an early investigator of the value of clinical trials.

Yuhanna ibn Masawayh (9th century), known as Mesuë the Elder, was a Persian Christian physician, translator of Greek medical works and tutor to Hunayn ibn Ishaq. Human dissection was banned but Mesuë became well known for anatomical studies of apes.

Abu al-Qasim al-Zahrawi (936–1013) was known as *Albucasis*. Under the reign of Caliph Abd al-Rahman III (r.912–916) Cordoba became the leading European cultural centre, with many physicians and a reputed 52 hospitals. Prominent in the medical field was Albucasis, who became the most famous surgeon of Islam. He wrote a 30-volume encyclopaedia *Kitab al-Tasrif*, embracing both medicine and surgery, containing much detailed information with observations that could only have been made by a skilled surgeon; he described many new and novel surgical instruments. He was influenced by the 7th-century treatise of Paul of Aegina, preserved in Byzantium. He recognised that Galen was relied on too much; a greater knowledge of anatomy was needed. He was the first to understand haemophilia and the first to use catgut as a surgical suture. Albucasis told surgeons 'God is watching you and knows if you are operating because surgery is really necessary or merely for love of money.' His work was translated to Latin by Gerard of Cremona in the 12th century and read in Europe throughout the Middle Ages, as the most important surgical text.

Ibn Sina (980–1037), known as Avicenna, was of Tajik origin. He was the most famous scholar and giant of Arab learning, a physician, a philosopher and thinker. His masterpiece work was his *Qanun fi al-Tibb* (*Canon of Medicine*), which was his listing and classification of medical knowledge. Avicenna attempted to blend the medical doctrines of Hippocrates and Galen with the biological doctrines of Aristotle. The *Canon* consists of five books: 1 main doctrines, diseases and symptoms, hygiene rules and treatment; 2 pharmacological overview largely based on Dioscorides, together with 'new' medications; 3 pathology with good disease descriptions; 4 contagious diseases, surgery and cosmetics; 5 preparation of medications, this became a universally used *materia medica* text. The book was translated to Latin in the 12th century by Gerard of Cremona and together with Galen's works dominated medical thought in Europe in the Middle Ages, serving as a textbook in European medical schools. Avicenna's other important work was *Kitab al-Shifa* (*Book of Healing*). Not a medical work but a brilliant philosophical overview, covering many topics including mathematics and physics. He was much influenced by Aristotle and the book was held to be of great significance in the West for many years. Avicenna had a controversial personality and was in frequent disputes, said to be the reason that he changed location frequently.

Ibn Zuhr (1094–1162), better known as Avenzoar, lived in Seville in medieval Andalusia (Spain), at the same time as Averroes. A renowned physician, his clinical emphasis was for a more rational, empirical basis for medicine. He was critical of both Galen and Avicenna, whose work he described as 'rambling'. His major work was *Al-Taysir fil-Mudawat wal-Tadbir* (*Book of Simplification Concerning Therapeutics and Diet*), the Latin translation was widely read. Avenzoar was important in both surgery and medicine. He was probably the first to perform procedures on animals before attempting them on humans: he practised the tracheotomy operation on a goat and proved that tracheal intubation could be successful. He also appears to be the first person to identify the cause of scabies as being a mite (*Sarcoptes* spp.). Both of these advances were equally of value to veterinary medicine.

Ali ibn Isa lived in Baghdad in the first half of the 11th century. The oldest Arabic ophthalmic work is attributed to him – *Tathkirat al-Kahhalim* (*Notebook of the Oculists*) which details the anatomy, physiology, diseases of and medications for the eye. He is also credited with being the first to make a copy of a Greek astrolabe.

Ibn Rushd (1126–98), known as Averroes, was a jurist, theologian, philosopher (with Aristotelian thoughts) and physician to the caliph; was regarded as a heretic by both Muslims and Christians, but exerted influence as a leader in the Cordoba medical environment. He discovered the role of the retina in sight, and observed that smallpox never attacks the same person twice. His best known medical text was an encyclopaedia in the Galenic tradition known as the *Colliget* or *Collection*, this was more concerned with the theory than the practice of medicine. Averroes' most famous pupil was Maimonides.

Musa ibn Maymun (1135–1204), better known as Maimonides, was a Jewish philosopher and physician, who trained under Averroes. A prolific author, he was influenced by Avicenna and followed Aristotle in trying to reconcile faith and reason. Of his ten surviving medical writings those on diet and hygiene were translated into Latin in 13th century. He reasoned that the practice of medicine should be founded on understanding the knowledge from the past, together with the experience of meticulous observation of the patient. He made no new discoveries but emphasised clinical study, and in his patients studied the psychological and spiritual aspects of healing. His most famous work, *Dalalat al-hairin* (*The Guide for the Perplexed*) written in 1190, sought to reconcile Aristotelian philosophy with Hebrew Bible theology, to minimise the ever present conflict between faith and reason.

Ibn al-Nafis (1210–1290) was a Syrian Arab Muslim physician and researcher, who studied anatomy, physiology, ophthalmology and surgery. He worked in Cairo and made important studies on the pulmonary and coronary circulations and compiled one of the largest medical encyclopaedias. Most well-known work was *Sharh Tashrih al-Qanum* (*Commentary on Anatomy in Ibn Sina's Canon*); recognised as a polymath with many interests including philosophy and Muslim theology.

Islamic Medicine

Islamic medicine was originally based in the teachings of the Koran together with the *Hadith* (the record of the Prophet's advice and conversations). As Greek medicine and Aristotelian philosophy was absorbed and rationalised with Islamic belief it became mixed with ancient herbal medications, folk remedies and occult beliefs. In time, two names dominated Islamic medicine: Avicenna and Rhazes.

While Avicenna became the dominant medical leader, not only in the Islamic world but also in Europe, current analysis has resulted in a more critical appraisal. His medical texts were essentially an attempt to reconcile the views of Galen and Aristotle. A close study of the work shows that it is essentially a rehash of Galen, including his anatomical errors, together with his bizarre concept of using geometric polygons to determine the healing of wounds, and astrology when selecting dates for bleeding and predicting a prognosis. Avicenna valued logic and reasoning and tended to guide the reader of his medical work away from personal clinical experience, which is the real basis of understanding disease. One 20th-century medical comment was, 'the *Canon* . . . seems an obscure hotchpotch from which no useful deduction can be made for the sick' (Sournia 1992, p. 130).

Rhazes was above all else a clinician: he understood the value of meticulous observation of the patient. His treatise on smallpox was a result of careful clinical study and recording. His being responsible for hospital management and seemingly the first person to utilise clinical trials demonstrates his concentration on patient care rather than theoretical speculation. He doubted some of Galen's ideas, including the four humours concept and wrote 'medicine is easy for imbeciles, serious doctors always discover difficulties'.

In essence, of these two giants of Islamic medicine Avicenna can be remembered as a great philosopher, and Rhazes as a great clinician. The translated works of Galen were well regarded in Islamic medicine. Avicenna tried to reconcile them with the views of Aristotle, later this philosophical discussion was followed by Averroes in Spain and was transmitted to Islamic Sicily, and then to mainland Europe, where Aristotle had been forgotten after the Roman Empire collapsed. The Avicenna *Canon*, after translation, had 60 editions published between 1500–1674 (Masood 2009, p. 105). The text gave medicine a base from which to move forward that resulted in the four humours concept becoming the basis of European human and veterinary medicine up to the early 1800s. Now seen to have resulted in a neglect of the value of clinical observation and experience.

One of the most important influences on Islamic medicine were the Egyptian Fatamid Caliphs who ruled from 909 to 1171. In 969 they established *al-Qahirah* (Cairo) which grew to be one of the most important cities in Islam. The Fatamids were patrons of science, in particular medicine, being great believers in learning as an aid to missionary work. The most important caliph of the dynasty was al-Hakim (r.996–1021), who took a milder attitude towards religion and encouraged science; Avicenna lived in Cairo under his regime. Cairo became a great medical centre and three large hospitals were established, including the famous *al-Mansuri*, where Ibn al-Nafis in the 13th century was chief physician. His hospital had specialist physicians, surgeons and ophthalmologists, and advanced hospitalisation practices. The Fatamids also located the *Al-Azhar* University in Cairo in 971 and Caliph al-Hakim gave the city the *Dur al-Hakim (House of Wisdom)* for learning, particularly medicine and engineering. The university was one of the first in the world and is the only early Arabic one to still exist.

Islam from its inception embodied a philosophy of good health and hygiene: this was expressed in many ways including *sufism*, a deeply ascetic Islamic belief whose adherents live modestly as a route to good health and pleasing God. The majority of the Islamic peoples used a medical system based in Galen and Dioscorides as the major influences, but recognising Rhazes as the outstanding clinician. Islam encouraged wealthier people to pay for public doctors and health care. A sense of religious duty drew many people into medicine: there were many charlatans but also some very good physicians. The records show that animal and human medicine were regarded as two parts of one science. As a result, Avicenna, and others, had a strong influence on the development of veterinary medicine.

Islamic Veterinary Authors

The Arab interest in veterinary knowledge was driven by their horse cult and their passionate devotion to the equine animal. Their early agricultural texts mostly feature the horse, but the veterinary content is variable in length and quality. Non-Arabic speakers have difficulties in investigating this subject because of the lack of reliable translations from Arabic, not only in interpreting the meaning of words but also in the Arab way of expression. The earliest historian writing in the English language on Arabic veterinary medicine was Frederick Smith in 1912 (Smith 1976, pp. 60–61). He found in the British Museum Library a publication, not in English, by Dozy: *Catalogue of Oriental MSS. In the Library, Academy of Leyden* Vol. III (Veterinary) 1865 (ref BM No. Ac. 940.4). This lists some early Arabic manuscripts dating from the 6th century, before the Islamic period, one is a translation of a Latin agricultural work, the veterinary content is not known.

From the 7th century there appear to be eight known manuscripts, but four of these may be altered copies, which all deal with horses and their diseases. One was recorded as being held at Oxford (No. 368 [z] Uri) and one by the British Museum (ref BM Add. 23, 416); one (Leyden 1411) is stated to include material from Greek, Persian, Indian and Syrian veterinary authors – Apsyrtus, written as 'Astortus' is mentioned by name. There does not appear to be any original Arab veterinary authorship from this period. Smith also noted three treatises from the 9th century on equine physiology recorded in 1852 by De Hammer-Purgstell, the same writer also listed 25 other writers from the same period, related to mostly equine studies (Smith 1976, pp. 58–59).

Because of the limited number of suitably qualified translators, and the difficulty many had in producing an accurate representation of these texts, researchers in veterinary history have had a shortage of material to work from. The three principal investigators were all located in France. Nicolas Perron translated three volumes of Arabic treatises. This included the notable 13th–14th-century work of Abu Bakr al-Baytar, known as al-Nasiri. Published in French as *Le Naceri. La Perfection des deax artes, ou Traitè complet d'hippologie et d'hippiatrie arabes* (1852–1860) Vol. II, Paris: Vve. Bouchard-Huzard. Leon Moulè in his *Histoire de la Medicine Veterinaire* (1896) Part II, AD 476–1500, Imprim. Maulde, Doumenc et Cie., made a detailed examination of the translations available to him and provides a useful commentary on the Arab equine cult which drove their interest in veterinary medicine. He also includes a list of medieval Arabic treatises on veterinary medicine and agriculture. More recently, 1966, Francois Vire has undertaken a major study of Arabic veterinary treatises mostly devoted to falconry; these are discussed in Chapter 24. The most significant advance has been made by the 2013 publication of *Mamluks and Animals* by H.A. Shehada; this book provides a broad perspective of the veterinary records of the medieval Islamic period. His work provides the most valuable reference text to this subject.

An effort has been made to list chronologically the known authors of Arabic Islamic veterinary literature. Because of the variation between translations of both authors names and titles of treatises there may be some inaccuracies with Arabic words.

Mohammed ibn Yaqub son of master of the horse for Caliph al-Motathed and a 'veterinarian' composed a book on hippiatry in 695, it was based on Greek, Persian, Indian and Syrian sources.

Al-Jahiz (8th century) the author of *Kitab al-Hayawan*, the first Arabic zoology work.

Hunayn ibn Ishaq (808–873), also called Johannitius, was the most notable trans-lator of Greek and other texts. Wrote a handbook on ophthalmology, translated the works of Galen, Apsyrtus, Mesuë Sr. and the equine work of the Indian Hippocrates. He also translated the Greek treatise of Theomnestus, and so provided the only complete version of that text.

Akhi Hizam al-Furusiyah wa al-Khuttal wrote a treatise in about 866 on equine management and health. Thought by some to be the first significant horse book, *Kitab al-Furusiyah wa-l-baytara* is the earliest Arabic veterinary treatise. Seven diseases that hinder mobility are described.

Mahmud b. al-Hasan al-Katib, known as Kushajm, wrote a treatise in the 10th century on hunting including a section on falconry.

An anonymous author, falconer to Caliph al-Aziz billah, wrote a manual on falconry *Kitab al-bayzara* (*The Art of Falconry*) published in the 10th century. This was translated to French by Vire in 1966.

Kabus el Moali, king of Ghilan, wrote a book on hippiatry for his son, in about 1080.

Abu Zakaria ibn al-Awwam al-ishbili (12th century) wrote an extensive work, titled *Kitab al-Filahah* (*Book of Agriculture*). Following discussion of arable farming and crop selection, chapters cover health and disease issues in livestock and dogs. The work provides a useful summary of the state of veterinary medicine in this period, the coverage of dental conditions is original. A partial translation to Spanish was printed in 1802.

Abd al-Rahman al-Balal (13th century) wrote a treatise, *al-kafi fil-bayarah*, on falconry.

Al-Malik al-Ashraf (d. 1296) was a ruler of the Rasulid Dynasty, located in the Yemen region. He followed his father in the intellectual field and developed a spe-cialist interest in medicine including a veterinary text, *al-Mughni fi al-Baytarah*, which became widely read in the Islamic world.

Ahmed ibn al-Hasan al-Ahnaf is believed to be the author of *al-Kitab al-Bayta-rah* in 1209. This was essentially a work on the diseases of livestock and draught animals – mules, asses and cattle. The book had good illustrations and lists of herbal prescriptions.

Al-Sahib Taj al-Din (d.1307), author of *Kitab al-Baytarah* (*Book of Veterinary Medicine*); he had much experience of the use of the horse in war and emphasises this aspect of training. The book is based in Islamic tradition and heritage in particular in rela-tion to *Jihad*, holy war. The veterinary section for disease diagnoses and treatment is based on a compilation from multiple sources including both Indian and Armenian. The Indian material indicates that these authors were competent in their veterinary practice.

Al-Malik al-Mujahid Ali b. Da'ub b. Yusuf al-Rasuli (d. 1362), a Yemenite king and authored a veterinary treatise, dealing with equine management, training and health.

Abu Bakr al-Baytar or Baitar (1309–1340), master of horse and chief 'veteri-narian' to the court of the Egyptian Sultan al-Nasir Muhammad bin Qalawun. The author of a 1331 treatise termed *Kashif hamm al-wayl fi akhbar al-Khayl* or *Kamil al-sinaatayn filbaytarah wal-zartaqah* but more usually known as *al-Nasiri*, a title to honour his master, the sultan. One of his epigrams was 'The veterinarian is always an equerry and the equerry is always a veterinarian.' The translation to French by Nicolas Perron is known as *Le Naceri*.

An anonymous work of 1327, *Kitab al Akual*, contains descriptions of diseases of all domestic animals, in particular the camel and elephant.

Kemal ed Din al Damiri (1394–1405) wrote a zoological work of interest; it contains descriptions of numerous animal diseases including rabies.

Al-Ghatrif (attributed), wrote in the 15th century *Kitab Dawari al-tayr* a treatise related to falcons, management and disease.

The above listing identifies a collection of Arabic Islamic texts related to veterinary medicine: it is probably neither complete, nor fully representative. Shehada (2013, p. 18), in his study of the veterinary literature of the Mamluk period, noted that in the Cairo National Library alone he was able to find 23 veterinary treatises attributed to that period. It is obvious therefore that there is much more work to be undertaken in translation to obtain a definitive picture of Arabic Islamic veterinary medicine.

Islamic Veterinary Medicine

The most important feature of Islamic veterinary medicine was that there was no difference between humans and animals. At the time that the Islamic belief was spreading, Europe was developing a stronger Christian faith, which at that time separated animals and humans based on the concept of possessing a soul, this belief took precedence over what had been conventional medical practice under the Roman Empire. A second factor was the passionate Arab love of the horse, which drove veterinary medicine as a part of equine care. A similar interest was in falconry where health care was most important. Both of these creatures were primarily owned by the wealthy or noble classes: while they were able to afford specialist care and the associated workers, they also created a culture of animal care.

In the pre-Islamic society the words *baytar* and *mubaytir* (derived from the Arabic *batara* root word meaning 'to cut or dissect'), were in use as designations for those persons responsible for animal healthcare, including farriery. As specialisation developed, while *baytar* indicated a 'horse doctor', words such as *kalbadhah* were used for dog specialisation and *bayzarah* for those who dealt with training and treatment of birds used for the hunt, with a *bazyar* being a specialist in the care and treatment of such birds. Equine specialisation was termed *zardaqah* (Shehada 2013, pp. 1–3). The interest in, and work on, veterinary subjects can be determined by the volume of literature that was produced: two main centres progressed the veterinary tradition. In the west in the land that became Catholic Spain the word *albeitar* was given to veterinarians before the creation of veterinary schools, and in Ottoman Turkey in the east the word *baytar* indicates a veterinarian.

One of the earliest works known to have been translated from Aramaic to Arabic, under the title *Nabatheen Agriculture*, attributed to Shanak, only had a limited text on veterinary matters, but did contain many details of talismans: how to make and use them, in particular for protection against poisoning. The exact date of this translation is unclear, initially it was thought to be 6th century, but is possibly 9th century. Copies are held in Paris, Leiden and Uppsala.

The early creation of the Arabic horse cult meant that there was a constant regard for the health and well-being of their animals. Healing was based in folklore and astrological predictions together with use of herbal medications. The knowledge that expanded Arab veterinary medicine was based mainly in the translations from the Greek, but also from Indian, Persian and other sources. Equine diseases, which form the bulk of the Arabic work were grouped according to body regions – eyes, nose, teeth, head, neck, extremities and so on. They were aware of contagion, but not of causation of infection.

Specific disease entities were described, some can be recognised but others have names that in translation are confusing, the term *malleus* (as in the Byzantine literature) continues to be used for a range of diseases. Equine adenitis is well described as also is epizootic lymphangitis, termed *kould* and treated by cautery. Anthrax was well known, but its pathogenesis was not. Dourine, and its transmission by coitus was understood but because of the disease characteristics, which were not known, they were unable to develop control measures. Abdominal intestinal conditions were studied in detail, in particular colic and diarrhoea termed *albagar*: both ailments were obvious problem conditions. Rabies was well described and its transmission by bite understood: while Avicenna did not write on veterinary topics he described rabies in the human and the role of the dog, as well as proposing herbal medications.

While the contributions to specific disease elucidation knowledge by the Islamic world were small they did aid 'the golden Arab horse hippiatry age' (Karasszon 1988, p. 126). The level of veterinary medicine (equine) was raised to that of medical science. Horses were separated from camels and livestock, specialist equine *baytars* were recognised. Diseases were considered to be species-specific – cattle, camels, elephants, horses, mules and asses were all treated separately. At the same time, the art of hippology – the management, breeding, training and feeding of horses – was equally recognised. Equines were important in Arab society, they even painted some animals, white hair was blackened with a mixture of henna and indigo.

In Arabic therapy purgatives, skincare, bleeding and cautery were the major treatments together with an extensive range of medications. These ranged from the rational to the totally (by today's standards) irrational. Ingredients such as pigeon and fox blood, baked frogs, staghorn, excrements, saliva, urine, egg yolk, honey, salt, alum, ash, borax, lime, saltpetre, sulphur, arsenic, zinc oxide and many more were used. As well as these there was a previous tradition of herbal medication which was enhanced when the work of Dioscorides was translated and widely utilised. Later Islamic researchers did significantly advance the science of pharmacology and the preparation of medicines.

Bloodletting was a widely accepted procedure with detailed instructions for use of the lancet on the jugular vein, or veins on the face, elbow, hock or spur (translated as a leg site). Islamic veterinary surgeons became proficient: abscesses were opened, osteal growths resected, cataract extractions performed as well as routine castration surgery. Skin grafting was performed using tissue from a recently slaughtered animal (this appears to have been more used, and successfully, with valuable falcons). Repair was also undertaken on the plantar surface of the hoof using either tissue from a slaughtered equine or metal implants. Bandaging and splinting of lower limbs for both fractures and injuries was undertaken, using similar techniques to those of human medicine. Bandages and sutures were in general use. Teeth were both extracted and filed. Slings were in use in treatment of leg injuries. Use of the cautery was frequently indicated by either puncture, needle or linear burning.

The Islamic period lasted several hundred years and the introduction and use of new procedures were spread across this time, frequently following human surgical advances. From the 11th century significant veterinary and agricultural treatises were produced in Spain, as it moved to become the leading European cultural centre. In the 12th century Ibn al-Awwan al-Ishbili wrote his notable *Book of Agriculture*, this includes much veterinary material with disease descriptions and treatments, almost all related to farm livestock in the Middle Ages. It was the first significant Islamic work devoted to livestock. He reviews the ancient Greek and Roman sources and cites Arab authorities to discuss breeding, rearing, nutrition and management. The horse receives one chapter, where he lists over 100 ailments described by the regions of the body; surgical procedures are discussed, in particular castration and casting techniques, and the related risks. Interestingly he covers the rearing and management of poultry and diseases of the chicken. Cattle and sheep are rather briefly discussed (but as this was Islam, not the pig); there is also a short section on diseases of the camel. The book suggests that there was a defined veterinary culture in Spain at this time. Later it was partly translated into Spanish and in 1864 to French.

Of the many veterinary related treatises written in Arabic the most notable one to survive was compiled by Abu Bakr al-Baytar (c.1309–1340), he was the son of a veterinary man and followed that vocation to become master of the horse to Sultan of Egypt al-Nasir Muhammad bin Qalawun (d.1341). Abu Bakr named his 1333 work *al-Nasiri* in honour of the sultan. His father Badr al-Din known as al-Baytar, had worked in the service of the sultans and was a major source of information on veterinary care of horses for his son (Shehada 2013, p. 163). Several copies of the text exist in different libraries. The first translation of the work, to French, was made by Nicolas Perron in 1852–1860 and it has been studied by several other translators in later years. A more recent and particularly useful review and explanation of the book has been made by Hakimi and Degueurce (2004, pp. 46–53). These authors examined the ten sections of the book to identify the most significant parts, for both scientific and poetic value.

The book, of over 300 'chapters' arranged in ten sections, is mostly devoted to the horse, with some content also dealing with donkeys, mules and other animals. The total equine coverage is very wide ranging from dealing, selection and purchase of animals, breeding, rearing, feeding, training for both combat and ceremonial duties and with a concentration on the art of horsemanship. Care, recognition of disease, treatment and medications are discussed in some detail. The work was well received at the time and Abu Bakr was widely respected. Some reviewers have stated that there is little in the text that is original and much is derived from the Byzantine authors, as well as Indian, Persian and Arab sources. Others disagree quoting the many examples in the text where he is critical of previous authors and either their medications or claims. It is obvious that Abu Bakr was a practical man who practised a hands-on approach to his subject and wrote with personal equine experience. This section of the text is described in detail by Shehada (2013, pp. 165–67) listing many of the diseases, with symptoms, by their Arabic names. Diseases are grouped according to the regions of the body. The treatment of skin diseases and wounds are discussed in detail, indicating that these were important problems, and also that this was the organ of the body that the author was most confident with, having little knowledge of the internal organs. Afflictions of the limbs and locomotory disorders are well covered, including shoeing. Both dental and eye conditions receive attention. Most medication is with herbal derived products.

In the Islamic years, there were advances in areas such as equine dental care and surgery; diseases of the limbs and feet and correction of shoeing faults and obstetric knowledge, particularly of the mare. Eight diseases were recognised to be of a contagious nature, however there was no real progress in understanding disease causation, and most importantly, because of religious taboos no dissection was allowed and therefore no advance in understanding of anatomy and physiology. Therapeutic methods did progress and medications (slowly) became simpler and more rational.

The camel was a most important animal for the Arabian people, but less so as Islam spread out of the desert regions. Several writers address management and diseases, but there appears to be little mention (or recognition) of the many varieties of the species that exist in the Middle East, each of which have evolved in accordance with their environment: the Egyptian Nile Delta camel is a very different creature compared with the Arabian desert camel. The majority of texts deal with the desert competent animal, which is recognised as being important in sandy, arid regions having an ability to cope with thermal stress, and reduced or nil periods without either water or food. The often difficult temperament of the male was noted. Their main use was for transporting loads and sometimes drawing wagons, resulting in attention being required for load bearing sores and abrasions. Skin disease, mostly mange, was a serious problem, as was foot care (the digits have evolved to undertake movement across sand). While not understood, problems now known to be caused by haemoprotozoa and bacteria were recognised.

The Iberian peninsula had been invaded by the Islamic Moors in the 8th century and by 726 they had conquered almost all the territory except for a small Christian state in the north. Under the then Umayyad Caliphate, *Al-Andalus*, a stable and economically successful country was created. The Moors continued with the agricultural land ownership system introduced by the Romans. This allowed for profitable and innovative farming to develop and enabled agrarian stability. Christians and Jews were allowed to practise their religions but were taxed as a lower grade of citizen. As the country prospered the capital, Cordoba, became the largest and richest city in Western Europe, with a well-developed appreciation of literature and science. This enabled a growing relationship with European Christian scholars, and medicine. The horse remained the most important animal and veterinary science developed well with the *baytar* a recognised professional group – to be continued in the later Spanish regime. In the succeeding centuries, the Islamic state fractionated, reunited and again split while the Christian forces began the slow *Reconquista* of Spain, with the creation of four Christian kingdoms (Aragon, Castile, Leon and Navarre). Following the unification, by marriage in 1469, of the two major kingdoms of Aragon and Castile, the Islamic army was defeated in 1492. This created the basis for the unified country of modern Spain.

The veterinary knowledge that had accumulated in Cordoba and the Moorish culture was to prove to be of value in hastening the veterinary medical renaissance that was to start in Western Europe. This was transmitted by important authors such as Juan Alvares de Salamiella and Marshal Don Manuel Diaz, both writing in the 15th century.

Islam and Judaism

Islam and Judaism enjoyed a similar culture, while the Jews were a minority group they also shared with the Christians a common god, and the followers of the three religions were regarded as 'People of the Book'. The Bible in fact provided a very strong link between Islam and Judaism and many of the key tenets of Judaism were adopted by Islam, such as a prohibition on consuming pork, ritual animal slaughter methods and a banning of idolatry. In these early days Islamic–Jewish relations were ones of toleration. Jews were able to prosper, even though second class citizens in the Muslim countries.

Jews tended to be better educated and had acquired a reputation as translators (of texts from other languages) and also had developed a special place in human medicine. Their physicians were well regarded and valued in the Muslim world: rather than concentrating on finding a cure, as was the usual practice, the Jewish physicians believed that prevention was the better method of approach to disease control. Initially this relationship worked well, in particular in the Spanish lands where they became very involved in Arabic life. This was partly due to their importance in the acquisition of knowledge. In this environment some eminent individuals evolved, such as Maimonides (1135–1204) the Jewish philosopher and physician, a pupil of Averroes in Cordoba, and Ali ibn Sahl (c.838–870), a Jewish convert to Islam and leading physician, who became tutor to Rhazes.

Ritual Slaughter

The Laws of Moses, as defined in the Bible, illustrated a concern that the followers of Judaism should be supplied with hygienic food. This was provided by instituting a strict ritual for the selection of animals for consumption, the method of slaughter and the inspection of the carcase before it was allowed to be eaten. This meant that their rabbis became familiar with certain parts of animal anatomy and abnormalities caused by disease or damage, mainly with beef cattle. The *Talmud* includes a section termed the *Mishnah*, compiled in AD 189, which contains the rules for inspection and control of the meat, these were largely adopted by Islam. The instructions for ritual slaughter (*sechita*) and the meat control procedure (*bedikah*) are very specific and pre-cise. They detail the place and method of killing, procedures for securing the animal, ensuring that it is fully conscious and the killing knife is checked before and after use. The five main errors of cutting are listed together with the definition of 'clean' or 'unclean' animals or meat. The law also decrees the penalties for the consumption of blood in any form.

These early Jewish food hygiene procedures, mostly adopted into Islamic practices, were the starting point for veterinary meat inspection procedure and public health measures. The controls as prescribed in the *bedikah* gave particular importance to examination of the lungs with actions to be taken based on lung colour, damage and specific lesions. Examination of the lungs for lack of any lobes, or presence of *sercho* (pseudo-membranes) or *bnos* (purulent cysts) is detailed (these specific requirements have been interpreted as a recognition of tuberculous lesions). Other instructions deal with the meat of animals killed by accident or outside of a prescribed premises and use of the meat of an unborn foetus. The consumption of any organ supplied with blood from the abdominal aorta was forbidden. Following examination by the rabbi, meat was either declared *kosher* (suitable) or *trepha* (unsuitable) for consumption.

These procedures not only resulted in an accumulation of pathological knowledge in the Jewish community but it also stimulated an interest in undertaking post-mortem examination of human cadavers.

The Kabbala

The Kabbala (also called Cabbala) began as an oral tradition of an occult Jewish belief, the word has been translated to mean 'tradition' or 'correspondence'. It is a creed 'only available to the chosen' and has existed for centuries: it is essentially a system of esoteric theosophy. Based on a mystical method of interpreting the Bible it was first spread orally and by using ciphers. The belief reached maximum influence in the Middle Ages and peaked in the 12–13th centuries in Spain and southern France. There was also a Christian sect who adopted a form of the teaching.

One of the tenets of the belief relates to healing and it is noteworthy that interest in the Kabbala was greatest in the time of the mass epidemic diseases that swept across Europe. One of the features of the tradition was a concentration on the significance of words, and the use of talismans. Horses and other domestic animals wore amulets or had written text hung around their necks with the magic word *abracadabra*. It was believed that Kabbalists had the power to cause illness and to heal humans and animals. This veterinary application of Kabbalist animal healing is well explained by Karasszon (1988, pp. 130–132). The belief is still maintained by Hasidic Judaism.

References

Al-Khalili, J. (2010) *The Golden Age of Arabic Science*. London: Allen Lane
Hakimi, M.M. and Degueurce, C. (2004) Le Traite des Deux Arts en Médecine

Vétérinaire ou 'Le Naceri': Presentation de sa Traduction. *Bull.soc.fr.hist.méd.sci. vét.* **3** No.1

Hourani, A. (2010) *A History of the Arab Peoples.* London: Folio

Karasszon, D. (1988) *A Concise History of Veterinary Medicine.* Budapest: Akadémiai Kiado

Lyons, J. (2009) *The House of Wisdom.* New York: Bloomsbury Press

Masood, E. (2009) *Science and Islam: A History.* London: Icon Books

Maxwell-Stuart, P.G. (2010) *Astrology: From Ancient Babylon to the Present.* Stroud: Amberley

Shehada, H.A. (2013) *Mamluks and Animals: Veterinary Medicine in Medieval Islam.* Leiden: Brill

Smith, F. (1976) *The Early History of Veterinary Literature*, Vol. 1. London: J.A. Allen

Sournia, J.-C. (1992) *The Illustrated History of Medicine.* London: Harold Starke

CHAPTER 7

East Asia: China, Indo-China, Korea and Japan

CHINA

To study Chinese medicine history requires an appreciation of the many inherent complexities in the national culture. It is now the most populous country in the world, with about 1.4 billion people, and has one of the longest continuous civilisations, beginning in the Northern China Plain in the fertile basin of the Yellow River.

The landscape and climate present extreme differences – from mountains, to tropics, to deserts and river basins; the major population regions have dry seasons and wet monsoons. There is an extensive biodiversity with over 32,000 species of plants recognised and over 10,000 recorded species of fungi. The country has a shortage of arable land, only 15% of the total area can be cultivated; farming traditionally has always been labour intensive. There have been periods of famine and China has a chronic food shortage problem.

There is no agreement for the date when agriculture commenced in China, estimates range from 11,500–6200 BC. Millet was the first domesticated grain, followed by rice, believed to be cultivated from 5700 BC and later by beans and other food crops. From 3300 BC agriculture became intensified, and with this developed advanced technology for irrigation and for lifting water above river levels. By the 2nd century AD there was a national granary system. Domestication of the silkworm moth was early, as widespread sericulture was present by 3500 BC. This is discussed in Chapter 26.

Food plays an important role in Chinese culture: rice is the staple food in the south, and wheat bread and noodles in the north, together with beans and vegetables, with fish and seafood from rivers and coastal fishing. In ancient times meat was only eaten on special occasions. Today there is a large livestock population of pigs, mainly in Yangtze River region: pork now comprises three-quarters of total meat consumption with the rest being mainly poultry and in some regions beef, sheep and goat meat.

Traditionally the livestock population was focused on the horse for warfare and ceremonial uses, with mules and donkeys used for transport. In the west of the country sheep, goats and camels were important, with nomadic herders; yaks have always been the main livestock in Tibet. Water buffalo are traditionally the work animal of the rice farmer, with cattle in the grassland regions. Dairy cattle are of lower importance with about 90% of the population still having some degree of lactose intolerance. Aquaculture is important, providing about one-half of China's fish consumption, mainly in the Yangtse Valley and Zhu Jiang Delta.

Background to Chinese Medicine

The basic medical concepts used in both Chinese human and veterinary medicine are not only unrelated to those in the Hellenic-European region but they are totally different.

The earliest records indicate that shamans (frequently of Mongol descent) were the healers. They possessed mysterious powers and used incantations, herbs, ritual ceremonies and some body treatments, such as massage. Medical texts can be traced to at least the 2nd millennium BC, these were oral folklore until the *Nei jing* treatise, dated to possibly the 3rd century BC. This detailed text provided the first written compilation of the earlier orally transmitted knowledge.

The great characteristic of Chinese medicine is the influence and involvement of numbers: used to index, classify and identify almost every aspect of the subject. This is probably a natural consequence of the very early, and widely practised custom of numeromancy: divination by numbers. This was one factor in the concept of the world being governed by two universal principles – *yin* and *yang*, with humans being just one element in this world. While these two principles are opposites, they are not seen as being in conflict. They are complementary and are seen essential for the movement of the stars, the climate, the rhythm of the seasons, and for life.

The attributes of the *yin* are negative, passive and feminine, and those of the *yang* are positive, active and masculine. The teaching also embraces the five elements – tree, fire, earth, metal and wood. The earth produces water, water extinguishes fire, fire melts metal, metal cuts tree and tree grows out of the earth: this demonstrates a complete cycle and can be related to living organisms. These teachings are connected in a complex nature-philosophical principle that underlies the ancient Chinese medical approach.

The five elements are seen to be in close interaction with five (named) planets, the five airs, the five (not four) seasons, the five parts of the day, the five main colours, the five tonalities, the five cardinal points and the five main compact organs or *Tsang* – liver, heart, spleen, lung and kidney which are related to the *yin*. These organs are also related to the five types of pulse, five odours and five types of appetite. The hollow organs or *Fou* – stomach, gall bladder, intestine and urinary bladder are related to the *yang*. This latter organ group control the functions of absorption, transformation and elimination.

Astrology was also thought to be important in the regulation of human and animal life with the movements of even the most remote heavenly bodies being believed to govern every activity, action and organ of human and animal kind. Together with a study of nature the teaching linked each plant, stone, animal and human to a precise place in life. When disease occurred the principles of *yin* and *yang* could be applied to adjust and correct the balance.

The Chinese concept of the origin of the world was quite unlike the ideas that had been adopted by other cultures. They had no invented gods to regulate the universe, instead there were legendary figures to whom certain doctrines are attributed. Later the teachings of Confucius and others were seen as a guide to social and family behaviour and political ethics, and Buddhism was a code of conduct, and not a practice founded in a sanctified text. They did, like other cultures, believe in the invincible powers held by spirits and demons whose actions caused typhoons, earthquakes, thunderstorms, rain and drought. However, the teaching was that these forces obeyed a universal order.

It is claimed that Shen Nung, who was said to have ruled 2838–2698 BC, was the inventor of medicine, under the inspiration of Pan Kua who according to Taoist legend created the world. By his acts chaos was overcome and order was established, on the basis of keeping a balance between the two opposite poles – *yin* and *yang*.

As all health issues were examined through *yin* and *yang* principles the structure of the body and bodily organs was not considered. What was important was how the human or animal functioned in the great universal scheme. This resulted in an ignorance of anatomy and the function of organs – until the beginning of the 15th century AD. Chinese teaching had an imagined plan of bodily structure and function. A body was said to have three regions, five organs, six receptacles and three cauldrons, with 360 bones (equal to the days in their year). These 'structures' were believed to be connected along invisible channels. Arteries, veins, lymph vessels, nerves and tendons were not identified. Each organ had its own *yin* and *yang* and its own *k'i* or *ch'i* (the mystical second circulation) with a systems of channels.

This believed bodily arrangement provided the basis for acupuncture therapy. Every part of the body (human and animal) is said to be associated with a clearly defined area of the skin. Precise points are identified and action can be taken by application of the necessary needles. Acupuncture, either alone or with moxibustion (producing a mild blister), developed to both an art and possibly a science. The purpose of Chinese medical intervention was to ensure that all the forces were acting in total equilibrium, as any breakdown of this equilibrium would result in disease (Sournia 1992, pp. 202–205).

Examination of the patient – as prescribed for a human, but also used for animals (chiefly horses) – began with a careful examination of the subject. The doctor would study complexion, breathing, tears, saliva, nasal secretions and examine hands and nails. The mouth, tongue and nostrils were all checked, as this is where the *yang* leaves the body. This external examination with many questions and study of excretions was very thorough, but was of limited value as the internal organs were not understood. There was no attempt to listen to either the heart or the lungs, or to investigate and consider the patient's previous medical history. Considerable time, however, was devoted to study of the pulse, twelve different pulse rhythms were described and examined using the left and right wrists, and each had a significance. The pulse indicated the flow of the vital element (the *ch'i*) formed from the union of *yin* and *yang* with the blood. There were many treatises on rhythmology and the relationship to numeromancy.

The object of Chinese medical intervention was to return the patient to perfect health, and the teaching was that this only happened when there was 'hygiene' in the individual's social and private life: there were seven emotions which needed to be understood. Before any treatment or medication was started there had to be an examination of the diet: it had to be varied, with no excess of meat or alcohol. Moderate physical exercise was advocated together with breathing exercises, baths and massage. A programme of behaviour was also introduced – of discipline and etiquette. The aim was to restore the whole being to their place in society, a psychotherapy application. Chinese procedure resulted in a prognostic rather than a diagnostic conclusion. While they believed that fate was predetermined, they also believed that they could intervene and change it by careful therapy.

The only practical preventive medicine procedure that was used was a form of variolation to prevent smallpox. Scabs from a clinical case were ground to a powder and inserted into the nose (left nostril for boys and right for girls), or pus from a patient was introduced into a small scarification (Margotta 1996, p. 19). Care was taken that the recipient was in good health and that the scabs or pus were from a mild case of smallpox. The methods were widely used by the upper Chinese classes from the 11th century onwards. Later Silk Road traders took the knowledge to Turkey from where it eventually reached Edward Jenner in England, who publicised the procedure and encouraged its widespread use in Europe.

The *Huangdi Nei jing*

This medical treatise, generally referred to as the *Nei jing*, is unquestionably the most important early Chinese medical work. For many centuries it was the main information source for both human and veterinary medical practitioners. The work is mentioned many times in the following text, these mentions are based on the contemporary literature being discussed in that period of history. These are sometimes confusing in both attribution and application. The following gives a summary of the probable history and content of the work and should be referred to should later comments require clarity.

Named after the Emperor Huang Di, the *Huangdi Nei jing* or the Canon of the Yellow Emperor has been regarded as the fundamental Chinese medicine text for well over 2000 years. There is a long history of this work being transmitted by oral tradition for possibly 2000 years before the written version was made by Confucian scholars in the Han Dynasty period, 207 BC–AD 220. Dating, content and attribution all vary by source and scholar's opinion.

The *Nei jing* consists of two texts, each of 81 'chapters' mostly arranged in a question and answer format.

- The *Suwen* (*The Basic Questions*) covers the theoretical basis of Chinese medicine and diagnostic methods. This includes Taoist (Daoist) theory and lifestyle: a teaching similar to Confucianism, but without rigid rituals and a strong belief in compassion, frugality and humility. The *Suwen* is the part usually cited or quoted.

- The *Lingshu* (*The Spiritual Pivot*) describes the pulse, details acupuncture, the points, the meridian lines and its application and interpretation. Includes probably the first description of the circulation of the blood: 'All blood of the human body is under the control of the heart and regulated by it. The blood current flows continuously in a circle and never stops; it cannot but flow ceaselessly like a current of a river or the sun and moon in their courses.' The circulation description and the relationship to the heart is fairly accurate, but as Chinese knowledge of anatomy was negligible (dissection was generally prohibited) it is possible that there was some lucky guesswork. Examination of the pulse and its variations formed the basis of prognosis for man and animals.

The work is important as it was the first that ignored shamanistic belief in devils, demons and magic. In its early oral form, it described what was to become the basis of Chinese medicine: an emphasis on diet, lifestyle, emotions, environment and age. These were seen as the major factors in maintaining health. The universe was seen as the macrocosm in which man was seen as a microcosm, but mirroring the macrocosm. Keeping the balance and harmony within this system was the *yin–yang*, the five elements and environmental factors (hot, cold, wind, wet, and so on). Disease in both humans and animals was seen as a result of the balance and harmony being disrupted; the medical procedures were to correct this and restore normality.

The influence of the philosophical teachings of Confucianism and Taoism is important as it is recognised that these placed wisdom above knowledge and slowed the development of medicine. Two other medically related treatises existed at the same time as the *Huangdi Nei jing*, the *Mingtang* and the *Taisu* but only fragments have survived.

Ancient Chinese Veterinary Medicine

A problem with Chinese studies is that it can be difficult to place accurate dates on early texts, successive rulers liked to destroy existing classic texts to hide the achievements of their predecessors. As a result, some of the earliest records are not only difficult to date but appear as a mixture of legend and fact. Much of the very early material was saved by the activities of the historians of the Han Dynasty (207 BC–AD 220). As very few texts, in particular from the early years, have been translated by veterinary medicine specialists it is believed that not only are many items open to closer scrutiny, but that there is still more material to be read.

In very early Chinese social structures shamans or priests held great power, it was believed they could placate the evil spirits that caused disease and disasters. This belief caused large numbers of animals to be slaughtered (cattle were the favoured species) to obtain their scapulae, these were grooved and scorched by fire and then the cracks were read by diviners. The carapace of the turtle or tortoise was treated in a similar manner. Both human and animal sacrifice was practised: the corpses were burned; the meat was not eaten. Because of the importance of horses in these early societies it was recorded that there were 'horse priests' to care for these animals.

The detailed and complex Chinese mythology also includes one Fu-hi, possibly the first emperor: the first basic principles of *yin* and *yang* were also attributed to him in the doctrine of Pan Kua. Another legendary emperor was Da Yu who is credited with draining the waters of the Great Flood. He is also attributed to outlining the basic nature-philosophical principles which provide the basis for the *yin* and *yang* concept.

Emperor Shen Nung was said to have compiled a three-volume herbal work, the *Pen-tsao Ching* (*Materia Medica*) with 365 identified plants, plus lists of prescriptions and poisons. While this work was only known of by quotation it apparently recognised many specific medications for humans and animals including opium (narcotic), rhubarb (laxative), artemisia (anthelmintic), rauwolfia (sedative), kaolin (diarrhoea) and ephedrine (asthma). It is questionable that this work actually existed as a book, it was more likely as oral transmission, however a pharmacology treatise of the same name appeared about 30 BC covering the same subjects and classifying plants as medicines; the 347 preparations listed are of plant, animal and mineral origin.

It would appear that the horse, *ma*, has been domesticated in China from about 4000 BC with evidence of animal husbandry and veterinary practices going back to that date: excavations have unearthed animal bones, stone knives and needles. It was stated that the legendary Emperor Huang Di (2698–2598 BC) had a 'horse doctor' named Ma Shihuang, who cured diseases of 'dragons' by using herbs, including a liquorice decoction, accompanied by acupuncture. From the very early times the major animal health interest was the horse, it was the vital factor in prestige and warfare.

The Development of Chinese Medicine: Human and Veterinary

This is best described in the chronological context of the dynastic rulers and periods of the country. Some of the names and titles of texts cited have been difficult to express in a consistent manner. Before 2209 BC is considered the Neolithic period, followed by the Xia Period 2209–1776 BC, but this date is questionable. From 1776 BC information is more reliable.

Yin and Shang Periods c.1766–1122 BC

During the Yin and Shang periods (the Bronze Age) a system of character writing developed and the mythological dragon became established. The dragon has a relationship to river valleys, water, food and festivals. It is more usually seen as a friendly symbol and not as an unpleasant creature. The vocabulary expanded with words for stable, cowshed and piggery. Livestock numbers were few in the main rural river basin areas: water buffalo were used for draught and family pigs were kept, as they did not require land, and could be fed on by-products and household scraps. Ducks raised on ponds became a popular food source. The Tibetan, Manchu, Mongol and Turkic peoples in the mountainous and arid areas of the boundary lands depended on yaks, sheep, goats and camels for both food and transport.

The horse had become a significant animal, used for drawing chariots and hunting; mainly owned by the nobility and ruling classes. The introduction of metallurgy allowed the invention of metal stirrups and ploughshares, two significant advances. Donkeys were the ubiquitous transport animal. Dogs were obviously commonplace as their bones have been found from the earliest Chinese settlements, along with those of pigs. The role of the dog at that time – food or friend – is not clear. Equine veterinary medicine was developing using the same beliefs and procedures as its human counterpart.

During the Yin and Shang periods the *yin–yang* teaching with the five elements was further developed and increasingly accepted by the people. These concepts, which emphasised ecological relationships and the balance within the body and environment, constituted the philosophy of human and veterinary medicine in China for centuries (Sun and Chen 2009, p. 73).

West Chou (Zhou) Dynasty to Spring and Autumn Period (c.1000–476 BC)

Precise dates for the Chou period are difficult to establish, reliable history does not go back further than 722 BC (the dates represent the middle of this period). The total Chou Dynasty is recognised as being one of the most glorious periods of Chinese history: 'literature, art, philosophy, religion, government . . . all flourished and reached a high degree of development' (Edwards 1945, p. 600). This was the age of Confucius, Lao Tzu (the guiding figure of Taoism/Daoism) and Mencius (philosopher, believed to have been a pupil of Confucius's grandson) whose writings and influence, in the Chou late period, reached every branch of literature and learning. The effect of these philosophic and aesthetic teachings was, however, harmful in the long term, to the advance of human and veterinary medicine. The emphasis became increasingly on 'wisdom' rather than knowledge, the former was deemed to be the basis of human happiness. Chinese society began to be organised, government was in the hands of scholar-administrators selected early in life, with the rest of the population remaining as labourers and craftsmen. The study of medicine became dominated by, 'the scholastic subtleties of visionary philosophers and was characterised by reverence for authority, petrified formalism, and pedantic excess of detail' (Wong and Wu 1932, pp. 40–45).

Before the decline, in the later years of the Spring and Autumn Period and into the Han Dynasty, medicine had become highly developed. Medical and veterinary practice were well organised with deliberate reference being paid to hygiene and public health. Four categories of the medical profession were recognised: ranked as nutritionists, physicians, surgeons and veterinarians. There was a form of examination and those who passed were recognised as 'doctors' and classified as either high, middle or lower grade. These were listed in the *Zhou li*, a government book detailing official personnel. In the veterinary listing an individual is named as 'one who cares for military horses': indicating this function as a state priority.

The system had a headquarters, and a number of regional units (no total figures available), each with a superintendent's office with clearly defined duties. The objective was to maintain health and the emphasis was on this aspect rather than on the treatment of disease, the occurrence of which was regarded as a failure. The performance of the veterinarians was examined and judged on the mortality of the animals that they examined. Salaries were related to what was judged to be the standard of work of the doctor; money was withheld from those who performed poorly.

Each unit had five departments, ranked in seniority these were:

- superintendent's office: 2 high grade and 4 lower grade doctors, 2 clerks and 20 servants
- dietetics department: dieticians (*she-yi*), 2 middle grade doctors
- medical department: physicians (*tsi-yi*), 8 middle grade doctors
- surgical department: surgeons (*yang-yi*), 8 lower grade doctors
- veterinary department: veterinarians (*sheu-yi*), 4 lower grade doctors.

The ranking of the departments shows the relative importance given to the different branches, with dietetics listed first and surgery and veterinary medicine being dealt with by practitioners of seemingly lower proficiency to those in human dietetics and medicine. An interesting rank order, because this differentiation in prestige evolved in a cultural world isolated from that in Western Europe, where in the 17th and 18th centuries exactly the same attitude had developed.

Some animal diseases, rabies, cysticercosis (tapeworm) and sarcoptic mange, were recognised and documented. Herbal medications were in routine use, veterinary surgery was mostly limited to castration (Sun and Chen 2009, p. 73). Castration was dated from before 2200 BC, it was most widely used with pigs and horses, draught animals and cockerels; sows were also spayed. The creation of eunuchs for service in the emperor's palaces was a well-established procedure (and much more radical, involving the removal of all the external genitalia) with many specialist surgeons. Tradition was that a 'whole' human had to be buried to enable the person to continue the cycle of life. Eunuchs preserved the result of their surgical intervention, to be buried with them. Because no dissection was allowed and therefore knowledge was lacking, surgery made little advance in the early Chinese medical system. A conservative attitude was expressed towards equine castration, but not for pigs and poultry.

It is notable that diet was seen as the most important aspect of this medical culture. A quotation from the *Suwen* illustrates the philosophy, 'The sage does not treat those who are ill but those who are well.' As already mentioned this was to become a problem because the abstract philosophy of Confucius and Mencius gradually overruled the increasingly talented medical groups who were developing a scientific approach to disease and its control. At the same time, the *yin–yang* concept of the balance of nature was increasingly employed; this resulted in a decline in the role of the shamans/priests. Towards the end of the Chou period, (in the Spring and Autumn period) lived Sun Yang, also called Bai Le (659–620 BC), who had legendary skill in horse care and advocated meticulous study of the patient. Described as the 'father' of veterinary acupuncture he named 77 sites on the body, 8 on the forelimbs and 8 on the thighs.

In the later Chou period animals that died while under care were counted and recorded against the supervising veterinarian; farmers were compensated for their loss. The key role of the veterinary department was healing equine diseases: very careful examination of patients was mandatory, together with topical herbal washes to ease pain, and gentle exercise followed by careful examination of the pulse. Herbal medications were used but nutritional care and controlled diets were the major factors in both disease prevention and treatment. By this time castration was a regularly practised procedure in horses and other species, but with the caution noted above. During this period aquaculture was being developed with the creation of ponds for carp culture.

Warring States Period (475–221 BC)

There were developments in Chinese medical science, two notable treatises began to be widely used that not only generalised the development of medicine in China but also confirmed the principles of human and veterinary medicine. The *Nei jing* (already discussed) organised the teachings of the *yin-yang* and five elements concepts, and established acupuncture and acupuncture points, and the *nun jing*, a book of medical lore based on the use of the pulse for diagnosis and prognosis. The origin of this second text can be traced back to 2500 BC and preserved by oral tradition.

Acupuncture and its use with moxibustion (mild blister) as a practical means of restoring the *yin–yang* balance had come into near-general use. The old habits of magic and mystery had fallen out of favour and the basis for human or animal medicine relied on reading the pulse for diagnosis and prognosis plus acupuncture, simple herbal therapy, nutritional attention, rest, quiet, comfort and nursing care.

The role of the horse veterinarian was becoming better defined. It was written that Shun Yeng, also called Pao Lo, born c.480 BC was the first full-time veterinarian and the father of veterinary medicine – such statements have to be taken with caution, almost every dynasty or period like to claim father figures. Zao Fu and Wang Liang were also named as being well-known practitioners of the veterinary art. During this period, a law requiring the cleansing of the wheels of all visiting vehicles was introduced, to prevent the spread of horse diseases: contagion was being recognised, but little preventive medicine was applied.

Qin and Han Dynasties (221 BC–AD 220)

Modern China has its origins in the Qin Dynasty (221–207 BC) founded by Emperor Qin Shihuangdi, following his unification of the regional warring states. During the following 2000 years the country has divided and unified more than once, nonetheless, it is possible to trace a continual thread of culture through most of these changes because Emperor Qin, who termed himself the first emperor, was a significant legislator. China takes its name from this dynasty, Qin is pronounced 'Chin'.

He imposed a single script on his diverse kingdom, an act which was key to establishing a core identity. He aimed to unify and to promote commerce – weights, measures and currency were all standardised, aided by the uniform system of writing. He also created a remarkable and large centralised bureaucracy, and with a strong military ended the conflicts between the regional states. Qin was a practical and thoughtful legislator – wheeled transport had become popular as people preferred a carriage to riding: one of his laws decreed a standard axle length to allow for easy use of bridges and roadways.

Qin's philosophy of 'legalism' in practice meant obedience to authority – his war tactics were ruthless. Confucianism was suppressed and books were burned. In the later Han period, it was recognised that Qin used violence to change the world, but in the words of the Han historian, Sima Qian, the 'accomplishments were great'. It is also important to understand that in China there is no tradition of individualism, the individual's life belongs to the collective state – central governance has a long history in Chinese culture and accounts for the relatively easy institution of universal concepts, but also the rejection of new ideas.

Veterinary medicine developed rapidly in this time, influenced by the growth of horse breeding, specifically for the army. Animal care was regarded as important, a law on horse husbandry which was issued in the Qin Dynasty (221–207 BC) was revised in the Han Dynasty (207 BC–AD 220).

Medical knowledge expanded in the Han Dynasty, there was greater use of the *nun jing* (*Classic of the pulse*) which was widely read, as was the *Nei jing* which included the doctrine of the dual circulation of the blood, with the concept of a mystical second circulation called *ch'i*, a *yang* attributed form of energy, that circulated in invisible tracts. The circulating blood was the *yin* element. These works, in particular the *nun jing*, began to circulate outside of China and were of influence on Persian and Arabic medicine. Chinese medicine was exploring the concept of biorhythms long before the idea had developed elsewhere.

These approaches to diagnosis and therapy were utilised in both humans and animals, in particular the horse. Surgery, however, remained essentially limited to wound treatment and castration. Two medical treatises were produced during the Han Dynasty, the *shén nóng ben cao jing* and *shang hán zá bing lun*, they described hundreds of medicinal herbs with comprehensive guides to diagnosis and treatment, of both human and animal diseases. Also surviving from this period are veterinary formulae and medicine bills inscribed on bamboo slips. Probably near the end of the Qin and Han Dynasties (China was riven by divisions for a period and dating is unreliable) more formularies and herbal medicines for animal use were described in books such as *zóu hou bei ji fang* and *qi min yao shu*. The latter text proposed 48 measures for the treatment of 26 animal diseases including isolation procedures for the control of infectious disease. Hoof cutting was also presented as being useful for the prevention and treatment of foot problems.

The cultivation of fish had been developing slowly for some 500 years but advanced in the Han period when it was recognised that fish in paddy fields could help in mosquito control. Goldfish culture also progressed (Chapter 25).

Sui Dynasty (220–618)

During the Sui Dynasty a special agency, *Tai-Pu-Shi,* was established by the central government: this was responsible for the administration of animal husbandry including horse breeding and employed some 120 veterinary scholars. It was recorded that books on diagnosis, herbal formulae, and animal acupuncture were published, but are now lost (Sun and Chen 2009, p. 74).

Tang Dynasty (618–907)

In the Tang Dynasty many disciplines flourished; printing was invented. It was documented that there were 600 veterinarians, 4 veterinary teachers and 100 veterinary students in the *Tai-Pu-Shi* organisation.

During this time the first comprehensive veterinary textbook was published, the *Si mu an ji ji* edited by Li Su (c.783–845), the title translates as 'The Collection of Ways to Relieve the Suffering of a Horse'. In four volumes it listed 76 serious diseases and 36 causes, and could be the first work to discuss veterinary differential diagnosis. The book proved to be very popular in China and Japan for several centuries: in the Song and Yuan Dynasties it was progressively expanded to eight volumes.

In 659 the emperor issued a book, *Xin xiu ben cao,* which is considered in China to be the earliest pharmacopoeia for human and veterinary medicine, it describes 844 different medications. There is evidence that science was making significant advances: a technique had been described as early as the 2nd century BC for the isolation of what we now term gonadotrophins and sexually active steroids, from human and animal urine, over 1500 years before the West. Diabetes mellitus was recognised and dietary control used; thyroid gland from rams was used to treat cretinism before 700; seaweed was recognised as an iodine source to correct nutritional deficiency.

Other literature sources indicate that in the Tang Dynasty acupuncture was widely used on horses, and all animals including elephants. A treatise on diseases of dogs and their treatment was written by Wang Tao. Many other texts on veterinary medicine appeared; one reason for this flourishing of the veterinary art was due to the value of horses, not just in commerce, but in particular in war. The looming threat of invasion on the northern frontier (which was to eventually cause the destruction of the dynasty) required large numbers of men and horses to guard the border.

During this period, the farming of the common carp was banned (due to its Chinese name sounding like the name of the emperor). Other members of the Cyprinid (carp) family were then used in extensive pond polyculture. Grass carp fed from the surface, silver and big head carp at mid-depth and mud carp fed on the pond bottom. There was a rapid increase in aquaculture.

Song Dynasty (960–1279)

When central government had again been restored, state veterinary hospitals were established, these each comprised separate clinics for moderately sick and for severely sick animals, a pharmacy and a post-mortem department. This latter inclusion is important to note as it shows a developing interest in internal anatomy, pathology and the causation of disease.

Books continued to be published, of which the most important was one of veterinary prescriptions, *Am ji yao fang*, followed by a pharmacopoeia, *Zheng lei ben cao*, which included 1558 'kinds of medicine'. These two books were said to have been published by order of the government (Sun and Chen 2009, p. 74). A military encyclopaedia published about 1004 described diseases of the horse including management advice, prescriptions, therapy, acupuncture and treatment of war wounds.

Yuan (Mongol) Dynasty (1280–1367)

The dynasty was established after the Mongol invasion: the emphasis remained on the horse. A 'famous horse veterinarian' (believed to be K'a Kuan Lon) produced a book, *Quan ji tong xuan lun* (*A Description of the Treatment of Sick Horses*) on equine disease with a particular emphasis on lameness. In about 1330 'beri-beri' (a lack of thiamine) was recognised as a nutritional deficiency disease in humans.

Ming Dynasty (1368–1644)

Progress continued with the government supporting private veterinary education facilities, which accepted 'only intelligent students'. In 1608 the veterinarian brothers Yu Ben-Yuan and Yu Ben-Heng wrote *Yuan heng liao ma ji* (*A Treatise on Horses*), which was a highly regarded work on equine diseases; a significant part of the content deals with acupuncture, illustrating the major points and meridians. New editions continued to be published up until 1957 and it remains widely respected in Asia. About the same time Yang Shih Ch'ao edited three books: *The Book of the Horse*, *The Book of Cattle* and *Prescriptions for Horses*. Additionally, *Ben cao gan mu* (*The Great Herbal*), compiled by Li Shi-Chen (1518–1593), was published in 1552, this detailed 1892 types of medications and 1096 prescription formulae, of which 229 were for animal diseases. In 52 volumes it was said to have taken 27 years to write.

Qing (Manchu) Dynasty (1644–1911)

In this, the last of the Chinese dynasties, there was a decline of both the standards and status of veterinary medicine; strict controls were placed on ownership and breeding of horses. Traditional Chinese medicine was being superseded by Western medical concepts, in particular after the Opium Wars in the mid-19th century. Society no longer regarded veterinarians as a respected profession.

In 1680 a book (title unclear) containing a compilation of texts relating to cattle and water buffalo appeared. The acupuncture points were detailed and a diagnostic procedure outlined which followed, in almost every action, that as prescribed for the human, including an examination of the animal's environment. Emphasis was given on reading the pulse, to be taken at the base of the tail. The detailed protocol was external examination only. Many diseases were described including bloat, lameness and infertility. The only surgical procedures were castration and abscess lancing. The treatments listed were all herbal medications. The first Chinese book on pig diseases, *Complete Collection of Pig Diseases* was produced in 1900 by Ju Jing Ta Qiuan: particular problems identified included diarrhoea and joint disorders. There was little indication of infectious disease, reflecting the housing of pigs in small family units.

In 1905 the Baoding School of Horse Medicine was opened, the first veterinary school modelled on Western teaching, with both traditional herbal remedies and acupuncture also being taught and used.

The establishment of the Republic of China in 1912 and the appointment of Sun Yat-sen as President heralded a new system of government. The first modern veterinary school was established later that year.

Since the 1949 Mao Zedong communist takeover 60 universities and colleges have been established providing veterinary education. They retain links to their traditional medicine past. In 1956 dedicated veterinary journals were introduced and by 2000 small animal practice had become significant.

Traditional Chinese Veterinary Medicine

The characteristics of traditional Chinese medicine (TCM) differ in almost every way from that of the West: being practised within a belief system that is unlike that in other cultures. It has a philosophical origin based on their observation of the world, and the way in which it is structured and is said to operate. Because of this the traditional practices have proved very resistant to Western concepts and developments in medicine. The belief in the *yin–yang* concept and the five element theory are deeply embedded in the culture as a way to correct the imbalances that cause disease.

Another important difference between Western and Chinese practice is the importance given to social well-being, for animals their welfare, and to diet. This was much related to the teachings of Confucius and Taoism, related to happiness as the basis for human health. This meant that the first concern of all medicine was the maintenance of health rather than the treatment and prevention of disease. For veterinarians this meant that their performance was judged by the mortality of their patients. From the historical record it can be seen that China has been much more progressive in its attitude towards medicine than other cultures. More than 2000 years ago veterinarians were listed as one of the four medical professions, with nutritionists, physicians and surgeons, entry to which was by a state examination system and grading of the graduates. The recognition of veterinary medicine as part of a total medical doctrine enabled a more rapid advance than that adopted in the West.

While Western medicine has become the lead influence in Chinese medical and veterinary practice, TCM remains as part of total medicine as well as being used in the less well populated areas of this enormous country. The extent of this inbuilt practice was demonstrated by the publication in 1970 of *A Barefoot Doctor's Manual*. The term 'barefoot doctor' was used for the paramedical assistants who supplement the professional staff. The book, in a translation of 960 pages, covers TCM and Western medicine with particular attention to herbal medicine, as well as acupuncture and moxibustion. These practices and many of the 522 listed herbs are also used in traditional veterinary practice (*Barefoot Doctor's Manual* 1974, pp. 75–695).

Nineteenth-Century Chinese Veterinary Medicine

Two reports by Western visitors are of interest. George Tradascant Lay (1841) obtained a copy of Chinese books which detailed veterinary practices and listed the principal ailments of the horse, water buffalo, sheep, dog, pigs and poultry; one book also discussed diseases of the camel. Forty-eight diseases were qualified by an illustration of the sick animal to show the visible symptoms. Twenty-nine diseases were considered incurable.

Medications included orpiment (arsenic sulphide), linseed oil, ashes of snakeskin, and a decoction of tobacco leaves for skin problems. The author added that most of the medicines used were unknown to the West except for alum for foot diseases and liquorice; he observed that to make a draught palatable, medications would be mixed with milk, wine or honey. The horse texts emphasised great care in judging the pulse with directions for the manner in which the middle three fingers of the right hand were to be applied to the artery, usually that on the neck. Fifty places were marked for acupuncture with some 'distinguished by very quaint epithets'. The use of the probang was listed for clearing oesophageal obstructions. Two types of cataract were described with two modes of operation, one using a 'needle with a small shaft' inserted into the upper part of the eyeball to remove an opaque lens. The author, a botanist and explorer, wrote in a very belittling, but probably Victorian, way of Chinese culture.

The other author, a British Army veterinarian on duty in China, wrote of his travels in the Manchu (Qing) Dynasty lands in 1861 (Fleming 1863, pp. 400–408). He describes meeting a *yima* or horse doctor, a 'well-to-do and intelligent personage' who ran a lively business. He was accompanied by a 'coolie' who carried his implements and medications. In Fleming's words,

> *he had a lot of idle notions, vague traditions and mouldy recipes . . . approved modes of performing operations handed down from experience of generations. His surgical instruments were in a brown leather case with two thongs to suspend it from his girdle belt. The instruments were carefully treasured . . . of great age.*

His practice was based (in Fleming's description) on the *yin* and *yang* together with beliefs in the celestial and the material worlds, and that all animals and inanimate nature may be divided into masculine and feminine. The *yima* cited the words of a learned author of a work on veterinary medicine written 'more than five generations ago' to the effect that:

> *though the forms and natures of the horse, ox and camel be so dissimilar, and so different from man, yet they are all equally amenable to the influences of the yin and yang; for as in him, it is only by a harmonious and due union of them in their proper proportions and qualities, that those sensitive conditions on which utility so much depends can be developed and maintained; when this is departed from disease is the result.*

Fleming noted that the horse doctor had a very poor knowledge of anatomy, but he did understand the arterial pulse at various points on the body and was interested in both the frequency and the force of the pulsations. He believed that the body was mapped out into 'gates of access' with names such as 'the golden gate' and 'the gate of life' and that these lead to various organs. When one is diagnosed as being in a morbid state he would 'stick a plaster or application' over the gate. (This appears to be describing the acupuncture meridians and points but in Fleming's description neither that word nor needles are mentioned.) If the condition was bad a little medication was given by mouth. Gentle methods are used but if these did not work there are more potent inducements. A head collar on a rope was slung from a tree branch and then slid on to the horse who is also fitted with a bent gag iron bit termed a *Tian chiau* or hanging bit. The rope was then pulled down to elevate the head and keep the mouth open, if this did not help accompanied by patting and so on, the *Nyng-tsz* or twister (in the West, a twitch) was used on upper or lower lip and a semi-liquid medication (said to be unpleasant) was given by a drenching horn.

The collection of instruments are described, of interest was a tube 'like a canula, made of goose or eagle quill with holes in the circumference at the round end. If a horse has a distended gut a cut is made over the large intestine and the tube introduced to release the gas'. For venesection in the jugular a barb shaped lancet is used with a little wooden mallet: but the doctor did not believe in bleeding, he did not think it was of any value. A seton was used, in the shape of a sailmaker's needle, to open abscesses and to leave in a medicated hemp thread for a period.

In discussion Fleming noted the doctor appeared to know 'a large class of diseases . . . including glanders' and expressed his ability to treat them. Should a horse eat from a pig's trough it was believed it would contract disease. If a serious disease outbreak occurred the custom was to burn incense to exorcise evil spirits or appease an angry god, but it was not thought wise to go after the good will of the god when all was well! Fleming was told that at that time there were no veterinary schools. In Beijing there was a Medical Hall but thought to be of little value, and an Imperial Academy in the capital claimed to teach medicine, but again there was little evidence. A final comment of interest, hippophagy was considered good human medicine, best from white horses. All parts of the horse had a medical use, except it was believed the liver was poisonous as it does not have a gall bladder. This report indicates that there were some deviations from TCM and not only a return to some of the shamanistic beliefs, but little or no advance in science. No new texts were known to this man, no veterinary education and little human medical education.

Current Chinese Veterinary Medicine

A more recent review of the medication products in use in Chinese veterinary practice (Bishop 2008, p. 98) notes the importance of herbal medications, which remain significant in Chinese pharmacy. Each herb is considered to be either *yin* or *yang* and to have a specific flavour and 'temperature', which determines its use for acting on specific organs. The example given is the plant *huo xiang*, an annual herb (*Agastache rugose*) and used to treat diarrhoea, vomiting or coughing. This herb is listed as number 514 in the *Barefoot Doctor's Manual*. The emphasis on herbal products, while founded on centuries of empirical experience is also based in the early Chinese belief that there was a plant to cure every disease. Tradition is a strong feature of Chinese behaviour: a 1955 book by Kim Chung Tze, *A New Treatise on Horses and Cattle*, using Western terminology was based on the Yu brothers notable book published in 1608 (in the Ming Dynasty), always highly regarded throughout Asia.

The current situation with the veterinary use of traditional medical procedures in small animal practice was investigated in 2014 (Kimm 2015, pp. 22–25). As many wealthy younger Chinese are acquiring pets, particularly dogs, there is an increasing demand for quality veterinary care, which is seen to be Western medicine. The investigation was centred at the Zheijang University Animal Hospital (ZUAH). The staff said that acupuncture was now only used occasionally, but the library held a number of very detailed veterinary acupuncture books. There was an electro-stimulation apparatus, used to activate relevant acupoints by either AC or DC current, but it was said to be little used. While moxibustion was no longer used at the ZUAH some older graduates would inject herbal extracts at the acupoints to increase the effects.

The university gave students thirty-two, forty-five minute lectures on traditional medicine, of which about 90% was on herbal medication and 10% on acupuncture. However, students expressed little interest in the subject, apart from passing the examinations, thinking it to be outdated. It appears that only at the Chinese Agricultural University was there active interest in acupuncture: they also taught a yearly course on the subject – for foreign veterinarians! The one part of TCM that has always attracted the most attention has been acupuncture: to the uninitiated, a rather unique mixture of intricate detailed procedure and mystical magic. In the period 1522–1800 some 920 Jesuit missionaries visited and collected Chinese knowledge to bring back to Europe – publication of their findings in technologies, art and medicine were avidly read. Acupuncture was a particular interest and was taught in the early veterinary schools in France, Germany, Austria and Eastern Europe. Its use gradually declined but had the greatest influence in France. The interest has existed however, exemplified by the studies in 1958 by Wolfgang Jöchle in Berlin who was able to demonstrate, by electroconductivity methods, the existence of the meridian lines in the horse, donkey, cattle, pigs and dogs.

Herbal medicine products are widely available in China and used, mainly by farmers for pigs, cattle and chickens. The principle indication appears to be as immune stimulants for treating viral infections, fever control, upper respiratory tract infections and hepatic stimulation. The ZUAH held eight different herbal medications, many of which were purified and injected intravenously. One herbal medication called *Shuang Huang Lian* contained honeysuckle (*Scutellaria baicalensis*) and *Forsythia Suspense Vahl*. It is given intravenously to both animals and humans to control fever and pneumonic infection.

It is possible that the use of traditional medicine in Taiwan differs from that in mainland China because there was a report of the use of acupuncture to induce the onset of oestrus in pigs (Hsia and Lee 1988, pp. 374–376). It was stated that this intervention was commonly, but not widely, used in the Taiwanese pig industry. Two needles are inserted at named (*pai hui* and *wen ken*) acupoints and activity stimulated by one or more of four methods, either rotated by hand to produce the necessary stimulation, used with *moxa* (dried herb) fixed on the needle shaft and ignited, used with glucose solution injected at the acupoint or by electro-acupuncture being applied at low intensity. Choice of method is either that of the operator preference or the operator deciding the degree of stimulation required. Oestrus is produced in about seven days after treatment. The records shown in the paper indicate a 60–80% success rate (lowest in gilts, highest in sows) and is usually required in the summer months when anoestrus can be a problem. No details are given of the history or discovery of this procedure: from the English-language literature surveyed this appears to be a unique example of this procedure being used to act as a hormonal stimulant rather than an ailment treatment.

INDO-CHINA

Vietnam is the largest, and a coastal, territory of the region once known as Indo-China that has always been influenced by China. This influence, in its most direct form, was being coming under Chinese rule for over 1000 years (197 BC–AD 937). Vietnamese traditional medicine has a history dating back over 2000 years, always with a dominating interest in herbal products. As a tropical country there is a very diverse range of plant species: some 1300 plants/shrubs/trees have a claimed medical therapeutic use.

Traditional medicine is a major factor in folklore beliefs (which are still followed by much of the population). Two types of traditional medicine, *Y hoc co truyen Viet Nam*, are recognised: *Thuoc Nam* or southern medicine or herbology and influenced by Chinese medicine, and *Thuoc Bac* or northern medicine or herbology, which is essentially *Trung Yi*, TCM. The southern medicine protocol relies totally on indigenous Vietnamese ingredients: these are either used fresh or dried, unlike Chinese preparations which are mainly used as decoctions. The local procedures are much simpler than the complex Chinese preparations. Following the Chinese influence acupuncture features as a part of Vietnamese medicine.

Traditional Vietnamese medicine dates back to the Hung Vuong Dynasty, over 2000 years ago. The acknowledged 'founder' of this medical doctrine was Tue Tinh (c.1330–1385) a Buddhist monk, who wrote an 11-volume work titled *Nam duoc than hieu*, included in the text are recommended herbal treatments for animal diseases. Several veterinary treatises were known but due to the tropical climate little of the early documentation has survived. During the next century (c.1428) the first Vietnamese pharmacy book was produced, listing the indigenous plant materials used in medications. Veterinary medicine appears to have become a recognised art by the 18th century. Herbal treatments have been, and still are, a major feature of the traditional human and veterinary medical practices in Vietnam. An old saying in the country is *Doi rau dau thuoc*, 'when hungry eat vegetables, when sick take medicinal herbs'.

The two smaller territories, now known as Cambodia and Laos, were in earlier times part of the Khmer or Angkor Empire, which also reached into present-day Thailand. Chinese influence was not as pronounced here as in Vietnam.

KOREA

A country with a most difficult and complex history, having to cope with varying degrees of Chinese occupation and influence together with an early period of three independent states (Korea, Kudara and Shiragi) until unification in AD 676. Japan invaded in 1592 and 1597 followed by Manchu invasions in 1627 and 1637. Finally, Japan began to exert its influence from 1871, forcing out China and then annexing the country in 1910, until it was freed at the end of the Second World War in 1945.

Through these many vicissitudes a highly sophisticated culture evolved (in 1234 they developed the first moveable metal type). Like many civilisations they had a 'golden age', this centred around the reign of Sejong the Great (1418–1450), in the Joseon Dynasty in the 15th and 16th centuries. The Korean alphabet was created and advanced printing. Particular progress was made in meteorological studies, ceramics and agriculture.

Traditional Korean medicine, called *Hangul* or *Hanja* can be traced back at least 3000 years, with a strong basis in the use of herbal medication and diet control to maintain health. There has always been a determination by Korean rulers to build and keep a separate national identity. In medicine this is shown by the early creation of their own herbal listing which included wormwood and garlic – both entities not recorded in the Chinese treatises. In the Three Kingdoms Period (AD 892–935) there was much influence from Chinese medicine, but this was followed by the Goryeo Dynasty when there was intensive study of herbs. Books were written, in particular including those herbs felt to be indigenous to Korea. During the Chinese Song Dynasty (AD 960–1279) there was a significant importation of Chinese medical texts. Korean medicine developed with its own individual methods, but the Chinese influences remained.

Medicine flourished during the Joseon Dynasty (1392–1897), a notable text *Hyangyak Gugeupbang* (*Prescriptions Using Native Ingredients*) was written and both doctors and nurses were trained. Sejong the Great took a particular interest in medicine and developed the use of Korean medical ingredients. This enabled the publication of the *Hyangyak Jipseongbang* (1433), which listed 703 native remedies, to break away from Chinese influence. Later a book by Heo Jun, *Dongeui Bogan* (c.1590s) integrated Korean and Chinese medicine procedures and treatments.

Two major influences on Korean medicine were Confucianism (which replaced Buddhism), and the *Sasong* typology which identified four main human body types and advocated specific treatment methods for each type. This was related to the link between health and the state of mind of the patient – a strong Confucian influence. Traditional Korean medicine is based in native herbal therapy, with the group including not just plants and their parts but also decoctions from shrubs, trees, moss, lichen, fungi and seaweed. Acupuncture and moxibustion are included. All were used in what was known as the Sasong Constitutional Medicine framework concept.

Korean Veterinary Medicine

Korean veterinary medicine was based in the same concept as human medicine and had the horse as its initial and primary interest. The oldest known Korean equine text *Sin pyeon jip seong ma ui bang* (*New Compilation of Prescriptions for Horse Diseases*) was written in 1399. This book is thought to have a strong relationship to the Chinese treatise of the 9th century, *Si mu an ji ji* (*The Collection of Ways to Relieve Suffering of a Horse*) edited by Li Su. The other Korean horse classic is *Ma kyeong eon hae* (*A Collection of Ways to Heal Horses*) produced in 1635 by I Soe; this is essentially a translation of the book by the Chinese brothers Yu Ben-Yuan and Yu Ben-Heng written about 1608, in the Ming Dynasty.

Korean veterinary practice was strongly influenced by TCM; taking the *yin–yang* belief they developed their own system using similar concepts to reach a diagnosis and determining a treatment programme. A wide variety of herbal medications with acupuncture and moxibustion were used. The veterinary practitioners had little understanding of anatomy and physiology but they did acquire some comparative anatomical knowledge. Surgery was limited to castration and abscess treatment.

Recent studies of the texts translated from the Chinese by Korean scholars (Chun and Yang 2007, pp. 24–31) have noted that the work was conducted by Korean Confucians, whose teachings regard sexual desire as a rudimentary animal instinct, therefore any subject involving the topic was seen as immoral and shameful. As a result, in the translation of the two equine texts there is very little information on gynaecology and andrology. The authors conclude that as those who cared for horses were well acquainted with these problems the knowledge was transmitted by word of mouth.

Livestock Husbandry

Livestock husbandry has traditionally been based in cattle, pigs and poultry with only marginal interest in sheep, goats and silkworms. The consumption of dog meat has a long Korean history, it is believed to have medicinal properties, but is now declining in popularity. Currently while pork remains popular, both poultry and beef are becoming important. Extensive aquaculture has a long history and in recent years intensive systems have been introduced as the demand for seafood increases. Arable farming is limited due to the mountainous terrain: rice cultivation is the major segment of the industry, assisted by a novel system of utilisation of animal wastes following treatment with local anaerobic micro-organisms to produce enhanced soil structure and fertility. As in other countries, pet keeping, in particular of dogs, is increasing. Currently there are 10 veterinary schools in the Republic of Korea (South Korea).

There is little knowledge of veterinary practice in the Democratic People's Republic of Korea (North Korea). Reports have identified animal waste seen in the streets and examination of defectors to South Korea have revealed high levels of helminth infestation – suggesting that anthelmintic availability is limited. It is noted that the Chief of State, Kim Jong-Un, in 2016 praised the eating of dog meat as a way to improve stamina.

JAPAN

Located off the eastern coast of Asia, Japan comprises 6852 islands, with the four largest, Honshu, Hokkaido, Kyushu and Shikoku, forming some 97% of the land area. Human habitation has been dated to the Upper Palaeolithic period (between 50,000 to 10,000 years ago), with the first written mention in Chinese texts (*The Book of Han*) from the 1st century AD. Chinese influence has played a significant role in Japanese history, Japan has also had several periods of self-imposed isolation.

The islands are a volcanic archipelago, the terrain is mountainous and forested with about 12% of the land suitable for agriculture. Most available land has historically been used for rice cultivation. Livestock populations, mainly pigs and poultry, have been small, cattle were originally only used for draught and there are few sheep and goats. Horses were the most important animals for ceremonial, war and transport. Seafood has always been a major part of the diet.

Ancient Japan was ruled by many small clans and kingdoms, which were frequently in conflict. There was periodic immigration from China, introducing rice, its cultivation and metallurgy. In the Kofun period (AD 250–538) the country gradually unified to a single state and kingdom. From this the Japanese imperial family trace their origin, making it the world's longest dynastic house.

The first clearly defined cultural structure was the Asuka period (538–710) when the *yin–yang* and five elements medical concepts were introduced from China. At the same time Buddhism was introduced from Korea and became a widespread teaching, but sharing importance with Shinto, the traditional Japanese religion noted for its ritual procedures. This was followed by the Nara period (710–794) during which a centralised state evolved with an imperial court and emperor. In the Heian period (794–1185) a clearly defined Japanese culture emerged, which became dominated by the *samurai* warrior cult. During this time Japan was blighted by a smallpox outbreak (812–814) said to have killed over one-third of the population.

As a part of establishing a definite culture there was an early wish to codify laws. This was eventually achieved in 927 with the formulation of the *Engishiki* statutes. From 1185 until 1600, in the Kamakura, Muromachi and Azuchi-Momoyama periods, the country, with a declining Chinese influence, was troubled by competing warlords. Following the decisive Battle of Sekigahara, Japan was ruled by feudal military *shoguns* acting in the name of the emperor. This Edo period (1600–1868) was one of stability and isolation, ending in 1854 after the US fleet pressured the Japanese rulers to open the country for trade with the West. In 1868 the imperial court regained full power, termed the Meiji Restoration. Following a unification of all sectors of the country under the rule of the emperor, there was a sudden movement to become 'Westernised'.

Western Influences

Contact with the outside world, and in particular Western civilisation, had been resisted by successive rulers until the 19th-century American intervention. Previous contacts had been limited to two encounters, the first in 1542 when Portuguese traders landed at Tanegashima island. They introduced guns to the Japanese and also made them aware of Western medicine, which attracted much attention. In 1549 Francis Xavier the Jesuit missionary landed at Kagoshima and began his mission, but within a year his work was banned. The Portuguese were instrumental in founding the port of Nagasaki and later developed an Asian slave trade, but were expelled in 1638.

In the 17th century other traders arrived, the English soon withdrew but the Dutch prospered following their arrival in 1641. As with previous visitors the Japanese avidly adopted the new ideas they brought; Calvinism replaced Catholicism, a Germanic language replaced a Latin one, and in particular, Western medical practice was adopted. Western sciences (*rangaku*) developed rapidly, based in the Dutch enclave or *dejima,* established on an artificial island in Nagasaki bay. The island was originally constructed to house the Portuguese traders and had been created as a method of constraining the activities of foreign traders (and their believed wider influence). It became the Dutch trading post from 1641 until 1853. During the Edo period this was the sole contact that Japan had with the outside world.

Japanese Medicine

Traditional medicine (*kampo*), as still practised in Japan, derives from the original input from Chinese medicine. The influence began in the 4th century AD when Chinese culture entered Japan and their medical practice supplanted the native medicine. Little is known of the pre-Chinese period; legends indicate that there was only rudimentary anatomical knowledge, with disease beliefs based on evil spirits and divine influence.

Initially the influence came with the importation and translation of early texts, in particular *Shen Nung Pen Tsao Ching*, the herbal classic. The first contact was when a Korean doctor from Silla visited in AD 414 and introduced the Korean practice, based on Chinese medicine. This was followed by another Korean doctor from Kokuryo in 459, who lived in Osaka, and then by Korean herbalists from Kudara in 554.

In 608 two Japanese students were sent to China at the time of the Sui Dynasty (AD 220–618) to study TCM. This produced national interest and in 701 the first Japanese medical system – the *Taiho* statutes – were formulated. In 753 a celebrated Chinese priest-physician, Chien-Chen, came to Japan and trained students.

Japanese medicine began to establish its own character and in 808 the first pharmacopoeia of Japanese medicinal plants, the *Daido-Ruijuho*, compiled by Manao Abe and Hirosada Izumo, was published in 100 volumes. Next in 982, Tambo Yasuyori produced the 30-volume *Ishimpo*, the oldest existing Japanese medical treatise, based on the Chinese *yin–yang* and five element concepts; Menase Dosan wrote several medical works, of which *Keitekishu* (1574) (*A Manual of Medicine*), was highly regarded. In the 16th century Nagata Tokohun, a reformer and physician, started to reduce the emphasis of Chinese medicine on Japanese practice: his two most well-known works were *I-no-ben* (1585) and *Baika Mujinzo* (1611). This latter treatise held that the aim of medical treatment was to support the 'natural force' and therefore the doctor had to understand the patient.

The arrival of the Portuguese in 1542 introduced the concept of Western medicine. Once the Dutch traders had established their position medical ideas began to transfer, initially through a German physician, Engelbert Kempfer, who came to advise the Dutch community. In 1722 the *Wayaku Aratame Kaisho* was created to check the quality of locally made pharmaceuticals – the origin of the Institute for Drug Inspection. The first Japanese publication on Western medicine, *Kaitai Shinso* (1774) in five volumes, based on anatomical studies, was compiled by Genpaku Sugita, and in 1805 the 48 volumes of *Honzo Komoku Keimo*, an *Encyclopaedia of Medicine* by Shokko Ono was published.

Japan soon adopted Western medicine. Smallpox had been a recurring problem in Japan with several severe epidemics. European vaccination procedures were introduced by a Dutch physician and in 1850 a vaccination institute was established, national programmes soon brought about eradication of the disease. The first medical school and teaching hospital was established in 1857 headed by a Dutch physician, Dr Pompe van Meerdervoort. The government sent Japanese students to train in European medical schools, and then built a number of medical schools with German, English and American aid. However, Japanese doctors and the public both kept an interest in traditional medicine.

Livestock Husbandry in Japan

Domesticated animals had a different place in Japanese culture compared with other countries. The first and, for a long period, the most important aspect was silkworm breeding, discussed in Chapter 26. Veterinary care did not develop until horses were imported in the 5th century AD from Korea. These small Mongolian animals provided the stock from which local breeds were evolved and the horse soon became a symbol of the state, and warfare in the Samurai period, until in the years of war from the 16th to 17th centuries when active interest in breeding declined. Following the 1868 Meiji Restoration large numbers of European and American horses were imported with a consequent increase in equine breeding and development.

Horses have always been important in Japan: the large Buddhist temples kept white horses as they were considered holy, they were well fed and had long lives. Horses were also valuable as pack animals in the mountainous regions, and when Westernised technologies were introduced Tokyo established a tramway system which at its peak employed some 600 horses. Horse racing was introduced by European settlers and soon became popular with the public. The army was slow to introduce cavalry but by 1888 had some 10,000 horses.

Cattle were imported between 300 BC and AD 300, but following the introduction of Buddhism the eating of meat was not encouraged and cattle became of minor importance, except as draught animals. From the first Portuguese traders who slaughtered cattle for consumption (to the amazement and consternation of the Japanese) the consumption of meat grew very slowly. Eventually in 1866 Tokyo opened its first slaughterhouse to supply foreigners and in 1882 meat was included in the army diet. Japanese cattle were not dairy breeds and milk production animals were imported, mainly from the USA. By 1890 the Tokyo area had 214 farms with 2000 dairy cows. Butter and milk sales grew slowly (limited by lactose intolerance); cheese was not acceptable to the Japanese taste. Sheep and goats have always had a minor role in Japanese farming, and pig breeding was only developed in the later 19th century. Poultry have been bred since very early times and later improved by imported breeds. Rabbits were introduced in 1873 (Janson 1892, pp. 321–335).

Veterinary Medicine in Japan

From very early days animals were second place as a food protein to seafood – the dominant influence in the Japanese diet. From ancient times the horse was the primary veterinary interest, for warfare, ceremonial uses and transport. Following the introduction of Buddhism in AD 538 imperial edicts were published prohibiting the slaughter and consumption of meat from cattle, horses, dogs and poultry. Eggs could be consumed and milk, but lactose intolerance and the lack of dairy breeds constrained this; there was little impetus for veterinary practice.

The development of veterinary medicine has a mythological beginning. In the *Kojiki*, the oldest Japanese historical work, the story is told of a god named Ookuninushi-no-Mikoto finding a hare which was crying because its hair had been removed and its skin was sore. Apparently the hare had jumped on the backs of a line of sharks by a trick, as a way to reach an island. The angry sharks reacted by plucking the hare. The helpful god suggested the hare should wash its body in clean water and then wrap itself in the flowers of *gama* (a bulrush), the hare recovered (Katsuyama 1994, p. 453).

In AD 595 a Korean Buddhist priest who was said to be 'well trained in horse veterinary' visited Japan on the invitation of Crown Prince Shotokutaishi. He taught Tachibana-no-Ihitsu the veterinary art. Later the first veterinary school, *Taishi-ryu*, was established in Japan, presumably teaching the arts of acupuncture and moxibustion. The Emperor Bunbu issued the *Taiho* laws in 701; in these are listed the medical department employees and naming the official ranks of masseur, veterinarians, pharmacists and milkmen. The imperial stables were shown as having 50 milkmen and four veterinarians on the staff. Records also show that in the reigns of Emperors Gansho (718) and Shomu (749) court veterinarians were listed as civil officials of good professional standing (Burns 1948, p. 226).

During the reign of Emperor Kammu a member of the imperial court, Taira-no-Nakakuni, was sent to China in 805 to study Chinese veterinary medicine. When he returned to Japan a school was established in his name, *Nakakuni-ryu*, and with his two sons he also wrote a book *A Hundred Veterinary Questions and Answers*; later the school's name was changed to *Kuwajima Ryu* (Burns 1948, p. 227).

The role of the veterinarian, for the care of horses, remained of importance in the imperial court and in 827 an official number of staff veterinarians was established. In 877 a report to the emperor on the number of horses treated was made by veterinarian Kotaku Kiyo-uchi, and when the Emperor Daigo visited the Hirano shrine in 898, one Shinto priest and one veterinarian were included in his party. Some old records of the feudal civil wars mention that every warlord was accompanied by a veterinarian, described in a book, *Bogu Yosetsu* (*War Equipment*).

In 1207 a treatise variously named *Bai Soshi*, *Umai no Soshi* or *Bai Zukan* (*The Scroll of Horse Doctors*) was written on the instruction of Sei-a, a priest and horse doctor, to instruct his son Tadayasu. The scroll is notable for its superb drawings of horses as well as portraits of one Hakuraku and nine other prominent horse doctors. Seventeen herbs for equine medication are listed.

Doha Hashimoto translated a Chinese veterinary treatise in 1604 and published it in 12 volumes as *Kana-Anki-Shu*; the work includes illustrations of equine anatomy together with many recipes for equine prescriptions. The medications were described in detail with quantities of each ingredient (almost all herbal) and doses for horses according to their body size. The Chinese medical principles together with the use of acupuncture and moxibustion are all described. Other texts published in this period were *Yoba-Higoku-Shu* (*Secret Methods Essential for Horses*) in 1688, *Ryoyaku-Baryo-Benkai* (*Explanation of Useful Medications for Treatment of Equine Diseases*) in 1705 and *Buba-Hitsuyo* (*Essentials for Military Horses*) in 1717 (Katsuyama 1994, p. 454).

During the 17th century, Shogun Tsunayoshi showed genuine welfare concern and had a stable constructed at Yotsuya (Tokyo) to accommodate sick horses within the area. He was particularly notable for issuing dog protection laws, 'anyone who injures a dog shall be given the death penalty, and anyone who kills an animal shall be beheaded and exposed at a public place, and become an object of severe public criticism and contempt'. Many provisions were made in the laws covering such issues as whelping care, canine diet and exercise. How comprehensively these laws were obeyed, and in which regions of Japan, is unclear. In this period veterinarians who were on the government staff had power and dignity and were always attended by six retainers. The animal welfare laws were abolished in 1704, after nearly 30 years, at the accession of Shogun Ineroi (Burns 1948, p. 227).

A small animal specialist, Heisuke Imagawa, living in the 17th century was celebrated due to his therapeutic methods, and his development and use of a 'plaster' made from red beans and urine. If this failed to cure a decoction was made from dried grass soaked in urine for 100 days, then washed in water for three days and dried. It was applied topically and given orally. He was said to achieve an outstanding recovery rate, the medication was also used as a human therapeutic: he accumulated great wealth.

The Influence of Western Veterinary Medicine

Following the introduction of Western medicine veterinary textbooks were obtained from Dutch traders and translated, and human medicine developments were studied. In 1725 Hans Jurgen Keijser came to Dejima, he was a keen equestrian and brought five European horses and a collection of Dutch veterinary books to Japan. He visited the shogun and presented the books, which were translated to Japanese, but remained in government hands and were not circulated. In 1840 Kikuchi Tosui, known as 'the old curesmith of Yedo' taught many students and in 1852 wrote a book *Kaiba-Shinsho* (*New Book of the Anatomy of the Horse*). This publication has been described as the start of a new age in Japanese veterinary medicine (Janson 1891, pp. 61–80).

The veterinary culture in Japan at this time was almost totally devoted to equine work and part of a structure that was controlled by the imperial court. Horseshoes had not been invented in Japan and when required hoofs were protected by straw sandals. In 1858 the British ambassador arrived bringing with him some 25 horses as mounts for his bodyguard, with shoes. This created great interest followed by the development of a Japanese version – powdered iron was mixed with powdered bracken, placed on the ventral surface of the hoof, covered with sheets of paper and then had a hot iron applied until the mixture solidified (the procedure may be lacking in description). It apparently gave some protection (Burns 1948, p. 228). About 1861 the system of feudal government ended with the last days of Shogun Keiki. The establishment of government retainer veterinarians and official state stables were abolished, and with it much of the pageantry of Japanese government.

With the Meiji Restoration in 1868 Western veterinary education began. In 1870 Japan sent two officials to the USA to be trained in animal husbandry; following their return Dr George A. Etchall came to Japan and established an experimental farm at Komaba, a Tokyo suburb, to deal with the importation and breeding of purebred horses. In 1872 the Ministry of Education proposed a veterinary school curriculum based on three years preparatory work and two of veterinary medicine tuition. Schools were established in Tokyo and Sapporo. Overseas scientific staff were sought (Burns 1945, p. 227).

In 1874 Lieutenant Auguste D. Angot of the French Army Veterinary Corps became the first foreign teacher at the Tokyo Komaba Agricultural School in the newly formed veterinary department: he taught equine veterinary medicine to military horse doctors until 1878. In 1876 he was joined by John A. McBride, an English veterinarian, who remained there until 1879: he founded the first veterinary school at Komaba, which produced the first 15 graduates in 1880. The head of the veterinary department was a physician, Dr Sugita who had been taught by two German physicians. Later the school became the veterinary department of Tokyo University Agricultural College.

In 1880 after McBride had left, two Germans joined the staff, Johannes Ludwig Janson, a royal Prussian veterinary officer and Carl Troester, a junior veterinarian. From December 1880 they taught at the Komaba school, in 1882 another 20 students graduated (they had been taught by McBride for one year, Japanese teachers for one year and two years by Janson and Troester). In June 1883, 31 graduates received their *Jui Gakusha* diploma with the same status as all other Tokyo university graduates. Between 1883 and 1890, 107 veterinarians graduated and the faculty included five Japanese professors and assistants. At that time there were eight other veterinary schools, official figures show that about 3000 veterinarians were working in Japan (Janson 1891, pp. 61–80).

In May 1890, the first veterinary congress was held in Tokyo with 200 participants. The veterinary school under Janson's direction was highly successful: the preparatory three-year agricultural training included anatomy and Latin tuition for the future veterinarians. The three-year veterinary course did not include food and slaughterhouse hygiene but otherwise followed the teaching at the Berlin School.

Janson was also active in the broader environment. While epidemic disease control was well run with reporting, slaughter of infected livestock, disposal of cadavers and hygiene there was no import control and rinderpest spread to Japan from Korea in 1890 and 1893. Janson described two outbreaks of what he called Oriental Cattle Plague on the island of Honshu, following importation of Korean cattle: he described it as 'no more dangerous than influenza'. Among his own studies he investigated dog parasites, in particular heartworm (*Dirofilaria immitis*), a widespread problem. Janson also had an interest in both the Chinese and the Japanese veterinary medicine literature and understood the difficulties in translation. In 1891 he published a critical review of the texts (Janson 1891, pp. 347–357). He was part author of 16 volume *Kachiku-Ihan* (*Standard Textbook for Animal Medicine*) 1887, written by the staff of the Komaba school (Kast 2010, p. 113).

Janson (1849–1914) was an impressive pioneer of Western medicine in Japan with many of his graduates achieving high office. Following his 22 years of work he was decorated and received the honorary title of professor emeritus at Tokyo University and uniquely was honoured with a bust, now preserved in the Tokyo Veterinary School. He married Haruko Taniyama and is buried in her hometown of Kagoshima (Kast 2010, p. 110).

Rabies was recognised as a disease, with a description and treatments included in *Ishimpo* (AD 982) the oldest existing Japanese medical treatise, mostly translated from the Chinese. But neither this nor other texts record the real existence of the disease until many centuries later. The first case of canine rabies was reported in 1732 in Nagasaki, the only port in which overseas ships were allowed to dock in the Edo period (1639–1854). The outbreak spread to Hiroshima and reached Tokyo in 1736, then taking 29 years to reach the north of Honshu Island. Following the Buddhist belief, dogs were generally allowed to roam free and in 1873 there was a severe epidemic in Tokyo, and again in 1892 and 1893. An infectious diseases law was passed in 1897, from that time cases were reported and recorded. Another epidemic in 1907 was followed by a particularly bad outbreak in 1924, then vaccination was introduced. Eradication was finally achieved in 1957, but compulsory vaccination of dogs is still enforced (Kurosawa et al. 2017, pp. 240–243). Rabies is also mentioned in *Kyoken Kosho Jiho* (1756) by G. Noro, *Keiku Shoko* (1836) by M. Hara and *Kenku Yochiku Den* (1847) by A. Kanenari.

Japan has played a role in the global progress in immunology and microbiology. Led by Shibasaburo Kitasato (1851–1931) who cultivated the cholera bacillus (*Vibrio cholerae*), produced the first pure culture of the tetanus bacillus (*Clostridium tetani*) and was co-discoverer of the believed plague bacillus (*Yersinia pestis*). He worked under Robert Koch and Emil von Behring in Germany and established the Kitasato Institute in Japan with a Veterinary Division. His work advanced worldwide veterinary vaccine development.

Traditional Japanese Veterinary Medicine

Four significant influences can be determined in Japanese veterinary practice: initially in the early years, animal disease was attributed to evil spirits or gods, and cures to divine intervention. This was followed by, in AD 595, the importation of the Korean version of veterinary TCM, which was well accepted until the introduction of Buddhism in the 6th century. Finally, the Meiji Restoration in 1868 was followed by the rapid absorption of Western medicine.

One of the most potent reminders of the early shamanistic times has remained as a strong folk memory: horse owners were afraid of the god Daiba, as should a horse become possessed by this god they would die instantly – this was said to occur outside most likely when acting as a pack animal or on a mountain trail. In some districts Daiba would appear as a goddess, dressed in scarlet and riding a multi-coloured horse. Should a horse be attacked the owner had a, very slender, chance of saving its life if the ear of the horse was cut, as Daiba disliked the sight of fresh blood. Remedies for treatment at this time also included prayers, spells and the use of certain herbs (Katsuyama 1994, p. 458).

Following the introduction of Chinese medicine, while the panoply of *yin–yang* and the five elements played a major role in human practice, the veterinary use concentrated more on the application of acupuncture and moxibustion, usually only for horses and cattle. In Japanese use the acupoints were known as *tsubo* and the meridians *keiraku*. The needles used were, as in human medicine, of various sizes and metals. For moxibustion the most frequently used moxa was from *Artemisia moxa*. The use of herbal medication expanded with much investigation of native herbs.

As Buddhist practice spread in Japan it coexisted with the native Shinto belief. Two guardian deities were celebrated: *Dainichi Nyorai* (Buddha) for cattle and *Bato-Kannon* (a Buddhist saint) for horses. Statues or monuments to the latter were frequently erected at crossroads or where horses had died. Straw sandals, then used on both horses and cattle, were given as a votive dedication when praying for cattle health to *Dainichi Nyorai*. Up to the present time at the temple to *Bato-Kannon* in Kamioka (in Saitama prefecture), on festival days bamboo grass and *ema*, a votive tablet of a horse, are presented as a charm against *Daiba*, or when an owner is praying for the health of their horse. In other similar temples bamboo grass plays a role in prayer for the health of horses and cattle. In some districts of Kyushu an abalone shell may be hung over the entrance to stables or cattle housing, as a charm to protect the animals. In the 12th century the Chinese god *Bareki-Shin*, the guardian of the stable, was introduced and is frequently depicted in statues (Katsuyama 1994, pp. 459–460). Venesection was also practised, both to protect against *Daiba* as well as a belief that regular bleeding would help to maintain cattle and equine health. Villages would have a specific enclosure for the annual practice which would be conducted by the *hakuraku* or *bakuro* (horse doctors).

There is little literature on early canine medicine. One book *Kenku Yochiku Den* (1842) details a variety of treatments: for mange, washing with extract of 'good quality' tea was said to be effective; for flea and lice control the application of camphor was used. A recommendation for wound treatment was the feeding of adzuki or soya beans. The feeding of shrimp was not advised as it would cause leg weakness and intoxication. It was recorded that puppies should be treated as children.

At the time of writing Japan has 16 universities, institutions, colleges and schools awarding veterinary degrees. This has resulted in a debate on the number of graduate veterinarians that will be needed for the country's projected requirements.

References

Anonymous (1974) *A Barefoot Doctor's Manual*, published by Institute of Traditional Chinese Medicine, Hunan Province 1970. Translated and published by US Department of Health, Education and Welfare: DHEW Publication No. (NIH)

Bishop, S. (2008) Traditional Chinese Veterinary Medicine. *Veterinary History* **14**

Burns, K.F. (1948) The History of Veterinary Medicine in Japan. *Journal American Veterinary Medical Association* **113** No.838

Chun, M.-S. and Yang, I.-S. (2007) Gynecology and Andrology, Reluctant Themes in Traditional Korean Veterinary Medicine (Conference Proceedings). *Geschichte der Gynäkologie und Andrology*. Hannover: Deutsche Veterinärmedizische Gesellschaft

Edwards, J.T. (1945) A Short History of the Veterinary Art in Antiquity. *Veterinary Record* **57**

Edwards, J.T. (1945) Eminent Veterinary Clinicians of the Past. *Veterinary Record* **57**

Fleming, G. (1863) *Travels on Horseback in Mantchu Tartary: being a summer's ride beyond the great wall of China with a map and numerous illustrations*. London: Hurst and Blackett

Hsia, L.C. and Lee, J.H. (1988) Inducing Oestrus in Sows by Acupuncture. *Clinical Insight* **3** issue 8 [reprinted from *Pig International* April, 1988]

Janson, J.L. (1891) Chinesis-Japanische Veterinärmedizinische Literatur. *Arch. wiss. prakt. Tierhlkd.* **17**

Janson, J.L. (1891) Tierheilkunde in Japan. *Arch. wiss. prakt Tierhlkd.* **17**

Janson, J.L. (1892) Haustiere in Japan. *Arch. wiss. prakt Tierhlkd* **18**

Kast, A. (2010) Johannes Ludwig Janson, Professor of Veterinary Medicine in Tokyo 1880–1902. *Acta. med-hist Adriat.* **8** (1)

Katsuyama, O. (1994) Veterinary Folk Remedies in Japan. *Rev. Sci tech. Off. Int. Epiz.* **13** No.2

Kimm, J. (2015) Acupuncture and herbal medicine use in animals. *Companion* June

Kurosawa, A., Tojinbara, K., Kadowaki, H., Hampson, K., Yamada, A. and Makita, K. (2017) The Rise and Fall of Rabies in Japan: a Quantitative History of Rabies Epidemics in Osaka prefecture, 1914–1933. *PLoS Neglected Trop. Dis.* **11** No.3

Margotta, R. (1996) *History of Medicine.* London: Hamlyn

Sournia, J.-C. (1992) *The Illustrated History of Medicine.* London: Starke

Sun, Y. and Chen, J. (2009) History of Veterinary Medicine in China. *Veterinary History* **15** No.1

Tradascant Lay, J. (1841) The Veterinary Art in China. *Veterinarian* **14**

Wong, K.C. and Wu, L.T. (1932) *History of Chinese Medicine.* Tientsin: Tientsin Press

CHAPTER 8

South Asia: India, Pakistan, Bangladesh, Myanmar, Sri Lanka, Malaysia and Tibet

The first three countries listed only appeared as separate entities in the mid-20th century following independence from British rule. They now coexist but are reviewed under India. Myanmar (Burma) and Sri Lanka (Ceylon) similarly obtained independence but are reviewed separately. Malaysia (Federated Malay States) was under British control at the same time as India. Tibet, now under Chinese control, had developed a veterinary culture founded in its relationship with India and a shared Buddhist belief, as well as its proximity to China.

INDIA

The subcontinent, bordered by the Arabian Sea on the north-west, Bay of Bengal to the east and Indian Ocean to the south, forms a separate and distinctive part of Asia. The Himalayan mountain range effectively delineates the north and east and the Iranian plateau in the west. The region is sufficiently supplied with natural resources within these boundaries to develop with a degree of isolation.

The land mass, essentially in the arid zone, is strongly affected by the monsoon rains. These are the common factor in the climatic variety. The north and west have six seasons of climate variation which affect both agriculture and health. Rainfall is excessive on the west coast, and in Bengal and Assam, but deficient on much of the Deccan plateau in the south and in Rajasthan (between Delhi and Karachi).

Agriculture has always been important in the Indian economies, with the emphasis on crop farming; currently arable land represents about 53% of the total while permanent pasture is less than 4%. The main food products are rice, millet and vegetables. Due to religious taboos meat consumption has been traditionally low: buffalo are used for agriculture (and limited milk production), sheep, goats, poultry and fish are farmed and of great value to the subsistence farmers. Donkeys are widely used for transport and horses have a long history of importance for warfare, status and ceremonial. Elephants have importance in certain areas for logging and ceremonial; in earlier times they were much used in war. For India, the population of some 200 million cattle preserved for religious reasons are within economic terms, a liability.

India (the country today) is the world's seventh largest and the second most populous with 1.3 billion people. The core of the population live in the north, in particular in the Ganges river valley basin. There are twenty-two official languages but English is in general use. Religion is an important factor across the whole region. While Pakistan and Bangladesh are essentially Muslim countries, India has Hinduism as the main religion followed by Islam, with Sikhism mainly to the west and north and Christianity more diffusely spread. The differing religions all have dietary rules and practices which influence the need for and use of veterinary care.

Historical Background

The Dravidian Civilisation

Archaeological evidence indicates that the earliest humans were present in the sub-continent 30,000 years ago; rock carvings have been dated to slightly later than this. Evidence of constructed buildings, production of food crops and the domestication of livestock has been found dating back prior to 6500 BC. This culture existed for several thousand years.

The Vedic culture

Migration by Aryan tribes from the north-east into the Indus valley in the 3rd and 2nd millennium BC established one of the world's oldest and most important civilisations. During this period the *Vedas*, the oldest Hindu scriptures, were composed and major conurbations were constructed (Mohenjo-daro and Harappa) creating the first urban society in southern Asia. The relationship between northern India and the Middle East continued for many centuries. Increasingly waves of Aryan tribes infiltrated from the north-west, moved south and by 1500 BC had merged with the existing society, and began to create a new culture based in the early Aryan rituals. Social stratification began with the evolution of a hierarchical caste system of priests, warriors, free peasants and the indigenous people who were classed as 'unclean'.

The Late Vedic Period

In the 6th century BC the civilisation moved into the Ganges valley and the smaller states consolidated to form sixteen major oligarchies. At the same time two non-Vedic (Hindu) religious movements evolved: Jainism following the teachings of Mahavira, and Buddhism following Gautama Buddha. These beliefs attracted significant adherents, but not from the wealthier classes, both religions advocated 'renunciation' with humility and frugality, which did not suit those with money. The new beliefs, in particular Buddhism, established a long-lasting monastic tradition with both beliefs being very strong advocates of animal welfare. This influenced meat and animal produce consumption, placing slowly evolving veterinary medicine in an interesting situation. Contact was established with the Greek world, following the travels of Alexander the Great (326 BC), with horses and elephants becoming animals of importance in the Indus valley.

The Mauryan Empire

Created by the consolidation of smaller states during the 4th century BC. By the start of the 3rd century BC, under King Ashoka Maurya it reached its height, stretching across the Indian subcontinent to Kandahar in Afghanistan in the west and the Himalayas in the north. Ashoka (r.268 BC–232 BC) was a remarkable man. He governed by moral force and turned Buddhism (to which he was converted in 262 BC) from a minor sect to a major faith. He managed public life, renounced militarism and advocated the population to follow dhamma (the Buddhist 'truth'). The Ashoka edicts, carved on pillars and rocks still exist in many places, mostly in the Prakrit language, but there are two surviving in Greek and one in Greek and Aramaic, an indication of the strong relationships that had been created with Greece and the Middle East. Ashoka controlled more of the subcontinent than any subsequent ruler until the advent of British control. He died in 232 BC and the empire disintegrated with a final collapse in 184 BC. Ashoka is an important figure in the history of both animal welfare and veterinary medicine. He greatly strengthened the already prevalent custom of animal protection from Hindu beliefs: the killing of all animals was forbidden and hospitals for humans and animals were established throughout the empire. Some of the animal sanctuaries (pinjrapoles) still exist under the care of the Jains.

The Imperial Gupta Empire

There was a period of small states and kingdoms until in AD 319 Chandragupta II founded the Gupta Empire which spread in power to embrace northern India and later further into the central regions of the continent. In AD 455 the Gupta Dynasty declined to make way for later Guptas, their rule ended in AD 606. The Gupta period was a 'golden age' with the flowering of art, architecture, poetry, literature, mathematics, astronomy, science and medicine. Buddhism and Jainism had been important throughout the period but began to decline towards the end as Hinduism had again risen in popularity.

The Muslim Influence

Following raiding parties to destroy 'infidel' temples from about 1001, in 1192 Islamic forces of Turks and Afghans arrived. Within 20 years they had control of the Ganges basin and established the **Sultanate of Delhi**. The size of this territory varied with each ruler, but then declined until the **Moghul Dynasty** was established in the early 16th century by Emperor Babur (r.1526–1530). The dynasty reigned under six emperors for almost three centuries. They constructed some of the great buildings of India, including Shah Jahan's Taj Mahal. Art and literature flourished as well as religion, the emperors were all Muslim and while respecting other religions, they destroyed many Hindu temples, replacing them with mosques. From 1707 the dynasty declined with weak rulers; small states were established as well as the Europeans, who had arrived in the 16th century. In the 19th century the British became the dominant political power: India become the 'Jewel in the Crown' of the **British Empire** which imposed Western culture and products on the country. Medicine in particular was gradually dominated by British methods, but traditional practices survived in rural areas.

The south of the continent developed under different influences. Hinduism was the main religion and prosperity was related to the trading links with other countries. Both the Egyptians and the Romans had early links and trade also developed with the islands of South-East Asia. Christian missionaries arrived (St. Thomas the Apostle is said to have visited Kerala in AD 52) and the Cochin Christians developed their community in the 2nd century AD. Several local empires rose and fell, two of the most important were the Chalukyas, and the Rashtrakutas who lasted until 1190: these empires also had 'colonies' in Sri Lanka, Sumatra and the Malay peninsula for periods. Eventually southern India also came under British rule.

Religions and Beliefs

The British objective was to make money in various ways from the lands now under their control. The complex of religions existing were of no interest, although Christian missionaries were allowed to enter. Because the Indian subcontinent has a greater diversity of religions and religious sects than any other country it is important to identify these, as they have an impact on behaviour towards animals and animal use, as well as having an effect on both human and animal medicine.

Hinduism

The early religion that developed from the Vedic culture dating from 500 BC–350 BC embraced a broad range of philosophies. Brahma (known as the self-borne) is said to be the creator, via human mediation, of the four books of the *Veda* (knowledge), the *Rigveda, Samaveda, Yajurveda* and *Atharvaveda*. These books, along with the *Upanishads*, were composed to provide an ethical guide for the world. The exact dates of these texts is unknown but could date back to 2000 BC, except for the *Upanishads* which were probably written between 600 BC–200 BC. The texts are an important part of the religion and form the basis of Indian/Hindu philosophy. There are also prose commentaries, the *Brahmanas*, which describe the role of the priestly class. The texts cover a wide range of subjects from which most aspects of Indian culture can be traced including science, medicine, mathematics and wellness. Texts of particular interest are *Charaka Samhita* a medical text, *Tattiriya Brahmana* a commentary on

Hindu sacrificial rituals, and *Atharvaveda* a collection of texts about Hindu medicine and magic: of which there are nine *Shakhas* or schools. These early texts form the basis of *Ayurveda*, a traditional Indian medicine practice, used for both humans and animals.

Hinduism is the main Indian religious belief, with one of its major precepts being a respect for all animal life. Some animals are given a sacred status because they are believed to have a closer contact to the gods, or possess a particular virtue. The most important of these are:

- **Elephant:** Ganesha, a god with a human body and head of an elephant, who overcomes obstacles and adversity and is considered a symbol of good luck and fortune.
- **Monkey:** Hanuman the monkey god, represents strength, knowledge and loyalty. Monkeys are seen as the allies of humans.
- **Cow:** the sacred animal designated *aghanya*, a manifestation of the mother-goddess and regarded as a gift from the gods; in Hinduism it is a sin to eat beef. Killing a cow is morally wrong and strongly condemned. Cows signify abundance, fertility and motherhood. The cow also accompanies Krishna, as the divine shepherd thus demanding complete respect.
- **Indian Cobra *(Naja naja)*:** known as Shiva's cobra, recognised as very poisonous and closely related to Shiva, the lord of creation and destruction. Cobras are seen to protect water sources and therefore life. As they shed and renew their skin they also represent life and death.
- **Bengal tiger *(Panthera tigris)*:** the national animal of both India and Bangladesh. The Hindu tradition of Shaktism focuses on the supreme goddess Durga, who rides on a tiger (or a lion) when she goes to war – it represents victory over evil forces.
- **Dogs:** occupy a special place in Hindu mythology. *Shvan*, the Sanskrit word for a dog, occurs in many places in the Vedic texts and Hindu folklore. Several gods had a dog as a companion, most notably Shiva.

Hinduism is both a religion and a way of life with a belief in the reincarnation of the soul. The believers have a respect for all life because they hold that divinity permeates all beings, including animals and plants. Many Hindus are vegetarians (possibly up to 40% of the total) out of respect for the other forms of life, and will not eat meat, fish or eggs. No Hindu will eat beef. *Tihar*, a five day Nepalese Hindu festival celebrated in Nepal, Assam, Sikkim and Darjeeling in West Bengal, features dogs, cows and crows and ravens as four creatures that have an intimate relationship with humans. The raven symbolises sadness and grief.

While animal sacrifice is now rare in India it is still practised by some Hindus, such as those in the *Shaktism* tradition which exists mostly in the eastern states and Nepal (and in Hindu ritual in Bali, Indonesia). The slaughter is by the *Jhatka* (Sikh method) and very rarely by strangulation or by driving a wooden stake into the heart. The meat is eaten as ritual food. Other Hindus, following the Vaishnava tradition, vigorously oppose animal sacrifice. Overall current practice indicates that animal sacrifice in Hinduism is now very rare. The fundamental Hindu beliefs are important for animal welfare and also for the use and application of veterinary medicine. Hindus have a respect for animal life.

Jainism

Jainism is a most ancient non-theistic Indian religion said to date back to the 8th century BC, but with its ethical principles defined by Jina Mahavira in the 5th century BC. While believers do not believe in a creator god they do worship deities. The word Jain is derived from the Sanskrit word *jina*, meaning victory in crossing over life's stream of rebirths. Jains lead a spiritual ethical way of life. Of their several religious precepts the most important are non-violence and asceticism.

Jains live a vegetarian lifestyle that avoids any harm to animals or their lifecycles. Meat and eggs are prohibited but they will accept milk if it is proven that no violence has been involved in its production. This rule even applies to foods – no root vegetables (potatoes, onions, and so on) are consumed as insects and other life forms will be harmed by pulling the plant out of the ground. Jains are recognisable by their use of mouth masks to prevent the accidental inhalation of insects and will carry a small broom to gently sweep away any in their path. Jainism is a small religion within Indian terms. Their members are in the wealthiest class in the country with the highest literacy rate and university education. Their attitudes and beliefs are good for animal welfare.

Sikhism

Sikh is a Punjabi word meaning seeker or learner. The religion Sikhism originated in the Punjab in the 15th century and is based on the teachings of Guru Nanak (1469–1539). The sacred scripture is the *Granth Sahib*. The original intention of Sikhism was to bring together the best of Hinduism and Islam. There is a belief in one creator and a teaching of divine unity, with honest conduct and equality to all humankind. Sikh men are instantly recognisable by their turbans (they do not cut their hair) and characteristic dress. They are opposed to the caste system, they practise tolerance and extending hospitality, and they cremate their dead. As a community Sikhs have a reputation for good quality work and technical skills and tend to be one of the wealthier groups in Indian society.

Sikhs observe several prohibitions, such as cutting hair, intoxication, smoking and priestly classes. They also ban the eating of meat that has come from Muslim *halal* slaughter. This is related to the procedure of cutting the throat (exsanguination) while saying the name of Allah. In Sikh slaughter, termed *jhatka*, the animal is killed by a single strike of an axe or sword to sever blood vessels, nerves and frequently the head; no prayers are said and the method is said to cause less suffering. Sikhs are not habitual meat eaters and one branch of the belief are strict vegetarians; beef consumption is a strict taboo. The ban on *halal* meat probably results from the oppression that Sikhs suffered under Mughal and Afghan rule. Sexual relations with Muslims is also prohibited. The Sikh religion is favourable for animal welfare.

Buddhism

Now one of the world's leading faiths, Buddhism was founded in north India about 450 BC when Siddhartha Gautama achieved enlightenment. It is not a religion, it is a teaching for a way of life with a system of philosophy and a moral code which is the ultimate aim of every Buddhist, after passing through the cycle of reincarnation. Buddhism was founded at about the same period as Jainism, both beliefs advocated simplicity, frugality and humility and both have established a long lasting monastic tradition. The word *Buddha* is Sanskrit for an enlightened person.

The Buddha did not write his teachings (*dharma*), they were transmitted by oral tradition. Centred on the Four Noble Truths, the Buddha's belief is that all life is suffering, but by following his path of moderation one can be led through the cycle of rebirths until the goal is reached. There are three important books in Buddhism: the *Tipitaka*, the earliest texts; the *Sutras*, more than 2000 sacred texts, and *The Book of the Dead*, a Tibetan text in great detail, on death. The belief has two main schools of practice: *Theravada* and *Mahayana*. Buddhism is important for animal welfare as the belief includes a prohibition on the killing of living creatures. Many temples also acted as sanctuaries for animals, following the edicts of Emperor Ashoka which established animal hospitals and sanctuaries.

Islam

Muslims represent India's largest religious minority, and Islam is the state religion in Pakistan and Bangladesh. The background and practices of Islam have been discussed previously (see Chapter 6). In the 11th century north India fell under Muslim rule with the Mughal Empire eventually controlling most of the subcontinent. While conversion to Islam was not compulsory – the Hindu population was too large – the majority of the converts were of the lowest castes.

The principal practice of Islam affecting animals is their ritual method of slaughter, *halal*, previously discussed. Additionally they have a prohibition on the consumption of pig meat, and therefore pig-keeping, and frequently also regard dogs as unclean, although cats are generally liked. Horses are held in high regard, well cared for and have traditionally received veterinary care equal to that of human medicine.

Zoroastrianism

This is one of the oldest world religions established in Persia in 7th or 6th century BC by the prophet Zarathustra, as discussed previously (see Chapter 1). The belief is of one omnipotent and invisible god. The members of the religion are termed *Parsis* and the temples all have an everlasting flame with the worship of the fire, as a symbol of their god. Their main scripture is the *Zend-Avesta* (previously discussed) which covers medicine for both humans and animals. At one time the religion had a strong hold across northern India following persecution of its followers in Persia.

While there is a record of animal sacrifice in the past this now appears to be almost, or totally, absent. Two animals are particularly important – the horse and the dog. The latter is an important companion and in particular has a role in the last moments of a human life, which is regarded as a temporary state. There are similarities between Zoroastrianism and the early Vedic beliefs. Generally the religion can be seen to be favourable to animal welfare, and also receptive to veterinary medicine.

Christianity and Judaism

The religions of the European (or Western) world have only had a minor impact in the Indian subcontinent. They have, however, created long-lasting, but small, communities. St Thomas the Apostle is reputed to have arrived in Kerala in AD 52, where a local Christian community still exists, and the Portuguese traders have left a strong Christian community in Goa. Christian majorities are found in Mizoram and Nagaland, two small states. Indians who have converted to Christianity have generally been of the lowest castes. Small Jewish communities are found in several of the major cities, and there is also a group in Cochin, Kerala that claim to have arrived in the 6th century AD. Neither of these two religious groups have made any significant impacts on animal welfare conditions. Jews employ their ritual slaughter procedure (see Chapter 6) and eschew the consumption of pig meat.

Traditional Indian Medicine

The development of Indian medicine can be traced back to the Vedic culture to before 2000 BC in early Indo-Aryan texts written in Sanskrit. Some Hippocratic ideas can be determined in the original Indian concepts, and over the centuries there has been a constant interchange with Chinese and Western thought. The impact of Indian practices can also be determined on Islamic medicine.

The first medical texts arose following invasion of the Indus Valley. These *Vedas*, written before 1500 BC, are philosophical and religious verses rather than medical textbooks, but they provide one of the bases of Indian medicine: the impossibility of understanding the differences between the body and the soul, or of dissociating the visible from the invisible, as both are energised by the same life force. One of the Vedic books, the *Ayuraveda* (*the Veda of long life*), is concerned with medical matters. The books are sacred texts revealed by divine beings – the history of these is interwoven with legend.

It has been suggested that the basis for these original Vedic texts were part of the scriptures of the early immigrants and show the influence of the Persian *Avesta* and possibly early Mesopotamian ideas. These then become blended with the original

Indian Dravidian religious hymns. They are certainly dated to before the Greek/ Hellenic concepts. The main message is that disease occurs because the rules that govern the world have been transgressed, but that the deity who has been offended also has the power to cure the problem.

The Indian culture began about 1500 BC, followed by the Brahmanical period from the start of the 9th century BC which gradually evolved into Hinduism. In this period, in about the 1st century BC, there was a peak in Indian medicine with writings by two legendary physicians: Charaka and Susruta, who each wrote a *Samhita*. They explained the Ayurvedic doctrine which provided the groundwork for subsequent Indian medical writings. Charaka wrote eight books in dialogue form of a pupil and master. Susruta is not as accurate, but is more rational and shows a knowledge of anatomy and related to this, surgical procedures. The original concepts were passed down by oral tradition with the writing providing a culmination of a long period of observations and increasing medical knowledge. They present a logical and understandable whole of the physiological and therapeutic beliefs of their time; the *Samhitas* are in effect composite encyclopaedias. The gods, spirits and demons have a declining role compared to the earliest *Veda* texts. The basic concept still includes the original belief in the four elements of the Universe – air, earth, fire and water. A similarity with both the five elements of traditional Chinese medicine and the four humours of Hippocratic medicine.

It is difficult now to understand the physiological and pathological concepts or the rationality of the therapeutic approaches in treatises dating back to the 6th century BC. This was, however, a particularly interesting period in human evolution, a group of individuals had emerged with teachings that spread across the then known world – Aristotle, Buddha, Confucius, Hippocrates, Socrates and Zarathustra. The influence of all these can be found in the Indian developing medical thought.

Ayurvedism developed as Hindu medicine at the same time as Buddhist teaching, emphasising moral vigour and bodily health, evolved as a regime that demanded behaviour of a good standard, respect for others, modesty and virtue. This was combined with a lifestyle of strict bodily cleanliness and moderation in the pleasures of the flesh. The hygiene regime involved bathing, washing clothing, cleaning teeth and rinsing the nasal cavities. Brahmanism was also important in Indian medicine because of its strict hygiene rules, a largely vegetarian diet, and its emphasis on cleanliness, both personal and in the home (prompt removal of all waste and excreta from the house). The resulting Ayurvedic teaching was a philosophy of life and individual collective morality. A quite different approach to hygiene to that developed by the Salerno school in Europe (Sournia 1992, p. 192).

The beliefs of Buddhism and Hinduism did not always agree. Hinduism was regarded as the wishes of the god Shiva, supreme being, creator and patron of yoga, meditation and the arts. These were passed to humankind by his wife and partner, Parvati. As Indian Buddhism declined in influence their beliefs were adapted to Ayurvedism, which also included dietary taboos, in particular the ban on eating beef and the recognition of the cow as the sacred animal (which in no way conflicted with Buddhism). These Ayurvedic texts were passed down over the generations, being copied and including certain ideas and concepts from outside cultures. Later versions were translated into Pahlavi in Sassanid Persia, Chinese and Arabic (and used by Rhazes in developing his own Islamic teachings, see Chapter 6).

The basic building block of Ayurvedic medicine was that life was thought to be generated by the simultaneous action of wind, fire and water which was triggered by a 'breath' (similar to the Greek concept of *pneuma*). The human body was said to be composed of seven living substances – flesh, bone, marrow, fat, blood, chyle and sperm. Good health was maintained when these were kept in equilibrium, the art of the doctor was to correct imbalances to return to that equilibrium. Understanding of anatomy and organ function was confused and dissection was not allowed. The blood vessels and nerves and their purpose was not known. The heart was seen as the seat of conscience and was activated by the 'breath' that also made the blood move and produce a pulse. The 'breath' also digested the food in the stomach and controlled the bodily functions. The fundamental vital energy was believed to be fragile and as it moved around the body there were believed to be 107 points where it was thought to be unstable and in danger.

The diagnostic procedures as used by doctors were quite good (by comparable Western standards). First the patient would be questioned, the sound of the voice studied and movements watched. The skin and tongue would be examined and body odours checked. The doctor would listen to heart and lungs and would palpate the abdomen. Urine would be assessed by smell, colour and sometimes would be tasted. The pulse does not appear to have been examined until after the 8th century, probably due to Chinese influence.

Some of the old medical treatises include very good descriptions of tuberculous pathology and diabetes signs, as well as smallpox symptoms and lesions. It would appear that the relationship of mosquito bites and malaria infection was recognised and one Sanskrit text, predating Susrata, nominated rats as being a carrier of the plague (Margotta 1996, p. 17). Many diseases were attributed to an imbalance of the spirit, bile and phlegm as well as a disruption to the 'moral' state. The clinician had to assess the patient by the signs and symptoms of illness by relating these to the visible and invisible characteristics, and thereby establish a cohesion between the patient and their environment, and the greater cosmos. It could be suggested that there was a strong psychosomatic influence on the final diagnosis and prognosis.

A wide range of therapeutic procedures were used ranging from ancient magic to bloodletting by leech application, steam baths, inhalation systems and the use of induced sneezing – to clear the head. A range of therapeutic products was developed; this was notable for the purgatives, emetics and enemas that were used. The most comprehensive text lists over 400 plants, 64 mineral products and 57 animal derived products (all classified by therapeutic activities). Their use was based on identifying the vital elements of the body that were sent out of balance by disease and needed to be treated to restore equilibrium. Final selection was made on the basis of taste and flavour, the products were seen as sour, salty, sweet, bitter, pungent or astringent. Susrata listed some 750 medicinal plants which included *Cannabis indica* (Indian hemp) used for its soporific effects; *Rauwolfia serpentina* used to treat hypertension and *Atropa belladonna*, the source of atropine, a highly active alkaloid with several medical applications, but also is an effective poison.

The major limiting factor to early medicine was a lack of knowledge of the internal organs and structure of the body as dissection was banned by the religious laws. There was a period, however, when it was possible (in advice from Susrata) to place a corpse in a wicker basket, immerse it in water, usually from a riverbank, for five or seven days (the texts vary) and then poke the rotting remains with sticks to view the internal organs and structure.

In spite of this disadvantageous position Indian medicine was advanced in several surgical procedures, in particular rhinoplasty. In the Middle Ages of the Vedic period mutilation of the nose was very common, either for prisoners of war or delinquents (adultery) or as a result of leprosy or lupus. Susrata explained the technique of measuring the area of the face to be covered, cutting a plant leaf to that size and placing this on the cheek or forehead, removing a flap of skin of that size and then sewing it into position. Instructions were given on how to repeat the procedure should the first attempt fail and also how to cut two reeds to be inserted to enable nasal function to continue.

In the 4th century BC there was believed to have been a medical man, Divika, accompanying the Buddha on his travels. He left a treatise, now much augmented and updated, which detailed a variety of procedures – the treatment of superficial tumours, skin sores and malformations, as well as urine retention. There were also recognised procedures for the treatment of anal fistula, tonsillectomy, lithotomy, boil lancing, abscess treatment and amputation. The Divika text lists 121 instruments required by a competent medical practitioner: this includes knives, scalpels, bistouries, scissors, forceps for specific uses, needles and suture needles. Instructions were also written on fracture treatment with bamboo splints.

Ayurvedic medicine was the basis of Indian practice for almost 1000 years. There was a hierarchical structure of doctors trained by gurus who provided a well-rounded education (based on existing knowledge and beliefs) and always with a strict ethical code. This was a society that lived within its self-imposed caste system. The medical pupils either came from an existing medical family or were from the upper social caste. They were educated, literate in Sanskrit and could both read the old treatises, and converse in the local language. While not organised as a profession many worked in the households and courts of princes and rulers while others practised from healing centres financed by their patrons. There were also a wide variety of healers with a range of varying quality skills in every community. Ayurvedic medicine was regularly revised over some 15 centuries, to incorporate new plant species. Yoga developed alongside Ayurvedic medicine, but not for therapeutic purposes, it is a discipline based on the body and the mind: a well-trained yogi has a remarkable capacity to control the bodily processes.

The Muslim invasion from the north began in the 9th century and by the 16th century the Mughal Empire reached its height. This prevented the progress of Ayurvedic medicine as the new rulers introduced Islamic medicine, based in Hippocratic medical beliefs. While traditional medicine was not totally repressed its use was increasingly in the hands of local village healers rather than that of trained individuals.

In the southern Tamil regions neither the Hindu language nor Islam exerted much effect. Medical practice was conducted by *Siddhars* who were doctors, alchemists, mystics and religious figures. They provided a medical culture believed to have originated in the ancient Aryan Dravidian civilisation. It is claimed that they developed pulse reading as a diagnostic and Ayurvedic medicine may have copied them. They also had a Varman Dynasty text which identified specific points on the body which when pressed could be used as a medical treatment. A pharmacopoeia was also produced which included many mineral substances, that were classified as male and female.

Livestock Development in Ancient India

Archaeological evidence indicates that domestication of bovines, elephants, dogs and fowls occurred in India between 6000 and 4500 BC (Somvanshi 2006, p. 133) in the basins of the Indus river valley. Animals were important and both humped and humpless cattle, buffaloes, horses, elephants, goats, sheep, dogs and fowl were all domesticated. Fish was the main protein food, but mutton, beef, chicken and wild game including tortoise were eaten as well as milk, curd and ghee. Images from the excavations reflect the popularity of animals.

In the Vedic period the *Rigveda* was written. The text reveals animals were regarded as wealth, in particular cattle, who were grazed on pastures close to the houses and milked three times a day. Males were castrated and used for farm work. The buffalo was not in common use at this time. Sheep were kept for wool and goats for milk. Dogs were used as guards and also for hunting wild boar. The *Rigveda* listed barley, sugarcane and post-extraction sesame seed residue as animal feeds.

Cattle

The cow was already regarded as a holy animal and was designated *aghanya*, it was not to be killed. During this period philosophy teachers, who were searching for the secrets of life and the universe, developed what has been called a 'cow science'. The cattle family of animals was considered to be *gau vansh* and was essential for human life by providing protection, food and as an aid to development and culture. Bovine milk was believed to provide a special energy, strength and intelligence; manure and urine aided farming and oxen were a source of power on the farm; cowhides were a valuable product for the leather industry. In the Vedic period cows and their husbandry became the centre of both lifestyle and the economy (Somvanshi 2006, pp. 134–135).

Goats and Sheep

Goats were probably first domesticated in the southern part of the subcontinent in about 2500 BC, somewhat later than those in Mesopotamia. During the pre-Harappan period wild goats were present in Baluchistan and other regions. From seals excavated at Harrapa, goats appear to be shown and are assumed to have been a part of the early Indus Valley culture. Their value then, as now, is in providing meat, milk, hair, hides and horn; the goat has always been a significant animal to the poorer subsistence farmer. Sheep have been domesticated in India from the pre-Harrapan period. Based in the Urial stock (see Chapter 19) they appear to have come from Western sources. Similar animals were also kept in Tibet. While domesticated the sheep were herded by a traditionally recognised pastoral caste. Their value was seen as wool production but also from meat, hides and bones.

Poultry

Domesticated Indian poultry were derived from the red jungle fowl (see Chapter 24), and today's poultry industry can be traced back to these birds. They were well recognised in the Indus Valley civilisation; domesticated fowl bones and pottery images have been excavated in Harrapa. Initially it appears that these birds were kept and trained for sport – the origination of cockfighting. When the Aryans invaded India in about 2500 BC they discovered these birds, although it is unclear when they were bred for meat. While they are mentioned in the *Atharvaveda* and *Yajurveda* they are absent from the *Rigveda*. The birds later obtained a religious significance and in about 1000 BC the eating of their meat was prohibited. Following trade and personal visits the birds were taken to Mesopotamia and then to Europe, first for cockfighting entertainment and then during the Roman Empire their use evolved into a poultry industry.

Buffalo

The buffalo appears to first be recognised in the very early Indian literature as both a demon, *Mahishasur*, and as a tractable animal ridden by the death god, *Yamraj*. Domestication took place during the Epic periods of Ramayana (c.2000 BC) and during the later and post-Vedic periods of Mahabharata (c.1400 BC). They then began to play a significant role in the Indus Valley. The main species found is the dairy or riverine type. Those buffalo used for ploughing in southern India are characterised by their wallowing in mud ponds as a relief from high temperatures and work stress. The buffalo in southern India represented prosperity in the same way that the cow symbolised wealth in the north.

Horses

The original Indus Valley civilisation does not appear to have possessed horses, as judged from the images found in the excavations. It is stated in the ancient literature that possibly the first recognised horse was named *Ucchasrava*. Horses were introduced by the Aryans who used them for pleasure, sport and war – where their chariots and speed gave them advantages. In the Vedic period (1500 BC–1000 BC) the use of horses was documented, and in the later Vedic, Buddhist and Mauryan periods, from 1000 BC to 400 BC horses were well used and represented.

In the later Mauryan period equine husbandry reached a high point as a result of their use in war. The records of the royal stables have survived which list the place of origin, breed, age and markings and colour of each animal. The royal stables had a superintendent and nominated veterinary and equine training personnel. Horses demonstrated their superiority in war due to their speed and ability to act quickly against the slower elephants, and in the Gupta dynasty (AD 300–AD 550) they became the nucleus of the army of Emperor Samudragupta (AD 335–AD 380). By the 600s AD army horses were equipped with saddles.

Traditional Indian Veterinary Medicine

There is a strong mythological background to the development of Indian veterinary medicine, linked to the similar development of human medicine. The legend is that Brahma taught the knowledge of the *Veda* books to the other gods, including the Sun God and his twin sons, the Asvins, who became the custodians of the *Atharvaveda*, which contains the treatises on medicine. They thus became, 'the medical attendants in the hierarchy of heaven'. These twins were recorded as being borne of a god in the form of a mare – they were centaurs. Another legend is that the god Indra imparted knowledge of life and surgery to the miraculous horse, Dhanvantari, to whom the *Ayurvedic* (science of life) approach to medicine and health is attributed. Dhanvantari is also known as the 'father' of Indian medicine. These concepts echo the Greek mythology of the story of Chiron the centaur and his relationship to medicine and surgery. There has to be a connection between the Greek and Hindu myths: maybe Greek ideas were incorporated following the conquering of the Indus valley by Alexander the Great in the 4th century BC, or possibly there was Aryan mythology behind both Greek and Indian legends?

The *Atharvaveda* has not survived intact but it included animal ailments, herbal medications and the cure of diseases; fragments of knowledge can be recovered, one of which gives a treatment for cattle helminths. Brahma is also said to be the source for the writing of the *Ayurveda* with the object of giving detailed instructions to mankind on the treatment of disease. This was written at the end of the Vedic period and again most of the text has been lost; from the surviving fragments philologists agree that the *Ayurveda* represents the foundation of Hindu veterinary and human medical science. From Dhanvantari can be traced Susruta, the founder of surgery and Charaka, the founder of medicine: their *Samhita* texts contain mentions of veterinary medicine including canine rabies. The development of Hindu veterinary science was contemporaneous with the development of human medicine, driven by the belief that men and animals were deemed to have an identical destiny based on the philosophy (represented by the sign of the *swastika*) that expressed peace and goodwill towards the whole creation.

The Vedic period priests had the responsibility to maintain the health of cattle, acting as 'veterinarians'. Vedic hymns of the that time tell of the value of medicinal herbs which were presumably used by priests to both cure ailments and maintain health. The *Atharvaveda* covered the veterinary art and use of herbs and other medicinals. The *Mahabharata* (c.1400 BC) refers to the active involvement of the society with animals, listing cattle, sheep, goats, dogs, elephants and horses, together with their uses, giving particular note to the value of cattle dung as a fertiliser.

The *Ramayama* (c.2000 BC), believed to be the oldest Sanskrit literature, covers in detail the treatment of various ailments using medicinal herbs and surgical procedures. These are well described and include caesarean section and hysterectomy in humans, undertaken by trained *vaidhyas* (physician-surgeons). The herbal listing describes many recognisable and useful plants and were prescribed for treating and curing the diseases of humans and animals (Somvanshi 2006, p. 135).

The ancient veterinary treatises, in particular those of Shalihotra (c.2350 BC) and Palakapya (unsure date c.1000 BC–AD 1000) also dealt with surgical procedures. The detail covered included dressing and bandaging of wounds and examination of possible surgery cases, to determine a procedure and prognosis. The cautery was used, foreign bodies extracted, skin grafts performed, and fractures and dislocations corrected. The most remarkable of these at the time being the use of skin grafting (as in humans). The application of surgical procedures was well advanced in the Vedic period and these early texts detail both the procedures and the pre- and post-operative actions. The procedures would appear to be conducted without anaesthesia, but possibly pain control, using opiates, as in humans was employed.

As animals and humans were treated with equal care the veterinary art advanced with rapidity. The renowned *Charaka, Susruta* and *Harita* treatises all include sections on the maintenance of health, as well as treatment of disease in animals. In veterinary care Shalihotra is recognised as probably the first named veterinarian; in ancient India, some men specialised in one species, others took a wider remit. Other named veterinary authors were Nakula and Sahadeva. While there does not appear to be organised veterinary education, the standard of care was good.

An important genre of ancient Indian literature are the *Puranas*, a genre of scriptures in which many include prescriptions for the treatment of animal disease. Written mostly in the so-called Golden Age of the Gupta Dynasty between 300 BC–650 BC some of the most important ones in this category are the *Skanda Purana, Devi Purana, Matsya Purana, Agni Purana, Garuda Purana* and *Linga Purana*; two of the known authors of *Puranas* with a veterinary content were Vaisampayana and Vyasa.

The Vedic literature, in particular the *Atharvaveda* is a recognised repository of what has been termed ethnomedicine, for use in both humans and animals and describing the value of medications for curing diseases. The *Yajurveda* provides much information on the use and cultivation of medicinal plants. A wide variety of diseases and ailments of animals and their treatment are detailed in these texts. These include infections of the horns, ears, teeth, throat, heart, navel, joint and muscle pain, haemorrhagic enteritis, dysentery, alimentary tract ailments, cold, endo- and ectoparasitic diseases, stomach helminths, rabies, treatment of abscesses, anaemia, wounds, urinary retention, constipation, arthritis, rhinitis, haematoma and dermatoses. The use of medication to improve milk production is also described. The coverage of diseases entries and veterinary needs is extensive (Somvanshi 2006, pp. 136–139).

The Elephant

Elephants of the Asian race were found in large numbers in the Indian subcontinent and Sri Lanka in ancient times. There is evidence to show that they extended as far west as Assyria and other Near East countries, as well as to Persia, Afghanistan and South China. They were hunted by the Kings of Babylon and Assyria. At the present time Asian elephants exist in greatly diminished numbers in the jungles of South India, Bengal and Assam. They are also found in Sri Lanka, Myanmar and Thailand, some are found in Laos, Cambodia and Vietnam and smaller numbers are found in Malaysia, Borneo and Sumatra.

The ancient Indian and Sinhalese writers described the characteristics of the races of elephants in the different regions and countries. They were classified according to adult size, the tusks and their colour, and also by their intelligence, docility and longevity (Deraniyagla 1955).

Manuscripts by the early Sanskrit writers are the first to discuss elephants. Muni Palakapya wrote the *Hastya Ayurveda* or *Gaja Ayurveda* in the Rigvedic period. This treatise, dedicated to Lord Ganesha, deals with elephant medicine and is presented in four sections and 152 chapters: the *Maha Rogasthan* on major diseases; the *Ksudra Rogasthan* covering minor diseases; the *Salyasthan* on surgery and a fourth section on medications, diet and hygiene. Ailments and diseases were classified as either *Adhyatmika* (physical), or *Agantuka* (accidental and incidental). The physical class of ailments were grouped as *Dosaja* – caused by an imbalance of bodily humours, the *vata* (air), *pitta* (bile) and *kapha* (phlegm). The treatise also includes sections on elephant anatomy, treatment of various diseases, training and a classification of elephants based on certain characteristics (Somvanshi 2006, pp. 137–138).

Ancient Indian Veterinary Authors

There was a vast knowledge of Hindu veterinary medicine existing in written, frequently illustrated, early Sanskrit texts. In the already cited *Atharvaveda* a cattle helminth medication is described and in the *Charaka Samhita* the manufacture of enemas for use in elephants, camels, cows, horses, sheep and goats are detailed. Other authors such as Parasara describe the care of cows in pregnancy and diseases. Many of these works are ascribed to *rishis*, or other holy or saintly individuals. Of the many named authors, at least thirty have major works attributed. In the Mahabharat period Nakul wrote the *Ashva-chikitsa* on diseases of the horse, and Sandev was named as a cattle specialist. Many of these have been preserved: particularly valuable collections are held in the Government Manuscript Library, Chennai (Madras) and the Tanjore Palace Library. Only a selection of these have been translated, mostly into either English or German.

Quite apart from the still untranslated manuscripts it is believed that there are more still to be found. The Brahmans who have custody of this literature have always had a reluctance to let it go outside of their own circle. There is also believed to be material in Kashmir, Nepal and Tibet, some of the latter has been identified, but not translated. One of the oldest extant veterinary manuscripts, held in the Chennai Library, called the *Asvayurveda* (knowledge of the life of horses) is an exhaustive treatise, in 820 pages, on the characteristics and diseases of horses. This was translated into both Tibetan in the 11th century and Farsi in the 14th century.

Of the many authors of veterinary works there are two names which are particularly prominent: Shalihotra and Palakapya. Their writings, which appear to date from the Vedic period (but may be of a later date), are some of the earliest examples of species specialisation. Palakapya wrote on the elephant, an animal of great importance to both the early Indian armies and princes. Shalihotra was devoted to the horse, from which is derived the word *Salihotriya* which is now reduced to *Salutri*, an Indian designation for a veterinarian. There has been debate over the word Shalihotra that this might not have been a single individual, however some of the original Sanskrit writings in this name are preserved. Similarly the work by Palakapya has been, by some, identified as being by Dhanvantari (*vide supra*). Since these texts coincide with both the invasion of the Sanskrit-speaking Aryans and the Vedic age it would indicate the works would not be earlier than 1800 BC. One Indian author, however, states that Shalihotra is mentioned in a Sanskrit text of 2350 BC (that is, at least 4300 years ago). It has to be noted that calendar interpretation difficulties are a problem with all old texts: however, there is no doubt of the antiquity of the Shalihotra writings.

Shalihotra has attracted much interest, with the suggestion that he could be the earliest known named veterinarian. His *Samhita* or encyclopaedia on the horse, but also including the elephant, covered anatomy, physiology, surgery, diseases, treatment and preventives as well as discussing body structure and ageing. Scholars also suggest that he was the author of *Asva-prashana* and *Asva-lakshana*, two related texts. The main *Samhita* was translated to Persian, Arabic and Tibetan. Shalihotra was said to have been the son of Hayagosha and to have lived in Sravasti (now Sahet-Mahet) in Uttar Pradesh.

British Jurisdiction

The British influence in India evolved in a complex and haphazard manner from the operations of the British East India Company which grew from being a trader in the 1600s spices market to an Indian operation with its own army. From the 1740s, it gradually acquired supremacy and, following the conquest of Bengal in 1757, became increasingly involved in politics. The Company became an agent of British imperialism in India, as well as generating large profits. At the same time there was an ever increasing British Army and British Navy presence in India, due to conflicts involving, in particular, the Dutch and the French.

In 1857 the Indian Rebellion erupted and was suppressed. A major cause of this had been the poor governance and local behaviour of the Company. In June 1858, the rule of the Company was transferred to the British Crown and in 1876 the territory was declared to be the Indian Empire. The capital city was Calcutta (Kolkata) until 1911, when it moved to New Delhi. The early British Indian veterinary picture is not a cohesive story, it was totally related to the needs of the Company, but its history has much interest.

Veterinary Administration

By 1770 the growing operations of the Company increasingly required horses for transport, their developing army and for personal use. There was a need to improve their quality, and also the quality of their cattle which, along with elephants and camels, were also used for transport. In 1791 the Military Auditor-General suggested a Board of Agriculture, based on regulations issued by Tippoo Sultan of Mysore for control of the breeding of horses, cattle and sheep, with the establishment of a series of stud farms; this was not approved by the British Board.

In September 1793 a Company report, by Lieutenant William Frazer, proposed a plan to establish a stud farm in the Ganges Valley to breed stallions and bulls. This plan also made the first recorded European mention of animal disease in India and the lack of veterinary knowledge. In 1794 he was appointed to purchase stallions, mares, bulls and cows for a stud farm at Pusa. In 1799 Captain Frazer reported progress and requested the services of a 'skilful veterinarian . . . to diffuse knowledge of the art' among local breeders. The London Directors said it would be difficult to find such a person.

In 1804 it was recognised that the Pusa programme was in trouble and needed expert help. The Court of Directors in London were using William Moorcroft as the veterinary adviser to their English stud farm in Essex. Moorcroft, who had an established equine practice in London, was medically qualified, had completed the French veterinary course and was the first British veterinarian. He agreed to replace Frazer and sailed to India in 1808 with the (then) large salary of £3000 a year plus expenses.

Moorcroft arrived in Calcutta, went to Pusa with a programme of management, feeding and disease control, and reduced the losses by 90% in a very short time. Deciding Pusa was too hot and humid he moved the stud to higher ground where he cooperated with local horse breeders. He calculated that he needed 120 stallions and 3000 mares to raise the 600 remounts annually required by the Company, mainly for their army. Moorcroft also realised that he needed better bloodstock to cross with the native horses.

The Company would not let him return to England to make purchases, so in 1812 he travelled and crossed the Himalayas to Nepal and East Tibet looking for suitable hardy stock. Describing his expedition in an 1818 article for *Asiatic Researches* entitled *A Journey to Lake Manasarovara in Undes, a province of Little Tibet* Moorcroft created his reputation as an explorer and ecologist, as well as establishing the role of the veterinarian in the economic development of India. He began a second journey in 1819, at his own expense, still looking for suitable equine bloodstock and pashmina sheep. He began this in Bokhara, and succeeded in purchasing some horses, but died in either 1824 or 1825 in unclear circumstances.

The London Veterinary College, opened in 1791, and under the second Principal, Edward Coleman, was producing the first British veterinary surgeons. There was an urgent need for these men in the army due to the wars with the French, and in 1796 he developed a three month veterinary training course for medical men and others. From 1797 these men became commissioned Veterinary Officers. At the end of 1799 five of these went to their regiments in India – Joseph Erratt arrived first, followed by Thomas Burrows, James Grellier, Richard Davies and Samuel Newman. Later Davies and Grellier were invalided back to Britain. While in Madras (Chennai), in 1802 Grellier wrote and published the variously titled *The Elements of Veterinary Science* or *The Veterinary Art in India*. This was the first English-language Indian veterinary publication, and it dealt with the physiology and pathology of the horse (Grellier 1842–1844, serialised).

By 1820 more British veterinary graduates were beginning to arrive in India and the Company was anxious to include a veterinary service for their growing army. In 1821 J T Hodgson MRCVS, who was with the Governor-General's Bodyguard in Calcutta, was instructed to arrange for apothecaries to be employed by the corps of Indian cavalry, as veterinary assistants. He did not agree, saying that they should be qualified veterinarians; which eventually the Company agreed to employ. Hodgson was the first appointment in 1826 and then veterinary graduates from both London and Edinburgh Colleges were hired. By 1832 the three regional Presidencies of Madras (Chennai), Bombay (Mumbai) and Bengal had the required complement of 32 officers.

Veterinary progress was slow, due to Company policy. Hodgson was dismissed in 1834 and the Company stud farms had no administrative control. There were an increasing number of papers being written in British veterinary publications and Calcutta medical journals, with major topics including *Kumri* (cerebral nematodiasis), *Bursati* (cutaneous habronemiasis) and 'worm in the eye' in horses, as well as canine distemper in dog packs (imported from England for hunting). By 1853 the profession in India was restless due to the lack of a senior veterinarian to oversee the service. The Company issued orders for the adoption of the 'mulling' method of equine castration in the Bombay army – maceration of the testicles as practised in India since very early days. This resulted in strong objections by J H B Hallen MRCVS, and the order was withdrawn.

Following the Indian Rebellion and the amalgamation of the Imperial and Company armies in 1859, there was little change until the Bombay Presidency appointed Hallen as Principle Veterinary Surgeon (PVS). This was followed by the Bengal Presidency appointing two Inspecting Veterinary Surgeons and then in 1866 R J G Hurford was appointed the first Indian PVS. Meanwhile in 1862 Hallen had established the Army Veterinary School at Poona (Pune).

At last, interest was developing in livestock disease. Dr K McLeod, a Civil Surgeon in Jessore, Bengal published a report in 1867 on diseases of cattle, recognising rinderpest, foot-and-mouth disease (FMD) and haemorrhagic septicaemia (HS). Following this, in 1869, the government of India formed the Indian Cattle Plague Commission, with Hallen as President. The brief was to cover India and epidemic diseases, in particular those affecting the supply of meat and milk to Calcutta, the hides industry, cattle poisoning, veterinary education and cattle breeding. The report, published in 1871, identified the cattle diseases that required special attention as rinderpest, FMD, hoven (bloat), quarter-ill, pleuro-pneumonia, purging, cystic disease and malignant sore-throat (HS): this created an awareness of animal disease and the role of the veterinary profession in its control. The report did not include anthrax, but a few years later it was seen to be so serious as to consult Pasteur. Hallen published *More Deadly Forms of Cattle Disease in India* in 1871. This text was translated into many vernacular tongues and was in great demand as the first Indian veterinary text.

The governmental response to the Report was slow and it was years before most of the recommendations were acted on. In 1888 the Central Bacteriological Laboratory was, with Hallen's involvement, established at Poona with Dr A Lingard appointed Director. In 1892 Hallen was appointed Inspector General of the Civilian Veterinary Department, but unfortunately had to retire four years after his appointment, reaching the age of 65. His contribution to developing veterinary services in India over a 44 year period had been impressive, eventually reaching his aim of a unified structure.

The Indian Civil Veterinary Department, renamed the Indian Veterinary Service in 1902, had 17 army officers transferred permanently to its staff, together with four from Britain. There were still not enough staff to cope with the enormous Indian cattle population and gradually control of livestock and horse breeding establishments moved to the provincial governments. Very slowly, due to the combined effects of staff shortages, the sheer size of India and the livestock populations, the difficulties of dealing with provincial governments (in many differing vernacular tongues), together with a general lack of serious interest and funding by central government, the veterinary services achieved a fair measure of effective control and understanding of the livestock disease problems.

Animal Disease Control

Following the 1871 Report of the Cattle Plague Commission the government had their first definitive listing of the major cattle disease problems and a list of requirements needed to enable a successful programme of controls. Reaction was slow due to poor governance, the immensity of the problems and limited funding. The Pusa stud was closed in 1894. While the central government had delayed on the many proposals in the report there was a movement by the Presidency provincial governments towards the development of horse, mule, cattle, sheep and shawl (pashmina) sheep breeding establishments. These proposals embraced improved feeding and fodder production as well as health controls. In 1876 Surgeon Major John Shortt, both medically and veterinary qualified, published a book on Indian cattle and sheep in which the generally poor husbandry by villagers was described along with the diseases listed. In 1880 Griffith Evans, an army veterinary officer, while investigating surra in horses identified a trypanosome as the causal organism, named *Trypanosoma evansi*. This was the first pathogenic trypanosome identified.

Colonel A.E. Queripel succeeded Hallen as Inspector General in 1896 and tried to move the veterinary emphasis away from the horse towards cattle, but found that cattle supervision in India was 'a herculean task', and more veterinary officers were needed. The Punjab led the way in creating a new start. Rinderpest was recognised as the major problem and Queripel tried to get the Bacteriological Laboratory involved. The Punjab government took action to administer the Glanders and Farcy Act passed in 1879 and raised with the government of India the question of vaccinating cattle against anthrax and other diseases, as demonstrated by Pasteur.

Hallen had always advocated veterinary education in India as a means of resolving the manpower problem of depending on British graduates. He had started the educational process by creating the Army Veterinary School in Poona in 1862. He advocated an all-Indian veterinary school, and started the Harpur School in 1877, then moved it to Lahore where it opened in 1882. The Ajmere School opened in 1881 but in 1902 joined with Lahore to create Lahore Veterinary College. Veterinary lectures were now also being given in several agricultural colleges.

The presidencies were concerned that government funding was not available for veterinary schools. In Bombay aid was provided by the Society for the Prevention of Cruelty to Animals (SPCA), who also allowed use of their buildings. In 1886 the Bombay Veterinary School started and established a three year course in veterinary science. Another veterinary school was opened in Simla in 1888 but this only had a short life. Further veterinary schools opened in Bengal in 1893, Madras in 1902 and finally Patna in 1930 with a three year course. These five colleges were thought to be sufficient to provide replacements for the total veterinary staff of 2500 men.

The initial task of the Central Bacteriological Laboratory was to investigate surra in horses and cattle – a disease of great importance to the army. As the Poona climate was humid it was decided to move the laboratory to Mukteswar in the Kumaon Hills. After many delays, the move finally took place in 1895. Queripel, when he took over from Hallen, made efforts to move rinderpest research into the lead place because of the importance of the cattle industry. Lingard had enlarged the surra studies and now commenced on rinderpest and other cattle diseases. In 1897 a branch was opened at Kurgaina, near Bareilly, the forerunner of the Izatnagar Institute.

Professor Koch visited Mukteswar in 1897 to help in the rinderpest control programme and demonstrate his method of protection by an injection of bile from an infected animal. It was decided not to use this method, which involved sacrifice of the bovine donor, as it was thought to be unsuitable for India, due to the Hindu respect for cattle. Eventually it was decided to use either antiserum alone which would give five months protection or sero-virus immunisation, but this resulted in some casualties. At that time Mukteswar was becoming difficult to organise with a major research programme into rinderpest, anthrax, surra, epizootic lymphangitis and strangles. In 1907 Lingard retired and was followed by J D E Holmes from Britain who purchased an 800 acre site at Izatnagar to enable an expansion of the research work.

In 1912 the Indian government placed Mukteswar under the administration of the Agricultural Advisor to the Government, until 1929 when the Indian Council of Agricultural Research was established. Mukteswar was growing rapidly with increasing work in producing biological products for disease control. In 1921 J T Edwards had arrived from the United Kingdom (UK) and made every effort to revive Mukteswar as a research centre. The name was changed to the Imperial Institute of Bacteriological Research. The demand for rinderpest antiserum was rapidly increasing and production was moved to Izatnagar. In 1925–1926, five million 5cc doses were produced; the disease was gradually being brought under control.

Mukteswar expanded the programmes into HS and blackwater vaccines, bovine tuberculosis, coccidiosis and piroplasmosis. In 1926–1927 the successful use of Bayer 205 (Naganol) for the treatment of surra in horses and dogs was announced. Also in 1927 the first description of Newcastle (*Ranikhet*) disease in poultry in India was made and the first successful cultivation of FMD virus on the plantar pads of guinea pigs. Most notable was the achievement of Edwards in fixing the rinderpest virus in goats, and using the blood from these animals with the attenuated virus, as a safe vaccine. It could be used with or without simultaneous serum. Rinderpest at last was coming under control.

The post of Animal Health Commissioner was created and Colonel A Olver MRCVS was appointed in 1930. Under Olver's rule from 1930 the Institute was reorganised, research flowered and in 1934, building on Edwards' work, a goat spleen rinderpest vaccine was developed. This was most effective on all indigenous stock, but not safe for European imports. Mukteswar's research also identified new parasitic problems, as well as studying warble fly control and nutritional diseases. There was now considerable veterinary research in provincial units. This type of work is illustrated by a paper by Vancheswaran (1945, pp. 410–414), graduate of the Madras Veterinary College, writing on rinderpest immunisation studies undertaken with goat adapted virus at the Madras Serum Institute. Izatnagar expanded to both agricultural and veterinary research with an emphasis on nutritional disease. Beekeeping, silkworms and fisheries research were all placed under this control. The importance of livestock production was being realised.

During World War II (1939–1945) funding for research work was difficult but Mukteswar was able to keep eight projects in progress. In 1945 he created an animal genetics section at Izatnagar for nationwide bovine artificial insemination.

A notable event was the publication in India in 1882 of *The Quarterly Journal of Veterinary Science and Animal Management*. The Editorial Board was made up of Charles Steel (Editor), Fred Smith and J H Steel; all army veterinary officers with Charles Steel at the Army Veterinary School, Poona. J H Steel was the son of Charles Steel and Fred Smith was to become Major General Sir Frederick Smith, head of the Army Veterinary Service. The journal was aimed at the military, its contributions were both of a high standard and covered a wide range of veterinary and welfare topics. After Smith was moved back to Britain in 1890, and J H Steel died in 1891, the journal ceased production. Before his death J H Steel had published four books in India on diseases of dogs, sheep, elephants and camels, with advice on management for the last two.

In 1906 a journal of veterinary science for India was published. The four editors of *The Journal of Tropical Veterinary Science* were all members of the Civil Veterinary Department. The journal attracted attention and did much to stimulate interest in tropical diseases. In 1909 editorship was taken over by the Inspector General of the Department, but when this post was abolished a few years later the *Journal* closed. India was again without a veterinary scientific journal until in 1924 Indian workers in Madras launched the *Indian Veterinary Journal*, now the official organ of the Indian Veterinary Association and the oldest veterinary journal in India. The Council, to aid the increasing research output, in 1930 instituted the *Indian Journal of Veterinary Science and Animal Husbandry* which attracted an immediate input of scientific papers. This publication has been replaced by the *Indian Journal of Veterinary Science and Biotechnology*.

Indian Veterinary Practice Under the British Raj

The *Raj*, a word literally meaning 'rule' in Sanskrit, was the term given to the British government in India between 1858 and 1947. Western medicine became the accepted solution to veterinary problems. The British veterinary graduates who staffed the growing number of veterinary services and research facilities soon faced a manpower shortage. The Indian veterinary colleges were opened. Their graduates filled posts in the government services and opened private veterinary practices. With an increasingly affluent population two groups of veterinary service providers were active: the new Indian graduates trained in western medicine, and the traditional veterinary healers known as the *Salutri*. This name was also taken by many of the College graduates as it explained their role to the population.

The comments from papers cited below are all from European authors and unfortunately most express a rather derogatory attitude towards the Indian practices and *Salutri*. A book on the treatment of cattle diseases, translated from the Tamil language of southern India was reviewed by Mills (1894, pp. 100–104). He noted that the work opens with prayers to the God Vishnu and that the author had a knowledge of 48 different plants used for medicinal purposes. Each disease was listed with symptoms and treatment with selected named herbs. In his review Mills provided a translations of the local disease names – *mannadappan* (malignant sore-throat), *pinn adappan* (splenic apoplexy), *tharian* (malignant catarrh), *kolli* (anthrax in the jaw) *vackey* (rinderpest), *padoovon* (inflammation with swelling), *alaripadoovon* (inflammation with burning sensation), *gunni novoo* tympanitis, *vakuti novoo* (phrenitis). Medications for administration by nostril and applications to eyes attacked by flies or injured are suggested. In a second article (Mills 1894, pp. 182–184) continues with the listing of diseases and medications including those used for aborting a dead calf, treatment of sores, medications for animals weakened by poisons, cracked hoofs, prescriptions to improve cows' milk flow and taming a vicious animal. The author of the two articles is unfortunately dismissive of them providing any value to western medicine, without, it appears, any effort to identify the many named plants. Of interest is the number of diseases recognised and described by symptoms, which indicate a level of knowledge and proficiency.

Throughout the Indian indigenous population there were strong beliefs regarding the hairmarks on horses and cattle. The positioning of these was thought to indicate good or bad luck to the owner and his relatives, with the saying,

a man may face a rifle fire and may escape, but he cannot avoid the luck, good or evil, foretold by hairmarks.

A purchaser would first consider these marks, if seen to be propitious all other features of conformation or soundness would be ignored. These beliefs were more strongly held in southern and central India; less stress was placed on them in cattle than in horses. They were not considered in a cow, as the animal was held to be sacred and in a bullock born and bred on the farm the hairmarks were not considered as important. There were six lucky hairmarks for horses and thirteen unlucky marks. Cattle also had a series of nominated marks as well as good and bad features resulting from horn shape. Superstition was widespread for cattle and a purchaser of a bullock which had cut only seven permanent incisors was advised to have his coffin ready! (Holmes 1903, pp. 175–179).

The use of animal features or behaviour to determine the fortunes of the owner seemed to have been widespread. There were also a series of superstitions related to foaling, in particular related to the time of day or time of year. If a mare should foal in *Chitra* (April–May) the lifetime of the owner was believed to be shortened, his poverty increased and all kinds of sorrow would befall him. To prevent these happenings the owner was advised to either cut the ear of the foal, or give it as a present to a fakir. These practices, and the Indian system of aging horses by their teeth up to 31 or 32 years, have been discussed in greater detail in the book *Lucky Marks of the Horse* (Mills 1904, pp. 24–27).

An anonymous paper (Anon. 1913, pp. 421–424) reviews the methods employed by the graduates of the veterinary colleges when they set themselves up in private practice. Advertisements were described as,

highly imaginative and illustrative of wonderful operations performed and cures obtained

and accompanied by testimonials to give authenticity.

One practitioner, Mr Ayoub Khan, inserted the following statement into his advertisement,

NOTICE.
No Cure no Pay. I am not responsible for the Death. The undersigned is the qualified Salutri of Babugarth department. Fee of treatment depends on examining the sickness of animals . . . (fees are listed) Yours faithfully, AYOUB KHAN SALUTRI.

Each illustration included in the advertisement was captioned, for example,

A fibrous tumour was taken out from the bitch of Capt. H. Brokesmith Esq., 7th R.F.A.

It was apparent from the illustrations and testimonials he used, that Mr Ayoub Khan had a distinguished clientele of army officers, local Indian aristocrats and at least one judge. The unknown author of the paper wrote,

Apparently for a Salutri with good shrewd common sense and a natural aptitude for veterinary work, there is an excellent chance to make a good living in India.

It is not known how widespread this type of practice was, probably mostly in urban areas, dependent on the wealthy upper classes and British residents. The traditional veterinary medicine therapies based in the *Ayurveda* have continued to be practised, in particular in the rural areas, for many hundreds of years (Mazars 1994, pp. 433–451).

Veterinary Medicine in India: Historical Overview

Many early studies into the history of Indian medicine, both human and veterinary, were poorly made and derogatory. Much of this was due to an ignorance of Indian history and an indifference to a culture that was subsumed by British domination. An assumption was made that before this it was a 'farrago of myths and legends'. These words by Peter Johnston-Saint (1929) are in the opening paragraphs of one of the earliest and best overviews of the subject, written in 1929 when he was working at the Welcome Historical Medical Museum following service in the British Army in India. He notes that one of the reasons for this ignorance were that the early Sanskrit treatises were little known and western education was devoted to ancient Greece and Rome, with Hippocrates as the founder of medicine. Another, and more important reason was that Indian medicine, at the time of British control, had fallen to a low level. The Hindu beliefs and practices had been depressed by the introduction of Buddhism and then pushed to one side by the Muslim invasion and introduction of Islamic medicine based in Galen/Hippocrates concepts.

While presented over 80 years ago the Johnston-Saint overview provided an excellent summary of the early mythology of Indian medicine, to its commencement based on the *Ayurveda* with the Susruta and Charaka *Samhitas* defining Indian surgery and medicine. While reviewing the herbal medication treatment routines he also examines and illustrates the remarkable collection of Indian surgical instruments and their incredible similarity to modern instruments – and also to Roman instruments, all following a similar pattern and a probable genealogical descent to our present day. Veterinary medicine is discussed,

> *Under Buddhism veterinary science . . . reached an enormously high level and infinite pains were taken for the care and treatment of animals*

and

> *Animal hospitals managed for the most part by the state and staffed by the state's own veterinary doctors . . . it was the Apotheosis of the animal world.*

The value of the ancient Indian veterinary literature is now being recognised. Many of the Vedic treatises were destroyed, looted or burned following the Islamic invasion, but there are still more to translate and more widely read. While the direct scientific value of much of this is possibly of little relevance there is an historical interest to trace how many diseases, infections in particular, were recognised and to examine the treatments then employed. It is notable that tuberculosis in the elephant was well described in ancient manuscripts (Palakapya). Other relevant topics that are extensively discussed are animal husbandry, dedication of bulls for breeding, farming, cattle feed and the nutritive value of dairy products. There is also much information, frequently illustrated in colour, of various breeds (54 for horses) conformation, hairmarks, temperament, measurement and many other observations.

There is extensive literature on the indigenous medications, mostly herbal derived. This details activities obtained from roots, bark, stem, leaves, seeds, unripe and ripe fruits – in several cases these have been examined and the active alkaloid identified, but there are many more that have not been examined. It has to be also noted, as in other early civilisations, that both urine, excrement and magic was also used. From ancient days there was a certain anatomical knowledge based in dissection. The ageing of animals – horses, elephants and cattle – by examination of the teeth was practised. There was use of firing, blistering, cautery, bleeding and treatment of fractures and dislocations. Dosing techniques included the bolus/ball, drenches and enemas. The stomach tube was described and used. Over 100 surgical instruments were described and available, most were also used in human practice. It is difficult to understand how competent the art of diagnosis was, but as noted tuberculosis was a recognised disease, with many others including rinderpest, rabies, anthrax, piroplasmosis and dysentery (without understanding the causation).

The Vedic interpretation of medicine, that man acquired the art by observation of animals and birds, not only resulted in veterinary medicine being held in high esteem in the Hindu culture, but also determined that veterinarians need to be experts in health, rather than the emphasis being on disease. The establishment of Buddhist beliefs then introduced the concepts of benevolence and moved towards the prevention of suffering in both man and animals. This meant that the Indian veterinary medication and care system blossomed under the reign of King Ashoka (r.268 BC–232 BC) and survived for over 1000 years until it was largely destroyed following the Islamic invasion.

In comparison with other chapters in this book, this discussion of the development of veterinary medicine in the ancient Indian subcontinent and adjacent territories might seem to be excessive. The reason is, following research, it would appear that the concepts and practices that evolved from the Indus Valley civilisation are probably the earliest recognition by humans of how to approach the subject of ill health. And from this to advance progress towards a logical and scientific discipline of medicine – which was seen as one subject with two clinical end points, in animals and humans. This recognition stems from the Hindu prayers in which animals received a prior mention to humans and in the Laws of Manu (c.200 BC) where animals were as equally protected as humans. Indian civilisation and culture is one where animals and humans are seen to have the same destiny, as a result veterinary medicine has always been held in high esteem. For further elucidation and study a selection of authors, papers and translations is given below.

An important contribution in the history of Indian veterinary medicine is found in papers written by Indian nationals, both before and after British control. Three papers by A. Krishnaswamy, a Madras Veterinary College graduate, are noted (he uses the word 'Iyer' as a surname, this indicates his caste as a Hindu Brahmin, usually of Tamil origin). The first paper (Krishnaswami Iyer 1937, pp. 717–724) provides a listing of ten ancient treatises starting with the *Asvavaidyaka*, an important early work on equine medicine and then discusses the elephantology work of Palakapya and his recognition and description of tuberculosis and its varying forms.

His second paper (Krishnaswamy 1945, pp. 388–410) is a good introduction to the ancient authors, the value of their work, early systems of animal husbandry together with a translation of an early book, *Sukra-Niti* with much interesting content. A further paper (Krishnaswamy 1950, pp. 507–520) provides a closer study of the authors and the value of their work (in relation to later western veterinary medical studies). An in-depth discussion is also given of the activities and value of many of the herbal medications, by virtue of their specific alkaloid or other content.

A useful historical overview is given by S Datta (1948, pp. 115–121). He recognises the very significant contribution made by Hallen in the struggle to establish India-wide veterinary services, and provides a valuable summary of research and other developments up to the time of independence. Of particular interest is the work by D V S Reddy (1945, pp. 320–324), based on the *Arthasastra* written in 4th century BC by Kautilaya, on the administrative code and record of the Mauryan Regime. Several segments of the treatise detail the care and treatment to be given by the state veterinarians to the elephants and horses used by royalty and the army. Another section covers the care and treatment of cattle, 'for the benefit of Agriculture and the sake of milk products'.

The listed procedures include diets, medications, care of elderly animals, slaughterhouses and welfare. Cruelty to animals was to be punished. It was stated,

Whoever hurt or caused another to hurt a cow was to be slain.

One of the most important and earliest (and undated) Sanskrit treatises was the *Asvavaidyakan* or *Book of Equine Medicine*. The author of the work is given as Sri Mahasamant Jayadatta, who, according to the custom of the early Vedic years would have been a rishi or saintly being. The work was translated by Nripendra Nath Majundar, of the Bengal Veterinary Services and published in the *Indian Veterinary Journal* (Jayadatta 1926, pp. 64–123). The book includes practically everything relating to horses that was known at that time. The 68 chapters cover the parts of the body, treatment of sterility, cauterisation, phlebotomy, administration of enemas, care following exercise, treatment of *mrgroga* (?glanders), description of diseases, and prognosis of curable and incurable diseases. The complete translation is published in 12 sections and includes fascinating detail, demonstrating both significant knowledge and equine expertise. Finally, T Mayer, a British veterinary surgeon obtained a copy of *The Veterinary Art in India* written by J Grellier (mentioned earlier) and published in Madras in 1802. Grellier was a qualified surgeon and veterinarian and able to present an interesting review of principally equine, practice in India. The book is published in several sections (Grellier 1842–1844, serialised from pp. 25–28).

BURMA (MYANMAR)

A country bordered by India and Bangladesh to its west and Thailand, Laos and China to its east and north. In the 16th century under the Taungoo dynasty the country was briefly the largest empire in the region. Following the Burmese Wars between 1824 and 1888 the country was annexed to become a British colony. Initially administered as a province of India, then as a separate territory until independence. With a typical tropical climate the environment is humid. The coastal regions have an average temperature of 89.6°F/32.0°C while the cooler north averages 70.0°F/21.0°C. The northern region is mountainous and the country's structure is dominated by three main rivers, each in a mountain valley and bordered by fertile plains. The longest river is the Irrawaddy at 1348 miles: the majority of the population live in this river's valley. Much of the land is still undeveloped with large areas of teak and bamboo forest, swampy delta regions and a wide diversity of wild animals and plant life.

Compared with other Asian countries, Myanmar is undeveloped with a dominant traditional rural structure. The Theravada Buddhism belief is currently held by about 85% of the population, with practically every community being based around a monastery. Other religious groups are small, some 6% Christian, about 4% Muslim and a few traditional or Hindu followers. The Muslim group, the Rohingya, are ethnically different, having arrived on the west coast some 1000 years ago. Speaking their own language, they are currently denied citizenship and have been subject to persecution and attack for many centuries.

Agriculture and Livestock

Rice has always been the main agricultural product and currently accounts for some 60% of the cultivated land area; the second major crop being opium. Livestock populations are small, with water buffalo and oxen being the primary draught animals. Sheep, goats and cattle are mainly kept on the drier lands to the north of the country. Chickens and pigs are ubiquitous in the numerous peasant farms. The equine population is very small, due to difficulties in maintaining health. In 1928 it was estimated that there were about 3600 domesticated elephants; another report stated that in the 1930s there were between 7000 and 10,000 working elephants. Currently there are some 5000 domesticated elephants, the largest global captive elephant population. The country is believed to have the second largest total elephant population.

Within the Buddhism belief livestock products play a small part in the national diet. Fish, both freshwater (for the inland communities) and sea (for coastal), provide the main protein intake – either as a sauce (*ngapil*), fermented seafood, dried or salted fish or prawns. Inland, and further north, pig meat and chicken are eaten as peasant food. Rice is the main vegetable. Most milk comes from goats, and most cattle and buffalo are used for farm and transport work.

British Jurisdiction and Animal Health

Following progressive annexation the British authorities began to institute veterinary controls. The first of these followed the 1869 *Report of the Indian Cattle Plague Commission* when an attempt was made to create a Burmese Civil Veterinary Department.

Prior to this, veterinary work in the agricultural sector was carried out by army veterinarians, in addition to their military duties. The first of these was a veterinary officer named Thomas Parinder Gudgin who assisted the civil government in controlling rinderpest outbreaks. Gudgin was mentioned in a letter of 1873 dealing with the 'cattle murrain' outbreak, where it was stated,

> *Mr. Eden would like much to have a really intelligent veterinary surgeon attached to this province for a few years, that he might give practical instruction.*

This was a rather severe judgement on Gudgin, who graduated from London in 1850, was commissioned into the army in 1854 and had a long career in the Crimean War, the Indian Mutiny and the South African Wars. He had been single-handedly trying to deal with the rinderpest outbreaks that occurred in the country before and shortly after the onset of the monsoon season.

In January 1874 Samuel Robert Sartin, veterinary officer, was placed at the disposal of the Chief Commissioner of British Burma. Sartin had graduated from London in 1869. His instructions included,

> *open a veterinary class and instruct young men, natives of Burma, in the art, in the districts in which cattle disease exists.*

There was slow progression towards the creation of a veterinary structure in a country with a population that had little understanding of disease control. It was not an easy project.

Veterinary Administration

Sartin made observations on FMD, but there is no record of any teaching work. In 1876 he was replaced by Robert Frost Veterinary Officer, an 1870 London graduate. Frost remained in post until 1890 with six major roles:

1. Veterinary Instructor for the province. He travelled the country giving advice on cattle disease control and stressing the value of such procedures. Also advised the Forest Department on elephant diseases and Police Department on the purchase and care of ponies.
2. Teacher at the veterinary school. Enrolling students for training for the three-year course was difficult as they could not see themselves making a livelihood as private veterinary practitioners. Frost then made their training suitable for

appointment as cattle market superintendents. This attracted students and by the end of 1840 there were eighteen qualified veterinary assistants and fifteen students.

3. Superintendent of Veterinary Practitioners. Frost travelled and supervised the local assistants' work and enabled the supply of free medicines if required. The diaries kept by the assistants enabled the spread of rinderpest outbreaks to be monitored.

4. Superintendent of Pony Breeding Operations. This resulted in stallion care and a free breeding service for mares, pony numbers grew and health improved.

5. Veterinary Surgeon to Transport Department. This additional post meant that all health care issues in the country were coming under one control, and provided transport officers with help in both purchasing animals and health care advice.

6. Veterinary Surgeon to Rangoon (Yangon) Municipality. In 1879 the Glanders and Farcy Act was extended to Rangoon town, Frost was appointed Official Veterinary Surgeon under the Act. The municipality was then able to advise on veterinary issues.

In 1885 Frost investigated a severe outbreak of rinderpest in the Arakan district, which eventually resulted in the 1894 Segregation Rules, defining the duties of the village headman in control of outbreaks of cattle disease. Veterinary assistants were trained, posted around the country and provided reports on disease outbreaks as well as giving some treatments. Frost returned to the Army Department in 1890.

G H Evans, from the Army Department succeeded Frost in December 1890 and held position as Head of the Veterinary Department for thirty years. The training school was reopened as the Rangoon Veterinary College in 1891 with a veterinary officer from the Bombay Veterinary College, J S Batlivla, on the staff: the course was fixed at two and a half years. In 1891 care of the Military Police ponies (2918 in thirteen battalions) was passed to the Veterinary Department and in 1893 Bhagwant Singh, a graduate of the Lahore Veterinary College, was appointed for this post. In 1897–1898 Evans was sent on special duty to Mukteswar, India to attend the demonstration by Professor Koch of his rinderpest control measures. On return to Burma he introduced the methods, with initially good results.

Evans developed the Burma Veterinary Department along different lines to those in India. He did not introduce full veterinary training but used the Veterinary College to provide a rather elementary course. Burma was a difficult country in which to work: communication between the many towns and adjacent territories, and regulation of the land frontiers with Thailand and China to supervise for disease control was difficult. Rinderpest control was a major issue and the vaccine methods available only partially successful. Anthrax, in particular in elephants, was found to be a significant problem. Endemic disease control was difficult in the humid, warm, tropical climate.

Evans became an authority on elephants and wrote *Elephants and their Diseases* 1901, reprinted in 1910; it remained an important reference work for many years. Evans also wrote a *Veterinary Materia Medica* which was translated into Burmese as well as a handbook *Directions for the Prevention of Contagious Diseases among Cattle in Burma* and a shorter booklet, produced in English and Burmese on FMD.

Thomas Rennie, an 1881 Glasgow graduate, was appointed in 1902 as Deputy Superintendent, and in 1920 he replaced Evans. Rennie served for 25 years as Superintendent of the Veterinary Department and Agricultural Advisor to the government. When he retired there were 168 veterinary assistants, 24 inspectors and an assistant instructor. Within the British colonial service Burma was always known as a 'difficult' territory – it was not like India and there was much underlying tension within the Indian-Burma relationship.

Animal Disease Control

Control over epidemic diseases was gradually achieved and legislation was introduced, notably in 1879 when the Glanders and Farcy Act was extended to the Rangoon region. Introduction of the Segregation Rules for cattle in 1894, greatly aided rinderpest control. Village headmen in Lower Burma were supplied with forms to record the deaths of cattle, buffaloes and horses, and by 1894 these were being well kept. Each form had notes describing the symptoms of rinderpest, anthrax and FMD to enable accurate reporting. It was not until 1922 that these forms were used in Upper Burma, due to great local opposition.

The Koch rinderpest vaccination method was introduced to Burma in 1900–1901 when 173 bovines were immunised, followed by 4006 in 1902, increasing annually. In 1903 anthrax was diagnosed as a significant cause of death in elephants, a disease well described in the novel *The Glass Palace* (Ghosh 2000, pp. 92–97). Veterinary assistants were issued with microscopes in 1908 and by 1911 there was confirmation of trypanosomiasis in elephants, HS (*Pasteurella boviseptica*) in cattle, buffaloes and elephants, and piroplasmosis in several species. By 1915 the presence of filariasis, anthrax and epizootic lymphangitis were all confirmed. FMD was an annual problem when Shan caravans from China arrived every winter. Controls were introduced at the frontier.

The veterinary school was moved to Insein, north of Rangoon, in 1908 and a hospital established in 1911 which helped in the education of the students. Anthrax, rinderpest and HS were the three major diseases; in 1927 local veterinary research began, based at new buildings in Insein. An anthrax vaccine was produced to combat the heavy losses in the elephants working in the timber industry. In 1930 a total of 1247 elephants were immunised. An elephant sick camp was established in 1931 and used to test anthelmintics as well as study wound treatment, parasites, general care and management. In the same year, an attenuated anthrax vaccine for equine use was developed. Rinderpest became the subject of research to find new and safer vaccines.

Later an anthrax vaccine was produced for cattle and the anthrax strain vaccine was developed successfully for immunisation of elephants. Investigations into elephant diseases remained a major part of the local research programme, with financial support provided by the timber companies. In 1936 an innovative rinderpest desiccated goat spleen vaccine was developed for use in cattle, but this was less successful in buffaloes and mythun (a semi-domesticated variety of bison). A simultaneous anthrax and HS immunisation vaccine was developed for cattle use.

Equine diseases had always been a serious problem in Burma, surra (*Trypanosoma evansi*) was enzootic in many areas and early work had begun in the 1930s with Naganol as a preventive. *Kumri*, dry coat and osteoporosis were also significant causes of loss. The cause of *Kumri*, a word derived from Hindustani meaning 'weak back', initially clinically termed lumbar paralysis, was eventually solved and described as cerebrospinal nematodiasis, frequently *Setaria (Artionema) digitata*, but other nematode filarial stages may be involved.

In 1941 Japan invaded Burma and with the evacuation of most senior staff, research ceased. War ravaged the country until the cessation of hostilities in 1945. The situation slowly returned to pre-war normality, to then be continued by the national government following independence in 1948. Today Myanmar has one veterinary school, the University of Veterinary Science, located at Yezin, near Naypyidaw. Tuition is given in the English language.

This text is partly based on *A History of the Overseas Veterinary Services: Part 1*, 1961, British Veterinary Association, London. Chapter 2, Burma, by S.R. Rippon

CEYLON (SRI LANKA)

Sri Lanka is an island country in the Indian Ocean near the southern tip of India, with the Bay of Bengal to the east and north and the Indian Ocean to the west. The total land area of the island is 66,610 square kilometres (about 25,000 square miles). Over the centuries there has been a continual struggle between rulers, religions and those who could see the strategic advantage of possession of the island. It has good harbours and is well placed for controlling sea trade between Asia and Europe. The northern land area is flat with extensive plains, with a high land mass in the south-central region. About 5/6th of the total land area has agricultural use. The climate is tropical with a humid, warm climate and a wide diversity of both plants and animals.

Historical Background

Cave excavations have provided evidence of early humans about 28,500 BP, with suggestions that they were engaged in agriculture and used dogs to drive game for hunting. The original people were the indigenous *Vedda*, who now only represent about 1% of the population.

The ancient Greeks, who knew of the island, and the Roman Empire had trading links transporting cinnamon. There is documented history detailing events for some 3000 years, this is based on 'chronicles' which were probably written about the 4th century AD. These ancient *Sinhala Ola* (palm leaf) manuscripts were in Sanskrit; they demonstrate that care and treatment of elephants was practised in the early civilisation. It was recorded that there were 'veterinary officers' in the elephant establishment of the court of the Kings on the island (Deraniyagala 1952). The early systems for preventing and treating animal disease on the island, including the first recorded treatment of an elephant in c.150 BC, are recorded (Piyadasa 1994, pp. 471–486).

Sri Lankan history is essentially one of a series of invasions, inevitably resulting in conflict and wars. The first and still the most significant were the Indo-Aryans, probably from the northern region of the Indian land mass, who invaded in 500 BC. This created the language, Sinhalese, and introduced Indian knowledge and culture, but with a different identity. This invasion also introduced Buddhism, which is now the belief of about 75% of the Sri Lankan population. Later there was an invasion by the Tamil people of southern India, speaking Hindi and holding their beliefs, now about 13% of population and finally the Muslim group with about 8%. These three groups represent some 96% of the current population – and each group has their own approach towards animal welfare and meat consumption.

The Portuguese arrived in 1505 and established themselves in Colombo in 1517, gaining control by 1619. They were followed by the Dutch who obtained effective control with the Dutch East India Company. When the Napoleonic Wars began the British were concerned that the French might try to achieve occupation and with the agreement of the Dutch they took over in 1796. This was followed by the annexation of the Kingdom of Kandy, with the British achieving complete control by 1815.

The population mix of indigenous *Veddas*, ethnic Sinhalese, Tamils, plus Europeans, Malays and Chinese has created a rich culture. The series of kingdoms and Buddhist beliefs has created a strong identity to this culture. There is a tradition of indigenous curative health care as well as practitioners of traditional *ayurveda* medicine (now outnumbered by western medicine). Records exist of a very early hospital, built at Mihintale in the 4th century AD. European medicine was introduced by the Portuguese in the 16th century and has been a significant factor in human and animal healthcare for many centuries since.

Agriculture and Livestock

From early times crop production has been the leading agricultural activity, supported by a remarkable sophisticated system of dams, canals and reservoirs constructed in the reign of Parakramabahu (1135–1186); the remains of which can still be seen. Agriculture has been based in plantation cultivation, initially of cinnamon, then rubber, coconuts and tea. Rice is a major crop for local consumption, with vegetables, and fish in coastal regions. Livestock populations are not large, but there are a significant number of elephants, both domesticated and wild.

At one time there were many cattle and buffalo used for draught work and ploughing in paddy fields. These functions are now mechanised except for the family farm units. Agricultural land usage is unchanged with about 70% used for crop production and 30% for mixed crop and livestock (mostly peasant farms). This ratio was probably much the same in the earlier years. Due to widespread Buddhism and

Hindu beliefs very little beef is eaten. Cattle produce milk, but goat milk is equally popular, as is their meat. Pig and sheep numbers are small. Poultry are important for eggs and also meat. Fish is widely consumed from rivers and the sea. Currently total livestock production is less than 1% gross domestic product (GDP).

British Jurisdiction and Veterinary Administration

Following the British gaining complete control in 1815 there does not appear to have been any recorded immediate veterinary activity. It would appear that the situation was satisfactory until a severe rinderpest outbreak in 1888–1890 killed some 40% of cattle and buffaloes.

In 1891 Charles Augustus Lye, an 1888 London graduate, was appointed as Veterinary Instructor to the School of Agriculture and, 'his services were available to the community at large'.

In the same year, a veterinary scholarship was offered, and W A de Silva went to the Indian Bombay Veterinary College. Following his graduation in 1894 he returned, to become Acting Government Veterinary Surgeon following Lye's retirement.

G W Sturgess then arrived as the Government Veterinary Surgeon and de Silva assisted him, before he became Colombo's first Municipal Veterinary Surgeon (later he became a politician and Minister of Health, dying in 1946). In 1895 E.T. Houle, another Bombay graduate, was appointed to assist Sturgess. By 1906 the Colombo Municipal Veterinary Department, headed by de Silva had six full-time veterinary assistants, an organised cattle market and a quarantine station: de Silva had done excellent work. In 1926 there were extensive rinderpest outbreaks resulting in the resignation of veterinary staff and the appointment of M Crawford as government Veterinary Surgeon – he totally reorganised the department and rinderpest was controlled. By 1933 fourteen Bombay graduates had joined the department. One graduate of the Bombay Veterinary College, Mohamed Zakriya Mahamooth GBVC, went on to the Edinburgh (Dick) Veterinary College, to graduate in 1937 as the first Ceylonese MRCVS.

Under Crawford's direction much progress was made in disease identification and control. In 1935 the Veterinary Department was absorbed into the Department of Agriculture. They moved to Peradeniya in 1936 where they became the Animal Husbandry Department headed by the Government Veterinary Surgeon. In 1944 Crawford retired after 21 years' service and was succeeded as Government Veterinary Surgeon by T M Z Mahamooth. In 1947 the Faculties of Veterinary Science and Agriculture were established in the University of Ceylon at Peradeniya. The first Professor of Veterinary Medicine was appointed in 1948.

Animal Disease Control

The 1888–1890 rinderpest outbreak was not only serious in causing the loss of some 40% of cattle and buffaloes, but was a disaster for the local indigenous people who were themselves suffering from poor health with malaria, intestinal parasites and yaws. It was soon recognised that rinderpest and FMD were the two major problems. Augustus Lye had identified another lethal cattle disease called *kandamale*, but which he termed *pharyngo-laryngitis contagiosa* (possibly localised anthrax or pasteurellosis). A cattle ordinance in 1891 had little effect in controlling rinderpest and prior to 1893 few preventive measures had been introduced. Sick animals in the villages were treated by local animal healers called *vederalas*.

In 1896 Sturgess reported that over 13,000 cattle and 4600 buffalo had FMD. The disease was endemic and had probably been so for centuries: it was mild in indigenous cattle, severe in European breeds and rare in sheep, goats and pigs. Control was difficult as pastures were unfenced and a potential disease reservoir existed in the wild deer, pigs and buffaloes. A slaughter policy was felt to be impractical. Sturgess visited South Africa to talk with D Hutcheon, Principal Veterinary Surgeon of Cape Colony, about rinderpest control. While there he noted 'three-day fever' in cattle, similar to a syndrome in Ceylon and studied Heartwater, the rickettsial infection of sheep and goats as it was similar to *koopooduwan* disease in Ceylon. He also described a then unknown disease of cattle (Sturgess 1906, pp. 209–303). In 1901 control measures for rinderpest control were drawn up, but they failed to be effective.

Crawford was appointed as Government Veterinary Surgeon in 1926 and following a total reorganisation rinderpest was eradicated by 1934 (but did reappear again in 1942). Crawford made an intensive study of local animal diseases. Many horses had been imported for racing or riding; no African Horse Sickness, glanders or epizootic lymphangitis was reported but osteoporosis was a problem – Crawford identified the calcium: phosphorus imbalance in the diet. *Kumri* was recognised (as was 'goat paralysis'). Later studies revealed the condition to be cerebrospinal nematodiasis. In 1922 Newcastle Disease of poultry was identified, fowl pox outbreaks were controlled by pigeon pox vaccine. In 1932 Crawford also identified *Plasmodium gallinaceum* as the cause of malaria in imported birds. Later he found *Aegyptianella pullorum* (or a similar organism) in imported birds.

A 1933 report noted that bovine tuberculosis was uncommon in Ceylon and had only been seen in imported cattle, a rabies vaccination programme was started. In 1934 *Oestrus ovis* was identified and a microfilaria was found in fowls, causing elephantiasis of the wattle. Many cases of FMD were reported in 1935–1936 causing severe losses in European cattle. Rabies incidence rose in several species, and *surra* was found in a dog, which was treated with Naganol. 1942 was a difficult year as many controls had been relaxed due to wartime restrictions. Rinderpest was reintroduced by goats imported from India, and was suppressed only to appear again in cattle. In 1944 the goat virus vaccine was introduced and with movement controls the disease was finally stamped out in 1946. Crawford retired in 1944. The majority of the disease identification studies and effective control programmes were due to his work and initiative.

In 1947 the Veterinary College was established in the University of Ceylon with the first Veterinary Professor appointed in 1948. The Faculty currently teaches a four year course with tuition in Sinhala, Tamil and English. Independence was granted in 1948, and in 1972 the country name was changed to Sri Lanka.

This text is partly based on *A History of the Overseas Veterinary Services: Part 1*, 1961, British Veterinary Association, London. Chapter 3, Ceylon, by C. A. McGaughey

MALAYSIA (MALAYA, SINGAPORE, BORNEO)

Territories now included in Malaysia, a country in Southeast Asia, are Peninsula Malaysia (the southern part of the Malay Peninsula south of Thailand and north of Singapore), and East Malaysia (the eastern and northern sectors of the island of Borneo, and bordering Brunei and Indonesia). The parts are separated by the South China Sea.

Historically the Malayan peninsula was dominated by the Malaccan Empire. In 1511 the Portuguese established a trading base. They were replaced in 1641 by the Dutch who occupied Malacca to obtain access to the tin mines. Following the Napoleonic Wars Britain took control of Malacca in 1829 and began progressive control over the States in the peninsula. By 1819 Stamford Raffles had acquired Singapore, then a desolate island. Within the British Empire the Malay States were one of the most profitable territories due to the tin mines and rubber plantations.

Agriculture and Livestock

The total land area of 127,355 sq.ml (329,847 sq.km) with a long coastline, is dominated by a mountainous range frequently topped by cloud. The climate is tropical with a high rainfall and two monsoon seasons producing a year-round average humidity of 90%. There are few hurricanes or droughts. The population traditionally lives in the river valleys in the mountains in local communities (*kampongs*) and on the coastal plains.

The traditional Malay peasant small farm agriculture was mainly rice padis and dependent on buffalo for ploughing and oxen for transport. Following British annexation, plantations of rubber trees, palms (for oil) and coconuts became dominant. Fruit production is now profitable for small farms and Chinese farmers specialise in vegetable and poultry. Logging is found in the heavily forested tropical regions.

Diet is based around rice, seafood, vegetables, poultry meat and eggs. Meat consumption is related to the several religious beliefs. Religion is dominated by Islam (well enforced) at about 61% of population, Buddhism is followed by 20%, Christianity 9%, Hinduism 3%, traditional Chinese 3%. Poultry is mainly eaten by the Chinese community, beef and mutton are not major foods. About 80% of total population live in Peninsular Malaysia.

British Jurisdiction

Following the acquisition and creation of the Straits Settlements (Penang, Singapore and Malacca) in 1824, the British influence extended until, by 1914, all of the Malay

States had come to be under British protection. Agriculture was at a subsistence level throughout the region and food requirements were supported by hunting and fishing. There was a traditional feudal structure, strongly based in the Muslim religion and a low level of agricultural economic activity due to the difficult environment, and widespread disease in animals and humans.

British veterinary activity was seen first in Singapore. Major Low wrote in 1840–1841 that buffalo and oxen are used mainly for draught, but are subject to frequent murrains. He also noted 'some black cattle and ponies and masses of anomalous breeds of dogs'. The first horse race meeting was held in 1843 (the British always rank their priorities) and a serious 'cattle murrain' was observed in 1873.

Charles Emmerson, an 1860 graduate from the London College, came to Singapore in the same year, but set himself up as a hotelier. In 1870 H Abrams arrived, he was recorded as a veterinary surgeon but no record of his qualification exists in the UK. He founded the Abrams Horse Repository in Singapore and was reported to have employed three veterinary surgeons. None of these men were in government employ. However, British records do list a Charles Abrams qualified in 1898 as being in Singapore.

Veterinary Administration

The Malaysian veterinary service commenced in the Straits Settlements and gradually extended to operate in the Federated and Unfederated Malay States. In most States this began as a branch of the Medical Department. The exact starting date is unclear but there is a record of L Burghope, (qualified London, 1884) employed as Government Veterinary Surgeon at Penang in 1888, with one local inspector. Rinderpest was a great problem; a cattle quarantine station was opened in 1896.

By 1895 all the Federated Malay States had an operational veterinary branch, the first traceable veterinary surgeon was G Moir, qualified from Edinburgh in 1896 (but listed as being in Malaya in 1893), who remained for 29 years. He became a Fellow of the Royal College of Veterinary Surgeons (FRCVS) in 1906 following his thesis 'Note of Rinderpest in Perak'. By 1920 every state had a professionally qualified veterinarian from either Britain or India. In 1905 the Veterinary Police Force was formed and by 1910 had 45 men who acted as the 'eyes and ears' of the veterinary departments and were a great help in detecting disease outbreaks. The Force was finally disbanded in 1955.

Singapore Municipal Veterinary Department began as an SPCA (Charity) clinic in 1876 before being taken over by the city in 1901. Singapore had its first government Veterinary Surgeon appointed in 1893, P S Falshaw, who served in that post for 30 years, as well as undertaking Municipal Veterinary Department duties. He identified *Trypanosoma falshawi* (now known as *Tryp. theileri*). The Department had purpose-built premises in 1904 and today has both a clinic and a hospital.

In 1930 the post of Principal Veterinary Officer Straits Settlements and Federated Malay States was created, allowing harmonisation of disease control programmes.

The title was amended to Director of Veterinary Research and Veterinary Adviser, Malaya in 1933 and eventually in 1953 a central laboratory was established.

Animal Disease Control

In 1888 it was reported that 'cattle disease appears year after year with fatal regularity and causes great loss'. Control was difficult as there was much cattle trading and no reporting of disease. It was recorded that canine rabies was common in both Singapore and Malacca. A major rabies outbreak had occurred in Singapore in 1884, resulting in a dog tax being introduced, stray dogs being captured (and drowned), together with a Superintendent of Rabies being appointed, who was also in charge of the Fire Brigade! Muzzling was then enforced and rabies was reported to be stamped out by 1892.

An 1889 report noted again that livestock disease was prevalent and widespread in the Malay States. Particular mention was made of both FMD and rabies. In 1895 the Veterinary Branch reported epidemics of glanders, FMD, swine fever and some anthrax. By 1896 swine fever and rinderpest were found to be widespread – reports from 1897 also reported widespread rinderpest, FMD, swine fever, glanders and rabies. In 1899 there was a major rinderpest outbreak, 'thousands of buffaloes and many bullocks have succumbed'. In the nineteenth century rinderpest was almost worldwide in its occurrence.

A 1900 review confirmed that livestock disease was rife throughout the country with particular mention made of epidemics of rinderpest and FMD as well as swine fever, glanders and rabies. There was, however, a growing awareness that some of the 'rinderpest' and 'anthrax' cases were actually HS. Additionally in 1903 surra was diagnosed in horses. There were only four veterinarians in the whole territory, and they were in a minor branch of the Medical Department, which was trying to cope with a similar onslaught of human disease.

France, in the neighbouring Indo-Chinese lands, was more advanced in tropical disease studies and had established the Saigon Pasteur Institute in 1889 with a second Laboratory at Nha Trang in 1895. Schools of Tropical Medicine had opened in Britain in 1899 and the Kuala Lumpur Institute of Medical Research (IMR) established in Malaya in 1901. As the Nha Trang Pasteur Institute was producing anti-rinderpest serum it was decided to purchase some, but first wanted to confirm the Malayan diagnosis. The Director of the IMR cooperated with the Nha Trang Director, who knew of the severe losses of cattle and buffalo in the past and mentioned a mortality of 30% in imported Indian cattle and 80–100% in local buffalo. He described symptoms and post-mortems and wrote 'the epizootic in the Malay Peninsula is not rinderpest but haemorrhagic septicaemia'. Subsequent events however proved him wrong – while there obviously was HS present the major disease was rinderpest. In 1902 it was established that rinderpest was caused by a virus and a 1903 investigation with the Royal Veterinary College, London proved the existence of rinderpest in the Malay Peninsula; anti-rinderpest serum was obtained from India and used as a preventive.

Surra was becoming a serious equine problem and an IMR study in 1907 identified Tabanid flies as the main transmitters of the disease. Gradually animal diseases became controlled or eradicated, but in 1930 outbreaks of rinderpest and FMD still occurred and were suppressed; there was also a constant underlying problem with swine fever, rabies, pleuro-pneumonia in goats and surra. It was very difficult to get Malay cattle owners to accept western medicine and sera, vaccines and medicines were frequently rejected. There was a strong belief in traditional medicines provided by shamans of various beliefs such as the *bomohs*, *pawangs* and *dukuns*.

By the late 1930s the disease control emphasis centred around rinderpest, poultry diseases, blood parasites and 'equine anhydrosis'. With strict quarantine, outbreaks of FMD and rinderpest became fewer. Animal husbandry work began as the importation of cattle, buffalo, sheep and pigs became controlled and monitored by quarantine checks. Small trial farms were created to upgrade indigenous stock, and improve poultry, which had become important.

The Japanese invasion in 1941, and British surrender in 1942, ended European control but a reduced service continued to operate with Asian staff until the Japanese surrender in 1945. Post-war British Army veterinary officers took control until a Director of Veterinary Services was appointed in 1946. In 1948 the Malayan Federation (now including Borneo) was formed and the Veterinary Department became a Joint Federal Department, this was followed by a difficult period of communist insurgency. A few years after its suppression independence was declared in 1957.

Post-war controls enabled the claim that rinderpest, FMD, HS, glanders and epizootic lymphangitis were all eradicated by 1946. Rabies in dogs remained a major problem as did Newcastle Disease (ND) in poultry, but this was soon controlled by vaccines imported from India, enabling rapid growth of the mostly Chinese owned poultry industry. The rabies problem was attacked by compulsory vaccination with Flury Strain chick embryo vaccine and the destruction of all stray dogs. Eradication was achieved by June 1953.

In 1953 the Veterinary Research Institute opened at Ipoh in Perak State providing vaccines for ND, fowl pox, contagious ecthyma and HS as well as a good diagnostic service. The research programme identified pullorum disease, infectious laryngotracheitis, brucellosis, moniliasis in poultry and pigeons, avian leucosis, *Vibrio foetus*, listeriosis, infectious canine hepatitis, trichomoniasis in pigeons and *Mycoplasma gallisepticum* in chickens.

The first Malay citizen to graduate in Britain was H.H. Tunku Abu Bakar of Johore, the son of the Sultan, in 1919. He became the first State Veterinary Surgeon of Johore in 1920 and after war in 1946 was made Chief Animal Husbandry Officer. A man of great humanitarian principles he devoted his life to improving the lives of the people and the animal husbandry of his country; he retired in 1952.

When independence was declared in 1957 there was the almost unique situation of a colonial tropical country with freedom from all major diseases and with almost all senior staff in the Veterinary Department Malaysian-born.

Veterinary Faculties with a full veterinary education degree course are available at two Universities: Universiti Putra Malaysia at Selangor and Universiti Malaysia

Kelantan at Kelantan. Depending on the syllabus being taught, courses last between five and seven years.

Independence Day on August 31, 1957 resulted in the Federation of Malaya, uniting all the States on the Malay Peninsula. In 1963 Singapore, and Sarawak and North Borneo (both on Borneo Island) also became independent and joined to become the Federation of Malaysia. In 1965 Singapore left to become an independent State.

North Borneo had the status of a British chartered company and colony until 1946, but Sarawak had been obtained by James Brooke, a British explorer, and been governed by the Brooke family from 1841 to 1946, when it became a British colony and then joined with North Borneo to enter the Malaysian Federation.

Information on the early veterinary history is limited. In 1914 J P Swan, a British veterinarian began to work on the island, but resigned in 1915 following 'friction' with the authorities. Other early records have been lost. It is known that surra was recognised in the territory in 1937 and had reached epidemic proportions by 1941. Following the Japanese surrender S R Rippon was appointed Veterinary Officer – his reports noted that working on the island was difficult but that surra was a major problem together with endemic ND in poultry. A programme of poultry vaccination brought ND and fowl pox under control and the last case of surra was treated in 1956. A survey then showed the territory was free of tuberculosis, rinderpest, swine fever and bovine pleuro-pneumonia. With the major diseases controlled efforts were made to reduce the helminth burden in all livestock. Borneo was always an area with difficulty in obtaining staff.

This text is partly based on *A History of the Overseas Veterinary Services: Part 1*, 1961, British Veterinary Association, London, Chapter 4, Malaya, by W.E. Lancaster and *Part 2*, North Borneo by E. H. Holland

TIBET

The country covers an area mostly on the north side of the Himalayan mountains. Until the late 1940s Tibet was regarded as an independent, semi-autonomous region in the fastness of the high Himalayas; somewhat of a religious curiosity. In 1951 the local government was obliged to sign an agreement of peaceful liberation by the Chinese State, being then occupied by the People's Army followed by renaming in 1956 as the Tibet Autonomous Region of China. A rebellion followed in 1959 with the Dalai Lama, the putative head of State, fleeing to safety in northern India. The Chinese Communist Government then took over total control.

Agriculture and Livestock

The Tibetan region is a vast, mostly inhospitable, territory between India and China. Agriculture is reliant on pastoralism with the animals that are supported on these lands: they provide subsistence and a mode of travel and transport. Animals have always played an important part in Tibetan culture. The principle livestock are yaks, *dzo* (yak/cattle cross), bullocks, cows, goats and sheep, there are also horses and a small population of indigenous pastoral pigs. Most fieldwork is performed by the *dzo* crosses. Cows provide milk and butter, and sheep provide milk, butter and wool. There is also the Tibetan mastiff, a particularly large breed of dog.

Farming is essentially high altitude plateau animal husbandry with sheep, goats and yaks the most important species. The majority of the population have always been traditional small holding or nomadic farmers. Most crops are grown in south Tibet: *gingke* highland barley and wheat. In the north, farmers are either nomadic shepherds or yak or horse breeders. Farming has always been difficult due to the altitude and the severe weather; frequent blizzards can result in serious livestock losses. It has been a custom for herders, if the flock is felt to be too large for available pasture, to free a certain number to go wild. This is believed to earn the herder merit in the next life.

Traditionally communities were self-sufficient and associated with monasteries and feudal landlords (now changed under Chinese communist rule). For centuries, the general population has been poor, at poverty level and usually with a food deficit. Human diet is based in local grain crops and potatoes with various meats when available. Fish is eaten only rarely.

Tibetan Culture and Medicine

Tibet has a long and complex history, that part of its culture related to medicine is slightly less complex and can be related to certain specific factors, of these the most important have been the influence of India and the arrival of Buddhism.

The medical texts of Tibet illustrate the multicultural character of their medicine which can be traced to the three major medical traditions (in order of influence) Indian, Chinese and Greco-Arab. These are expressed in the Four Tantras, the native Tibetan books that incorporate these important teachings. Early medicine, human and animal, was based on shaman practice and supernatural beliefs, but then influenced by the introduction from India of the Vedic *Ayurveda* as well as Chinese acupuncture with moxibustion. Texts from both countries dating back to 2000 BC were translated and used in both human and veterinary medicine practices.

Traditional Tibetan medicine, also termed *Sowa-Rigpa*, like other Asian medical systems first makes a specific definition of health and then works to maintain a balance in the three principles of function (or humours). Translation is difficult but these can be described as *rLung*, the capacity of the body to circulate blood, energy (nervous) and thought, *mkhris-pa*, related to heat, and *Bad-Kan*, related to cold. There is also much use of astrology, herbal medicine and amulets. Tibetan medicine pays great attention to practical skills. Diagnosis is by observation, consultation, smelling, questioning and reading the pulse. Both human and veterinary practitioners are skilled in acupuncture, moxibustion and simple surgery. The available translated literature indicates that veterinary practitioners had a good reputation within Tibetan society.

Buddhism arrived in Tibet from India during the reign of King Thothori Nyantsen (AD 245–AD 364) and was soon incorporated into all aspects of Tibetan culture as Lamaism, or the Mahayana School of Buddhism. This is seen in the principle Tibetan medical text, the *rGyud-Zhi* and in the Four Tantras, possibly written in the 12th century, and forming the basis of Tibetan medical practice. Following this religious introduction was the use of Buddhist literature, in particular the *Abhidharma* and *Vajrayana Tantras*, thus influencing the Tibetan *Bon* tradition. The Buddhist belief that illness results from three 'poisons' – ignorance, attachment and aversion, became incorporated into Tibetan medical practice. This also follows the Buddha's Four Noble Truths which apply medical logic to suffering. Later in the 11th and 12th centuries AD, more Indian culture of all types was introduced and well accepted, this included many medical and other texts that were translated and circulated.

One characteristic of Tibet is the many taboos that have developed over the years. Most of these are related to religion and range from the almost obligatory require-ment to turn prayer wheels when passing them – but remembering that it is forbid-den to turn them counter-clockwise. The Buddhist belief means that the followers are forbidden to kill, and all animals, birds and fish have been protected in some way for centuries, thus restricting meat consumption. Tibetan history, culture, Buddhist introduction and beliefs are both complex and interwoven. The above presents a very brief introduction.

In 1696 the fifth Dalai Lama supported Desi Sangye Gyatso in founding the Chagpori College of Medicine, located on Chagpori Hill (the Iron Mountain) in Lhasa. It was a monastic medical and astrological school, later renamed the Men-Tsee-Khang Medical and Astrological College by the thirteenth Dalai Lama (1873–1933).

The College was destroyed by the Chinese People's Liberation Army during the 1959 rebellion. It has been re-established by the fourteenth Dalai Lama at Takdah, Darjeeling, India and opened in 1992 as the Chagpori Tibetan Medical Institute. Students take a five-year course in Tibetan medicine (as practised in Tibet, Nepal, Bhutan and other Asian countries), this is based in the traditional *Sowa-Rigpa* with inclusions from the Ayurveda, Siddha and Unani systems of medicine.

The Dunhuang Manuscripts

In 1900 a collection of some 20,000 ancient manuscripts were found sealed in one of the Mogao Caves at Dunhuang, an oasis on the Silk Road, in Gansu Province, Western China. The site is a crossroads with one leading to Lhasa. Dated between the 5th and 11th century AD, the manuscripts are a mixture of religious and secular texts. The religious ones are mostly Buddhist in content but the others are Nestorian Christian, Daoist and Manichaeistic. Most are in Chinese with some in Sanskrit, Tibetan, Hebrew and other ancient languages. Many of the Chinese manuscripts are now held in Beijing, but several thousand of the other folios, many in Tibetan, are now in museums and collections around the world. They contain some of the best examples of Tibetan writing. Many reasons have been suggested for the hiding of these manuscripts but none have been confirmed.

Studies in the 1970s–1980s revealed a series of medical manuscripts, many of which were written in Chinese. Examination suggests that the accepted dominant place of the medical *Huangdi neijing* text in early China should be reassessed. At the time of writing it is estimated that there are about 100 medically related manuscripts of varying content, some have been examined in depth. In 1994 the International Dunhuang Project was established to allow global scholars access to the scrolls.

In one Tibetan series of six medical texts (dated between the 9th and 10th century AD), three were devoted to moxibustion use and three to various treatments and prescriptions. They are mostly practical manuals with the main therapeutic method employed being moxibustion (*me btsa*) with both cautery and various herbs or woods. Acupuncture gets very little mention. Bloodletting, cautery by iron, fumigation, massage and cupping (using cattle horns) are all described. In the materia medica prescriptions most medications were herbal based.

Many mentions are made of other countries, in particular Persia and India, as is the use of both camphor and *theriac* (a medical mixture devised in Greece in the 1st century AD, with many ingredients it was considered to be a panacea). These were very rare and costly in Tibet and used for ceremonial and medical purposes. Astrological readings and supernatural beliefs also played a role in diagnosis and prognosis.

Much of the above content is derived from two studies: (Lo and Cullen 2005) and (Lo and Yoeli-Tlalim 2014).

Tibetan Veterinary Medicine

Little is known of traditional veterinary medicine in the early years of Tibet, as further documents are translated hopefully more will be revealed. It is stated that the early animal healers were very proficient and highly regarded. As animals for transport, food and fibre were of vital importance to such an isolated community it would follow that healthcare would have been a major concern. Treatments, where used, appear to have been mainly bloodletting, the use of the cautery and moxibustion (but like medical practice little mention of acupuncture) and herbal medications. Influencing all procedures was a magico-religious perception of the nature of both illness and healing (Hefferman 1997, pp. 37–59). The nomadic herders continued to use traditional treatments and herbal medications up to recent years.

Translation of a Tibetan veterinary equine manuscript, found in the Mogao Caves (Blondeau 1972); indicates that foot problems, lameness, urethral calculi and management issues related to the high altitude (exhaustion and malnutrition) were the main problems. Among the procedures mentioned are bleeding, use of the cautery, rectal examination and as an aid to move bladder calculi. Moxibustion was obviously a significant treatment for many conditions and herbal medications were in frequent use. Treatment of loadbearing sores and injuries are also discussed. The emphasis of the text is on medications to cure, rather than prevention.

From extant manuscripts it is noted that the Indian *Veda* texts of Salihotra were recognised and translated to Tibetan. There is very little known of veterinary care or health problems of other livestock.

Animal Disease

Studies, following Chinese annexation, have revealed that Tibetan livestock have a serious disease burden. It had been known for some time that brucellosis is endemic in the yak population and that parasitism is widespread. Cestode infestation with *Cysticercus tenuicollis* was found in 45% of pigs sampled, with the main definitive host for *Taenia hydatigena* being farm dogs.

From published papers it is obvious that there are now serious studies being undertaken, under Chinese veterinary direction, to determine the state of Tibet's livestock. In 2018, peste des petite ruminants (PPR) was identified in sheep and goats in the Ngari region; Chuzan virus (CHUV), reputed as a cause of reproductive organ disease, found in yaks on the Qinghi plateau; pseudo-rabies virus (PRV) found in pigs in the Nyihgchi region; and bluetongue virus (BTV) found in 20% sheep and 13% yaks in several regions. In 2019 *Enterocytozoon bieneusi* has been recognised in pigs as a cause of diarrhoea and enteric disease, and African swine fever (ASF) found in several regions in Tibet.

Of public health consequence has been the recognition in 2018 of human plague (*Yersinia pestis*) bacteria in sheep on the Qinghi plateau, the originating host is believed to be wild marmots. A more serious problem is with humans being intermediate hosts for two *Echinococcus spp* tapeworms: *E. granulosus* as hydatid cysts and *E. multilocularis* as alveolar hydatids. In both cases farm and livestock herding dogs are the definitive hosts in what has been stated to be a major zoonotic problem.

While it is conjecture, it would appear that most of the currently significant animal health issues in Tibet have existed for centuries. However, bearing in mind the relative isolation of the region, until the mid-20th century, it may be that some of these diseases are recent introductions to a highly susceptible animal population.

As there is no veterinary school in Tibet, students are trained in one of the several Chinese Universities with a veterinary faculty. The Xizang Agricultural and Animal Husbandry College at Linzhi in Bayi District south-eastern Tibet, houses the Laboratory of Clinical Veterinary Medicine. There is said to be a Central Veterinary Station in Lhasa with branches in 70 of the 71 regions.

References

Anonymous (1913) The Many-Sided Duties of a Certified Salutri. *Veterinary Journal* **20**

Blondeau, A-M. (1972) *Materiaux pour l'etude de l'hippologie et de l'hippiatrie tibetaines*, Hautes Etudes Orientales 2. Paris: Librairie Droz

Datta, S. (1948) The Nature and Significance of Veterinary Problems in Ancient and Modern India. *Indian Veterinary Journal* **25**

Deraniyagala P.E.P. (1952) *Sinhala Ola Manuscripts*, National Museum Manuscript Series, Vol II, Veterinary Science (Elephants) Vol. I. Columbo: Ceylon Government Press

Deraniyagla, P.E.P. (1955) *Some Extinct Elephants, Their Relatives and two Living Species.* Colombo: Ceylon National Museum Publications, Government Press

Ghosh, A. (2000) *The Glass Palace.* Delhi: Ravi Dayal Penguin Books India

Grellier, J. (1842–1844) The Veterinary Art in India. *The Veterinarian* **15**, **16**, **17** (serialised from part 1 in **15**)

Hefferman, C. (1997) Tibetan Veterinary Medicine. *Nomadic Peoples* **1** No. 2

Holmes, J.D.E. (1903) Native Beliefs Regarding the Hairmarks on Horses and Cattle. *Veterinary Journal* **8**

Jayadatta, M. (1926) Asvavaidyakan Trans by N.N. Majundar. *Indian Veterinary Journal* **3**: 64–67 and 118–123 (and in 12 sections issued up to 1940)

Johnston-Saint, P.J. (1929) An Outline of the History of Medicine in India, *Journal of the Royal Society of Arts* (July 12) pp. 844–870

Krishnaswami Iyer, A. (1937) Veterinary Science in India, Ancient and Modern, with special reference to tuberculosis, in *Agriculture and Livestock in India.* New Delhi: Government Printer

Krishnaswamy, A. (1945) What a Veterinarian Can Learn from a Study of Ancient Indian Veterinary Lore, *Indian Veterinary Journal* **21**

Krishnaswamy, A. (1950) Is a Study of Our Ancient Veterinary Literature Necessary to Us? *Indian Veterinary Journal* **26**

Lo, V. and Cullen, C. (Eds.) (2005) *Chinese Medicine in the Dunhuang Medical Manuscripts*, Needham Research Institute Series. London: Routledge & Curzon

Lo, V. and Yoeli-Tlalim, R. (2014) Travelling Light: Sino-Tibetan Moxa from Dunhuang. Proc. 12th Biennial Conference of Asian Studies. Haifa University, Israel

Margotta, R. (1996) *History of Medicine.* London: Hamlyn

Mazars, G. (1994) Traditional Veterinary Medicine in India. *Review Science Technology* **13** No.2

Mills, J. (1894) The Native Treatment of Cattle Diseases in India. *Veterinary Journal* **38**

Mills J.B. (1904) Lucky Marks of the Horse. *Veterinary Journal* **9**

Piyadasa, H.D. (1994) Traditional Systems for Preventing and Treating animal diseases in Sri Lanka. *Review Science Technology* **13** No.2

Reddy, D.V.S. (1945) Veterinary Medicine in Mauryan Times. *Indian Veterinary Journal* **21**

Somvanshi, R. (2006) Veterinary Medicine and Animal Keeping in Ancient India. *Asian Agri-History* **10** No.2

Sournia, J.C. (1992) *Illustrated History of Medicine.* London: Harold Starke

Sturgess, G.W. (1906) Observations on a Curious Disease affecting Cattle in Ceylon. *Veterinary Journal* **11**

Vancheswaran, S. (1945) Rinderpest and its Control Methods employed in the Madras Presidency. *Indian Veterinary Journal* **21**

CHAPTER 9

The Americas: North, Central, South

The American continent contains lands of great contrast from ice-cold tundra to steppe, to extensive grasslands, forests, dense jungles, deserts and volcanic mountain ranges. The land was unpopulated until the first migrants were believed to have crossed a land bridge from Siberia to Alaska over the Bering Strait (dates vary from 40,000 to 10,000 years ago). Several animal species also migrated, notably the progenitors of the buffalo, bighorn sheep and the horse, but the latter became extinct. Moving along the coasts and into the interiors the migrants are estimated to have reached Tierra del Fuego, the most southerly point, possibly earlier than 9000 BC.

Following the end of the last glacial period about 12,500 years ago, a wide range of cultures developed throughout the United States of America (USA). The first migrants were nomadic hunter-gatherers but by about 5000 BC some of the peoples had discovered edible plants and began cultivation. Some also domesticated animals, but very few compared to other continents; there was either little inclination to domesticate, or they did not find suitable species. In North, Central and South America widely differing cultures and civilisations emerged, but with certain shared similarities and with demonstrable links to Siberian people through dialects and blood types.

NORTH AMERICA

North America is a northern hemisphere land mass, today shared between the USA and Canada. This land mass is bounded by the Pacific Ocean to the west, the Atlantic Ocean to the east, the Caribbean Sea and Mexico (Central America) to the south, and the Arctic to the north. The Rocky and Sierra Mountains dominate the west of the land and the Appalachian Mountains the east. Between these are the vast expanse of the Great Plains. Both east and west have coastal plains. In the east these terminate in southern subtropical Florida. Plains stretch north to the Canadian Shield. The southern regions are characterised by arid lands and desert. The central basin is drained by the Missouri/Mississippi river complex.

Indigenous Peoples

Some initial nomadic hunter-gatherer tribes continued this lifestyle on the Plains, but others settled by rivers or fresh water, and began arable cultivation. In the southern and western more arid and mountainous regions, a pueblo culture evolved with multi-storey dwelling conurbations on hill tops or below protected rock overhangs, and the use of irrigation in their crop production. The number of tribes (linked by language groups) existing before the Europeans arrived has been estimated at some 2000, of which today only 570 are known.

Agriculture, Livestock and Wildlife

From their early origins as hunter-gatherers the tribes' diets were centred on meat: predominantly this was the buffalo (*Bison bison*). They were expert trackers and to kill their prey they would herd them into or over traps, or stampede a group over a cliff edge. Depending on the region the target animal could change. In the north deer (caribou, moose or white-tailed) were targeted and in the mountains this changed to bighorn sheep, as well as many species of bears, wolves, racoons, cats, rodents and beavers. All of these animals could have been hunted for food or fur.

There was no domestication of animals except for dogs (used in hunting and as pack carriers by some tribes) and wolf derived sled dogs by Eskimo tribes. There was some minor interest in fowls in the pueblo culture. With the introduction of horses by the Spanish, the plains tribes soon learned how to catch, break and ride: the horse becoming a major and important part of their life for both hunting and war. The European demand for fur, in particular from the beaver, gave the native population an additional income source through trading the furs for goods.

Birds were also hunted for their feathers and skin to be used in headdresses as well as for ornamentation. Some birds were regarded as sacred and the eagle was greatly revered. The turkey was generally not eaten as most tribes regarded the bird as a coward – the belief was that if consumed the person would also become cowardly.

Crop production became important for those tribes in permanent settlements. The most important crop was maize which, with beans and squash, made up the basis of most diets, together with meats and supplemented by wild rice, herbs, seeds, honey and maple syrup. Other crops included pumpkins, tobacco and cotton. Much ceremonial ritual accompanied every stage from planting to harvesting.

The buffalo was the most valued animal. Hunting of this creature was restricted to absolute needs. In a way the tribes managed the herds to achieve maximum production. Some followed the migrating herds but others lived on the borders of the plains sending out hunting parties as required. The main killing period was in the autumn when the buffalo were fat from summer grazing. The men killed and the women then butchered the carcase taking the meat for food, hides and hair for ropes and ligaments for twine. The skins were used for clothing, shoes, tipis (tents) and cured rawhide as armour (for both men and horses), the bones were used to make tools, the hoofs for glue and the dung collected, dried and used for fuel.

While animals were slaughtered as a source of meat, fur, hides and so on, there was also a feeling of relationship. Probably the strongest emotion that the native Americans had was a feeling of mystical communion with the earth, sky and animals. Many animals featured in their art, as seen in rock carvings as well as interesting land sculptures or earthworks. One of the most notable examples is the great serpent in Adams County, Ohio – a twisting mound of yellow clay and stone with a coiled tail and head, and a believed egg in its mouth. This sculpture is over 400 yards long and dated to about 2000 years ago. The shape and moulding is perfect when viewed from the air. Equally impressive are the extraordinary groups of earthen sculptures of various animals and birds found across areas of Iowa, Wisconsin and the upper Mississippi valley often on high plateaus. These shapes are only raised a few feet above ground level making it impossible to see the whole of the group except from the air – and then only when a low sun casts a shadow. Equally unexplained are animal and human outlines cut into rock with characters that look as if someone was using a language, but for which no one has ever been able to translate the 'text'. The most intriguing of these is the Dighton Writing Rock in the Taunton river, Massachusetts.

Animals were highly regarded in tribal cultures, but not so much in the animal welfare sense of the European world. However, the killing of any creature other than for necessity, namely for food or to protect oneself, was not practised. For further study on this topic, the *Encyclopaedia of Native American Culture* (Nozedar 2012) is instructive.

Beliefs, Religion and Medicine

The tribal societies of North America produced a wide variety of cultures, but were unified by possessing a broad range of interrelated beliefs. Religion is probably an incorrect word: to these people life was spiritual and this spirituality was the basis of their beliefs. Native Americans thought with their emotions rather than their minds and had an integrity of spirit that was deeper than conscious reasoning. The essence of this was a love of their homeland which developed into a mystical identification with it. One of their leaders said, 'I was born by these waters, the earth is my mother' – the belief was a spiritual essence of the landscape and its many creatures, with a mystical connection to the earth, sky and animals. The spirituality created and aroused was stronger than the religious teachings of the immigrant Europeans, and both groups failed to recognise the others' convictions.

One fundamental native American concept, which Europeans neither appreciated nor understood for a long time, was that land belonged to everybody. There might be 'tribal lands' but everybody had a right to use it as the 'creator' had made it for everyone. Tribal beliefs were based on traditions and customs which had evolved over thousands of years and could be monotheistic, polytheistic, pantheistic or animistic. The beliefs were passed on orally and were engrained in the peoples.

Tribal life was dominated by ceremonial rituals, which included special clothing, fasting, singing prayers, drumming, dancing and sacred objects – these formed the core of the tribal identity. In some regions there were sweat lodge ceremonies which created ritual cleansing, and with the heat and darkness allowed intensified sensual experiences, in a state of heightened awareness. Spirituality dominated the culture; dreams and visions were very important for obtaining a message, which then had to be obeyed.

Medicine, in the context of native American cultures, is a word that means various concepts related to spiritual efficacy. Medicine was the 'power' in an object or substance used in curing or in another beneficial way. It did not have to have attributes of a pharmaceutical nature, only the capacity to harness and direct spiritual forces. The ingestion of herbs or other substances, or the smoking of a sacred pipe, might either provide or be good medicine. An important role in the tribal structure was played by the medicine man, or woman, who was a major figure in the spirituality of the tribe: in some cases it was the chief, notably Sitting Bull of the Sioux. A valuable guide to these beliefs and practices is *Mythology of the American Nations* (Jones and Molyneaux 2009, pp. 10–14).

Traditional Medicine

Tribal medical practice involved the medicine man, both a traditional healer and a spiritual leader. Very little is known about their work, as the position was usually passed from father to son, or daughter, with little revealing of the knowledge or success of their activities. It was recorded in a journal written by early European travellers that they were amazed at the successful cures that were obtained, but no further details were given.

It would appear that there was a whole range of holistic treatments plus an emphasis on the promotion of health and well-being, defined as a bio-psycho-socio-spiritual approach. The objective was to obey the 'laws of nature'. Advice given included taking a run each day to greet the dawn to provide exercise plus a spiritual uplift. Herbal medication was used, as were sacred herbs: sage and sweet grains (orally), tobacco (in the pipe), mescal (agave) a potent fermented drink, and peyote (cactus) which could be taken as a drink or eaten raw. Both mescal and peyote could be used as agents to induce a trance. Manipulative therapies, ceremonies and prayers were employed with much symbolic healing that might be spread over days or weeks, as a community effort. These would involve many objects held to be deeply sacred – crystals, stones and natural remedies (herbs, roots or plants).

Medicine men were recognised as healers and people of wisdom who kept the sacred knowledge. They would advise hunters before they left camp, but their value was in maintaining the health of the tribe – they would exorcise demons with rattles and drums as well as providing treatments by using suction cups, purging, setting bones and acting as midwife and counsellor. Aside from any traditional or ceremonial dress, a medicine bag was always carried by the medicine man: frequently this was hidden under exterior clothing. It was a most secret and precious possession containing sacred items. The identity and purpose of these items remains unclear as owners invariably refuse to discuss the contents, but it is understood that these could include stones, bones, crystals, roots, herbs, feathers and fetish objects.

Traditional medicine, however, was of little use when the indigenous peoples came into contact with the diseases carried by the Europeans. Smallpox arrived in North America from Central America in 1525, before the Spaniards had themselves arrived. It was a disease that swept through a population with no immunity. With successive arrivals more diseases arrived: typhus in 1544, influenza and smallpox in 1558, smallpox in 1559, diphtheria in 1614 and measles in 1618. All of these diseases, as well as bubonic plague, mumps and whooping cough, came to the USA in the century after the first landing by Columbus, to be later followed by cholera, malaria and scarlet fever.

There is no definitive estimate of the size of the North America population before this onslaught of disease. One researcher (Dobyns 1966, pp. 395–416) estimated that during the first 130 years of contact with white men about 95% of the native population died. This figure has been questioned, but as estimates of the original numbers range from 3,800,000 to 18,000,000 and even higher, the only valid conclusion is that the disease losses probably represent the worst demographic catastrophe in history.

As there were no domesticated animals, except for dogs, there was no tradition of veterinary medicine. The introduction of livestock from Europe included horses. Some escaped captivity from the Spanish in 1540 and bred well in the Great Plains. The local population soon became proficient horsemen which totally transformed the native culture, in particular that of the Plains tribes. It is important to remember that although the people did not domesticate animals these creatures were a major part of their culture. In 1855 Chief Seathl of the Duwamish tribe said,

What is man without the beasts? If all the beasts were gone, men would die from great loneliness of spirit, for whatever happens to beasts also happens to man. All things are connected.

The full story of the life and ultimate tragedy of the native American peoples can be read in *A History of the Indians of the United States* by Angie Debo (2003).

European Arrival and Colonisation

The first known European to set foot on the North American continent was the Norse explorer Leif Erikson (c.AD 970–c.AD 1020). It is believed, from the Icelandic Sagas, that Erikson established a small, but short-lived settlement on the Newfoundland coast, but there was no evidence that he took animals on these visits.

As there was no tradition of animal farming in the existing tribal population, the story of veterinary medicine in the continent has to start with the importation of livestock. It should be noted that there was a difference between the Spanish (and in South America the Portuguese) and the British, French, Dutch and Swedish colonisers. The Spanish had one overriding interest – gold and plunder for items of wealth.

The other Europeans aimed to establish a New World, and farming was a major objective. Their reasons for migration were influenced by a wish for a better life, religious freedom and land to farm.

Shipment of animals across the Atlantic between the 15th and 16th centuries could not have been easy as the larger species such as horses and cattle, would require ships with special holds, and smaller species, in particular swine, were regularly enshipped as a living meat larder.

The chronological record of these new species arriving in the continent reflects the purpose of the people on board the ships.

1493 Christopher Columbus (on his second voyage to the USA) brought horses from Spain to his previously established settlement at Santa Domingo on Hispaniola Island. On his fourth voyage in 1502 he visited Honduras in the mainland of Central America, but no horses are mentioned.

1527 Cabeza de Vacca, a Spanish explorer with the Narvaez expedition, landed on the west coast of Florida with 42 horses. Following conflict with the local population most of the men and all the horses perished.

1539 Hernando de Soto, a Spanish explorer and Conquistador landed near Tampa Bay, Florida with a private army of 620 soldiers, together with 220 horses and 300 pigs. Over a period of four years he wrecked and rampaged his way through the South and South-West regions of the country – the objective was gold and plunder. Many of the pigs escaped to the wild, and some horses to be the progenitors of the mustang.

1608 M. L'Escarbol, a French lawyer, brought horses to an early French colony in Quebec. They are believed to be the ancestors of the Canadian pony.

1609 Jamestown, the British colony in Virginia received 100 pigs and a 'few' sheep from England (in 40 years the sheep flock had increased to 3000).

1610/1611 Jamestown received a major shipment of 100 cows.

1626 In New Amsterdam (later New York) the Dutch colony imported sheep, most of which fell prey to wolves and dogs.

1633 Massachusetts imported their first sheep from England. By this time, the livestock industry was becoming self-sufficient.

Horses were very important for the early settlers as they were the only means of travel between towns, they were kept by all except for the poverty-stricken. Most haulage work was done with horses, but oxen were used for the heavy work in the cities. The horses in the original thirteen colonies came from England and Flanders.

The cattle shipments were initially seen as most valuable, due to the need to build up the herds. In Jamestown, the death penalty was introduced for anyone found killing a cow or heifer calf; and for being an accessory, the punishment issued was the burning off of the right hand. Imported cattle were recognised by breeds, all other cattle were known as 'scrubs'. Improvement by selective breeding did not really commence until 1810, but it was recorded that one 'fine bull' was imported in 1785 (Merrilat and Campbell 1935, pp. 51–53).

The first pigs arrived in Florida from Cuba with de Soto in 1539. Those in the northern colonies came from England and the Netherlands, and were described as 'long-legged, large boned, slab-sided, flop-eared, unprofitable and unsightly beasts'. They habitually ran at large in both towns and country. The de Soto pigs escaped to the wild during his expedition, which might have had unexpected consequences (Mann 2005). René Cavelier was the first observer to visit the Texas/Arkansas border area, where de Soto had found cities 'cheek-by-jowl', over 100 years later. He canoed through the area and found it deserted; it looked like an epidemic disaster. Mann's study suggested that the de Soto group was too small to be an effective biological weapon and there was no mention of illness in his men. He postulated that the pigs, who breed rapidly, could have acted to transmit disease to other wildlife. In this way influenza, anthrax, leptospirosis, tuberculosis, trichinosis and taenia could all have spread, killing both wildlife and humans. It was estimated the native American population fell by nearly 96% to about 8500 people: possibly by animal transmission.

Sheep were important and recognised as a necessity for the new colonists and nearly all farms had a small flock. Home-spun was the universal clothing type in the rural communities and a cloth trade also developed for urban clothes. In 1793 William Foster of Boston imported the first fine-woolled sheep from Spain.

The Development of Livestock Farming

The Spanish invasions into the USA, driven by a search for gold and wealth proved highly successful, but did also bring cattle, first as meat-on-the-hoof for the ship journey and then they were released for wild ranching, to be harvested later for their hides and tallow (leather and candle making were important industries). This happened first in California and in the south-western areas (present-day Texas). As land ownership changed, the cattle became the foundation stock of the early cattle herds of Texas longhorns. This was followed later by low-grade sheep that were driven from Mexico to California (at that time all this region was under Spanish control), later these were upgraded by breeding stock. Texas Longhorns were exploited to produce a cattle population of considerable size, becoming the main beef source for the USA until the dawn of the 20th century.

Along the eastern seaboard, colonies were established by England, France, Holland and Sweden; following the first successful English colony at Jamestown in 1607 these had all come under British control by 1763. The livestock industry developed in New England, Pennsylvania and Virginia utilising horses, cattle, sheep and pigs.

Colonial New England, especially in the Connecticut valley, was important for horse breeding while Massachusetts developed a strong horse and cattle industry: both of these before the Revolutionary War of 1776. During the period 1717–1775 some 200,000 emigrants from the German Palatinate (in the Rhineland) arrived and settled in the Allegheny Foothills. These were mainly people seeking religious freedom, many of Lutheran or German Reformed churches, but also many Anabaptists including the Amish and Mennonites. They all promoted a simple hardworking lifestyle and their farms soon featured as well run, well stocked livestock enterprises. Later named the Pennsylvania Dutch, they tended to keep to their own communities and promoted good farming practices. The English settled in the Virginia valley, the French in Maryland and the Scots-Irish in the Piedmont, a plateau region between the Atlantic coastal plain and the Appalachians. These all created viable farming and livestock structures, led by equine management, and raising horses. In New England, some horses escaped captivity and began to breed in the woodlands.

Livestock Production Increases and Health Risks Appear

For the early colonists, the loss of a single animal was serious. There were no epidemic diseases and little spread of disease, as livestock were widely distributed on isolated farms. The major problem was predation – either from wolves or the resident native American tribes. Any veterinary care needed was provided from old family almanacs brought from Britain and the woods were searched for medicinal herbs and roots (Bierer 1955). Pig production soon exceeded local needs and by 1627 Jamestown was palisaded to keep them out, whilst the local tribes also fed on them. Within a few years the colony was exporting pork and lard to the West Indies in exchange for sugar and rum. The Connecticut valley became the livestock centre.

The attitude of the early United States (US) farmer towards diseases of live-stock was 'remarkably complacent and self-confident' (Campbell 1934, pp. 48–52). Religious belief was strong in rural society. Death was attributed to an act of God, and sickness in man and loss of animals was evidence of a Divine wrath. This religious attitude even permeated livestock breeding. For hard work the mule was better suited than either the horse or ox, but the mule was unpopular and hardly used in the northern colonies, and only bred a little in the southern ones. The mule's lack of popularity was seemingly due to the Biblical injunction, 'Thou shalt not let thy cattle [animals] gender with diverse kind' – an attitude that still prevailed up to the time of the Civil war. Veterinary care was provided by the colonial farmers, and later supplemented by farriers or cow-leeches, usually unfortunately as both were as ignorant as each other.

Colonial growth and spread of agriculture to the West and South was led by farmers with cattle, who were always at the outer edge of expansion. In the Texas region there was a concentration of cattle farming based on local stock and the Texas cattle herds and sheep flocks have historically been among the USA's largest. A sales pattern developed in which cattle were gradually moved in groups and herds from the south to the towns and cities of the rapidly growing North along named 'trails'. This movement caused disease to be recognised in cattle. In 1766 the Colony of North Carolina passed laws to control the movement of cattle from South Carolina and Georgia. This was because it was seen that while the southern cattle being driven remained healthy a fatal disease developed in the local northern cattle. The inhabitants wanted the movement stopped.

There was seen to be a need for veterinary medicine and in 1785 the Philadelphia Society for Promoting Agriculture was organised. In its memoirs there were many articles on animal disease including the earliest recordings of ergotism and what came to be known as Texas Fever of cattle, as well as articles on diseases of sheep, pigs and horses. This was the beginning of veterinary medicine in the USA. The story is continued later in this book (see Chapter 15).

CENTRAL AMERICA

Also termed Mesoamerica, Central America is a geographical area as well as a cultural concept, and is recognised as one of the six areas of the world where an independent and distinct civilisation evolved, and one of the four which first independently developed a system of writing. The region is defined by mountain ranges, deserts, central plains, tropical forests, grasslands and marshes, and within broad geographic terms it includes the lands of Mexico and south to Costa Rica and Panama.

Indigenous Peoples

Many peoples, cultures and languages developed with a unifying factor in primary cultural characteristics, in particular maize (corn), agriculture, long distance trading, stepped pyramid temples, hieroglyphic writing, written texts on deer skin or bark paper, basic mathematical principles and ball courts. The evolving civilisations all developed around large urban conurbations, with well-defined social systems and complex religious beliefs with many gods and goddesses, invariably utilising human sacrifice.

The major civilisations, which overlapped each other in time and geography were:

Olmecs, 1600 BC–AD 400, who influenced all later cultures with their rigid social castes dominated by priests. Their two most important symbolic creatures were the jaguar and the plumed serpent (Quetzalcoatl) which were present in all following cultures. They were fine builders and stonemasons with an important class of pre-Olmec farmers dating from 4000 BC, who were also skilled in irrigation.

Mayans, c.AD 750–c.AD 1450 (but most dominant in AD 300–AD 900). They created 'city states' and were great builders, astronomical observers, mathematicians, calendar creators and has a sophisticated style of writing. The Mayans also had a rigid social class system and produced good farmers.

Toltecs, c.AD 1000–c.AD 1300 gave an impetus to the declining Mayan culture. They were great builders and developed agriculture and new strains of maize and cotton. They also made excellent fabrics and devised hieroglyphic writing. Eventually this civilisation collapsed possibly due to disagreement over human sacrifice.

Aztecs (or Mexica), at their peak of power between AD 1200–AD 1500. A warlike people, the Aztecs gradually took control of central Mexican valley. They were good farmers (used water well with artificial islands), constructed a great city, Tenochtitlan, acquired much wealth by the conquest and taxation of conquered peoples. The Aztecs had the most extreme nature of the Mesoamerican peoples in the sacrificing of humans to satisfy their god of war, Huitzilipotchli, who appeared as a great hummingbird. They established a strict hierarchical system with an emperor and priests at the apex and treasured a folk image of an eagle. The Aztecs have been brilliantly described and illustrated in their painted pictographic writing manuscripts.

Agriculture, Livestock and Wildlife

The successive cultures in Mesoamerica were all based in agriculture. The people were effective farmers, practised the 'slash and burn' approach, used irrigation well and also made floating vegetable and flower gardens. The main crop was maize (a plant with many religious connotations) but beans, tomatoes, avocados, squash, chilli peppers, amaranth, sage, sweet potatoes and some cacti (for making alcoholic *pulque*) were all cultivated. The word 'tomato' is derived from the Aztec Nahuatl word *tomati*.

The wildlife in Mesoamerica was extensive due to the differences in topography and climate. To the native peoples the animals and birds were fundamental elements of their religion, either to represent the gods or for use in everyday language to describe days or weeks. The most important were the jaguar, the serpent and the eagle. Other creatures used in their language and mythology included deer, rabbits, monkeys, dogs, lizards, crocodiles and birds. Among the birds, the vulture is frequently listed.

Diet was mixed with a strong plant and seed input. Maize was the staple food with vegetables and fresh fruit. There were well-organised daily markets in every town supplied by local farms. Meats of several types were eaten either from the 'domesticated' species of turkeys, Muscovy ducks and small dogs, or from the hunting of deer, rabbits or fish. The cacao bean was also harvested and used for stews, sauces and a drink known as *xocalatl* which later became known as hot chocolate in Europe. The water supply to the region was good, with the bigger cities being supplied by aqueducts (Thomas 1993, p. 35 and pp. 312–313). Dogs occupied an interesting position, they lived as part of the family but were usually kept fat and then eaten at some point. It was an accepted custom to sacrifice a dog at the time of a human death so that it could escort the deceased person through the underworld.

Beliefs and Religion

A variety of beliefs were formed to meet a need to explain the universe, how it started and what the place of humans was. This developed with a mythology based in naturalism; these legends relate to the observable universe and helped to explain their place in this creation. The legends and beliefs formed the structure of their religion and allowed for an understanding of their place in what was seen as a mysterious universe. A more comprehensive discussion can be read in *Mythology of the American Nations* (Jones and Molyneaux 2009, pp. 10–14).

While the people felt that they had a measure of control of their environment through their application to agriculture and the construction of cities, there was always a preoccupation with death. If this occurred in battle, childbirth or sacrifice it was considered honourable, but was also feared. Sacrifice was of humans, also of some animals (mainly deer). Auto-sacrifice by deliberate bleeding from insertion of thorny threads through the tongue, earlobes or genitals was usually committed by the nobility. Blood was seen as essential in restoring the divine energy of the gods. Ritual sacrifice, by cutting out the living heart of the victim, was seen as necessary to protect their civilisation. This practice was most pronounced under Aztec rule. Cannibalism was also regularly undertaken, utilising the sacrificial victims on ceremonial occasions by the Olmecs, Maya and Aztecs. The flesh was cooked and was regarded as a communion with the gods.

Animals were more rarely used in sacrifice but they played a significant role in almost all other aspects of the beliefs – either as part of the legends or in figurines, paintings or stone carvings. Earth was believed by some to be resting on the back of a huge crocodile or caiman, lying in water. Another belief was that Earth was a huge house constructed of iguana bodies. Celestial deities were associated with individual birds. Animals were used both to represent individual gods and also as part of their symbolic written language: all creatures were seen as an important part of the Mesoamerican life.

When the Spanish Conquistadors arrived in the Aztec capital they were amazed to find that the emperor had a zoo, with a menagerie of animals and birds including jaguars, coyotes, rattlesnakes and the beautiful quetzal bird, whose long feathers were used in the headdresses of the state's royalty. The animals were fed with the hearts and flesh of sacrificial victims (Pohl and Robinson 2005, pp. 116–117). The emperor also had a private 'zoo' in which social misfits were kept.

Traditional Medicine

A notable feature of the Mesoamerican cultures was that the cities, roads and people were clean and tidy. Workers and others would wash several times a day. Steam houses were popular in towns and included birching and massage. Soap was made and used and hair was regularly washed. Public latrines were frequently sited alongside major roads, and the excrement used as a crop fertiliser. Apart from the last practice, which would enable transfer of gut helminths, the population, by good hygiene, did much to control any disease spread and epidemics were not known.

The most obvious feature of the medical system was that if one was ill the first treatment was to bathe. Hot baths were taken, followed by a cold one. The temples held a store of bitumen, regarded as 'divine medicine' and supplied by priests to be rubbed on the body. It was also used on open wounds, as was *pulque* an alcoholic drink made from the agave plant. A wide variety of more specific treatments were used, 1200 plants were reputed to be recognised for their medicinal properties. Tree resins were used for some skin diseases and crushed insects were incorporated into ointments. There is some evidence from the records of the early Spanish invaders that certain plants with a medicinal value were cultivated.

Disease was seen as being sent from the gods as a punishment for blasphemy. A principle cause of illness appeared to be related to either bad food or no food. Spanish records identified gout, cancer, lameness, blindness, paralysis, stomach disorders and inflamed glands.

The priesthood played a major role in medicine. To aid identification of the cause of a disease they used hallucinogenic plants to induce a trance to gain divine guidance in individual cases, these were also used together with smoking tobacco. Another diagnostic procedure used by local sorcerers was observation of the patterns created when maize seeds or beans were cast on to a white cloth. The god Macuilxochitl would punish with piles and boils those who broke the rule of sex abstinence during a fasting period. The rites associated with the goddess Xochiquetzal required everyone to bathe in a river, if not they could expect skin diseases and pustules (Thomas 1993, pp. 444–446).

While the basic rules for cleanliness and hygiene were sound, the medical practices used mostly fell into the category of witchcraft and black magic. Many of the herbal medications were based in long-standing usage with a recognition of benefits. There was a significant use of hallucinogenic substances such as *peyote* cactus, datura seeds and others. The upper classes would also relax by smoking a mixture of tobacco, charcoal and liquid amber resin. All, within a specific context, were believed to aid health. The system which existed with the priest structure, herbal medication and good hygiene appears to have been relatively successful. However, with the introduction of smallpox and other European diseases the population was totally susceptible and the fall in the numbers was catastrophic. As there was in effect no domestication of animals (except for some keeping of wild turkeys and dogs), there was no tradition of veterinary medicine.

European Arrival and Colonisation

In 1519 Hernando Cortez with 400 soldiers overthrew the Aztec empire using guns and horses, but in particular he allied with the subject peoples of the Aztecs. He was helped because the Aztec priesthood at first believed he was the god Quetzalcotl returning as predicted. The Spaniards looted and smashed buildings and temples for gold and precious metals and jewels, destroying books and artefacts, and imposing the Christian religion. The territory became the base for the Spanish annexation of California and the south-west region of North America; as well as providing the wealth to start the plunder of South America.

The Aztec society was brilliantly described and painted in the native pictographic writing shortly after the Spanish conquest. Several manuscripts were written and annotated in Spanish: they provide a unique authentic view of the civilisation that was about to be destroyed. One of the finest, the *Codex Mendoza* is now in the Bodleian Library, Oxford (Ross 1978). See also Chapter 15 for the beginning of veterinary medicine in Mexico (see Chapter 15).

SOUTH AMERICA

A continent joined by a narrow isthmus to Central and North America mainly in the southern hemisphere, South American is bordered by the Pacific Ocean to the west, Caribbean Sea to the north, South Atlantic to the east and Antarctica to the south. The topography is dominated by the Andean mountain range which runs the length of the western side of the continent. Climatically the range includes the tropical north and temperate pasture and grazing in the south, as well as arid and mountainous regions. The major river systems of the Amazon and Orinoco drain the north, with the River Plate in the south. The population is mostly found in the coastal regions.

Indigenous Peoples

The earliest people were migrants from the north. By 3000 BC agriculture had commenced in several situations and by 2000 BC there were many organised agriculturally based communities in existence. There is a long history of civilisation and culture evolution across the continent. Most of the growth and development of expertise evolved in the north and central western region between the coast and into the Andes. On the eastern side of the Andes in the tropical Amazon basin and coastal regions the development was more tribal and less sophisticated.

A series of cultures, which then grew to be empires, evolved and were characterised by monumental temple structures and developing agriculture. The principal civilisations all developed in the region now known as Peru: first was the Norte Chico c.3000 BC–1800 BC, and the last was the Kingdom of Chimor c.AD 1000–c.AD 1470. At the same time the related Muisca culture was developing in present-day Columbia, also known as the 'gold culture' due to the natural deposits and production of gold artefacts of all types, including the original Eldorado location (Jones and Molyneaux 2009, p. 195).

The Chimu reign ended when the Inca civilisation evolved to become dominant over the whole region in the early 13th century, stretching from present-day Ecuador to the north of Argentina. The imposing capital city of Cuzco in the Andes was connected to the whole empire by some 25,000 km of roadway and was characterised by massive buildings and magnificent stonework and masonry. As an agricultural society it was notable for the development of terraces to maximise the mountainous landscape, combined with innovative irrigation and water control systems. The population totalled between nine and fourteen million.

Inca society was planned so that no citizen went hungry, no one was without a house, land was owned communally, every person or family had a land allotment which was increased as the family grew, there was an equal distribution of food and there were state-run warehouses distributed throughout the land with food stores, should a harvest fail or there be an emergency. This, however, came with a high degree of regimentation: idleness was punished. The conquered peoples were not slaves, they were encouraged to join the Inca society. In many ways it was similar to a communist society.

The Inca dominance was rather short-lived, reaching its peak in the early 1500s, and being overthrown following the Spanish invasion in 1531. The last emperor, Atahualpa, only reigned for one year.

Agriculture, Livestock and Wildlife

Incan society was based on agriculture, but with stony soils, steep slopes and difficult irrigation; all of which were overcome by good management, strict controls and building expertise.

The types of crops grown would depend on the region and climate. The basic foods were maize (as a food source and for brewing *chica* beer), potatoes and manioc; others included squashes, chilli peppers, lima and haricot beans, sweet potatoes, groundnuts, tomatoes and avocados. Cotton, tobacco and *cuca* (called coca by the Spaniards) the source of cocaine, were cultivated too – the latter with great care for its use by the noble families and the priesthood (Métraux 1969, pp. 61–63). Seafood was eaten in the coastal areas, whilst the meat from llama and guinea pigs was eaten in the mountainous regions. The llama meat was also dried in the sun and used over a period of time.

Only two species of animals were domesticated: guinea pigs, which were fed on scraps and kept in the home to be consumed as required, and camelids. Of the camelids the llama was raised in large flocks in the Andes. While used as a pack animal, it could only carry minimal loads and only for short distances; they were not strong enough to take a rider. There was intensive breeding of the llama stock for wool on the basis of coat colour; white wool was the most valuable as many hundreds of these animals were needed for sacrifice in religious ceremonies. Other coat colours bred for included varying shades of brown, with the darkest being used for pack work. It is recorded that in Inca times 'enormous herds' of llama were farmed on the plains around Lake Titicaca. The related camelid, the alpaca was also bred for wool. Weaving was a major occupation in the Inca world – in every village and also in special facilities in major towns. Llama wool was used for everyday work clothes, alpaca wool for the noble and priest classes, and vicuna wool for the Emperor (the latter was said to weave like silk).

The people were good stockmen, most villagers had one or two llamas. When the Spaniards introduced horses, donkeys, cattle, pigs and sheep these were all welcomed. Sheep wool in particular was seen to be an easier commodity to produce and harvest than the wool from the camelids. Very good agricultural records were kept. While no system of writing had been developed a device termed a *quipa* was used, in every community. This was a system of knotted and coloured strings held on a loop, by which mathematical data could be stored, as well as historical and other information, and 'read' by expert users.

The wildlife in the coastal and Andes mountain regions was diverse. The camelid species were found in the pastoral regions of the Andes mountains; the llama and alpaca were most widespread and both were domesticated. The vicuna was less prolific and probably was not well domesticated; the guanaco, found in the more arid southern regions, appears to have remained in the wild. Guanacos were the parent species of the domesticated llama and the alpaca from the vicuna.

Other common species included deer, jaguars, pumas, bears, monkeys, foxes and wild cats as well as many snakes, and many species of bird. Both the eagle and the jaguar were revered. Jaguars were believed to have been masters of the Universe until humans appeared who then acquired the power of the jaguar to use for themselves. Animals, birds and 'serpents' were all important in Incan beliefs, religion and ceremonials. They all feature regularly in carvings, figurines and rock drawings.

Beliefs and Religion

The religious beliefs and deities were derivatives of those formed in the early Andean civilisations and included the rain forest and its animals, the movement of the heavenly bodies, lunar phases and so on. They were the forces of nature and were originally used to help explain the place of humans in the larger scheme of things: they provided a conceptual framework for living. Two mythical figures emerged and remained in the culture; one was Viracocha 'the creator' and the other Pachacamac 'the earth maker'. The gods were influenced by the rainforest animals – the jaguar, monkeys, serpents and birds. Feline-human hybrids, a feline face with human body, also occur in artworks; as do winged humans and falcon-headed soldiers.

The Inca religion was a fusion of beliefs gained from their conquered citizens. Viracocha remained as the creator, with a calendar of ceremonial rituals to be observed, based on the solstices, equinoxes, and lunar movements, which were all known. There were also auguries to be determined including planning the planting of the crops, the harvest and the days to go fishing. The stars were seen as marking celestial animals which all had earthly counterparts. Under Inca domination the main object of worship was Inti, the Sun, and the ancestor of the Inca dynasty (Métraux 1969, pp. 121–131).

A major part of all the ceremonial and rituals was sacrifice; mostly animals and birds, but also human (men, women and children). This was conducted by beheading, strangulation, clubbing or throat cutting (and is illustrated in murals, ceramics and carvings). The purpose of the sacrifice was to both secure the favour of the gods as well as enabling the congregation to commune with them. At major ceremonies, every household would prepare *sanko*, a paste of maize flour. Pure white llamas would be sacrificed at the holy place so that their blood would fall on some of the paste. The priest would taste this and put a curse on all those who took part in the ceremony with 'a divided will'. After tasting it was declared good and the paste was made holy by the blood, it would then be smeared on the body (of all people, children and invalids) and on the threshold of all buildings to 'expel diseases and weakness' (Métraux 1969, pp. 146–147).

The role of the (unfortunate) llamas was central to the rituals. The wool colour was important with pure white being the most sacred to the gods. The early records by the Spanish conquistadors stated that it could involve hundreds in one day for some ceremonies. A reddish coloured llama was sacrificed every day in Cuzco, the capital. The religious beliefs of the Incas and their subject people were complex, but they also served the purpose of applying a national system to the whole Empire. Many of the rituals were conducted directly or indirectly as an aid to preserve health and ward off illness and disease. In this medical attribution it was the priesthood acting as magic medical men.

Traditional Medicine

As the South American peoples had no written literature the actual practice of medicine is not well described: the following is derived from early Spanish accounts. The role of the priests was either in the use of ritual or prayers to ward off disease, or in their use of hallucinogenic substances which enabled them to enter the spirit world and to negotiate a cure or a cause of the problem. If a village or community had a health issue: the priest/shaman would speak to the spirits to ask them to send the illness from their village to that of their enemies. Animal sacrifice was also used to aid a cure. For any poor peasant who could not afford a llama, a guinea pig was used.

Many remedies of animal, mineral or plant-origin were used as medications, these varied between the differing ecological zones. Surviving reports would indicate that plant materials were the most frequently used. Three were determined to be the most valuable.

- Cuca – the source of cocaine. This was cultivated with great care, harvested as leaves and used both as a preventive and treatment (a coca leaf 'tea' is still taken to prevent altitude sickness). It was widely used as a preventive (believed to restore a body temperature) and also topically to treat bodily sores, in particular those that were maggot infested.
- Sayri – called tobacco by the Spaniards, which was used to promote good health.
- Sarsaparilla – valued by the Spaniards as a treatment for bubos (plague) and other infections.

Although the use of herbs was well-developed, Inca medicine was also strongly influenced by magic and incantations (Bernard 2001, pp. 148–153). While there was very limited anatomical knowledge it is recorded that trepanation was practised and that limb fractures were successfully splinted. Patients with broken bones, following reduction, would use coca to control pain.

There does not appear to be any surviving information on veterinary medicine. Presumably, efforts would have been made to help injured or sick domesticated llamas and alpacas, and the procedures used in humans would probably have been utilised. In the big llama raising region around Lake Titicaca there might even have been animal healers.

European Arrival and Colonisation

In 1531 Francisco Pizarro, with a small group of 63 horsemen, 200 infantrymen and horses, made his third voyage to Peru. He captured the Inca Emperor Atahualpa, whom he executed in 1533, travelled inland, took Cuzco the capital city and installed a puppet regime. By 1572 the last Inca stronghold was captured. Much of the agricultural structure remained but this gradually deteriorated over the years due to a lack of previous controls. The introduction of horses, cattle, sheep and pigs was well received by the local farmers and these all replaced the llama as the principle livestock animal. Pizarro and his fellow conquistadors succeeded in destroying and pillaging a culture and a country for gold, silver and personal wealth.

References

Bernard, C. (2001) *The Incas. Empire of Blood and Gold*. London: Thames & Hudson

Bierer, B.W. (1955) *A Short History of Veterinary Medicine in America*. East Lansing, MI: Michigan State University Press

Campbell, D.M. (1934) Development of Veterinary Medicine in North America. *Veterinary Medicine* **29**

Debo, A (2003) *A History of the Indians of the United States*. London: Folio (this edition of the 1970 text is based on the seventh impression published in 1983)

Dobyns, H.E. (1966) Estimating Aboriginal American Populations: An Appraisal of Techniques with a New Hemisphere Estimate. *Current Anthropology* **7** No.4

Jones, D.M. and Molyneaux, B.L. (2009) *Mythology of the American Nations*. London: Hermes House

Mann, C.C. (2005) *1491: New Revelations of the Americas before Columbus*. New York: Knopf

Merrilat, L.A. and Campbell, D.M. (1935) *Veterinary Military History of the United States*. Chicago, IL: Veterinary Magazine Corp

Métraux, A. (1969) *The History of the Incas*. New York: Random House

Nozedar, A. (2012) *The Element Encyclopaedia of Native Americans*. London: HarperCollins

Pohl, J. and Robinson, C.M. (2005) *Aztecs and Conquistadores*. London: Osprey

Ross, K. (1978/1984) *Codex Mendoza: Aztec Manuscript*. Fribourg: Libor (manuscript held at Bodleian Library, Oxford)

Thomas, H. (1993) *The Conquest of Mexico*. London: Hutchison

CHAPTER 10

Australasia: Australia and New Zealand

In geographic terms Australasia is a group of islands in the Southern Hemisphere. The principle islands are Australia with Tasmania, New Zealand (North and South Islands), and New Guinea with Melanesia. The two countries included in this study are Australia and New Zealand. Neither country had any domesticated animals nor any livestock farming before colonisation by Britain, starting in the late 1700s.

AUSTRALIA

Australia is the sixth largest island continent in the world by land area. It is bordered by Papua New Guinea and Indonesia to the north, the South Indian Ocean to the west, the South Pacific Ocean and New Zealand to the east, and Antarctica to the south. Topographically it is a flat country, with deserts in the centre, tropical forests to the north-east and mountains in the south-east. Australia is the driest continent. Rainfall is low and there are good grasslands to the south-east.

Indigenous People

First human habitation, by migration from Southeast Asia, has been dated back to over 50,000 years ago. The Aboriginal native culture is recognised as one of the oldest civilisations in the world. When the country was first visited by Europeans the people were mostly hunter-gatherers with complex tribal communities and relationships. It was not until 1992 that aboriginal ownership of land was made legal.

Beliefs and Religion

The indigenous people have a culture and oral tradition of strong spirituality, developed within an animist framework and with a particular respect for the land. The belief system is termed Dreamtime and dates back to when their first ancestors travelled the country. There are many ancestral spirits including the Rainbow Serpent, and others based on animals and birds. Many of these animals and mystic creatures feature in the ancient rock art and paintings, illustrating a close relationship with the natural world.

Agriculture, Livestock and Wildlife

The native people do not appear to have practised cultivation of plants to any discernible extent and had no domesticated animals with the exception of dogs (dingoes).

Types of wildlife found feature two groups of unique animals: the monotremes including the platypus and echidna, and the marsupials including the kangaroo, koala and wombat. Other native wild animals included birds such as the mu and kookaburra and, of particular importance, the several types of venomous snakes.

Traditional Medicine

Aboriginal people had a system of traditional healers, these men or women were known as *Ngangkari*. Their place in the tribal society was important as they were the respected keepers of the oral Dreamtime history.

The medical practice was a holistic approach involving the healers; plant and tree bark medications; communal healing dances and prayers. The medications have not been well described as the plant materials (known as bush medicine) in use vary between both tribal groups and ecological situations. There are no described veterinary medicine practices.

European Arrival and Colonisation

The first European arrival in Australia was by a Dutch ship in 1606. Later in the century the Dutch charted the western and northern coastlines: they named the land New Holland but made no attempt at colonisation. In 1770 James Cook mapped the east coast and claimed it for Great Britain.

In 1788 a fleet of eleven British ships under the command of Commodore Arthur Phillip arrived to set up a penal colony. The first settlement was Port Jackson at Sydney Cove. After roughly three years, as the European population grew, the indigenous people numbers fell drastically following the outbreak and spread of smallpox, a disease against which they had no natural immunity. A separate colony was later established on Tasmania in 1825 and as more convicts were shipped to Australia further colonies were settled on the eastern coast. Other migrant settlements were also created on the southern and western coasts; these were designated as 'free provinces' but later accepted convicts. As settlements and colonist numbers grew they formed the basis of the separate states.

Livestock Farming

With the first fleet of ships came the nucleus of a livestock industry. Sensibly it had been planned to purchase these animals in Cape Town, South Africa, which was then a Dutch colony. They did not have to undergo the eight month voyage that was endured by the convict passengers. According to *The Australian Encyclopaedia* (Vol 4, 1963) the stock shipped was one stallion, three mares, two bulls, seven cows, four goats, 44 sheep, 32 pigs and a 'large quantity of various kinds of poultry'.

As there were already animals on board the ships, both personal (horses) and others to provide fresh meat, these would have been included in a census made by Phillip in 1788; this listed five rabbits, seven horses, seven cattle, 19 goats, 29 sheep, 29 geese, 35 ducks, 74 pigs, 87 chickens and 122 'fowl'.

Livestock were important, the purpose of the settlement was to start agriculture to feed the settlers and to provide income. The plan was to make land grants, these were of a minimum 30 acres for convicts and free settlers, and 100 acres for ex-marines. Included in the early colonist group there would presumably have been farmers and men with knowledge of horses and livestock. One record in 1822 indicates that there were 14 farriers in the colony, possibly with veterinary skills of a sort. Almost certainly some immigrants would have brought books on farriery and family almanacs of recipes and treatments for both human and animal diseases. There would not have been any veterinarians: the London Veterinary College did not open until 1791.

A Need for Veterinary Medicine

Purchasing livestock in South Africa was fortunate as the diseases then rampant in Europe were not introduced. Further livestock shipments were made from South Africa, India and Southeast Asia: epidemic disease was not a problem in these countries. In 1800 the Governor of the now named New South Wales wrote, 'Where sheep were taken care of they do well' and in 1860 'No cattle in the world are less liable to disease than those in New South Wales' (Vallis 2011, p. 5). Colonisation of the continent progressed well and within a few years the territory was divided into states (New South Wales, Victoria, Queensland, Western Australia, Tasmania, South Australia, and Northern Territory), each with their own legislatures.

From the 1850s migration grew rapidly and food needs increased, more livestock were imported and production moved from extensive to intensive. Before any quarantine laws could be enacted the livestock were infected with diseases including tuberculosis, contagious bovine pleuropneumonia, foot-and-mouth disease and anthrax. Some diseases had already been recognised, in particular sheep scab (Psoroptes ovis infestation), this had become obvious in the early days, having arrived with the first fleet shipments.

Ecto- and endoparasitism, and foot rot were seen as problems, but sheep scab was the serious one. It resulted in the NSW Scab Act of 1832, the first animal disease legislation in Australia. This prohibited the owners of infected sheep from driving them on any road or turning them out onto others' property. Any male convicts found guilty could be, 'worked in irons on the roads for up to six months'. Soon the other colonies also enacted scab legislation. As this developed, scab inspectors were appointed with the power to seize, detain and destroy infected sheep. The first scab inspector was William Dumbleton, a former butcher, appointed in NSW in 1840. The wool industry had become the most valuable export from Australia.

In spite of the recognised seriousness of sheep scab there was little interest in obtaining professional veterinary help. The farming interests were mainly from wealthy graziers with enormous properties and big flocks: they preferred to find their own solutions, using a variety of topical acaricides and dips for the treatment. In 1864 legislation was enacted in NSW to make sheep dipping compulsory and this was regulated by the scab inspectors. This was soon copied by the other states and by 1896 sheep scab was declared eradicated from Australia. This success formed the basis of national disease control, the first step in the creation of a government veterinary service.

Each Australian state had a government stock department headed by a Chief Inspector of Stock. These were generally laymen, as veterinarians were not well regarded; if professional advice was sought it was medical men that were consulted. This may have been due to there being so few veterinary graduates available. One problem was that there was no system of control, anyone could call themselves a veterinarian, there were no veterinary publications and, most important, there was no veterinary school. It was not until the 1880s that the value of the profession began to be appreciated.

Veterinary Professionals Become Recognised

The first veterinary surgeon in Australia is believed to have been John Stewart. He graduated from Edinburgh in 1827, and on his arrival in Sydney in 1841 he set up a private practice. Stewart had been a teacher at the Glasgow Veterinary College and had authored two books on horses. In 1847 he was asked for help by the NSW government to investigate Cumberland disease in sheep; named after the region, southwest of Sydney, where it occurred. Affected sheep died quickly, as did some of the men working with them. An enquiry was commissioned with Stewart as a member of the team. The disease was recognised as being similar to a condition seen in Europe which was known as *milzbrand* in Germany and *maladie du sang* in France. Movement of infected flocks and herds was prohibited and all carcases of dead animals were burned. Later this condition was diagnosed as anthrax by Graham Mitchell, a veterinarian. While this use of veterinary expertise had produced effective controls the relationship with government was not followed.

In 1858 a Shorthorn heifer was imported from London to Melbourne and shortly afterwards was correctly diagnosed, by clinical symptoms and post-mortem examination, as having suffered from contagious bovine pleuro-pneumonia (CBPP) by Henry Wragge, a consultant government veterinarian. He recommended that the in-contact herd be slaughtered. The owner disagreed as did public opinion and Wragge's advice was ignored. Because of illness, it was decided 11 months later, to slaughter the whole herd. Three veterinarians, Pottie, Miscamble and Gribton all diagnosed CBPP by clinical symptoms and its presence was confirmed at post-mortem. Then in 1860 the disease broke out on a neighbouring property – to start what developed into the 'most devastating livestock disease in Australia'. The rapid spread of the disease caused the legislators in New South Wales, Victoria, Queensland and Tasmania to appoint veterinarians as consultants or inspectors.

As a result a Royal Commission was set up to investigate the disease and methods of control, but this did not include any veterinarians. The final report concluded that CBPP was neither contagious nor infectious and that preventive inoculation was of no value. Graham Mitchell, who had previously identified the cause of Cumberland disease strongly disagreed with the Commission's findings. Together with John Miscamble they adapted Willem's CBPP tail inoculation technique to produce a commercial vaccine product, which was well accepted by stock owners. In 1872 the Diseases of Stock Act was passed and in the following year Mitchell was appointed to the government service. He ensured that control measures for CBPP were soon in place across the state of Victoria.

Cattle imported into NSW in 1871 and 1872 were diagnosed as infected with foot-and-mouth disease (FMD) by John Pottie, a government consultant veterinarian. In 1872 an outbreak also occurred on farms in Victoria. The government inspectorate, now mostly veterinarians, advised a slaughter and disinfection policy which eradicated the outbreak. A further outbreak was diagnosed by Mitchell. He ensured a public outcry and Victoria banned the importation of cattle, sheep and pigs from Britain for seven years.

Veterinary influence, by the 'hybrid government-private' veterinarians such as Stewart, Pottie and Mitchell had changed official recognition of the value of the veterinary profession. This was aided by Queensland appointing James Irving, a British veterinary graduate who had migrated to Brisbane in 1873, to government service.

Veterinary Medicine Is Established

In the 1870s and 1880s there was growing recognition by the livestock industry of the importance of veterinarians in the control of disease in the livestock industry: both wool and meat were important economic exports. There were no veterinary schools, most veterinarians had either been trained in Britain or had been 'apprenticed' to an Australian practitioner. In 1880 there were only about 12 qualified veterinary surgeons practising in Victoria, but every shoeing forge called itself a 'veterinary shoeing forge'. This situation began to change with the arrival in Victoria in 1880 of William Tyson Kendall, a 29-year-old British graduate.

The small group of veterinarians began to organise themselves and build their professional image, while waiting for the government to take the lead and invest in veterinary education. In 1880 the Australasian Veterinary Medical Association was formed with Mitchell as president and Kendall as secretary, who also started publishing the Australasian Veterinary Journal in 1882 – both joint efforts with their New Zealand colleagues. Kendall became well-known for his high quality animal care as he worked to demonstrate the difference between qualified veterinarians and unqualified 'healers'.

Kendall, who worked with Mitchell, soon appraised the situation: in 1881 no veterinarians were employed full time by the government in any of the states. Many, if not most, of the stock owners and farmers had no experience of veterinary aid and guidance. In much of the country the farms were isolated and away from the towns where most veterinarians worked – and there was no government veterinary service to help them. Kendall found, that on slaughter for human consumption, about 25% of the cattle were infected with tuberculosis and there was no system in place to prevent cattle meat or dairy products being offered for sale. Kendall lobbied for a Royal Commission to examine this subject. He also found people would rather sell a sick or lame horse than pay for treatment.

By Kendall's efforts the Veterinary Surgeons Act 1887 was passed in Victoria, giving legal recognition to the veterinary profession. The Act required a four year veterinary education course, and also allowed registration of unqualified veterinary practitioners who had worked as such for five years before January 1888. Since before the Act was passed Kendall and others had unsuccessfully lobbied government to provide the resources for a veterinary school; they then felt more action was required. As a result Kendall bought a site for a privately run college.

This opened in 1888 as the Melbourne Veterinary College, with the expectation that government would take over, this, however, took time. The college produced 61 graduates between 1891 and 1909, when their 22 students passed to the newly established University of Melbourne Veterinary School. Having closed his college Kendall taught at the new school until 1918. In every one of the 20 years over which the school had been open, it had operated at a loss. Kendall had received no help – monetary or otherwise; as he wrote, 'My staff accepted moderate salaries'. Kendall was known as 'the father of veterinary medicine in Australia'.

Continent-wide Disease Control

Australia was a good environment for sheep, and later cattle farming. The livestock population grew rapidly, as did the export of wool, meat and dairy products, together with the imports of livestock which also brought a wide range of animal diseases to a country with few veterinarians and where stockmen ignored veterinary help.

Eventually the value of veterinary advice was recognised and a programme of disease control began. This was initially difficult because the different colonies did not always agree on legislation. New South Wales and Victoria led the way. The first Act, passed in 1830 was to control slaughter and prevent tuberculosis-diseased meat being sold for consumption. This was followed by the Meat Supervision Act of 1901, and the Milk and Dairy Supervision Act of 1905, both in Victoria.

Disease control began with the Sheep Scab Act of 1832 followed by further legislation in 1861, and the Diseases of Stock Act of 1872. By the 1890s most colonies had disease control legislation, and disease recognition moved quickly. Once diseases including FMD, CBPP, anthrax, bovine tuberculosis, brucellosis, cattle tick fever, sheep louse and ked, swine fever and Newcastle disease were discovered, control and prevention measures were introduced. Rinderpest, introduced on the west coast in 1923 was rapidly stamped out.

Rabbits became a serious pest and in 1887 NSW offered a £25,000 prize for a biological method of their destruction. The French Pasteur Institute needed money and sent a team to Australia – they failed to find a rabbit solution but did develop an anthrax vaccine in the 1890s, urgently needed to control the Cumberland disease epidemic (this was soon superseded by a locally produced vaccine). As a result it became obvious that regional bacteriological research laboratories were needed. The first of these was established in Brisbane, Queensland in 1893 and later a tick fever (Babesia bigemina) vaccine was developed there.

In 1908 the Federation of the Australian Colonies, now states, was achieved. The Chief Inspectors of Stock became Commonwealth Chief Quarantine Officers and the Quarantine Act 1908 was passed controlling importation of livestock (updated by the Biosecurity Act 2015). Over the next few years each state established a Veterinary Research Laboratory. Control of CBPP was the greatest problem but this was finally eradicated in Queensland in 1973; followed by bovine brucellosis in 1989 and bovine tuberculosis in 1997. In 1985 the Commonwealth for Scientific and Industrial Research (CSIRO) Animal Health Laboratory opened providing a central research facility, replacing the 1974 Bureau of Animal Health. A unique use of a biological disease control method has been the use of the myxomatosis virus to reduce the enormous plague-like rabbit population. Within a few months of its introduction in the 1950s the numbers were drastically reduced.

With the passage of Veterinary Surgeons Acts in NSW and Victoria in 1923, veterinary education could develop. Melbourne University had absorbed Kendall's school in 1909 and Sydney University opened a school in 1910. This was followed by the opening of veterinary faculties in Queensland in 1936; Murdoch University in Perth in 1973; Charles Sturt University in Wagga Wagga, NSW in 2006; James Cook University in Townsville, Queensland in 2006 and Adelaide University, South Australia in 2007.

Australia has become a global leader in animal disease research. It has not been an easy road for the veterinary profession. They have had to fight to get recognition by demonstrating, to the farming community and legislators, the value of veterinary medicine to ensuring a healthy livestock and export industry.

Writing this chapter, in particular the parts related to legislation, has been aided by reading an Australian Department of Agriculture publication on the history of the role of veterinarians in government (Vallis 2011).

NEW ZEALAND

New Zealand is a country comprising North and South Islands, and is located in the southwest Pacific Ocean about 1200 miles (2000 km) to the east of Australia.

Topographically it is a long and narrow country with the South Island being the largest part and the Southern Alps mountain range positioned on the east side. There are extensive grasslands and in most regions a temperate climate, but it is generally cooler in the South Island region. Rainfall is quite high and drought conditions very seldom occur.

Indigenous Peoples

Due to its geographical isolation, New Zealand was one of the last land areas to be occupied by humans. This allowed for a biodiverse and unique animal and plant environment to evolve. The first humans to colonise the country were the Māori who arrived from eastern Polynesia between 1300 and 1350. They developed a specific culture based on their religious beliefs. Life, however, was plagued by internal dissent between tribes.

Beliefs and Religion

The Māori people developed a belief system similar to that of their Polynesian homeland. The concept is one of every natural object and living thing being connected by *whakapapa*, a form of genealogy, and because of this connection everything possesses a *mauri* or life force. This life force is represented by three mythical personifications: *Tangaroa* for the oceans and origin of all fish; *Tane* for the forests and origin of all birds; *Rongo* for peaceful activities such as agriculture and the origin of cultivated plants.

Related to this belief system were sacred ritual procedures and practices called tapu and mana: essentially for the maintenance of a rigid social hierarchy. Elements of tapu continue to be used related to Māori illness, death and burial. Since there were no mammals in the New Zealand ecosystem, the creatures symbolised in their beliefs were mostly birds, of which there were a large terrestrial number.

Agriculture, Livestock and Wildlife

The Māori developed a village-based culture which cooperated in food production, both by plant cultivation and gathering seeds and other edibles. This radically changed when potatoes were introduced by traders. No animals were domesticated, but they fished for and ate seafood.

Wildlife presents an interesting diversity, notably for the absence of mammals, except for whales and seals in the coastal seas, and bats which will have flown there, but which live mainly on the ground. Places in the environment that could be utilised by mammals have been occupied by some insects but in particular by a number of flightless birds, such as the kiwi, weka, kakapo and the extinct moa. There are also many species of lizards, frogs and tuatara (lizard-like reptiles).

Following the arrival of humans many invasive species could be found. The original Polynesian migrants brought the Polynesian rat and the domesticated dog. Europeans added pigs, sheep and cattle (the pig was introduced by Captain Cook when he visited in the 1700s). The introduction of rats, cats, dogs, possums and deer (among others) have seriously damaged the natural fauna of the country. Under European farming the populations of sheep, in particular, and cattle have become major agricultural and export activities of significant economic value.

Traditional Medicine

The traditional medicine, termed *Rongoā* is basically an enhancement of wellness using a holistic approach embracing spiritual, psychological, physical and family elements. It has been transmitted orally over many generations. Considered to be *tapu*, the sacred knowledge was only passed to a select few who were trained by an expert *tohunga* or priest from the *whare wananga* – the house of knowledge.

There were four main elements to the practice:

1. Spiritual healing from a tohunga who would look for a mental or physical imbalance in the patient and remove the spirit that was the causation.
2. The power of *karakia* – Māori incantations and prayers.
3. The use of *mirimiri*– massage technique.
4. The use of *Rongoa rakau* – herbal medicaments.

A wide range of plants were used, collected and prepared according to sacred rituals. Both internal and external indications were prescribed. Sometimes bloodletting by skin cuts was used. Fractures were reduced and splinted. The transmission of the healing knowledge represented a preservation of the historic Māori culture (including their mythical personifications of birds and fish). There was no tradition of veterinary medicine as there were no domesticated animals, apart from dogs.

European Arrival and Colonisation

The first European to arrive was Abel Tasman the Dutch explorer in 1642, followed by James Cook who mapped the entire coastline in 1769. From the later 1700s visits were made by European and North American whaling and trading ships. They traded metal tools, weapons and other goods for timber, food and water. The introduction of the potato and the musket resulted in a total change in Māori agriculture and tribal strife, causing serious loss of life. From the early 19th century Christian missionaries began to settle in New Zealand and converted a majority of the Māori people.

When the colony of New South Wales Australia was established in 1788 the British government included the New Zealand islands in its draft, however there was little interest in any additional responsibilities. In 1833 James Busby was appointed British Resident in New Zealand to try to create order in what was becoming a complex situation. The New Zealand Company had been formed and was advertising for settlers, while at the same time it was buying land from the Māori at very cheap prices and selling this to new settlers.

In 1840 the Treaty of Waitangi was signed with Māori chiefs to bring the country into the British Empire. Due to differing interpretations of the text the New Zealand Wars erupted in 1845, ending in 1872. Extensive British settlement commenced in both islands in the latter half of the 19th century and in the early half of the 20th century. This resulted in the indigenous Māori people being both deprived of land and infected by European diseases (including influenza and measles), leading to rapid impoverishment.

A Need for Veterinary Medicine

Captain James Cook released a boar and two sows into the wild during his visit to New Zealand in the latter part of the 18th century; their descendants appear to have been free from any serious diseases before the large scale settlement of Europeans following the Waitangi Treaty. When the large sheep and cattle importations began in 1844 the country was disease free, but not for long as diseases were also imported and were not watched for by either the settlers or the Government.

In 1843, John Webster arrived from Britain and started a cattle veterinary practice in Petone. The next two arrivals from Britain were J Thompson who began to advertise his practice in August 1850, and J W Moorhouse who advertised that he was opening an equine and cattle hospital in the Hutt Valley in 1856. From that time there was a slow increase in British graduate veterinary numbers in the developing settlements.

As in Australia it was not long before sheep scab (*Psoroptes ovis*) was recognised as a serious problem, as was a condition of sheep called 'catarrh'. Legislation was passed to control these diseases. While catarrh appears not to have been dealt with, the scab legislation was both acted on and amended over several years. By 1889 there was a staff of six inspectors and 33 sub-inspectors, and from 1870 the incidence of the disease fell steadily until in 1891 New Zealand was declared scab free. In 1893 the national flock was 9.7 million head.

The control system was operated by inspectors using hand lenses to examine sheep, segregating the infected and in-contact animals, and instituting treatment. The treatment commenced with clipping and applying medicaments. Many substances were tried but few were really found to be effective until a tobacco-sulphur dip was introduced in 1854. By the 1860s the standard dip had become one of slaked lime and sulphur. In the 1870s Cooper's Sheep Dipping Powder (sulphur and arsenic) was officially approved for scab control.

Other diseases included 'catarrh' in sheep, probably caused by Pasteurella haemolytica; footrot in sheep which was reported in 1861 and CBPP in cattle which occurred in imported stock in 1880 but was rapidly eradicated (Fisher 2006, pp. 439–444). The Diseases of Animals Act was amended in 1881 with a defined list including FMD and other possible importations:

- cattle – catarrh, FMD, murrain, CBPP and rinderpest
- horses – glanders, murrain and pest
- sheep – fluke or liver-rot, FMD, sheep pox, scab and lice
- pigs – FMD and swine-pox.

Both bovine tuberculosis and sheep internal parasites had been noted in official reports.

Veterinary Profession Becomes Recognised

In 1888 J F Maclean was appointed government veterinary surgeon in the Livestock Branch of the Lands Department. He was the first full-time government veterinary employee; until 1893, when the Department of Agriculture was formed and three additional British veterinarians were appointed. It is estimated that there were probably no more than 17 veterinary graduates in the country. In 1890 Maclean studied bovine tuberculosis incidence and in 1892 reported on a series of disease issues in lambs and adult sheep in both islands. Following the Australasian Stock conference held in Wellington in 1892 a list of recognised diseases was compiled, and in 1893 two stock quarantine stations were established.

Meat and meat products inspection was recognised as an important veterinary function. The Slaughterhouse Act of 1877 consolidated Provincial Acts and in 1894 the Department of Agriculture provided the legislation to condemn diseased carcases and meat.

The salaried government veterinary staff were, however, poorly recompensed. In 1892 the Chief Veterinary Officer, responsible for the whole country, received an annual salary of only £300 while the lay Chief Stock Inspector received £500. This changed in 1893 with the formation of the Department of Agriculture and employment of additional veterinarians (Laing 1964, pp. 67–71).

Veterinary Medicine Is Established

Groups of farmers began to organise to obtain veterinary services and in 1903 the Southland Farmers Union employed a veterinarian at Invercargill. This was followed by a number of veterinary practices being established by farmers' groups and dairy cooperatives in the 1930s and 1940s each employing their own veterinarians. By 1909 the Department of Agriculture had 26 veterinarians, with 19 of them working as meat inspectors at freezing works and six on field duty.

The New Zealand Veterinary Association (NZVA) was formed in 1923. In 1943 the Dominion Federation of Farmer Veterinary Services was set up to coordinate activities of cooperative practices, but in 1946 the government took over the role with the Veterinary Services Council (VSC) which encouraged the creation of veterinary practices. By 1955 nearly all livestock farmers had access to veterinary services.

Education remained a problem, efforts to establish a veterinary school at Otago University in 1904 failed and the VSC provided funded help for students attending Australian schools. In 1962 the Faculty of Veterinary Science was established at Massey University in Palmerston North and has been most successful. By 1992 there were 830 veterinarians in clinical practice in New Zealand (Mavor and Gumbrell 2008).

New Zealand has an impressive record in animal disease prevention and control. It is free from all major epidemics. This record is well explored and explained by Davidson (2002, pp. 6–12).

References

Davidson, R.M. (2002) Control and Eradication of Animal Diseases in New Zealand. *New Zealand Veterinary Journal* **50** No.3 (supplement)

Fisher, J. (2006) The Origins, Spread and Disappearance of Contagious Bovine Pleuro-pneumonia in New Zealand. *Australian Veterinary Journal* **84** No.12

Laing, A.D.M.G. (1964) Some Historical Notes on the Veterinary Profession in New Zealand. *New Zealand Veterinary Journal* **12** No.4.

Mavor, H. and Gumbrell, B. (2008) Veterinary Services Early Veterinary Services, 1850s–1940s. *Te Ara – The Encyclopaedia of New Zealand* http://www.Teara.govt.nz/en/veterinary-services/page-1 and http://www.Teara.govt.nz/en/veterinary-services/page-2

Vallis, R. (2011) *A Veterinary Awakening: The History of Government Veterinarians in Australia.* Canberra: Department of Agriculture and Water Resources

CHAPTER II

Africa: South Africa and Colonial Countries

Africa is the second largest land mass after Eurasia with, in broad terms, a Mediterranean and Nile valley peoples and culture north of the Sahara desert and clearly defined African peoples and cultures to the south. The northern half of the continent, below the Mediterranean coastal region and Nile valley, is mainly desert, with over half of the area arid or dry land. The southern half ranges from tropical forest to savannah plains, with a volcanic valley to the east and mountainous regions in the south.

Indigenous Peoples

It is believed that the human species originated in Africa some seven million years ago. Diverse groups of people evolved and settled in the differing climatic zones of the continent. There were many early civilisation and cultural developments across all regions, most notably in the Nile Valley. South of the Sahara Desert a variety of tribal groupings and states evolved. Of significance is the early domestication of cattle, possibly by 7000 BC–8000 BC, followed by domestication of the donkey and screw-horned goat by the Nilotic people, in the north-eastern region. In almost all of these cultures cattle were the most important animal, not primarily for production but as a means of accumulating wealth – the number of animals owned counted for more than their quality or health. Of the other types of domesticated animals, depending on the region, goats, donkeys and some sheep had importance. Most agriculture was crop related as the primary food source and supplemented by meat, usually as a result of hunting.

The traditional religions (because of their great diversity, not discussed in any detail here) included the recognition of a creator, and a strong belief in spirits who sought to place humans in the role of joining the natural world with the supernatural. Magic played a major role in the early religious ceremonies and was also a key part of traditional medicine practice, with herbal medications. Currently some 40% of the population follow Islam, a result of the 6th century northern Africa Muslim invasion. In central and southern Africa the majority of people are now Christian, but there remains a strong recognition of earlier beliefs.

African wildlife is one of the most extensive and diverse of all global regions, and includes herbivores, carnivores, primates, snakes, crocodiles and birds. Animal sacrifice featured in religious rituals to honour and appease the gods. Animals, including birds, are strongly represented in early art, wood carving and sculpture, frequently showing relationships with divine spirits.

Animal Diseases

Africa is a prolific global disease centre; aided and exacerbated by the dual agencies of blood-borne parasites and insect vectors, such as the fly or tick. These diseases have required not only research but careful observation of the species involved to gain effective control.

First mention of such diseases appears in the records of the 1836 Great Trek when Afrikaner families left the South African Cape Colony, moving into the interior to preserve their traditional bible-following way of life. In these unknown lands their animals experienced what they called 'the mysterious disease'.

David Livingstone (1813–1873) on his Zambia expedition observed a sickness in livestock, noting that it related to the tsetse fly. In 1857 he wrote,

> *symptoms seem to indicate what is probably the cause, a poison in the blood. The poison-germ [is] contained in a bulb at the root of the proboscis. . . .*

When healthy horses and cattle enter tsetse fly country they will take several months to show trypanosomiasis symptoms. Indigenous Zulu Africans called it *anagana* a word that literally meant powerless, frail and useless (Chyzyaka 1991, pp. 81–98). The discovery of the causal trypanosome was made by David Bruce in 1894.

It was soon recognised that trypanosomiasis was a problem with a particular consequence in cattle and horses (and also humans). The disease is now controlled by mapping tsetse fly free areas and by the use of chemotherapy to treat or protect at-risk stock. As the disease occurs in many species of wildlife, control is a difficult exercise in most regions.

Parasitism is a major issue and with haemoparasites being the most difficult to control. East Coast Fever (ECF) caused by *Theileria parva* and vectored by ticks remains a problem in many regions. Anaplasmosis caused by *Anaplasma marginale* can be controlled by use of an *Anaplasma centrale* vaccine. Babesiosis, heartwater (cowdriosis), besnoitiosis and avian malaria are all found in different regions. A wide range of helminths, nematodes, trematodes and cestodes are of common occurrence.

Of other diseases, in the early days of colonisation, contagious bovine pleuro-pneumonia (CBPP) (Long Ziekte) was a serious cattle problem. Isolation of the *Mycoplasma* organism has enabled the production of vaccines and CBPP has now been mostly eradicated. Other bacterial diseases, such as clostridial, anthrax, brucel-losis, contagious caprine pleuro-pneumonia, haemorrhagic septicaemia (HS), skin and genital infections, and rickettsial diseases are all still found. The most serious viral diseases are African horse sickness (AHS) and rabies, both of which can be controlled through vaccination programmes. Other viral diseases found include African swine fever (ASF), classical swine fever (CSF), foot-and-mouth disease (FMD), lumpy skin disease, Nairobi sheep disease, pox diseases and Rift valley fever.

Using now well practised methods of control – vaccination, isolation, dipping and regular medication – livestock farming can be conducted in most areas of Africa but some, due to tick and fly infestation, are still unavailable.

Traditional Veterinary Medicine

Little is known of the ethno-botanical medications used in the tribal communities: as cattle were regarded as 'wealth', obviously measures were taken to protect them, such as the use of the CBPP vaccine. Magical incantations and dances were used to aid human health, and similar activities were used for cattle. Many animal diseases were traditionally treated with various plant preparations of unknown efficacy. One paper dealing with this subject is known, but the writer has been unable to trace a copy of the now defunct journal (Chavhunduka 1976).

The most serious problem that the African herders faced, and recognised, was bovine trypanosomiasis, now termed *nagana*. Diseases were named by a characteristic symptom, trypanosomiasis was known as *kaodzera* (Ngoni language) or *ndulu* (Chewa) both meaning to nod; or by the tsetse fly, as the relationship was recognised – *luuka* (Tonga), *tushembe* (Bemba), *kamdzembe* (Nsenga) and *zeze* (Lozi), (Chyzaka 1991, pp. 81–88). In West Africa, the trypanotolerant dwarf N'Dama humpless cattle evolved and were domesticated. This unique characteristic has been exploited by local peoples in areas where other cattle cannot be kept.

The other most serious cattle disease was CBPP, which could rapidly decimate a herd. Cattle owners in Mauritania, western Africa discovered that insertion of diseased lung tissue under the skin of the nose would produce an immunity, but not without side-effects. The disfiguration of the face was frequently accompanied by a boney exostosis resembling a third horn, when first seen it was believed that this was a new species of bovine (*Bos triceros*). The procedure frequently caused serious inflammation and oedema of the face, often barbarously treated by the cattle owner with a hot iron, usually making the condition worse. It was a method of producing a level of CBPP protection and its use spread to East Africa, and was still being employed within living memory (see Chapter 18).

When the rinderpest epizootic struck in the later 1800s it swept across the continent causing a catastrophe for cattle and other species, including wildlife.

Colonisation and Veterinary Medicine

There were no reliable records of animal diseases dated prior to the colonisation of the continent in the late 1800s. The major countries involved in the colonisation were Britain and France (much of the French territory was desert or arid lands); although Portugal, Germany, Italy and Belgium also had colonies. Ethiopia was not colonised, although it was influenced by Portugal in the early days. The best developed colonial veterinary services created by Britain and France, and Germany in their smaller colonial lands appear to have been very efficient.

The region now known as the Republic of South Africa has the best recorded history and is discussed first. The country overviews following are mostly derived from a series of reports on the history of British Overseas Veterinary Services (West 1961 and 1973). As these were located in most regions of the continent they provide a reasonable assessment of the total picture. The disease and country names used for each overview are as given in the reports.

SOUTH AFRICA

Originally a Dutch colony established to service their trading ships, the territory passed into British control in 1806, with the Republic of South Africa created in 1931. First record of disease problems was made by Jan van Riebeck at the Cape in 1654; legislation to control sheep scab spread was passed in 1693. Increasing numbers of horses, pigs and sheep were imported from Europe. Records show cattle deaths in 1661, with no causes recorded. AHS was first recognised in 1719, and during the years 1860–1907 CBPP (1853), Babesiosis, glanders (1844) and rinderpest (1896) were all diagnosed.

The first qualified veterinarians arrived with the British military in the mid-1800s, with Chief Colony Veterinary Officers appointed in the late 1800s. A Commission investigated cattle and sheep diseases in 1877. Rinderpest and AHS were the serious issues, one killed oxen (used for transport) and the other horses (used for combat), soon lamsiekte, babesiosis, blackquarter, CBPP and FMD were all recognised problems.

Wool exports were a major (farmer) income source and sheep scab was a serious problem. Following the first legislation in 1693 similar notices were issued in 1704, 1715, 1727 and 1740. Penalties were issued for non-reporting of cases, the slaughter of infected animals was required, along with the disinfection of animal housing. In 1789 the first Spanish Merino sheep were imported and became the basis (with crossbreds) of the South African flock. The disease was still a problem in the 1800s. In 1874 the first British Scab Act was passed but it was not fully successful; the 1877 Commission revised the Law with Scab Inspectors appointed in 1885 and compulsory dipping in 1894. By the 1930s it was thought the disease was eradicated, but it still existed at the end of the 20th century. CBPP was first recognised in 1853 and spread along the cattle transport routes. It created an economic disaster for the transport system and also for the Xhosa Nation people.

The importance of veterinary services was emphasised by the rinderpest outbreak in 1896. Two veterinarians were recognised for their heroic efforts to control the outbreak: D Hutcheon in Cape Colony and his assistant Jotello Soga (1866–1906), who was Xhosa-speaking and the first native South African to become a graduate veterinarian, from Edinburgh veterinary school in 1886. Hutcheon and Soga conducted their own research on rinderpest vaccination methods and treatments and as a result of their work, Rinderpest was finally eradicated in 1898. Although Jotello Soga had played a leading role in the rinderpest campaign, the Colonial Government denied him a permanent position because of his race. He continued to practice and was a sought-after speaker at Afrikaner farmer conferences; he was also a co-founder of the Cape Colony Veterinary Society in 1905.

State Veterinary Services Evolve

The evolution of veterinary services in South Africa was related to the colonial history. All of the early veterinary staff were in the British Army but were soon supplemented by British, Swiss, German and French graduates. The first Colonial Chief Veterinary Officer was W Wiltshire appointed to Natal in 1874, followed by other Officers appointed to Cape Colony in 1876, Free State in 1896 and Transvaal in 1897. These appointments were driven by the need to control AHS and rinderpest.

There was an urgent need for a research programme to enable effective disease control. Dr (later Sir) Arnold Theiler was appointed by the Zuid-Afrikaansche Republic (later Transvaal) to undertake this work; by 1908 he had the funding to build the first Onderstepoort Laboratory, which has expanded progressively over the years. In 1911 Theiler was made Chief Veterinary Officer for the country with C E Gray as the First Principal Veterinary Officer. The initial work plan was to control AHS and rinderpest, but this soon expanded to include many unknown diseases as well as those related to importation. At Theiler's request, John McFadyean at the Royal Veterinary College (London) demonstrated the viral cause of AHS. Next Theiler was able to prove the viral cause of Bluetongue disease (first described in 1880 by Hutcheon in Merino sheep, but probably endemic in wild ruminants). Theiler was able to develop vaccines against both diseases. The many haemoprotozoal diseases were studied including anaplasmosis and ECF. Theiler discovered the causal organism of ECF, now named *Theileria parva*. Both African Swine Fever and Classical Swine Fever have been studied with efforts at producing vaccines. A notable success was the discovery of the cause of *lamsiekte*, a cattle problem initially believed to be due to a dietary phosphorus deficiency; this was only part of the story, Theiler demonstrated that the actual cause was botulism (*Clostridium botulinum*).

In 1962 a national field veterinary service was established as a separate government activity. Many unknown animal diseases (frequently in the wildlife national parks) were studied, as well as the construction of a 2500 km stock-proof boundary fence completed in 1964 to prevent the reintroduction of FMD by game or livestock.

The Veterinary Profession Is Established

The Transvaal Veterinary Medical Association was created in 1903 and in 1920 merged with the Cape Colony and Natal Associations. In 1923 they joined together, becoming the South African Veterinary Association in 1971. They have published *The Journal of the South African Veterinary Association* since 1927.

In 1933 the Veterinary Act was passed to regulate the profession. This has been updated with the South African Veterinary Council (SAVC) being created in 1982 to oversee and govern the profession. Veterinary education commenced with a Faculty of Veterinary Science created in 1918 at Onderstepoort and run jointly by the Department of Agriculture and Transvaal University College, replaced by the University of Pretoria in 1920. A second school was established at Medunsa, close to Onderstepoort to train black, coloured and Indian South Africans. This was success-ful and the school was amalgamated with the Onderstepoort School in 1999 provid-ing a six-year course in veterinary medicine. The Veterinary Faculty cooperates with the SAVC on regulatory matters and the examination of foreign graduates.

South African Onderstepoort research into animal diseases, in particular those caused by haemoparasites, and its role as a major international vaccine producer and supplier, have been important. A series of papers read at the 30th World Veterinary Congress provide an overview of their development (South African Veterinary Medicine History 2011, pp. 136–142).

BASUTOLAND (LESOTHO)

Coming under British control in 1869, Lesotho's disease pattern was influenced by being an enclaved country within South Africa. Babesiosis in cattle was observed in 1891, followed by rinderpest in 1896 and again in 1900; Koch's bile vaccine was used for rinderpest vaccination. The 1902 veterinary report, from the Basutoland Veterinary Department, listed the main diseases as rinderpest, CBPP, anthrax, glan-ders and sheep scab; in 1906 quarter-evil was added and in 1907, AHS. In 1908 scab was the major problem and compulsory dipping began, leading to its eradication in 1934. Internal parasites were also a serious issue. In 1955 the first Lesotho citizen graduated in Britain as a veterinary surgeon. Independent in 1966.

BECHUANALAND (BOTSWANA)

Between 1885 and 1890 the territory came under British control. David Livingstone had written that tsetse-flies 'abounded the riverbanks' and that horse distemper 'abounded'. In 1886 rinderpest arrived followed by recognition of ECF in 1904 and CBPP which was widespread in 1905, but eradicated in 1926. FMD invaded in 1931. The first veterinarian was appointed in 1905. FMD was initially a major problem in this predominantly cattle country but was finally eradicated in 1965. The country became independent in 1966.

EAST AFRICAN PROTECTORATE (KENYA)

Occupied by Britain in 1895 and renamed Kenya in 1920. The Veterinary Department was formed in 1903 following the need for veterinary help in the con-struction of a railway from the coast to Nairobi and Uganda. Local cattle herd size was low due to outbreaks of rinderpest, CBPP and ECF. In 1907 enzootic lymphangitis, swine fever, canine babesiosis, glanders, dourine and internal parasites were all recognised. FMD, which was introduced from Uganda in 1917, became a major problem. A research laboratory was opened at Kabete in 1913 to study ECF and Nairobi sheep disease and to produce vaccines for the blackquarter and rinderpest diseases. The laboratory expanded in 1914 when the war started.

Following the rinderpest panzootic of the 1890s, control by vaccines was finally achieved in 1947. By 1907 CBPP was under control and by 1911 ECF 'clean' and 'dirty' regions were delineated, but control remains a problem. Trypanosomiasis and tsetse fly control has been followed since 1907 and still remains a problem today, as do babesiosis and anaplasmosis. AHS is now controlled by vaccination, but Rift Valley Fever, seen in 1912, is still a problem. Veterinary school opened at Kabete in 1962, in 1970 moved to a faculty of University of Kenya in Nairobi. The country became independent in 1963.

GAMBIA

A small country almost totally surrounded by Senegal, and absorbed into the British Empire in 1821. No knowledge of veterinary issues is held prior to 1921 but the country is known to have been regularly swept by epidemics of both rinderpest and CBPP. This area of West Africa, along with Senegal, is where the facial implantation of infected lung tissue was used to promote CBPP immunity. Severe rinderpest losses were suffered in 1880. Eventually, in 1929, efforts were made to control the Senegal border. Vaccine use began in 1933 with reasonable control of the disease being gained by 1945. A Veterinary Department was created and anthrax, blackquarter, HS and CBPP tackled. The Veterinary Department opened a laboratory and produced vaccines against blackquarter, HS and CBPP. In 1957 Dawda Jawara graduated as a veterinarian from the University of Liverpool in Britain. He returned to Gambia and took charge of their Veterinary Department. Jawara became the first Prime Minister of Gambia in 1962 and the country gained independence from the United Kingdom in 1965. In 1970 Gambia became a republic with Jawara as its first President.

GERMAN SOUTH-WEST AFRICA (NAMIBIA)

Africa's driest country, Namibia was colonised by Germany in 1884 and came under South African jurisdiction in 1915. Little veterinary information had been recorded until CBPP was diagnosed in 1859 and efforts were made toward its control. Colonial administration was created in 1884 and animal disease legislation passed in 1887, with Wilhelm Rickmann appointed as the first Veterinary Officer in 1894. Rinderpest disease was first diagnosed in 1897, and as a result a laboratory was established at Gammams, near Windhoek, in same year. A veterinary cordon line was created and replaced by a fence to control rinderpest. The fence was used to prevent movement of animals and to keep out rinderpest infected stock. FMD was diagnosed in 1961 and the cordon fence was strengthened and the protected area enlarged with a small efficient veterinary service. A veterinary association was created in 1947 and in 1984 legislation was introduced which established the Veterinary Council of Namibia. The country became independent in 1990.

GOLD COAST (GHANA)

Originally mostly Kingdom of Ashanti, Britain acquired control in late 19th century. Ghana's first veterinary officer was appointed in 1909, and determined the main disease issues to be CBPP, rinderpest, epizootic lymphangitis, equine trypanosomiasis, anthrax and internal parasites. Principle problem was bovine trypanosomiasis with transmission by the tsetse fly as well as *Stomoxys*, *Hippobosca* and other flies. The haemoprotozoan parasite Piroplasmosis was widespread mainly in cattle but also some other animals. In 1929 there was a major programme to vaccinate livestock against rinderpest and CBPP, but trypanosomiasis remained a major issue. Local dwarf N'Dama trypanotolerant cattle were well domesticated. Ghana became independent in 1957.

NIGERIA

Nigeria as a territory was occupied by Britain in the late 19th century, with its current borders being established in 1914. Before the introduction of rinderpest in about 1866 there were few major disease issues present in the country, except for trypanosomiasis. The trypanotolerant humped, dwarfed cattle were bred and in tsetse-free areas cattle flourished. Nigeria's Veterinary Department was created in 1914, and at the time was mostly occupied with attempts to control rinderpest. A veterinary laboratory was established in 1925 and a programme of sero-virus vaccination commenced, with the disease finally being brought under control by 1950. The CBPP nasal tissue implantation immunisation procedure was in use up to the 1960s. Vaccination 'camps' were held to vaccinate against rinderpest, CBPP, blackquarter and in some regions, anthrax. Outbreaks of HS were seen, as well as nutritional deficiencies in most livestock, poultry infected with Newcastle disease (ND), fowl cholera and pox, and canine rabies. Equine diseases diagnosed included: trypanosomiasis, AHS and epizootic lymphangitis. Parasitism was diagnosed across all species. The important hides industry had to cope with streptothricosis, demodectic mange and goat pox, as well as anthrax. Vaccines and diagnostic procedures developed at Vom by the Veterinary Department enabled satisfactory control of most livestock diseases but trypanosomiasis remains a problem.

Veterinary education began in 1930 with the Kano school, in north Nigeria, producing Assistant Veterinary Officers; this was moved to Vom and by 1957 students also sent to Britain. Relationships with neighbouring French territories were good, and resulted in the formation of the 1948 West African Institute of Trypanosomiasis which was a joint Franco-British venture. Nigeria became independent in 1960.

NORTH RHODESIA (ZAMBIA)

In 1888 the territory of Zambia was occupied by the British South Africa Company and became a British Protectorate in 1911. Located in central Africa it remained relatively undeveloped, apart from some mining activity. A Veterinary Department was created which surveyed the livestock. Initial diseases recognised included trypanosomiasis, tick infestation, CBPP and ECF, but rinderpest was not seen. The major problem was trypanosomiasis with heavy tsetse infestation. Blackquarter, anthrax and rabies were all subject to vaccination control schemes. Later lumpy skin disease, babesiosis and gall sickness were found in cattle, the main livestock species in Zambia. Independent in 1964.

NYASALAND (MALAWI)

Malawi came under British control in 1891, with the first Veterinary Officer being appointed in 1910. From 1910 there was a slow process of recognising and diagnosing the diseases. Trypanosomiasis in cattle and game animals was the main problem with other diseases recognised including piroplasmosis in cattle and dogs, glanders, AHS, fowl cholera and ECF. Later this disease list included rabies, FMD, AFS, lumpy skin disease, blackquarter and clostridial infections in sheep. Neither rinderpest nor anthrax was found. The main control programmes established were directed toward tick-borne diseases. By 1964 trypanosomiasis was under broad control. Malawi became independent in 1964.

SIERRA LEONE

Became a British Crown Colony in 1808. Initially the veterinary services were shared with Gambia. A survey conducted in 1942 showed that CBPP was widespread. A vaccine was introduced and the disease finally brought under control in 1958. There is no known history of rinderpest before 1949, but this disease was also eventually brought under control by vaccination. Rabies was endemic, and frequent outbreaks were seen of anthrax and blackquarter in cattle, along with trypanosomiasis in pigs. ND in poultry was controlled through a vaccination programme. Sierra Leone became independent in 1961.

SOMALIA

Somalia is a country created from the previous colonies of Italy and Britain. The camel is the most important animal. A study conducted in 1924 revealed severe trypanosomiasis and scab in camels, as well as trypanosomiasis, severe rinderpest, CBPP and anthrax in cattle. A further study conducted in 1925 revealed cases of

AHS, FMD, ECF, gallsickness, heartwater in cattle; biliary fever of horses; tetanus, blackquarter, pleuro-pneumonia of goats; HS, strangles and cutaneous habrone-miasis in horses; sheep scab and internal parasites. A difficult country due to the topography, climate and building a relationship with the nomadic population. By the time of Somali's independence in 1960, a measure of control had been achieved over sheep scab, along with rinderpest and CBPP in cattle.

SOUTHERN RHODESIA (ZIMBABWE)

Zimbabwe was incorporated into the British Empire in 1888. Their veterinary services department reported a rinderpest outbreak in 1896 and the disease was eradicated by 1899. Legislation to control CBPP and gallsickness was introduced in 1891. Problems with babesiosis, glanders (including farcy) and AHS identified, followed by recognition of trypanosomiasis. Vaccines were introduced to control glanders, CBPP and rabies, with topical treatment for sheep scab and dipping used for ECF. The role of tick-borne diseases and incidence of brucellosis in cattle were studied with the aim of introducing control measures based on the findings. Zimbabwe was declared free of rinderpest and CBPP in 1933. ECF continued to be a problem in livestock until it was eradicated in 1954. FMD first occurred in 1931, but remains a problem to this day. Tick-borne diseases such as babesiosis, gallsickness and heartwater all still cause issues for livestock farmers. At the time of independence in 1980, the major disease was trypanosomiasis found in cattle and some equines. Soon after independence a veterinary school was established at Harare and produced good graduates, but is now closed due to economic problems. For further information, the books *History of Zimbabwe Veterinary Service Parts 1 and 2* provide excellent coverage (Busayi 2006, Part 1 pp. 45–22 and Part 2 76–84).

SUDAN

In 1868 Sudan was occupied by an Anglo-Egyptian condominium with governance by Britain. A rinderpest epizootic began in 1896 and was still widespread in 1905, when vaccination programmes began. The British Army created the Sudan Veterinary Department in 1910 and began disease control, prioritising rinderpest, CBPP, trypanosomiasis, piroplasmosis, epizootic lymphangitis and AHS. Rinderpest, CBPP and camel trypanosomiasis remained serious problems, with a major rinderpest outbreak occurring in 1930. A difficult country in which to maintain satisfactory control measures. The Khartoum Veterinary School opened in 1937, and by 1950 it had become a Faculty of Khartoum University. In 1954 the Veterinary Council Bill gave statutory recognition to veterinarians. Sudan became independent in 1956.

SWAZILAND

Under British control from 1903 when veterinary work began: survey discovered ECF, rickettsiosis, FMD, sheep scab, rabies, tick-borne diseases (anaplasmosis, piroplasmosis) and later besnoitiosis (globidiosis) and lumpy skin disease. Control measures were established with dipping programmes to control tickborne infections and vaccines being used mainly for rabies but also some for clostridial diseases in cattle and sheep. Independent in 1968.

TANGANYIKA (TANZANIA)

Tanzania was originally a German colony in 1884, until its occupation by the British in 1918. A study conducted in 1909 indicated that the major diseases present were rinderpest, ECF, ovine pleuro-pneumonia and trypanosomiasis in cattle and horses. Following 1918 rinderpest and trypanosomiasis were widespread; but eventually rinderpest was brought under control through vaccination. Anaplasmosis, babesiosis and trypanosomiasis were the major issues but CBPP, ECF, anthrax, rabies, FMD, blackwater, brucellosis, ASF, epizootic lymphangitis, cutaneous streptothricosis, tuberculosis and gut helminths were also identified as problems. Tanzania's independence in 1961 was followed by unification with Zanzibar, the island veterinary issues then were cattle trypanosomiasis and ECF.

UGANDA

In 1894 Uganda came under British control. In 1909 veterinary measures were introduced to campaign against rinderpest and CBPP. Other diseases recognised included anthrax, tuberculosis, blackquarter, FMD and rabies together with the major issues of trypanosomiasis and tick-borne parasites, ECF, babesiosis, piroplasmosis, gallsickness, anaplasmosis – mainly in cattle but rabies, however, was a problem in dogs. Uganda became independent in 1962.

References

Busayi, R.M. (2006) History of Veterinary Services in Zimbabwe: Part 1. *Historia Medicinae Veterinariae* **31** No.2

Busayi, R.M. (2006) History of Veterinary Services in Zimbabwe: Part 2. *Historia Medicinae Veterinariae* **31** No.3

Chavhunduka, D.M. (1976) Plants Regarded by Africans as Being of Medicinal Value to Animals *Rhodesian Veterinary Journal* **7–8**

Chyzyaka, H.G.B (1991) The History of Trypanosomiasis in Zambia. *Historia Medicinae Veterinariae* **16** No.3 and **16** No.4

South African Veterinary Medicine History (2011) Abstracts of Papers read at the 30th World Veterinary Congress. Cape Town: South African Veterinary Medical Association

West, G.P. (1961 and 1973) *A History of the Overseas Veterinary Services: Part 1* and *Part 2*. London: British Veterinary Association

PART II

Europe Develops Veterinary Medicine

CHAPTER 12

The Middle Ages and Renaissance

The Middle or Medieval Ages were the years following the collapse of the Roman Empire (AD 476) followed by the onslaught of Islamism at its southern borders. European culture disintegrated and gradually evolved to a structure that produced the Renaissance, and the age of discovery.

The once dominant Roman culture decayed slowly. The loss created a governance vacuum with barbarian invasions and a struggle to create new fiefdoms. The Carolingian Empire was formed in the mid-8th century AD, and in AD 800 Charlemagne was crowned as emperor of the Holy Roman Empire. It has been said that this was neither holy, Roman, nor an empire, but it enabled the single most significant feature of the early Middle Ages – the establishment of a Christian Church that claimed with its spiritual power to inherit the role of Rome. This provided the one unifying factor for European people, who followed a powerful neoplatonic Christian belief developed by St. Augustine. The Church preached that this was the final age of the world, which would climax with the last judgement: a belief which lasted up to the 14th century.

There were many significant events, resulting from the conflict and violence that pervaded these centuries – the expansion of Islam, the Norman invasion of England and then Sicily and Italy, the Crusades, the slow reconquest of Spain and Portugal, the rise of the Baltic Teutonic Knights, the 100 Years War, the Black Death and the Gutenberg printing press with the first books in 1454. This achievement lit a light that opened the way for the Renaissance (Le Goff 1988).

Agriculture and Animals

Agriculture was the basis of medieval life. Over most of Europe there were agricultural settlements, in England these were known as 'manors' or 'estates'. These settlements included villages with a group of dwellings, each in a cultivated area comprising three or four large fields subdivided into parcels of land. Every villager with his oxen and plough had his share of the land spread among the fields, with one field being left fallow each year and used for grazing, as were the surrounding waste lands. Each settlement was under the control and ownership of a feudal lord, with his share of land – he ruled the community with most of the villagers his bond-men.

These settlements were part of a network including small towns with markets and fairs for trading in grain, wool and hides. The manors were, in a way, the living cells which formed the body politic (Given-Wilson 1996, p. 11).

Oxen were the work animals used for ploughing and transport. Cattle numbers increased gradually for beef, to satisfy a growing demand from a developing middle-class of traders. Sheep were particularly important where grassland was on well-draining soils. Pigs were not intensely farmed and mainly herded in woodland for pannage. Horses were mostly kept by the noble classes for combat; their use for transport only grew as roads improved. Wool production was the most important livestock product, Britain led in this field because it had the right grasslands and sheep breeds, Spain came second as they had merino sheep and a traditional farming method which produced high quality wool.

By the start of 14th century the feudal farming system had improved and was producing surpluses of agricultural produce. The demand for markets increased, towns grew and cities formed to become the birthplace of the Renaissance.

Medicine

Medieval medicine was based in Galenism and correcting the balance of the four humours to restore health. The initial patient examination was sensible but diagnostic, and treatment procedures were seldom logical. The diagnostic methods included examination of urine and taking the pulse to determine the internal factors, along with the use of astrology to determine the external factors. Treatment was based on diet with herbal simples and compounds for purgatives, laxatives and so on. Treatment also regularly included clysters (enemas) and bloodletting. However, medical care was restricted to the upper classes of society. The majority of people resorted to folklore medications and practices, both influenced by magic. At the same time, the Church was becoming more powerful and enhancing its own place in a society frequently ravaged by disease epizootics. Neither physicians nor healers were any help, but the Church offered sympathy, aid in infirmaries attached to some monasteries, and the hope of divine intervention by prayer. The congregations grew.

One factor that certainly influenced developed medicine was the Black Death plague epizootic (caused by the bacteria *Yersinia pestis*), which killed a third to a half of the European population, peaking between 1347 and 1351. Not only was it the most catastrophic disaster in Europe's history, but the plague also remained endemic for three centuries. This epizootic had important effects: the balance of power between the manorial Lords and peasants was altered; the ranks of clergy were decimated and religious belief declined as people no longer had confidence in the divine power of prayer (Gottfried 1983, pp. 1–40 and pp. 104–139).

Doctors, using the classically based medical corpus were perceived to be of little value. The Church was unable to control the desire for medical knowledge and in the late 14th century the first medical school started in Salerno, Italy with medical and surgical ideas from Islamic scholars in Sicily. Post-plague medicine changed and, by 1400, texts were being written in vernacular languages rather than Latin. Medical ethical codes evolved and the professions took shape, led by the physicians (Nicolle 2000, pp. 96–100). In the early 16th century medicine required a complex range of skills and knowledge; later in the century developments were led by Paracelsus and Vesalius, to influence both human and veterinary medicine.

Animal Disease

Historical records show evidence that from around AD 570 an increasing number of epizootic diseases ravaged European livestock. Some came in repetitive waves, but others lingered in certain regions. From the symptoms and signs described it would appear that rinderpest, foot-and-mouth disease (FMD), anthrax and a range of pox infections were all encountered, together with botulism, ergotism and many alimentary disorders. The effects on the cattle population were catastrophic. Some twelve epizootics have been estimated, of which six only affected cattle, two only affected horses and four affected both animals and humans. Earthquakes, floods, drought, comets and evil spirits were all blamed.

Specifically sheep diseases were recognised, due to the economic value of wool: scab, 'red death', pox, 'rotte' (liver fluke), 'husk' (lungworm), the 'pelles', worms and footrot. For all animals, the common epizootic disease name was 'murrain'. Pigs were relatively disease free (apart from epizootics) as they lived free range. Equine problems most frequently mentioned relate to hoof and limb lameness, colic, wounds and sores. Medication and treatment was mostly folklore, magic and hope for divine intervention. There was little concept of contagion, hygiene or the isolation of sick animals. Spaying of gilts and sows and the castration of piglets were all practised, frequently by a travelling gelder (Trow-Smith 1957, p. 252).

Veterinary Medicine Stagnates

As Roman influence declined, the lack of contact between regions meant that the exchange and use of knowledge also vanished. Rational and often logical treatments that had been evolved by the Romans were discarded in favour of superstition and magic. Veterinary practice seems to have been mostly concerned with the foot – for horses in particular and also for cattle. There was gradual development of the Roman *hipposandal* and *solea*, aided by a need in the Crusades (from 1095); by the 13th century the conventional iron shoe was widely manufactured. A similar demi *solea* was developed for cattle.

The medieval mind believed that plagues were sent as punishment for the sins of humans. The consequence of this belief was that no investigations of the actual causes of these plagues were made. The influence of the Church was pronounced: the lamp oil from Christian sanctuaries was valued as medication for topical application and for sprinkling on pastures as a cure and a preventive. Another sure preventive method to purify stock was to heat the Church key red hot and brand the animal's forehead. Religious belief became intertwined with sorcery – one mandatory procedure used to protect cattle was to take a knife with a cow's horn handle and trace the mark of Christ on the forehead and legs and then, in silence, pierce the left ear of the animal. Some of these procedures bear a resemblance to early logical Roman procedures, but this could be coincidental.

Huzard (see Introduction) noted several early Medieval manuscripts that mentioned veterinary matters. Within the Saxon communities scholarship began to develop and England exported information to the Franks and Germans. Animal diseases are specified in the English and Welsh Laws of the 8th and 9th centuries. Three manuscripts survive from this Anglo-Saxon period, the most important being the *Leech Book*, possibly written in the 10th century. The first owner was named Bald and the scribe Cild. It was written on parchment in Anglo-Saxon for medical readers. The first part deals with external diseases and injuries, the second with internal ailments and the third is described as 'monkish in character'. There are three veterinary references, all are a mixture of common sense and superstition – 'Leechdom for swelled legs in a horse, and if a horse be galled, and if a horse or other neat cattle be elf-shot'.

The treatments are mainly herbal but 'elf-shot' (thought to be acute tympanites), which the Church taught was attributable to an elf or demon, required a man to say twelve masses and put holy water on the animal.

The next manuscript is the *Herbarium*, dating is possibly 4th or 5th century but the authorship is questionable. The stated author is Apuleius Platonicus, but is possible that the actual author was Antonius Musa. The manuscript was copied from a Latin text written between AD 1000 and 1066. The first part is comprised of Anglo-Saxon observations on medicinal plants, described as 'worts': 185 plants are described together with the diseases each is prescribed to cure and every plant is depicted with a well-drawn, coloured illustration. There is only one veterinary reference – 'centimorbia' – which is a treatment for sore backs and open wounds. Frequent mentions of snake bite and mad dogs indicate problems, or fears, of the time. Part of the book is a translation of the Dioscorides *Materia Medica*.

The third text, accompanying the *Herbarium*, is titled *The Medicine of Quadrupeds* and is attributed to Sextus Placitus, a 4th century Roman physician. While of interest as an Anglo-Saxon document, it is also a collection of trivia from many sources from Pliny onwards and of which all are essentially based in folklore, superstition or magic. The Anglo-Saxon years were ones including beliefs and great use of charms, amulets and prayers for divine intervention. The three texts indicate the level to which veterinary knowledge had fallen, and the superstitions that existed were abetted by the Church (Smith 1976, pp. 62–71).

13th Century: The Veterinary Art Awakens

The renascence of veterinary medicine began in Sicily and Southern Italy. Frederick II of Sicily (r.1212–1250), of German origin, was interested in zoology and birds, and worked to build a culture of knowledge (Nicolle 2000, p. 100). He established the Universities of Padua and Naples and helped the emerging Medical School at

Salerno. While starting in a monastery dispensary it was not a Church institution, but did have contacts with the Monte Cassino monastery, which contained both a hospital and a famous collection of medical manuscripts, many of which discussed anatomy. The Salerno Medical School is considered to be the earliest European higher education establishment and accepted both male and female students. Anatomy was an important subject but, because human dissection was banned by papal edict, was conducted on the pig: this formed the basis of *Anatomia Porci* a text by Copho – a very early veterinary book. Frederick decreed in 1221 that no one should practise medicine until they were approved by the Masters of Salerno.

Through his animal interests Frederick began to investigate the veterinary art and sought information from Spanish Islamic scholars (although banned by the Church). He then instructed Jordanus Ruffus to translate the Arabic equine texts to Latin. These were not original, but mainly derived from Byzantine Greek sources.

Jordanus Ruffus was born in Calabria, Italy possibly at the end of the 12th century. He was employed by Frederick II as veterinarian to his court, and from contemporary documents was obviously Frederick's close adviser. Sicily at that time had a significant Arab population which must have aided his translation of the Byzantine manuscripts. He would presumably have known of the *Hippiatrica* but does not appear to have used it as his source. Ruffus, his background, and the history of his approximately 35 manuscripts has been extensively investigated. Most of his manuscripts are written in Latin and Italian and mainly held in Italy and Paris. The first printed edition of his work on equine medicine was published in Venice in 1492 titled *Hippiatria*.

Examination of this text shows that Ruffus was the first to use a definite system of nomenclature for horse diseases (many of the disease names are still in use, in particular in Italian). Equine breeding, domestication, care, selection, training, shoeing, bridles and bits are all covered, followed by a listing of diseases by bodily systems. The limbs, lameness, limb and foot ailments are well discussed but much less on alimentary disorders. While the work does not equal the Byzantine texts, he was an originator in this field and added his own observations. His book was widely read in Italy and neighbouring countries. He enabled the regeneration of the veterinary art in Europe.

Albertus Magnus, also known as Albert the Great (c.1200–1280), was a Catholic theologian, philosopher and prolific author on scientific topics, in particular zoology. He provided the link between the Aristotle writings on the natural history of animals and modern zoology. His writings are divided into 36 volumes, of which one is titled *De Animalibus* and deals with quadrupeds and birds; the first printed edition was from Rome in 1478. Albert discusses animal diseases and lists 25 equine ailments, as well as including a treatise on diseases of birds (mainly falcons and hawks). He studied infection and had quite advanced ideas on contagion and methods of spread. He considered inhalation and physical contact to be the most dangerous, but he also believed in the 'ill effect of moonlight on wounds'.

Other 13th century authors on veterinary topics, but without original observations, included Misser Boniface who wrote *Merescalaria of the Horse* which illustrated the parts of the body related to the zodiac signs. Jacob of Doria described a cure for farcy – a celebration of the Mass and the consecration of three Hallelujahs. Bishop

Theodore of Lucca wrote on medicine and surgery of horses and falcons. Petrus of Crescentius wrote on agriculture and discussed livestock diseases. Walter of Henley wrote his *Husbandry*, an excellent book on livestock management and husbandry and mentions a 'murrain' of sheep. Two other similar husbandry books were the *Seneschaucie* (Farm Steward) and the *Rules of Robert Grosseteste*. An interesting contribution was *The Properties of Things* by Bartholomew Glanville a Franciscan Friar, which includes a most accurate description of the signs and behaviour shown in a rabid dog. He could possibly be the first British veterinary writer. All these works have been described in detail in *The Early History of Veterinary Literature, Vol I (From the Earliest Period to AD 1700)* (Smith 1976, pp. 85–92).

As the Iberian Peninsula moved back into Christian kingdoms, veterinary manuscripts began to appear. Two are known to exist but some of their details are unknown: *The Six Books of the Veterinary Art* by an anonymous author, held in Madrid and *The Veterinary Art* by Mestre Giraldo, written in Portuguese.

14th Century: Veterinary Knowledge Is Recognised

An Italian man by the name of Laurence Rusius, is recognised as the only veterinary author of significance in the 14th century. Little is known of Rusius' early years, but he came to Rome to study equine diseases probably about fifty or sixty years later than Jordanus Ruffus, whose work he used in his own writings of a 181 chapter book. He wrote from a practical knowledge of the horse, advocating care in treatment and surgery and the use of medications for specific activities, rejecting empirical pharmacy. Rusius became widely known and respected, with his work being used in many compilations and by equine establishments. Many of his manuscripts exist in different languages with amendments and additions by later scribes. The first printed edition, titled *The Book of Marescalia* (farriery) possibly appeared in 1485, but a 1490 edition is better known; both bear the same title. A 1531 Latin edition, published in Paris, was titled *Hippiatria Sive Marescalia*: the contents listing follows that of Ruffus. In this book Rusius adds his own observations including the use of leeches to reduce inflammation and noting the transmission of farcy from horse to human – both first records. But he also believed in astrology and used the zodiac constellations to guide his prognoses. Rusius complemented the leadership shown by Ruffus and was a significant influence in the regeneration of the veterinary art.

There were other men who wrote on veterinary matters, these were mainly Italian, and some French; it showed that there was a growing group of 'veterinarians', all concerned with the horse. Of these, Dino di Pietro Dini (c.1350) a member of a Florentine family of such people, named many colleagues. Also the first known German veterinary author, Andreas Albrecht (c.1355), his work was printed firstly in 1498 titled *The Little Book of the Cure of the Horse* and then under several other titles up to 1612. There was little original content included in these reprints. These men, and others, together with several unpublished manuscripts, mainly discussing equine matters have been reviewed in *The Early History of Veterinary Literature, Vol I (From the Earliest Period to AD 1700)* (Smith 1976, pp. 99–103).

Juan Alvares de Salamiella wrote a treatise in the mid-14th century titled, *Libro de Marescaleria et de Albeyteria*. This Spanish text comprised two books – *Libro de Marescaleria* and *Libro de los Caballos*. The first discusses health of the horse – oral dosing, dental work, setons, shoeing, the foot, the limbs and lameness, bleeding, castration, reducing fractures, topical blisters, nasal medication and restraint methods. The second discusses the external features and management of the horse. The books are superbly illustrated in colour, surgery and the instruments are illustrated; they present a picture of the level of veterinary practice in Spain. Following the capture of Naples by Alphonso I of Aragon the Spanish were excited by the discovery of Italian advances in equine care and added their Arabic knowledge, in particular in ophthalmology.

Gaston III, Count of Foix (1331–1391), French nobleman and huntsman wrote, between 1387–1389, a treatise titled *Livre de Chasse*. This became the standard hunting text. The text was translated to English by Edward, Duke of York in about 1413. It was titled *Master of Game* and first printed in Paris in 1500. The treatise is outstanding for the illustrations of dog care showing 'dog valets' administering treatments, washing and grooming. The first such images seen in Europe (C. d'Anthenaise 2002, p. 25).

15th Fifteenth Century: Spain Emerges With an Islamic Veterinary Art

Veterinary medicine in this century made slow progress with little advances. Italy remained the centre of activity with clear evidence that there was an increasing number of men who could be termed veterinarians. Many of them were employed or sponsored by Kings or Nobles who had interest in developing studies. The knowledge that they worked with was still that derived from Ruffus and Rusius, which was essentially that of Byzantium. However, individual observations were being made and recorded. France, Germany and England were well behind Italy in understanding the issues, but in the growing kingdoms of northern Spain progress was seen.

Piero Andrea, Master of Horse to King Alphonso of Spain, wrote a *Treatise on the Veterinary Art*. The content is unoriginal, but the author disputes the belief in the harmful effects of moon rays and his text is free of superstition.

Manuel Diaz, Majordomo at the court of King Alphonso V of Aragon (1416–1458), at the instruction of the King in 1443 wrote *Libro de Albeyteria por lo noble Mossen Manuel Diaz* (*The Book of the Veterinary Art*). The book was first printed in Castile in 1495 and reprinted in later editions. The work was mainly based on the Ruffus translation of the Arabic Codex and the *Marescalia* of Rusius. This was also produced at the time of the establishment of the Spanish Riding School and the discipline of horse training and management. It was an important period in Spain which laid the basis for their veterinary profession. The men were termed 'albeytor' from the Arabic 'al-Baitor' or 'albeitar' meaning a healer of horses: the veterinary tradition derived from the Moors.

Another important text is the *Boke of Seynt Albans* (*Book of Saint Albans*) written in 1496. The text's authorship is uncertain, although it is credited to Juliana Berners who was born about 1388. The content covers hawking, hunting and fishing; mainly focussed on hunting with dogs and falcons, and their care. It is not a veterinary text but diseases and injuries are mentioned, as are the 'properties of good horses and grey-hounds'. It contains little original material but the book is among the first in English to mention these subjects.

There was little other activity in European veterinary medicine in the century. Smith (1976, pp. 107–116) reviewed a series of manuscripts held in the British library concerned with equine and animal health. They are anonymous 'mostly with appalling remedies, drivel and prayer'. England was hundreds of years behind Italy in the development of veterinary knowledge, Smith commented, 'One would have thought that Jordanus Ruffus had never lived'.

One very significant occurrence of the fifteenth century was the commencement of printing in Gutenberg in 1440 (and introduction in England 20 years later), this heralded the end of veterinary ignorance and opened the way to knowledge and understanding and learning. Italy adopted this new technology at once. Of the 10,000 books and pamphlets printed on all subjects (but mainly theological) in Europe before the end of the century, half were produced in Italy, Paris produced 750 and England only 140, but the Middle Ages were ending.

16th Century: Veterinary Medicine Texts In Print

This century is distinguished in European culture as being the early formative years of what was to be known as the Age of Enlightenment. In the 1500s the stimulus for change was the realisation of the importance of the printed word. Scholars of all disciplines worked to develop their literary skills – at last their work could be published and disseminated to a wide audience. Knowledge was sought and eagerly read.

For veterinary medicine there were many who needed help and advice but few who were able to provide it. Of the writers on veterinary topics, at least fifty are recognised from their surviving books; few, however, were veterinarians, many were simply compilers of previous texts and several were plagiarists. There are a few names that have to be remembered. Two of particular importance are Carlo Ruini, an Italian lawyer whose anatomical work was a masterpiece, and Thomas Blundeville, an English country squire and scholar, who produced the first printed veterinary book in English which dealt with the subject in a rational and scientific manner.

The century was also notable for the first printed availability of the veterinary books of *Vegetius* and of the *Hippiatrica*: both eagerly read for their 1000-year-old knowledge. At the same time Leonardo da Vinci was producing unique anatomical drawings, including animals, aiding an understand of anatomy and bodily formation. The century also produced several royal sponsors of veterinary studies, in Spain these produced an early flowering of the art.

The following review of the veterinary literature of the century identifies the names of those contributors who were able to offer the reader some benefit or interest. They are listed chronologically; there were many others and most are discussed in greater detail by Smith (1976, pp. 123–221).

Agostino Columbre dedicated *The Nature of the Horse and the Method of Curing its Diseases* to King Ferdinand of Aragon. It was published in 1518 in Venice and the author may have been Italian. The work is of interest because attention is given to equine anatomy, the influence of Galen is obvious and the early literature is well reviewed. He was possibly a physician, he also believed in astrology and similar doctrines, as was the common practice. Later editions of this text were published up to 1622.

Franciso de La Reyna was Spanish and the author of *The Book of Veterinary* which was first published in Alcala in 1522. The content includes the selection of horses, shoeing and diseases. There is little original content included in the text, but de La Reyna demonstrated that he had examined the circulation of the blood (some commentators felt that he foreshadowed William Harvey).

Sir Anthony Fitzherbert the English author of *The Boke of Husbandrie*, which is believed to have a publication date about 1523. It is an agricultural text but the diseases of sheep, cattle, and horses are all discussed with many of them named. Sheep were recognised as 'the most profitabilest cattle that any man can have'. Fitzherbert identifies 'scab' and the use of the tar box salve; describes the 'rot' and its relationship to white snails and recommends the castration of calves 'when the moon was on the wane'. He also names and describes many diseases including cattle 'murrain' (possibly rinderpest or anthrax), 'morefounde' (laminitis) and 'mourning of the chyne', which is stated to be incurable. The derivation of this strange term seems to be from the French *mort du chain*, the death of the chain, (spinal cord), which was corrupted into English as a diagnosis of (possibly) glanders. He does not suggest treatments as he thought this was not his occupation. While not a veterinary book it does indicate the state of knowledge in the mid-1500s, and would have provided useful advice for the livestock owner.

The decade 1528–1538 has to be remembered in the history of veterinary medicine. In 1528 the Latin work of *Vegetius* was printed in Basel, to be followed by the *Hippiatrica* in Paris in 1530 and then in 1538 the publication of the Byzantine *Geoponika*. (See Chapters 4 and 5.)

Henry Cornelius Agrippa (1486–1535), a German physician, alchemist and scholar. His book *Vanity of Arts and Sciences* c.1531, has a chapter devoted to 'The Veterinarian', praising the art and its value. He is said to have been an educational influence on Paracelsus.

Philippus Aureolus Theophrastus Bombastus von Hohenheim (1493–1541), better known as Paracelsus, was a Swiss physician, chemist and philosopher. He had a brilliant mind, renounced the ideas of Galen and the four humours, but believed in astrology and the occult. He held the Chair of Physic at Basel University and was also a traveller. His early alchemist studies as he prepared 'chemical medicines' led to serious chemistry and opened the way to pharmacology. He introduced laudanum (opium) to Europe, investigated mercury treatment for syphilis in humans, and arsenicals for glanders in horses (believing these to be the two most serious ailments). He was responsible for commencing the discipline of toxicology with his statement, 'solely the dose determines that a thing is not a poison'.

Paracelsus was eccentric in many of his views and behaviour, but is seen as a significant influence on the development of modern medicine (Webster 2008).

Of other authors Federigo Grisone (n.d.) is noteworthy as the founder of the Neapolitan School of Horsemanship and for his study of equitation and book *The Rules of Riding* 1550. This book reached fifteen editions in Italian and was translated to French, German, Spanish and English.

A Swiss man Conrad Gesner (1516–1565), was famed for his five-volume work *History of Animals* in which he discusses animal diseases. He created a bridge between natural history and zoology.

Thomas Tusser (1523–1580), an English agricultural writer in verse. His *Hundred Good Points of Husbandry* 1557 contained several items dealing with animal diseases and hygiene. The book was widely read.

An Italian man, known to Blundeville, Claudio Corte was born about 1525, studied equitation and came to England in 1565 to work for the Earl of Leicester. Corte wrote a treatise titled, *Cavallarizzo*, which was focussed on the training and management of horses. The text was widely read, and was published in Venice in 1562 and also in France and England.

John Phillip Ingrassia (1510–1580), an Italian physician who practised in Sicily. He wrote in Italian; *Veterinary Medicine* is formally one and the same with the better known human medicine, differing simply in the dignity or nobility of the subject, 1564. The book explains veterinary work, its history, relationship to human medicine and states the two vocations are united in one subject.

Thomas Blundeville (d.1605) was an English country squire. He was well educated, wrote on many subjects, and was a traveller in Europe, but little else is known of him. He wrote ten major treatises: two concerned animals, a translation of Grisone's book, retitled as *The Arte of Rydinge* 1560, followed by *The Fower Chiefyst Offices belonging to Horsmanshippe* in 1566, with further editions up to 1609. Blundeville gave credit to others, and wrote well: trying to write with accuracy and present his work in a logical manner. His work was the first of its type, but was, however, a compilation. Blundeville had little practical knowledge of the horse, unfortunately shown by his repeating of the errors of previous writers. Arranged in four sections directed at: the Breeder, dealing with selection; the Rider, covering equitation and breaking; the Keeper, concentrating on diet, hygiene and management and the Ferrer (farrier) discussing disease, for this part of the work he took information from Martin Shelley, the Queen's farrier. He had read and quotes from the ancient authors and tried to define disease and note the signs. Blundeville did understand the essential lesson that maintenance of health was the job of the keeper and that it was directly related to the prevention of disease and the work of the farrier. He advised annual bleeding to remove 'corrupt' blood after the winter, but generally gave sensible advice. Of the errors repeated, possibly the worst is where he states, 'a horse or a moyle [mule] hath no brains but in place thereof he hath, as it were, a bladder filled with wind and no brains within or other thing but like a white water'.

The book was an interesting contribution to the literature, but Blundeville was not a veterinarian.

George Turberville (?1540–1610) was an English poet and hunter, who wrote *The Noble Arte of Venerie or Hunting* 1570. This was the first English work to discuss diseases and treatments for dogs: specifically this was for hounds. A book of historical curiosity for the ancient and superstitious beliefs it contained. He did however reject 'the worm under the tongue' and its removal myth to prevent rabies, as well as the use of charms as cures. Turberville made a good attempt at describing the various forms of rabies. Spaying was obviously practised for hounds but the operation was only partially described. Wound treatment was a frequently mentioned procedure.

Leonard Mascall (n.d.), an English author who wrote in the later years of the 16th century; his six books had some 40 editions over a hundred year period. Nothing appears to be known of him or his life. He was a borrower and compiler; he copied some dreadful remedies including the Blundeville error on the brain of the horse. He did however have a great reputation, with the (untrue) claim that he was far-rier to King James I. Mascall published *The First Booke of Cattell* in 1587, *The Second Booke in treating the government of Horses, The Third Booke in treating of the Ordering of Sheepe, Goates, Hogges, and Dogs*. He had also previously published *The Husbandlye Ordering, and Government of Poultrie* 1581. His books had no merit, but did indicate the state of veterinary medicine in the 16th century.

Carlo Ruini (?1530–1598), Italian. Little is known of his life, except that he trained as a lawyer, inherited considerable wealth and lived well. He produced *Anatomia Del Cavallo, Infiermita et Suoi Rimedii* (The Anatomy of the Horse, Diseases and Treatment) in 1598, with editions up to 1618 and translations in German and French including a French version in 1647 (which used the original plates, reversed). The book was published just after his death. The work is in two parts, the first focussed on Anatomy and covers body systems, with much original content, and the second focussed on Diseases, which is mainly a reworking of the earlier Ruffus writings. Ruini had to have been influenced by the masterly human anatomy work of *Vesalius*, 50 years earlier. There is no mention of the artist who drew the plates, suggestions have been made that it was Titian, whom he could have afforded. Ruini probably made the initial drawings from which the final illustrations were made and then etched. There is little question that Ruini's book was a landmark text in the evolution of veterinary medicine: it set a standard. Not only did it spawn many followers, copyists and pla-giarists, but it opened the way to education by offering the first description of equine anatomy, the skeleton, muscles and circulatory and neural pathways, as well as show-ing the disposition of the internal organs and structures. While not totally accurate, it was used when the first veterinary school opened in Lyon, France 164 years later. A full description of the content is given by Smith (1976), who as there has never been an English translation, worked from a French translation of one in German.

By the close of the 16th century there was a growing awareness of the need to pro-gress from what was still considered the art to become a science. Ruini led the way but others also had similar ideas, including Volcher Coiter (1534–1600) who studied comparative anatomy and M. Heroard who published a partly plagiarised version of Ruini's work *Osteology of the Horse* 1599, in Paris: it contained original observa-tions. At the same time medical science was advancing in surgical techniques, led by Ambroise Paré (1516–1590) a French barber-surgeon who developed skills treating conflict injuries and gunshot wounds, also describing these in the horse. There was a path that medical and veterinary medicine was following.

17th Century: A Veterinary Knowledge Base Develops

From the 14th century Europe had experienced progressive activity in all forms of cultural, artistic, political, economic and scientific enterprise. This varied in intensity by country and interest, it was the rebirth of European culture and is known today as the Renaissance. Much was based in the rediscovery of the classical literature and manuscripts and an increase in secularism with a decline in Church influence. This was enhanced by the introduction of the printing press which allowed the democratisation of learning, and the propagation of ideas. The Renaissance began in Italy, spreading to Hungary, and France in the 1500s driven by the recovery from the Black Death. It then spread further to Spain in the Aragon Kingdom followed by the Netherlands, England by the 16th century and Germany in the later 16th century. By then all of Europe had become involved.

The medical disciplines began to build science foundations, initially in anatomy and physiology. Leonardo da Vinci aided anatomical interest with his graphic interpretations of animals. The work of Andreas Vesalius with *De humanis corporis fabrica* set the anatomical standard. The role of dissection, observations and anatomy began to explain how the body functions, to be followed by Ruini's equine anatomy. Guilio Casserio (1601) with his remarkable series of engraved plates illustrating the anatomy of the vocal and auditory organs, in the dog, cat, rabbit, pig, cattle and birds, also provided a first step in physiology. Hieronymus Fabricius (1533–1619) in his two treatises on reproduction followed on from Aristotles's original work, and William Harvey (1578–1657), one of his students, produced *Exercitatio Anatomica de Motu Cordis et Circulatione Sanguinis in Animalibus* (The Anatomical Study of the Movement of the Heart and the Circulation of the Blood in Animals) which provided a breakthrough for both medical and veterinary science, but one that was only slowly accepted. It was followed by numerous other investigations of mammalian physiology. These studies were building a knowledge base that would result in the Age of the Enlightenment in the 18th century and the start of veterinary education.

The 17th century produced many authors who wrote on veterinary matters, a few of them made original contributions to knowledge, many did not. Nine are worthy of discussion, each for a different reason.

Gervase Markham (c.1568–1637), one of the sons of an English gentleman who had lost most of his wealth. He was well-educated and a proficient linguist, and appeared to have been a prodigious worker; he wrote on almost every subject. However, hardly anything was original in any way: he was a copier and a plagiarist. Some 36 books were published under his name, some dealt with horses of which probably *Cavelarice* (1607) is thought to be his best work. *Maisterpeece* (1610) was his most well-known 'veterinary' book – he promised that all who read it would be able to perform 'invincible cures'. He was a believer in the puritanical religion of the time and so the cures that he promised were always due to the beneficence of God, (which would remove the blame from Markham if they did not work). The *Maisterpeece* went through 21 editions remaining popular for over 100 years. Smith (1976, pp. 222–284) wrote a most extensive review of all of Markham's work with a particular emphasis on his veterinary cures and observations in the *Maisterpeece*, he stated 'no work published in this country has done more damage to veterinary progress'. Not a good author to start the century with, but it illustrates the gulf between the animal owner and the few dedicated veterinary workers.

Thomas Spackman (n.d.), an English physician, wrote *A Declaration of such grievous accidents as commonly follow the biting of Mad Dogges* 1613. This is the first English text specifically dealing with rabies. It is a well-written account of hydrophobia, in particular, and rabies in the dog. While the author had many misconceptions it is a valuable description of symptoms and advice on treatment of dog bites.

John Crawshey (n.d.), an English veterinary practitioner with good powers of observation and author of *The Countryman's Instructor* 1636. He commented on some diseases, but the most interesting sections are his instructions for calving, undertaking a caesarean section on a cow, treatment of uterine prolapse, surgical removal of cysts from the brain in cattle and sheep, cryptorchid castration in rams and spaying in sheep. Remarkable procedures conducted without anaesthesia but no observation on the pain for the animal, and always the comment that the patient 'will do well God willing'.

Thomas de Gray (n.d.), English gentleman and breeder of horses, wrote *The Compleat Horseman and Expert Ferrier* 1639 in two books; one on breeding and the second on the maladies and diseases in horses which contained 'the secrets . . . [of the] . . . Horse-Leach'. In a lengthy dedication he explains that he wants to educate noblemen so that they can question the horse-leach to make sure he knows his job. The book is long-winded and includes superstitions and fallacious remedies, including one for the treatment of Wild Fire (possibly sheep pox) and based on a powder made from live toads, moles, ants, old shoe-soles, garlick, salt beef, oats, woollen rags, swallows' dung and living swallows. The book has interest but did nothing to advance veterinary medicine.

Sir Thomas Browne (1608–1682), a physician and polymath notable for his ability to devise new words as they were needed in an environment of expanding knowledge. In *Pseudodoxia Epidemica* 1646, a book devoted to removing superstition and errors, he used the word *veterinarian* for the first time. A milestone in veterinary history, the embryo profession now had a title.

William Cavendish (1592–1676), the first Duke of Newcastle, was not a veterinary man but devoted his life to equitation and the study of horsemanship. In 1658 he published his book in French (being in exile following the Civil War) and then in English in 1667: *A New Method and Extraordinary Invention to Dress Horses and Work them according to Nature*. The French book contains 43 of the most beautiful copper-plate illustrations. He discusses the European history of horsemanship and almost every aspect of management with a few observations on diseases. As a book it has to be every equinophile's greatest acquisition.

Jacques Labessie de Sollysel (1617–1680), French, studied horsemanship and in 1645 became Master of the Horse to French Ambassador in Münster, Germany. Met with local veterinary practitioners which started his interest in animal disease. Sollysel believed in study and kept up to date in physiology and chemistry developments. He was a good observer and a clear thinker, but as a man of his age his knowledge was permeated by a belief in astrology (he studied the phases of the moon for all he did) and superstitions such as the bite of the shrew-mouse.

In 1664 he published *Le Parfait Maréchal,* a book in two parts, the first dealing with care, management, shoeing, selection, breeding and bleeding. He was a master of the art, but also includes the old erroneous belief of the thickness variation of the hoof wall. The second part discusses diseases and their treatments and included many original observations: he described 'pointing' of the foot when in the stable, as a sign of lameness; recognised 'windsucking' as a vice and differentiated between 'roaring' and 'broken wind'; recognised strangles as a contagious disease; differentiated different types of colic, including volvulus; recognised different parasites. He did not mention the pulse and was cautious on the use of bleeding and purgatives. He made sensible recommendations for wound treatment and thought inflammation was a form of fermentation, but was not totally convinced. He also recommended only the simplest low-cost medications and wrote, 'despise not the herb which grows under your feet, but justly suspect all costly medicines'.

Sollysel's observations on glanders have to be the outstanding feature of his work. He identifies the features of the disease; states it is the most contagious disease of the horse; associates it with farcy; but does not mention its infectivity for humans. While he lists possible cures for the disease he also states, 'I might justly say is impossible'.

An English version was translated by Sir William Hope in 1696, titled *The Parfait Mareschal or Compleat Farrier.* It was costly, and an abridged version, *The Compleat Horseman or Perfect Farrier* appeared in 1702, it was much reduced and consisted mostly of the cures, as this was seen to be the market. Sollysel is remembered as an able, articulate, sensible and experienced veterinary observer and author who produced the best up-to-date book of its time. Many of his observations were ignored, the readers just wanted cures, they did not understand prevention. Sollysel worked with horses for 40 years, and died suddenly in 1680, aged 66. A full description of his work is found in Smith (1976, pp. 349–365).

Michael Harward (n.d.) an Englishman living in Ireland, published *The Herdsman's Mate or a Guide for Herdsmen* 1673 in Dublin. Possibly the most original veterinary work in English produced in the 17th century, little is known of the author, who states that he had had 30 years in practice. A small book, it opens with the comment that the local population, when confronted by disease in their livestock make use of 'charms, inchanted water, inchanted rings and bells' or drive their cattle miles to 'force them through a river they call a murrain ford and some lose more by badly driving'. Harward has to be remembered for his obvious surgical skills and his sensible advice to others proposing surgery, to visit a slaughterhouse first to see how the organs are placed in the abdomen. He discusses a range of diseases including canine rabies. Harward was a good clinical observer, and was interested in poisonous plants, various insects and 'worms'. The description of hydatid disease and surgical removal of the cysts through the cranium is written from experience, as is his treatment of abdominal horn wounds and hernias, including the return of the intestines. He had similar expertise with obstetric cases, describing how to tackle difficult parturition and the use of embryotomy. His methods and procedures would appear to have been developed as a result of his own studies. While much of his text is derived from others, and there are places where he follows some of the superstitions of the day including the believed shrew-mouse, his book is free of the appalling remedies and drivel in Markham's work. Unfortunately Harward had only a limited readership for such a progressive book.

Andrew Snape Jr. (1644–?), English and 'Farrier' to King Charles II. He was veterinary advisor to the King, who was keen to encourage science and medicine. The post was hereditary and had been held by his family for the previous 200 years. He was well educated and wrote that he wanted to see his vocation raised to a profession equal to human medicine. Snape recognised that to achieve this by education it was essential for people to understand anatomy, and the structure and function of the bodily organs. He has to be remembered as an original thinker. Snape's book *The Anatomy of An Horse* 1683, was the first on the subject to be written in English. It was expensively produced and with 49 copper-plates, which possibly explains why there were only two editions. It was also translated and published in France in 1733. The content was described as, 'An exact and Full Description of the Frame, Situation and Connexion of all his Parts with their Actions and Uses . . . [and] two Discourses: Of the Generation of Animals and the Motion of the Chyle and the Circulation of the Blood'.

The text is arranged in five books – *Of the Lowest Belly or Paunch; of the Middle Venter or Chest; Of the Head; Of the Muscles* and *Of the Bones* – in 237 pages of well-designed type and layout.

Snape endeavoured to not only describe the skeleton and the internal organs, but to also explain as much as he could of the current knowledge of physiology and pathology. He demonstrates his interest in the circulation of the blood, the nervous system and reproduction. He obviously read widely and quotes various Renaissance scholars in England and Europe who had conducted experiments on pancreatic function and the pituitary gland. He also describes the internal structures of the lung, kidney and spleen probably derived from the early microscopic studies of Marcello Malpighi (1628–1694). His observations on the muscles are rather brief, he admits this by explaining that it was a waste of time to translate all the names from the Latin when he was trying to educate farriers! He also does not expand knowledge on the hoof.

The one criticism that has to be made is that of the 49 plates that are used to illustrate his work, 22 are Ruini copies without acknowledgement; these plates he reversed and as a result transposed the viscera. He even copied Ruini in describing the horse's collar bones, which do not exist. Overall the work presented gives a good overview of current information and is readable; it includes a condemnation of Markham and his statement that the horse has no brain. Snape was a good clinical observer and a forward thinker. He mentions that he planned to publish a *Book of Cures*: unfortunately, it never materialised. The man and book are examined in great detail by Smith (1976, pp. 334–342).

The 17th century was when veterinary medicine began to crystallise into a definite discipline. Of the contributors Sollysel, Harward and Snape (apart from his Ruini blunder) have to be remembered. Also Sir Thomas Browne who gave the practitioners the title 'veterinarian'. For totally different reasons Markham has to be remembered, both for his dreadful book and also for the gullible readers.

Medical men were taking an increasing interest in animals: Sir John Floyer (1649–1734) an English physician, described the pathological changes in the lungs of a horse with 'broken wind'; Dr Richard Lower, (1631–1691) an Oxford physiologist described a *corpora nigra* in the horse and made studies on respiration; a paper by Sir Theodore Mayer, *An Account of the Diseases of Dogs* discusses rabies and its 'varieties'. These men all published their work in *The Philosophical Transactions* of the Royal Society, which also at the same time published a study on blood transfusion between dogs. The Age of Enlightenment had truly begun.

References

d'Anthenaise, C. (2002) *The Hunting Book of Gaston Phébus*. Texas: Hackberry Press

Given-Wilson, C. (Ed.) (1996) *An Illustrated History of Later Medieval England*. Manchester: Manchester University Press

Gottfried, R.S. (1983) *The Black Death*. London: Robert Hale

Le Goff, J. (1988) *Medieval Civilisation*. Oxford: Blackwell

Nicolle, D. (2000) *The History of Medieval Life*. London: Chancellor Press

Smith, F. (1976) *The Early History of Veterinary Literature, Vol I (From the Earliest Period to AD 1700)*. London: J.A. Allen

Trow-Smith, R. (1957) *A History of British Livestock to 1700*. London: Routledge Keegan Paul

Webster, C. (2008) *Paracelsus: Medicine, Magic and Mission at the End of Time*. New Haven, CT: Yale University Press

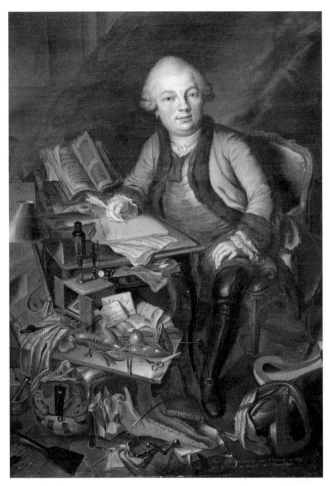

Claude Bourgelat (1712–1779). Founder of first veterinary school in 1761 in Lyon, France. In 1765 he moved to Paris region to establish and become Director of the Royal Veterinary School of Alfort. Portrait by Vincent de Montpetit (1713–1800). Image courtesy of Ecole Nationale Vétérinaire d'Alfort.

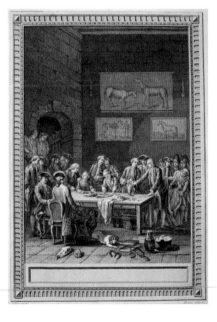

Frontispiece from *Cours d'hippiatrique, ou traite complet de la medicine des chevaux* 1772 by Philippe Etienne la Fosse (1738–1820). A two volume masterpiece with 65 engraved plates. Royal College of Veterinary Surgeons Historical Collection.

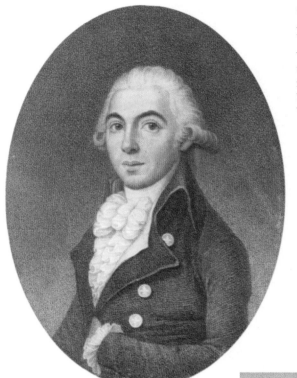

Charles Vial de Saint Bel (1750–1793). Appointed Professor of London Veterinary College in 1791, the first veterinary school in England. He unfortunately died in 1793, probably from glanders infection. Reproduced by kind permission of the Royal Veterinary College.

Engraving by Richard Lawrence, published in 1795, showing Saint Bel demonstrating to a shoeing smith in front of the London College, with 'Ignorance' in flight on the left. Reproduced by kind permission of the Royal Veterinary College.

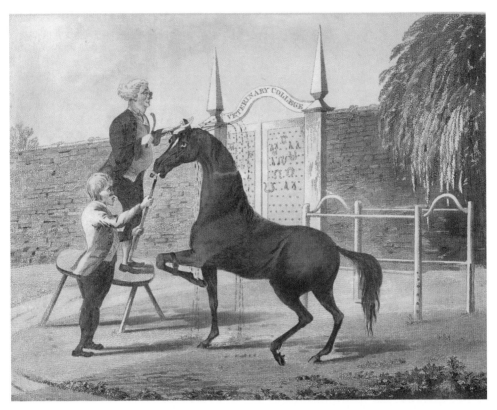

Cartoon 'Upon the improv'd mode of cropping' – one of a series published in 1792 as part of a campaign by farriers to ridicule the London Veterinary College. Reproduced by kind permission of the Royal Veterinary College.

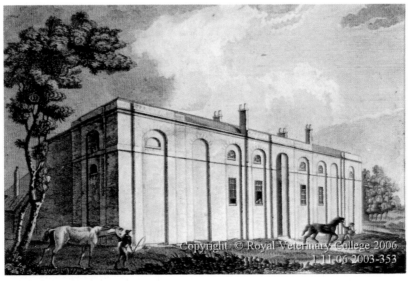

'Perspective' view of the front of the London College in about 1793. The height is greatly exaggerated in this engraving. Reproduced by kind permission of the Royal Veterinary College.

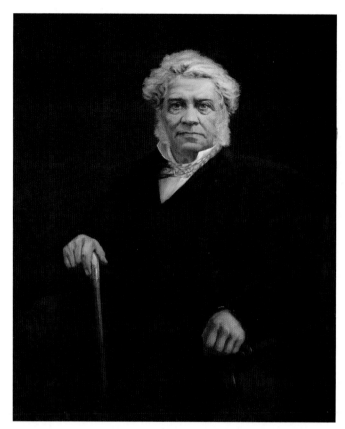

William Dick (1793–1866).
Studied at the London
College, returned to Scotland
and founded his own school
in Edinburgh in 1823. Now
known as the Royal (Dick)
Veterinary College. William
Dick by John Dunn (EU0932)
© University of Edinburgh
Art Collection.

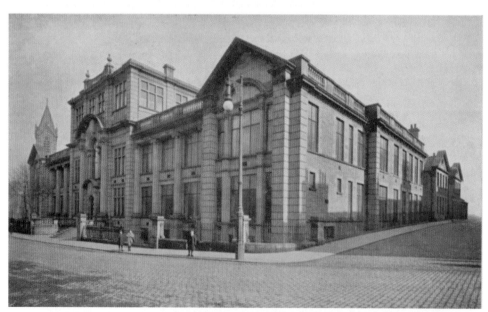

The Royal (Dick) Veterinary College building at Summerhall, Edinburgh. Incorporating part of the earlier Clyde Street building. Opened in 1917. The Veterinary School is now located at the Easter Bush Campus. Royal (Dick) Veterinary College Calendar 1916–1917 (0009663) © The University of Edinburgh.

Medicines for Horses: A Medieval Veterinary Treatise, 1468. The first page of the manuscript, discussed by G.R. Keiser (2004) *Veterinary History* **12** pp. 144–145. Veterinary Collections, Medical Sciences Library, Texas A & M University.

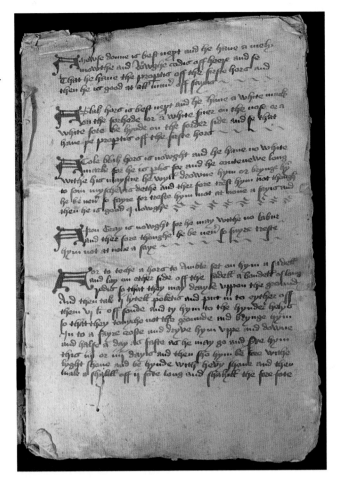

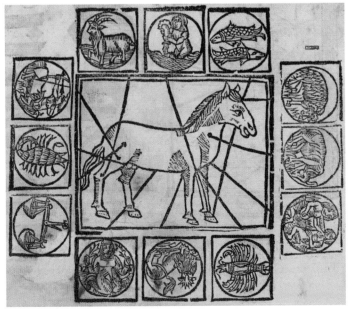

Woodcut from title page verso *Libro de Albeyteria emendado y corregido: y añadidas en el sesenta y nueve preguntas* (*Book of Veterinary Amended and Corrected*) by Manuel Diez de Calatayud, 1511, published in Toledo, Spain. One of the very earliest printed veterinary books. Veterinary Collections, Medical Sciences Library, Texas A & M University.

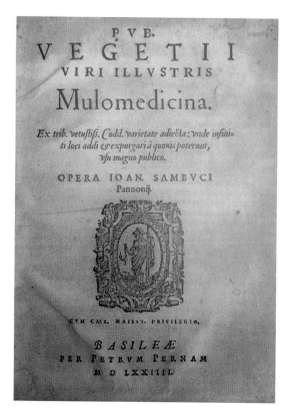

Title page of Publius Vegetius Renatus book published in Latin in Basel 1574, the usual title of *Artis Veterinariae Sive Mulomedicina* has been abbreviated to *Mulomedicina*. The diseases and treatment of mules was the main objective of the book. Reproduced by kind permission of the Royal Veterinary College.

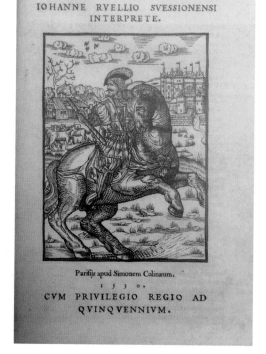

Title page of first printed edition of the *Hippiatrica* translated by Johanne Ruellius. Paris, 1530. Reproduced by kind permission of the Royal Veterinary College.

Illustration from *Gründlicher Bericht und ordennlichste Beschreibung der bewerten Rossärtzney* by Johann Fayser, 1576, Augspurg: Manger. The book deals with equine ailments and treatments. The drawing identifies the problem location and the related word either gives a name or page reference in text. Veterinary Collections, Medical Sciences Library, Texas A & M University.

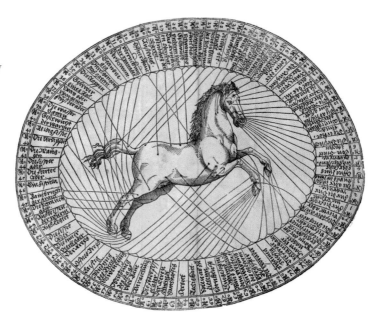

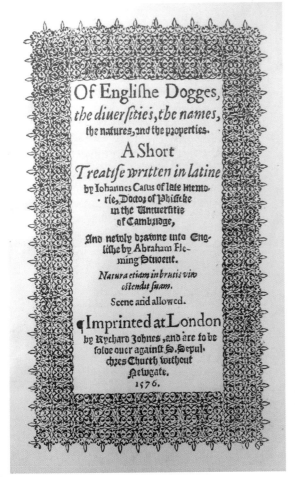

Frontispiece *Of English Dogges*, 1576, by Dr John Caius. The first book exclusively devoted to dogs in English language. Caius recognised 16 types of dogs, one the *Canis delicates* was the 'comforter' or pet. Private collection.

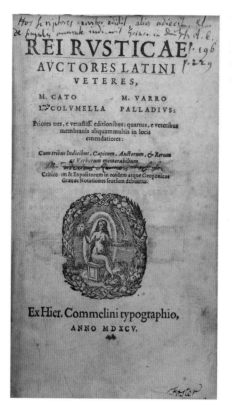

Title page *Rei Rusticae*, 1595. The complete Latin treatises of Cato, Varro, Columella and Palladius. Much read in 16th and 17th centuries for their advice on agriculture and veterinary remedies. Private collection.

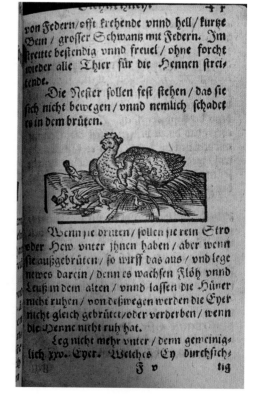

Woodcut from *Vieh artzney* (*Livestock medicine*), 1596 by Vincents Strach, published in Leipzig. A small book but details medicines 'for all ailments'. Text derived from 'Varro, Pliny, Vergilius, Palladius and others'. Veterinary Collections, Medical Sciences Library, Texas A & M University.

Title page of *Conocimiento de las diez aves menores de jaula* by Juan Bautista Jamarro, 1604, Madrid. This early Spanish book, *Knowledge of the ten smallest cage birds* describes breeding, singing and remedies for illness. The author was a Neapolitan surgeon-barber to King Philip III. Veterinary Collections, Medical Sciences Library, Texas A & M University.

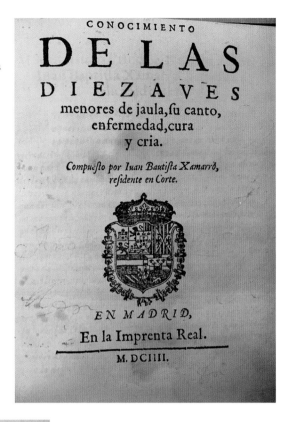

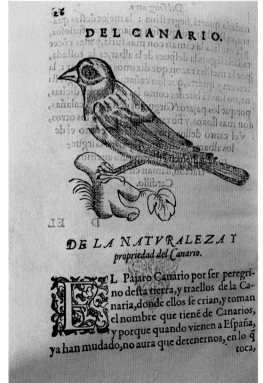

Canary image from Jamarro book. Each species was discussed and illustrated individually. The canary was probably the most popular caged bird. Veterinary Collections, Medical Sciences Library, Texas A & M University.

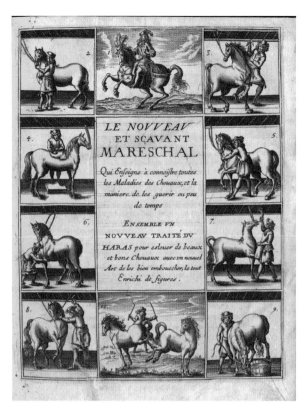

Title page of French translation of Gervase Markham's (c.1568–1637) *The New and Learned Marshal*, 1666, Paris. One of Markham's seven books on care and ailments of the horse, published after his death. Veterinary Collections, Medical Sciences Library, Texas A & M University.

Frontispiece of *The English Horseman and Complete Farrier: Directing all Gentlemen and others how to Breed, Feed, Ride and Diet all Horses, Whether for War, Race or other Service*, 1673, London. Almond stated that he was 'a well known and skilful farrier of the City of London'. Veterinary Collections, Medical Sciences Library, Texas A & M University.

Title page of English language translation of *Vegetius Renatus* treatise (translator unknown). Published in London, 1748, probably in response to rinderpest outbreak in Britain. Royal College of Veterinary Surgeons Historical Collection.

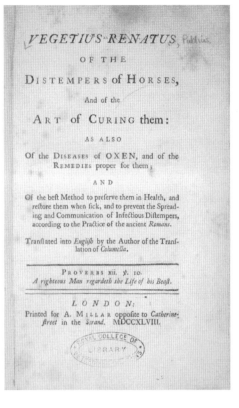

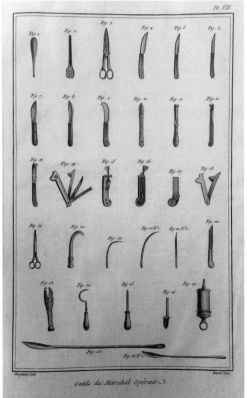

Page from the *Grande Encyclopédie* compiled by D. Diderot and J.R. D'Alembert. Printed Paris, c.1770. Showing instruments used by a *marechal ferrant* ('veterinary farrier'). Note the variety of fleams in third row. Private collection.

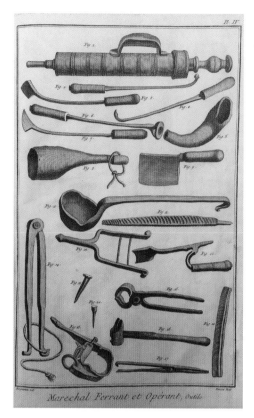

Page from the *Grande Encyclopédie* illustrating an assortment of equipment used in equine veterinary work including a clyster (enema) syringe, firing (cautery) irons, mouth gags, clamps, and mallet, axe and cautery iron used for tail docking. Private collection.

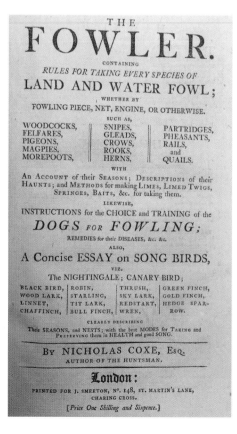

Title page of *The Fowler* (c.1794) by Nicholas Coxe (1669–1758). A superb listing of birds including cage birds and their illnesses and of the dogs used and their diseases and treatment. A scarce book due to the loss of printers stock by fire. Private collection.

Page from an undated Sanskrit Manuscript (c. late 1700s). One of 169 leaves bound wallet style in a single gathering. A total of over 400 drawings with descriptive verses covering recognition of breeds, characteristics, management and breeding, feeding and disease treatments. Veterinary Collections, Medical Sciences Library, Texas A & M University.

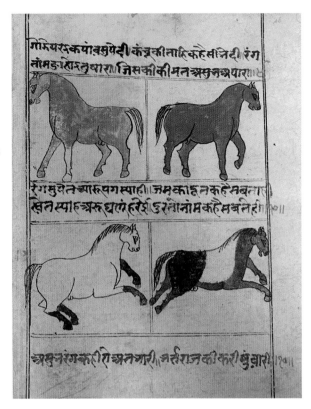

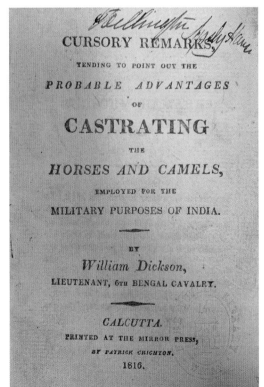

Title page of book, probably by William Dickson (1781–1828) a lieutenant in the 6th Bengal Cavalry. Printed 1816, Calcutta. A detailed, and surprisingly heartfelt treatise on the benefits to the British army in India of castration methods for horses and camels. The book seems to be unrecorded and not found in any veterinary listings. With the presumed signature of the Duke of Wellington, Apsley House. Veterinary Collections, Medical Sciences Library, Texas A & M University.

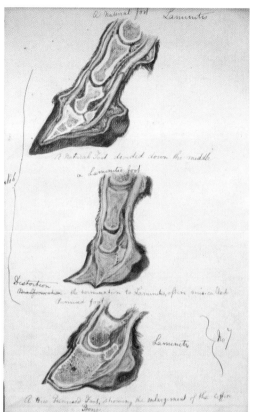

Watercolour painting by Edward Mayhew (1808–1868), English veterinary surgeon, author and talented artist. The illustration shows normal hoof and progression of the laminitis condition. Royal College of Veterinary Surgeons Historical Collection.

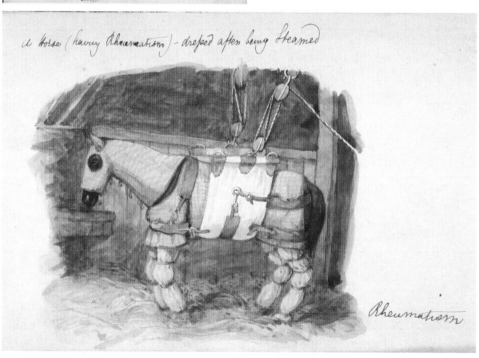

Watercolour painting by Edward Mayhew showing horse dressed after steam treatment for 'rheumatism'. Royal College of Veterinary Surgeons Collection.

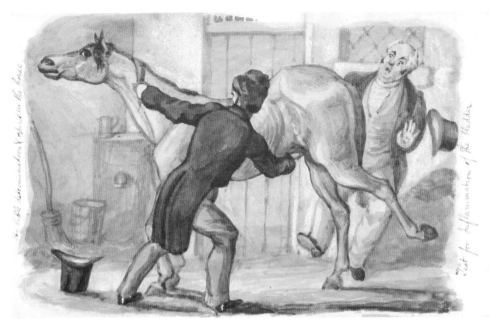

Watercolour painting by Edward Mayhew showing 'Test for inflammation of the bladder'. Royal College of Veterinary Surgeons Historical Collection.

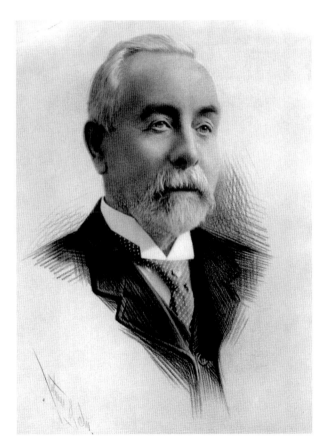

Duncan McNab McEachran (1841–1924). Edinburgh graduate and founder of Montreal Veterinary College in 1866. A pioneer in standards of veterinary education. The College closed in 1903 due to competition from low-cost private USA schools. Royal (Dick) Veterinary College Collection © The University of Edinburgh.

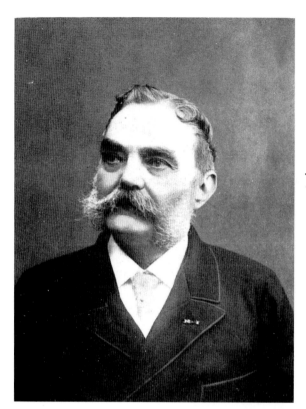

Alexandre Francis Liautard (1836–1918). A graduate of Toulouse Veterinary School, emigrated to USA in 1859 and became a major figure in the developing veterinary profession. Founder of the American Veterinary College in 1875 in New York, demanded high standards from his students. Founding Editor of *American Veterinary Review*, later renamed the *Journal of American Veterinary Medical Association*. Wikimedia.

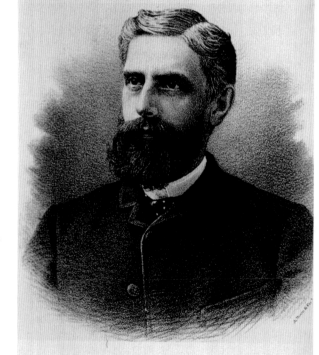

Daniel E. Salmon (1850–1914). First DVM graduate in USA, from Cornell University in 1876, taught by James Law. Organised and led the Bureau of Animal Industry, 1884–1906. The bacterial genus *Salmonella* is named after him. History of Medicine Collection, National Library of Medicine, Bethesda, MD.

CHAPTER 13

The Scientific Basis for Veterinary Medicine Evolves

The 18th century was the most important in the history of veterinary medicine. In 1791 the first European veterinary school was founded. It was a logical conclusion to the three important events of the century: the increasing development of universities; the catastrophic rinderpest plague affecting cattle, and others affecting humans, which swept the continent; the blossoming of medical research studies. These three events were a part of what is known as the Enlightenment; a movement which had grown out of the Renaissance.

The Enlightenment or Age of Reason

The movement was based in discussion groups, meetings, coffee-house gatherings, pamphlets and books. Scientific bodies were created and two of the most important were the French *Académie des Sciences* and English *Royal Society*. They were both established in the 1660s under royal patronage, but provided a base for the expression of new ideas. The activity was centred on the exploration of reason, the scientific method and reductionism. In turn, this progress in thought advanced ideas of freedom, liberty and the separation of Church and State. The movement achieved its objectives so well that it undermined the place of the Church and paved the way for the 19th century political upheavals.

One of the most important events was the publication, in France, of the *Encyclopédie* in 1751–1772 by Denis Diderot and Jean le Rond d'Alembert. This monumental work, conceived by the authors in the Parisian Café Procope, comprises 35 volumes in full folio size containing 71,000 entries. These volumes together were described as a dictionary of the sciences, arts and crafts, and provided an excellent overview of the state of available knowledge. A significant contributor to the text was Claude Bourgelat, who was to go on to become the founder of the Lyon, France veterinary school in 1791.

The Universities: The Medical Sciences Develop

The university structure had grown from the 13th century Salerno medical school which had been the first European higher education establishment. Universities can only start when economies have grown sufficiently to support and house scholars. Previously the seats of learning had been centred on cathedrals or traditional monastic schools. By the year 1200 the earliest universities were established in Bologna and Paris (essentially guilds of students regulated by masters). By the start of the 14th century there were six principal medical schools – Salerno, Montpellier, Bologna, Paris, Padua and Oxford. Bologna was a law and medical school (in 1260 Mondino de'Liuzzi, a member of the Bologna medical faculty, wrote *Anatomia* based on human dissection).

It had been realised that the grant of privileges from the Pope, or Emperor, King or commune was needed to develop a university (Mackay and Ditchburn 1998, pp. 241–243). Teachings started with separate faculties of arts and usually theology, canon law or Roman law, and medicine. Soon textbooks were written and reputations gained. By 1500 there were almost 90 universities in Europe, with the greatest concentration located in Italy, France and Spain. The Italian group of universities were particularly strong in the medical sciences while those in northern Europe tended to show more interest in theology (Macardle 2012, pp. 122–125). The Black Death plague (1347–1351) was important for medicine. The Black Death challenged medicine and the medicine profession, and the place of the physicians who never touched their patients weakened, as the second-class surgeons, whose knowledge was based on experience and who had physical contact in surgery and fracture fixation, were seen to be of increasing practical value (Gottfried 1983, pp. 106–107).

The Rinderpest Plague

Animal plagues had been a part of agricultural life for centuries. The Popes, as leaders of society through the medieval years, were of more hindrance than help in controlling the epidemics. The Church preached that the plagues were evidence of divine displeasure for the sins of the people, and so there was no effort to either understand or control disease. It was not until the cattle plague suddenly reappeared in Italy in 1709, and then in 1711, that Pope Clement XI acted and directed his court physician to investigate.

Giovanni Mario Lancisi (1656–1720) was an important medical figure in Rome. He was physician to the Pope, a professor in anatomy and Giovanni Morgagni's Master. Lancisi had a particular interest in human endemic disease and investigated animal disease. One of his equine dissertations was titled *Febris epidemica*, but he is best known for the treatise *De sede cogitantis animae* (1711), the first proper identification of rinderpest. The initial outbreak of this disease was seen in cattle owned by a bishop near Padua, who asked his friend Lancisi for help. Following Lancisi's study of these cattle he went to Padua University and talked to Professor Ramazzini who took over the work. Lancisi had examined the sick cattle and at post-mortem, described the disease, its signs and symptoms. He recommended strict quarantine measures, prescribed a rigid sanitary policy and advised that all diseased animals should be slaughtered as no medicine would help them and if left alive 'their very presence would assist in the diffusion of the contagion'. Lancisi presented his findings to the

Vatican Collegium Sacrum on 28th October 1711 and again to the Philosophical College on 9th November. The Pope then issued his *Edictum Pontificum* and ordered regulations to be brought in following Lancisi's advice, together with prayers for the forgiveness of sins. The movement of cattle was banned, dead animals were buried in quicklime unskinned, the meat trade was controlled and within nine months Rome was free of the plague, which persisted for several years elsewhere in Italy. At the same time that the Pope issued his Edict, Bernardino Ramazzini addressed the Philosophical College.

Bernardino Ramazzini (1633–1714), studied philosophy and medicine at Padua University, graduated in 1657, practised medicine in Rome then moved to Modena with a chair in theoretical medicine. He undertook a notable study on occupational diseases as well as investigating epidemic disease problems. In 1700 he accepted the chair of practical medicine in Padua. Ramazzini studied rinderpest at Lancisi's request: he confirmed his work and other research, proved transmission between animals, identified pathognomonic post-mortem findings and tried immunisation including a variolation method. Ramazzini not only demonstrated the value of diagnosis by post-mortem findings, but also proved the ineffectiveness of all 'proven' remedies including phlebotomy as a cure. He wrote his dissertation *De Contagiosa Epidemia* in 1713 (Karasszon 1988, pp. 299–300). The proceedings of the Rome meetings (1711) were sent to European medical bodies and in 1714 a meeting at the Medical Faculty in Paris agreed Ramazzini's findings and requested they be adopted in all countries. Ramazzini made a major advance in the understanding of how disease infection is spread.

Johann Kanold (1679–1729) at Halle University in Germany also emphasised the contagious nature of rinderpest and described how it spread from the Asian Steppes through Russia, Poland, Hungary, Transylvania to Italy and then across Europe. He stated the disease could not be cured and must be prevented. He also condemned magical and witchcraft remedies. He published his work in the 1721 text *Jahrehistorie von Seuchen des Viehes von 1701–1717*.

Thomas Bates (n.d.) was a Fellow of the Royal Society (FRS), surgeon to King George I, was requested in 1714 to report on a cattle disease that had appeared in London and to investigate if it was contagious. His final report appeared in *Philosophical Transcripts for 1717–1719, A Brief Account of the Contagious Disease which raged among the Milch Cows near London in the Year 1714*. Bates described the difficulty he had with both cattle owners and Cow-leeches due to their reluctance to talk, and their ignorance. Bates made post-mortem studies and showed that the disease was spread by both cattle and attendants. He recommended that entire herds be slaughtered, the owners compensated, the dead cremated, the cattle houses disinfected and left empty for at least three months, the quarantine of all new cases of the disease and the banning of secret sales. No action was taken and the disease spread rapidly. Eventually the authorities responded and having unwillingly adopted his measures, the epizootic was finally stamped out. It is not known if Bates was aware of the Lancisi dissertation, but he followed a very similar path with a clearly defined plan for control.

It was calculated that in the four years prior to Lancisi's report at least 1.5 million cattle died from rinderpest in Western Europe. Another Italian physician, Lanzoni, wrote in 1717, 'Fear took possession of the people in the provinces, lest the contagious epidemy of the year 1713 should appear in the bovine race' (Smithcors 1958).

Rinderpest did appear again in Italy in 1730 and again in 1735 – the two outbreaks lasted for nine years, only for it to be reintroduced in 1744. In Britain, rinderpest was imported in 1745 and Bates' advice was forgotten. The disease ran its course until 1756 with several hundred thousand cattle lost. It has been estimated that between 1711 and 1769 over 200 million cattle died of rinderpest in Western Europe. It was a terrible catastrophe. There would appear to have been three major panzootic episodes, which varied in duration and by region in the periods 1709–1720, 1742–1760 and 1768–1786 (Smithcors 1958, pp. 234–235).

Veterinary Medicine Begins to Develop as a Discipline

The advice given in the reports of Lancisi, Ramazzini and Bates was all forgotten and rinderpest continued to appear until stringent preventive measures were introduced. What was notable, in the absence of any veterinary leaders, was the presence of the medical men. These were the people the governments turned to, generally physicians dropped out and the surgeons took a continuing interest (Bates was a surgeon). These men also made increasingly valuable contributions to the literature. Many people were becoming authors, unfortunately many without the capacity to add to knowledge. There were several writers on rinderpest, most contributed little of any value but a few made very sensible suggestions on how the State should behave to control the disease. Those contributions of interest and value are identified below. A full review of many more contributors is available in *The Early History of Veterinary Literature*, Vol. II (Smith 1976, pp. 8–179).

William Gibson (?1680–1750) was a surgeon who served with the British Army and would have seen horses in veterinary care. He studied Sollysel and Snape and set up his own veterinary practice in central London, building a lucrative business. His early books, *The Farrier's New Guide* 1720, *The Farrier's Dispensatory* 1721 and *The True Method of Dieting Horses* 1721, were publications made before he had much practical experience: they helped to build his practice and ran into many editions. Thirty years later he wrote *A New Treatise on the Diseases of Horses* 1751, a book which displayed his skill as a clinician and observer; the book was published just after his death. It provides a good overview of veterinary medicine in the mid-18th century, but the content related to glanders and farcy, alimentary disorders and foot conditions is weak. He recommends training for farriers so that they can give reliable advice on equine ailments and management. He undertook bleeding for many conditions, but was moderate in the amount withdrawn: he believed in balancing the humours. Much of his writing is either with acknowledgement to Sollysel, or a simple condensation of his work. Gibson wrote well on diet and care of horses in travelling, and he is critical of road surfaces. His work basically was good common sense and he showed both a humane interest in animal welfare and a concern for the state of affairs with farriers' lack of knowledge. In 1759 George Washington

(1732–1799), the first President of the United States of America (USA), purchased a copy of the *Treatise* and used the medications recommended (Smithcors 1975, p. 28).

Daniel Le Clerc (n.d.), physician to King of France, published *A Natural and Medicinal History of the Worms Bred in the Bodies of Men and Other Animals*, translated to English in 1721. He recognised cattle warbles as being the parasitic form of a fly (*Hypoderma bovis*) and described parasites in sheep nostrils, probably *Oestrus ovis*.

William Burdon (n.d.), Cavalry Captain, published *The Gentleman's Pocket Farrier* in 1730. He urged that the study of animal diseases and their treatment is the province of educated men not ignorant farriers who pass on their 'secrets' to their apprentices. He stated that these men were not only illiterate but some were 'totally incapable of improvement'. Burden displays a good empathy and compassion for animal patients. He describes some of the 'surgical' methods used by farriers in treatment – disastrous interventions and cruel methods. He preached much common sense and expressed a humane approach to veterinary medicine. His book appeared in several editions published up to 1806.

Stephen Hales (1677–1761) FRS, was a curate and scientific explorer in physiology, chemistry, botany, hygiene and an inventor. He published *Statistical Essays Containing Haemostatics . . . Experiments Made on the Blood and Blood Vessels of Animals*, 1733. He was the first to study experimentally 'the force of the blood' and experimented on the arteries of dogs, horses and sheep. In the equine work he inserted a brass tube into a femoral artery connected to a 9 ft glass tube and saw the blood rise to 8 ft 3 in, and rise and fall with the heartbeat. He made other experiments on the heart rate and pulse: he calculated the pressure exerted by the left ventricle. Hales' record of studies in a wide range of subjects was quite remarkable.

Hermann Boerhaave (1668–1738), a medical teacher at Leyden University in the Netherlands, studied both rinderpest and rabies. He taught 'bed-side' thinking to his students and instructed them to look at animal diseases. Several of his students were to be influential in veterinary activities.

Henry Bracken (1687–1764) studied medicine in London, Paris and Leyden, where he was a student of Boerhaave. He returned to England and went into practice as both a surgeon and a physician. He was elected local Mayor but appears to have had a difficult personality – he denigrated physicians, surgeons, apothecaries, medical quacks and double-dealing horse-traders. Yet he also wrote of how to 'prepare' a horse for sale to hide any deficiencies. As a veterinary author his experience appears to be based on the information he obtained in his own horse-dealing, racing and the members of that fraternity. He did recognise the ignorance of most of these people and tried to expose their lack of knowledge. His books came to be well read. Although he was regarded as an authority, he was a compiler and a plagiarist. Bracken wrote five veterinary and three medical works. His most widely read books were *Farriery Improved* 1737, twelve editions; *The Traveller's Pocket Farrier* 1742, six editions and *Farriery Improved* Vol II, 1743, six editions.

An Essay on Comparative Anatomy, written by an unknown author, was published in 1744. This book contains lecture notes from the Professor Alexander Monro classes at Edinburgh University. These notes describe the anatomical variations between different species: the dog, cow, birds and fish are all discussed, and compared to man. The work is based on original dissections. A full description of this unique treatise is given by Smith (1976, pp. 4–7).

An Essay concerning Pestilential Contagion occasioned by the Distemper now raging among the Cattle was published in 1747. The unknown English writer was a country physician, he does not discuss rinderpest as a disease but examines its consequences, the poor response by government and advises that a Board of Health be appointed to control the outbreak and draft controls and regulations. In 1748 he expanded on his initial thoughts and demonstrated that he understood how rinderpest could be controlled: a practical approach that was urgently needed when the great British cattle plague epizootic arrived in 1865.

The English translation of the book *On the Distempers of Horses*, written by Vegetius Renatus some 1300 years previously, was published in London in 1748. The English translator felt that the book could be of value in helping to understand and control the 'murrain' (cattle plague) that was sweeping the country. This text was discussed previously (see Chapter 4).

Jeremiah Bridges (n.d.) was an Englishman who published a book with the (abridged) title *No Foot, no Horse, an Essay on the Anatomy of the Foot* in 1751. Bridges described himself as 'Farrier and Anatomist'. An unusual pairing of interests, but also that of Andrew Snape (see Chapter 12) whom he acknowledges. There is no information on his life except that he gave a course of lectures, and from the knowledge presented he had worked in practice in London. The purpose of the book was to investigate the anatomy of the horse's foot and is notable because it is a competent description and published a year before the well-quoted work of La Fosse. He explains the role of the laminae in weight support, and of the lateral cartilages in allowing elasticity. Bridges' book also includes a section on diseases and treatment. While this work is very similar to that of other writers, Bridges does deplore the extensive bleeding and purging of sick animals and advises that good nursing care and welfare must take the place of too liberal use of medicines. At the same time he promotes the use of his own medicine range, but not their ingredients. He also unfortunately, recommends that those that are administered orally should be used in a draught made from 'fresh wholesome human urine'.

J. Bartlet (n.d.) was an English surgeon who dabbled in veterinary work. His first book *Gentlemen's Farriery* 1753 was a compilation of work from previous authors – Gibson, Bracken, La Fosse, Sollysel and Burdon. Bartlet had little equine experience but refers to human ailments. Of the several surgeon authors on equine disease he shows himself to be the least competent. He does however provide a comprehensive coverage of the veterinary environment and does make some useful proposals to raise the quality and expertise of the farriers who practise the art. His second book *Pharmacopaeia Hippiatrica* 1764 (later retitled *Pharmacopaeia Bartleiana*) is essentially a repeat of his first work with the inclusion of a greater surgical content. He discusses the use of the cautery, by then largely removed from human practice, and also topical caustics, but adds no useful comment. Frederick Smith, in a lengthy examination of the books adds a summary, 'Bartlet, in other words, was a fraud' (Smith 1976, pp. 69–77).

William Gibson (n.d.), son of the William Gibson, published *Mr Gibson's Short Practical Method of Cure for Horses* 1755. This is a digest of his father's *Treatise* in the popular pocket size edition with little original content included.

Count de Buffon, George-Louis Leclerc (1707–1788) was an accomplished French naturalist and encyclopaedist whose works influenced later naturalists and evolutionists, in particular Jean-Baptiste Lamarck. Between 1749–1788 Count de Buffon published 36 volumes of *Histoire naturelle, général et particulière*: a notable link in the chain of studies starting with Aristotle, Alean, Magnus and Gesner that have led to the discipline of zoology. He had several collaborators including Daubenton (see Chapter 19). The chapters on domestic animals were translated to English in 1762. While Count de Buffon was not always accurate in his descriptions, his work advanced both anatomy and physiological studies. He does not discuss veterinary medicine but regrets that animals have 'been left to the care and blind practice of men destitute both of skill and literature'.

E.G. La Fosse (senior) (n.d.), farrier to the King of France, published his notable research work in 1754. This work was translated to English in 1755 and titled *Observations and Discoveries Made Upon Horses, With a New Method of Shoeing*. It can be described as the first attempt at recording veterinary scientific experimental work. The subjects included: The Anatomy of the Equine Foot; Observations on Foot Lameness, incorrectly diagnosed; Further Observations on the Treatment of Glanders; On a Method of Controlling Haemorrhage from Large Arteries, and On a New Method of Shoeing Horses. The translator is unknown but it has been suggested that it was Dr James Parsons FRS who had previously communicated with La Fosse and was anxious to see veterinary medicine taken from 'the most illiterate empirics' and placed into the hands of gentlemen (Smith 1976, p. 79). The most interesting and remarkable work reported was on the control of haemorrhage from large arteries. This was based on the use of the powder from the puff-ball fungus *Lycoperdon*. La Fosse applied the powder as a cone-shaped plug and found that within minutes bleeding was controlled, and this remained in place during healing. His experiments are described following amputation of limbs. It appears that this discovery was never adopted in either veterinary or human surgery. Other studies concern shoeing and, in particular, the bad habit of farriers in paring the sole and frog in the hoof, as well as listing a number of bad, cruel or ineffective practices employed by farriers.

William Osmer (n.d.) was a surgeon who practised in London as a veterinarian. He had a surgeon brother who worked with him and shared his interest in using rational medical treatments. He would appear to have been self-taught, but well read, in particular studying the works of La Fosse. His first book, with the abbreviated title *A Dissertation on Horses* . . . 1756 is difficult to understand. He obviously knew thoroughbred horses and tries to discuss their breeding, with his interest in the racetrack seemingly his incentive. In 1759 he published *A Treatise on the Diseases and Lameness of Horses*, with later editions published up to 1830. Again the main interest is thoroughbred horses and he is much concerned with body shape and form. The text covers shoeing and lameness, wounds and diseases: the latter topics are poorly discussed, with most information derived from other earlier authors, in particular La Fosse. On lameness he showed originality, otherwise his works added little original thought.

Daniel Peter Layard (n.d.) FRS, was an English doctor who published in 1757 *An Essay on the Nature, Cause and Cure of the Contagious Distemper among the Horned Cattle in these Kingdoms*. He wrote a well-constructed treatise on bovine anatomy and physiology, describing his dissections and post-mortem studies and reviewing the past literature. He believed, like Ramazzini, that rinderpest was a similar disease to human smallpox and investigated preventive measures. In a 1758 address to The Royal Society he provided evidence that there was no case of a cow contracting the disease twice, but was unable to prove that any preventive treatment had been effective. He argued that as long as cattle or their hides were imported to Britain the country would be open to disease.

John Wood (n.d.) is an English author of whom little is known, although he claimed that he had been groom to the King of Sardinia and others. His books contained nothing new and included much discredited old remedies. Wood is of interest because, along with five London farriers, he issued a public circular in 1758 proposing a hospital for horses. It does not appear to have been successful, but was the first public statement made in Britain addressing the need for such a facility.

Thomas Wallis (n.d.) was a surgeon who published *The Farrier and Horseman's Dictionary* 1759. This book was a compilation text which provided an overview of British veterinary practice in the mid-18th century, but Wallis had no practical experience to contribute.

Earl of Pembroke, Henry Herbert (1734–1794) was a significant man in the training, management and care of cavalry horses; he fought against the habit of tail docking. He wrote two books on military equitation and is listed here because during continental travels he established a friendship with Claude Bourgelat (the founder of the first veterinary school), referring to him as 'my ingenious friend'. This relationship might have included Bourgelat suggesting the opening of a veterinary school in Britain (Smith 1976, p. 99).

Daniel Peter Layard was previously noted for his observations on cattle plague in Britain. He published *An Essay on the Bite of a Mad Dog* in 1762. While this essay was written on the assumption that the outbreak described in London was rabies, it was almost certainly canine distemper. Layard had his own doubts and considered that it could have been related to human fevers. This could be the first description of the disease in Britain.

George Stubbs (1724–1806), an English artist and anatomist, particularly of the horse. In describing his equine work he stated that it was planned to be of use to veterinarians, comparative anatomists, horse owners and horse breeders. When he drew and painted his horse anatomy he knew that a veterinary school had opened in France. His anatomical study took 18 months of dissection and drawing – conducted in an isolated country farmhouse, no doubt due to the odour from his specimens. It took six or seven years to engrave the plates and 150 copies were published by subscription. The book was titled *The Anatomy of the Horse, Including a Particular Description of the Bones, Cartilages, Muscles, Fascias, Ligaments, Nerves, Arteries, Veins and Glands* 1766 and was reprinted in 1853. The 18 plates are remarkable for their clarity and accuracy but difficult to interpret as Stubbs used his own system of numbering rather than names. It is a perfectly executed work of superb draughtsmanship, while of little practical veterinary value, it did increase awareness of anatomy and its understanding as a basis for veterinary knowledge. Later in his life Stubbs commenced on a similar study of comparative anatomy using the human, tiger and fowl as his examples. The work was not completed.

James Clark (n.d.) worked in veterinary practice in Edinburgh but little else is known of his life. Described as farrier to the King of Scotland, he was well-educated, wrote well and tackled the problems that were impeding veterinary medicine. He read widely and was self-taught using the early veterinary texts, as well as texts on agriculture and the rapidly developing discoveries in medicine and physiology. Clark recognised the work of Bracken and Osmer but was determined to create his own medical philosophy and to do this from his own experience, studies and reasoning. Smith, in a detailed analysis of Clark's books, suggests that his anatomical knowledge was weak, but by undertaking post-mortem examinations his diagnosis was more precise (Smith 1976, pp. 112–113). Much of Clark's importance was due to his rejection of the current practices of indiscriminate bleeding, medicating healthy animals and always looking for a 'cure'. Clark stated that the practitioner 'must first investigate the cause, the nature and various symptoms . . .'; he also disputed any belief in the 'humours' and emphasised the place of gentleness and kindness in all procedures, as well as discussing the place of nursing of the patient.

Clark wrote three books. In *Observations Upon the Shoeing of Horses With an Anatomical Description of the Bones of the Foot of the Horse* 1770, he is highly critical of the then cruel manner of shoeing horses, and acknowledges the prior work of La Fosse and Osmer, but omits that of Bridges. He challenges both the current type of shoe and barbaric method of shoeing. The second book, *A Treatise on the Prevention of Diseases Incidental to Horses From Bad Management in Regard to Stables, Food, Water, Air, Exercise . . .* 1788, is outstanding. It introduces the concept of veterinary hygiene: fresh air in stables, cleanliness, balanced food and pure water. Smith described the book as 'a revelation'. It was published in Philadelphia in 1791 but not widely read in either the United Kingdom (UK) or the USA, and took many years to be fully recognised (Smithcors 1958, p. 284). The third book, *First Lines of Veterinary Physiology and Pathology* 1806 is totally different, as it was written as a textbook for a proposed veterinary school in Edinburgh, Clark adopts the title Veterinary Professor. The book is well presented for students as 'a necessary preliminary to the study of veterinary medicine'. A full review of each book is available in *The Early History of Veterinary Literature*, Vol. II (Smith 1976, pp. 114–130).

Clark has to be remembered as one of the most important men in the history of English language veterinary medicine. Early in his life he saw the need for veterinary schools to train young men, with the need for Professors of Anatomy, Materia Medica and The Practice of Physic. Clark also saw the need for state sponsorship and was a corresponding member of the Odiham Agricultural Society before Vial Sainbel made his second visit to Britain. After the London school was opened in 1791 Clark requested one for Scotland and said one had been approved, which was why he did not accept the invitation in 1793 to take the post of Professor at the London College following the death of Sainbel. He missed a great opportunity and the young College failed to get the leadership that it so urgently required.

James Blunt (n.d.), an English surgeon, wrote *Practical Farriery, or the Complete Dictionary of Whatever Relates to the Food, Management and Cure of Diseases Incident to Horses* 1773 (in different editions he is named Blount). Like Wallis, Blunt was not in veterinary practice, he simply compiled the work of others. It contains nothing new and much that is useless.

Francis Clater (1756–1823), English, wrote two books, *Every Man his own Farrier* and *Every Man his own Cattle Doctor*. He worked as a farrier in a country town and published the first book in 1783 aged 26, based on training by his uncle, a farrier, from whom he learned 'all the secrets of his profession'. In 1810 he published *Every Man His Own Cattle Doctor*. It is unclear if Clater had any actual clinical practice, he did however have a chemist and druggist business and lists some 140 formulations – his books, in particular the cattle one, were his advertising media. There is nothing original in the books. They were compiled from several sources, and contain much misleading content (some of which was corrected in later editions). The *Farrier* book had 20 editions published up to 1810 when the agreement with his publisher ended, with four more published before his death in 1823. Later ones were revised by Youatt and Spooner in 1836 and 1848 with a reasonable content. The *Cattle Doctor* had five editions published before 1823 and also in 1832, 1848 and 1870, again all revised by competent authors. Clater was listed in *The Dictionary of National Biography*, his books were published in the USA and the final editions published in 1919. No new knowledge was contributed, the books were mainly a collection of cures, but their publishing record was remarkable.

William Taplin (c.1740–1807), an English surgeon with interests in horse racing and hunting. His surgical career was short-lived and by 1770 he was developing an interest in horses and dogs (treating a case of canine distemper in 1781) and by 1789 appears to have moved his practice to animals. In 1788 he published *The Gentleman's Stable Directory* which ran to 15 British editions and at least three in the USA. His book was an advertisement for what he described as 'Genuine Horse Medicines' and in the text as 'reliable remedies'. These provided his main income, each bottle and pack sealed with a label bearing his signature; he established agencies throughout the British Isles. Taplin moved to London and built his 'Equine Receptacle' a prestigious building on Edgeware Road illustrated in one of his books. At this time, Taplin described himself as an Equine Physician, and his Receptacle, planned for sick and lame horses, also acted as a shoeing forge, stables for horses at livery and for sale on commission, and a place for horses to have a course of medication or bleeding. He also soon added a Dispensary for the sale of his 'Genuine Horse Medicines'.

In 1796 Taplin published *A Compendium of Practical and Experimental Farriery*. This was primarily an advertisement for his London premises and his medicines; it was based on the previous book, but reduced in content and size. In 1803 he published the *Sporting Directory* and the *Sportsman's Cabinet*, he had previously published *Observations on the Present State of the Game in England* 1777. There is a little mention of distemper in dogs in the text but otherwise they had no veterinary content. Taplin had strong ties to both the racetrack and hunting. He was a good writer and knew horses, the racetrack, hunts and hounds but his veterinary authorship only presents the views of others, seldom with any attribution. Other writers published very critical comments on Taplin, both on his veterinary competence and also on his character as a person (he could be a 'most vituperative writer') (Smith 1976, pp. 162–163). Taplin made no contribution to veterinary medicine but used it to provide a lucrative income and his books were widely read. One message that he did convey through his work was humanity and care in both handling and nursing sick animals.

Thomas Prosser (n.d.) was a British physician who also acted as a veterinary practitioner and who, in 1791, published *A Treatise on the Strangles and Fevers of Horses*. He reviews the writings of Bartlet, Bracken, Merrick and Taplin on strangles and disagrees with them. The book is rambling and does not provide any addition to veterinary knowledge.

Edward Snape (c.1728–1813) was 'Farrier to King George III' and the Life Guards, a London veterinary practitioner and claimed to be a descendent of Andrew Snape (see Chapter 12). He was described as 'ignorant and illiterate', he advertised himself at every opportunity and like Taplin sold his own prepared medicines. Snape did have a wish to progress veterinary medicine and issued a plan in 1766 for the establishment of a Hippiatric Infirmary, which followed on from John Wood's 1758 failed proposal for an equine hospital. His plan was to include a school to instruct students on the work of 'the profession'. He raised funds and opened the school in Knightsbridge, London in 1778. Shortly afterwards it closed due to lack of support. While Snape did little to contribute or progress veterinary knowledge, he did open the first veterinary school in Britain, thirteen years before the London School with Sainbel. Snape published *A Practical Treatise on Farriery* 1791. The content was deplorable – he had a remedy for glanders and a list of outmoded, many barbaric and illogical treatments, frequently to be given in a urine draught, a favourite liquid. He also recommends that the floor of stabling should slope towards the front of the standing so that the feet are bathed in urine. Snape added nothing to veterinary progress.

The 18th century was important. The medical profession had begun to appreciate that veterinary and human practice were in fact two clinical endpoints for one discipline. There were eight recognised medically qualified individuals who also entered the British veterinary world. They were mainly surgeons; human practice was still at the stage where physicians would only rarely, if at all, touch a patient – let alone a sick animal. Surgeons were hands-on people, and regarded as being of a lower order. Of our group Gibson, Osmer and Taplin all built lucrative veterinary practices, Bartlet and Bracken were in medical practice and dabbled in veterinary work. Blunt and Wallis remained in medical practice and compiled veterinary books. Prosser, a physician, of lesser importance wrote one, unreliable book. Out of the group of men discussed in this chapter, Gibson was the most competent practitioner, and wrote well. We know of these men because of their books, but there must have been many more who had ideas, or interests in animal disease.

The Enlightenment Enables Veterinary Education

The period known as the Enlightenment, came to its fruition in the 18th century. This was a time when many people investigated a diversity of sciences, many directly related to medicine – human and veterinary – and many more in the basic sciences which provided an understanding of so many factors that advanced medicine. It is tempting to use words like 'genius' and 'polymath' to describe the scientists as the intellectual environment of the time was outstanding. We have already noted the remarkable cleric Stephen Hales (1677–1761) and his measurements of blood pressure in animals, and Hermann Boerhaave (1688–1738), a leader in medical education at Leyden who encouraged his students to also investigate animal disease. One of these students was Albrecht von Haller (1707–1777), a Swiss man, who went on to become Professor of Medicine at Göttingen and lead the way in physiological studies. Another was Gerard von Swieten (1700–1772) who, with Boerhaave's help, was employed by Empress Marie-Theresa of Austria and became the president of the Vienna Medical Faculty and imperial physician. Under Swieten's guidance the Vienna medical school became one of Europe's leaders. He heard of the first veterinary school in Lyon in 1792 and considered starting one in Vienna but first instructed Paul Adami (1789–1772) to investigate animal diseases as rinderpest was a major problem in central Europe. Adami saw that the Lyon graduates were unable to halt the rinderpest plague in France, Denmark and Netherlands. He realised that this was not the time for lectures but his time was better spent collecting specimens and case histories, describing the epizootics, devising a control programme and starting veterinary education. Adami became a full professor of medicine in Vienna and was, after a political upheaval, in 1795 appointed Professor of Veterinary Medicine at Krakow (Poland). Not speaking Polish he lectured in Latin from 1804 and taught epizootiology, therapeutics and physiology. Adami's Polish assistant, A.A. Rudnicki, who acted as translator of his lectures in 1808 became the first Polish professor of veterinary medicine. Adami had been the first professor of veterinary medicine in Vienna and an initiator of veterinary education in Hungary. Krakow was ceded to the Warsaw Grand Duchy in 1809 and Adami retired to Vienna. Veterinary medicine had become important in Europe. There were many wars, horses were needed and needed veterinary care, and rinderpest was still uncontrolled.

The art of alchemy was giving way to the science of chemistry. Joseph Priestley (1733–1804) in England studied the air and isolated a pure form that he called 'dephlogisticated', noting that it supported respiration in animals. Antoine Lavoisier (1743–1794) in France, known as the founder of modern chemistry, studied both air and fire. He named Priestley's pure air 'oxygen' and with further study with hydrogen developed the concepts of combustion and respiration. Lavoisier also drew up a listing of 33 elements and evolved a system of chemical nomenclature. He had corrected an error in G.E. Stal's (1660–1734) original phlogiston theory, which was however the first to bring a system into chemistry (Karasszon 1988, pp. 296–297). Lavoisier had proved that the living organism utilised oxygen, from the air, to enable its vital processes. Regrettably, Lavoisier died at the guillotine following the Revolution in France. There was a rapid expansion of research in Germany in particular, much of it based in physiology following the teachings of Johannes Mueller (1801–1858), a gifted but enigmatic man who educated many eminent scientists including Henle, Helmholtz, Schwann and Virchow. Physiology also grew in a chemical direction to metabolic studies, led by Justus von Liebig (1803–1873), recognised as the founder of organic chemistry and biochemistry.

Biological studies advanced, particularly in Italy, with Giovanni Battista Morgagni (1729–1799), Professor of Anatomy at Padua University, seen as the father of the scientific discipline of pathological anatomy. Lazzaro Spallanzani (1729–1799) also at Padua University conducted experiments that rejected the theory of spontaneous generation, explored the activity of the gastric juices, and successfully fertilised fish, frog and silkworm eggs. In 1780, using artificial insemination, he impregnated a bitch with dog semen resulting in healthy puppies. On hearing of this work Empress Maria-Theresa doubled his salary and gave him long-term leave. Luigi Galvani (1737–1789) at Pavia University demonstrated that electricity was generated in the living animal. The activity was named 'galvanism' and aroused a great interest in human and animal electrical activity, which eventually proved to be of little value. Galvani also wrote on communicable diseases between animals and humans.

These individuals and their activities were just a few of the many breaking new ground in different areas of science. With a pattern of constant animal epizootics in Europe, in particular rinderpest in cattle, there was a growing recognition of a separate medical discipline – veterinary science. This required education to train the practitioners. In 1761 Claude Bourgelat obtained the licence to open the first veterinary school at Lyon, France. A veterinary profession was about to be born.

References

Gottfried, R. (1983) *The Black Death*. London: Robert Hale

Karasszon, D. (1988) *A Concise History of Veterinary Medicine*. Budapest: Akadémiai Kiadó

Macardle, M. (2012) *Timeline History of the Middle Ages*. Cambridge: Worthy Press

MacKay, A. and Ditchburn, D. (1998) *Atlas of Medieval Europe*. New York: Routledge

Smith, F. (1976) *The Early History of Veterinary Literature*, Vol. II. London: J A Allen

Smithcors, F. (1958) *Evolution of the Veterinary Art*. London: Balliere, Tindall & Cox

Smithcors, F. (1975) *The Veterinarian in America 1625–1975*. Santa Barbara, CA: American Veterinary Publications

CHAPTER 14

Veterinary Schools in France, Europe, then Britain

The start of medical education in Europe can be traced back to the first medieval period school at Salerno, Italy. By the 18th century there were many well established schools in universities across the continent, and as medical science advanced both physicians and surgeons became involved in trying to understand the problems presented by animal disease. In some countries there were individuals suggesting or starting veterinary schools but lacking expertise, financial support and patronage. Influential figures in this movement were the masters of riding schools and teachers of equitation, such as William Cavendish, the Duke of Newcastle (1592–1676) in England; Jacques Labessie de Solleysel (1617–1680) in France and George Simon Winter (c.1634–?) in Germany.

The establishment of a system of education brings about the beneficial processes of learning and teaching, but most importantly enables the creation of a discipline. It then becomes possible to craft a way of studying that particular discipline: the scientific method. Claude Bourgelat, a French citizen, had an educational idea and influential contacts. He became the enabler and catalyst for the initiation of the veterinary education process and the establishment of the veterinary profession.

The Lyon Veterinary School and Claude Bourgelat

Claude Bourgelat (1712–1779), scion of a wealthy noble Lyon family, received a classical Jesuit education. For a while he practised Law, but to pursue his profound interest and love of the horse, he joined the army. He became recognised by King Louis XV and Emperor Frederick the Great as an outstanding horseman. In 1740 Bourgelat was both appointed a royal equerry and became Director of the Lyon *l'Academie d'Equitation*. At the Academy young men were educated; taught the arts of equitation and swordsmanship; received tuition in music and manners.

This was Bourgelat's most productive period. He studied the works of the acknowledged masters of horsemanship: the Duke of Newcastle and Marechal Jacques Labessie de Sollysel, which led to the publication, in 1744, of his work, *Nouveau Newcastle: ou Traité de Cavalerie (A New Treatise on Horsemanship)*. With the aid of local surgeons he studied equine anatomy, physiology and pathology and published his three-volume *Elémens d'Hippiatrique* in 1750–1753, on the anatomy and form of the horse. For this he earned the distinction of *Correspondent de l'Academie de Science de Paris* in 1752 and membership to the Berlin Academy in 1763. In the following years he published six other equine/veterinary books and continued to study the principles of medicine.

Bourgelat's reputation grew, his position at the Academy together with his family background enabled him to form a large circle of friends. Of these the most influential was Henri Léonard Bertin, at first Commissioner of Lyon, but then promoted to Paris becoming Lieutenant of Police and later Comptroller General of Finance for Louis XV. Whether Bourgelat knew it at the time or not, Bertin's move to Paris (as ever the centre of influence in France) was to prove to be the key to his advancement. Bourgelat began to broaden his horizons, he mixed with the leading thinkers of France, corresponding with Voltaire and with Jean-Baptiste d'Alembert, the mathematician and co-editor of the great 28-volume *Encylopédie* with Denis Diderot. This particular piece of work is famous for portraying the ideas of the Enlightenment. Bourgelat wrote many articles for the work, he was moving towards the concept of veterinary education. In his *Elémens d'Hippiatrique* he wrote that without schools it would be difficult to acquire veterinary skills, but did not appear willing to risk any of his own money on starting a school. He must have discussed this with Bertin, now in Paris, who was instrumental in Bourgelat being appointed to oversee the Royal studs and equine breeding establishments in the Lyon area. The Court, with some 5000 horses and a magnificent new military school built near Paris in the mid-1700s, would have had an increased interest in improving equine medical care. In 1760 Bourgelat had an additional advance by being installed as Inspector of the Lyon Library.

There was increasing concern in Court circles about the losses in French livestock. In the 1710–1714 rinderpest outbreak, an estimated half of the cattle population died, followed by another outbreak in 1750, together with pleuro-pneumonia and anthrax in cattle, other epizootics in sheep and horses and the ever present challenge of rabies. Bertin had a major interest and concern for agriculture and promoted the need to control these problems. He proposed to the king that a school be established in Lyon to teach the veterinary art and that Bourgelat should be the director. As a result, on 4th August 1761, the Council of State issued a decree authorising Bourgelat to establish the school to 'teach the knowledge and treatment of the diseases of all domestic animals'. While the school was a private institution, retaining control of all fees collected, the Council awarded a grant of 50,000 livres, payable over six years.

Both Bourgelat and Bertin had what they wanted, while Bourgelat's focus had always been on the horse, he followed Bertin's broader interests. A prospectus circulated throughout the French Provinces in later 1761 to promote the new school, it carried the Royal insignia at the top and was titled *Art Vétérinaire ou Médicine des Animaux*. The opening lines stated that agriculture was a major concern of the government and expressed the opinion that teaching the veterinary art will help the situation.

In January 1762 *L'Ecole Veterinaire de Lyon* opened, the premises were a disused tavern with minimal facilities; in February six students were admitted, all of whom had to present a certificate of baptism. The entry requirements included the ability to read and write, but the many diverse French dialects created difficulties for some students. Bourgelat was a hard taskmaster; students were expected to work, behave, help with cleaning, and work in the forge and herbarium garden. They also had to write out Bourgelat's lectures and then learn them verbatim. Later he published these as textbooks to supplement the practical classes in dissection, botany, medicine preparation and caring for hospitalised animals. The number of students had risen to 38 by the end of the year. Bourgelat as Director appointed professors of anatomy and surgery, materia medica, skin conditions, as well as a forge master.

Bourgelat was not a natural teacher and was not well grounded in the sciences, but he was a good organiser and was determined to give his pupils both a scientific and well balanced education; he came into his own in creating a course for the new discipline. The course was well structured and covered the main subjects in line with current knowledge and thought: the main subject animal however was the horse; cattle knowledge was weak. Later, midwifery, human fracture and wound treatment, eye disease and certification of death was introduced: it was thought that the new *vétérinaires* could supplement medical services in country areas. This diluted the basic syllabus, was not widely accepted and was dropped after a few years.

The success of the school was recognised in 1764 when it was granted royal patronage, ensuring its finances and status. The first page of the new prospectus now carried a much larger royal insignia and was titled *ACADÉMIE Du ROI pour l'éducation des Gentilshommes tenue par M. Bourgelat* followed by his titles and details of the fees. Fortuitously the rinderpest epizootic died down, this reflected well on the new school, enhancing its reputation in France and elsewhere. Bourgelat then lobbied Bertin to move the school to the Paris region where, ever ambitious, he would be nearer the corridors of power. Bertin, who was still concerned with the poor state of health of the country's cattle and sheep agreed, but suggested it would be better to start a second school to train more graduates. The new school was established at Charenton in 1765, Bourgelat relocated to take charge, placing M. Flandrin in charge at Lyon. Soon he was able to move the embryo school to a large property nearby – the Chateau d'Alfort – naming it the Royal Veterinary School of Alfort.

Bertin had satisfied both his own vision and Bourgelat's aspirations. The King was delighted by the new school and took great pleasure in showing it to visitors. Bourgelat was given the post of Director and Inspector-General 'of all veterinary schools to be established in the Kingdom' (Bertin had hopes of several provincial schools, concentrating on livestock diseases), as well as Commissioner General of all breeding studs in France. He remained in these positions until his death 14 years later in 1779.

The move to Paris brought Bourgelat into close contact with his most serious rival, Philippe-Étienne Lafosse (1738–1820) the son of a distinguished father, E.G. Lafosse, Marshal of the King's equerries. Philippe-Étienne Lafosse was deeply upset because Bourgelat had moved on to his territory. He felt that he should have been the Director of the Alfort School: he had his own well-formed views on veterinary education. Lafosse was well-educated, had trained as a Marshal, produced work on anthrax, written a dissertation on Glanders in 1761 and even opened his own school in 1767 to compete with Alfort. He closed it in 1770 to complete his opus work *Cours d'Hippiatrique* 1772, a two-volume masterpiece with 65 engraved plates. This earned him fame almost overnight and the work was translated into German and Spanish. He followed this with a series of books on veterinary and equine subjects. Lafosse continued an unfortunate outpouring of criticism against Bourgelat and Alfort, for some thirty years after Bourgelat's death. He had no need to, his own fame and scholarly reputation were well established; he distinguished himself at the taking of the Bastille, was imprisoned for a year in the chaos of the revolution (1789–1799), but was then appointed Veterinary Inspector-General of Remounts.

After Bourgelat left Lyon the standard of teaching declined. It was bombarded in 1793 in the Revolutionary Wars, and in 1796 was rehoused in an ancient convent. In both French schools the teaching coverage concentrated on the horse, the army needed veterinary support in the wars and the course became shorter. Both schools attracted the enrolment of a significant enrolment number of students from outside of France, but they were generally disappointed that the course was mainly directed towards the horse. Progress in France was delayed by the Revolution years, but finally a third school was established at Toulouse in 1825 with a specific brief to concentrate on livestock diseases.

Bourgelat's fame, and that of the schools, spread fast. Many of his students, usually sponsored by their governments, played roles in the foundation of their own national veterinary schools. These early disciples at Lyon included William Moorcroft (1767–1825), becoming the first trained veterinarian in Britain, briefly being involved with the early London school, but preferring to work in his own practice. Other notable graduates were Peter Christian Abildgaard (1740–1801), who was an outstanding student but disappointed by the equine focus of the course and Bourgelat's 'arrogance and self-importance'. Abildgaard started the first Danish veterinary school in 1773 which gained royal approval in 1777. He was an outstanding scientist and teacher, having trained Erik N. Viborg (1750–1822), his successor, who studied glanders and strangles in horses and wrote the first reliable book on pig diseases. Peter Hernquist (1726–1808) selected by Carl Linnaeus in Sweden to go to Lyon was also disappointed in the course, and took extra tuition from Lafosse; opened private school in 1769, then granted official consent and opened state school at Skara in 1775; followed by Sven Erik Norling (1785–1858) also trained under Viborg in 1806–1807, then opened Royal School in Stockholm in 1821 which eventually moved to Uppsala in 1912. At Lyon in 1763 Ludovici Scotti (1728–1806) established the forerunner to the Vienna College, which opened in 1777 under Alfort graduate Johann Gottlieb Wolstein (1738–1820). Wolstein had also trained under Lafosse and helped to establish the Hungarian Budapest College, later headed by Ferenc Hutyra (1860–1934) a leading veterinary scientist, and Rector for 34 years.

The Continental Veterinary Schools

The genius of Bourgelat was that he established the first two schools of veterinary education. The European countries eagerly followed the French example, almost all with royal or government assistance. The spread of the veterinary schools was dramatic: Turin 1769; Copenhagen 1773; Skara, Sweden and Padua, Italy 1774; Vienna 1777; Hanover 1778; and Dresden 1780. Between 1762 and the end of the 18th century, 19 schools were established in Europe; the establishment of the Toulouse school in 1825 brought the European total to 30.

Britain, however, did not react in the same way, many people knew of the Lyon and Alfort schools and praised them, but there was no government support. King George III was also ruler of the Duchy of Brunswick, in which the city of Hannover was located. On July 18th, 1778, by royal mandate, he ordained that a veterinary school be created in Hannover. Either he was not aware of this or he had not been advised by his ministers, as there is no record of the subject being discussed in London. His British government had shown no interest. Leslie Pugh, who studied the story of the first school wrote, 'The explanation probably lies in the customary contrast between the benevolent despotism of the continent and the laissez-faire regime of eighteenth century England' (Pugh 1962, p. 6).

The London Veterinary School

In 1783 in a small English country town the Odiham Agricultural Society was formed. It was part of the 18th century British Enlightenment movement. Animals were beginning to be looked upon in a new light, not just the horse (still the engine of transport) but also the growing reputation of British livestock. The Society began to discuss matters of agricultural and social concern. One of these discussions was held in response to the perceived quackery and cruelty used in the treatment of sick animals. On 19th August 1785, the Rev. Thomas Burgess proposed a motion, his interest was probably more philanthropic than practical, campaigning for more humane treatment of sick animals. His proposal included the words, '. . . That the improvement of Farriery established on a study of Anatomy, diseases and cures of cattle particularly Horses, Cows and Sheep, will be an essential benefit to Agriculture. . .'.

No progress was made for two years until in 1787 Arthur Young, a celebrated English writer on agricultural matters, visited the Alfort Veterinary School, near Paris. His enthusiastic report probably influenced the society to decide, in 1788, to send two boys to Paris to study at the school. The idea of a veterinary education was not new in Britain: several proposals had been made since 1758. Granville Penn (1761–1844), grandson of William Penn, founder of Pennsylvania, was a well-educated bachelor with strong philanthropic leanings. His name appeared as an Odiham Society Member in 1789 when they formed a London Committee and he soon became Chairman. In the same year he happened to meet Charles Vial de Sainbel, an Alfort veterinary graduate who had just directed the dissection and measurement of the famous thoroughbred, Eclipse. Sainbel was canvassing for interest in starting a British school, but had failed, Penn urged him to try again, and said that he would organise the campaign. Penn ran a well measured campaign and redrafted Sainbel's plan which embraced opening a school, establishing a national system of animal hospitals and replacing farriers by trained veterinary men (Pugh 1962, pp. 17–130).

As there was no government support, Penn had to solicit funds. In January 1791, the London Committee resolved to establish a fund and create an animal hospital to provide education based on medical and anatomical principles. In February they renamed themselves, with Penn as their chair, The Veterinary College London Committee. Sainbel was appointed as Professor and rules and regulations were drawn up. It would appear that Penn selected Sainbel and had naively, and uncritically taken him at his own valuation. The College was established, but with no buildings, land or pupils: on 13th September, a house for Sainbel and six acres of land were leased at Camden Town (then a London suburb). A building was constructed for lectures and on 4th January 1792 Sainbel gave his first lecture. One of the most active and enthusiastic supporters of the new College was John Hunter, Fellow of the Royal Society (FRS), a leading surgeon and anatomist, who attended meetings and visited the new school. An infirmary was opened in January 1793 and the first British veterinary school was established (Cotchin 1990, pp. 12–65).

The College was underway, but with many problems ahead, some of which were in the immediate future. In June 1791 Penn obviously felt he had achieved his objective, he married and left for a three-month honeymoon. He soon retired from the scene, but for three years he had been the driving force in the creation of the College and the plan for the emerging profession. Granville Penn being named the 'Founding Father' of the British veterinary profession is justified.

The first Professor, who had renamed himself Charles Benoit Vial de Saint Bel, started well but in 1793 died, probably from glanders. This was a disaster, but John Hunter immediately granted the students free access to his lectures and requested other lecturers to give similar help. Not long afterwards Hunter also died. The College was in crisis, the finances were very fragile. There were two possible replacement candidates for Professor. One of these was James Clark in Scotland, but he declined hoping for fulfilment of a government promise of funding for an Edinburgh school – this was a tragic loss for the College. The other obvious candidate, William Moorcroft, the only British veterinarian, refused. As a compromise two Professors were appointed: Moorcroft and Edward Coleman, but Moorcroft soon resigned to return to his lucrative London practice. Coleman was left in charge; he had trained as a surgeon and had no veterinary knowledge.

Coleman remained as Principal for 43 years; the College became totally equine oriented, the curriculum was drastically shortened, education standards declined and graduate quality was very poor. The one bright spot was William Dick (1776–1847), an independently minded graduate who experienced all the failings of Coleman's school. He returned to Edinburgh and opened his own school in 1820, which became the Edinburgh Veterinary School in 1823 and produced broad-based graduates. Dick was an excellent clinician and understood the needs of livestock owners as well as the horse. He established an examining board and awarded certificates of competence; at that time Edinburgh was an important medical centre, which aided the development of the school. Today it is called the Royal (Dick) School of Veterinary Studies. Britain slowly moved ahead with other schools being established initially in Glasgow and Liverpool, then in Bristol, Cambridge, Nottingham and Surrey. And the London school, now named the Royal Veterinary

College, after its difficult start was ranked in 2019 as the world's leading veterinary school.

Mr Sainbel Becomes the First London Professor

Charles Vial de Sainbel (1750–1793) was born near Lyon, France as Charles Benoit Vial. He entered the Lyon Veterinary School in 1769 and was recorded as an excellent student, joining the Alfort School in 1774 as a junior Professor. Sainbel disagreed with Bourgelat and after a while he returned to Lyon in practice, before becoming a Demonstrator in Comparative Anatomy at Montpellier University. He was appointed an Equerry to Louis XVI and made Director of the Lyon Riding School. When he visited England in 1788 at the suggestion of his French patron, he made proposals to establish an English veterinary school, without success. He returned to France but as the political situation was becoming difficult, went back to England in 1789 where he was requested to undertake the dissection of Eclipse, the celebrated racehorse. Shortly afterwards the French Revolution began and he lost his positions in France and his income. He then met Granville Penn, as described previously, became the first Professor of the Veterinary College of London in 1791, publishing his *Essay on the Proportions of Eclipse* in the same year.

Sainbel began teaching with four students in January 1792. There were many problems but he hired an assistant, Delabere Pritchett Blaine, and in January 1793 the new hospital, for fifty horses, opened. During the year Sainbel published *Lectures on the Elements of Farriery, or the Art of Horseshoeing*, the college had fifteen students. Sainbel worked hard to establish the new school and also made his students work both in studies and in cleaning and running the school. On August 4th he was taken ill and died on August 21st, 1793, probably from glanders infection. The infant College had lost its Professor and its leading protagonist; Blaine had also left his post.

After his death, in 1795 for the financial benefit of his widow, *The Works of Charles Vial de Sainbel* were published. The third edition included his posthumous writing on *The Art of Veterinary Medicine* which detailed the equine problems of glanders, grease and colic.

Sainbel has to be acknowledged as a leader and the pioneer of British veterinary education. He did, however, have a strong personality and a reputation for being 'difficult', shown by his relationships in France and in Britain. He was a Frenchman in England at the time his own country was in the throes of a violent revolution – life could not have been easy for him. He was a hard worker, introduced a three-year course, knew he needed quality staff to educate the students properly and had a plan to create a veterinary profession. All of these ideals which were abandoned by his successor, Edward Coleman. A full review of Sainbel's life is available in *The Early History of Veterinary Literature*, Vol. II (Smith 1976, pp. 184–203).

The Discipline Expands

In the final years of the 18th century there were few notable veterinary advances, the schools were becoming organised and research studies started, with many by physicians and surgeons. The British environment was receptive to new ideas. Arthur Young FRS (1741–1820) the leading agriculturalist, enthusiastic about the creation of the London College, was made an Honorary Member of the Board in 1792: his writings demonstrated his veterinary interest. John Hunter FRS (1728–1793), a British surgeon and comparative anatomist, was a man who led in both surgery and anatomy, with several important treatises on both human health and veterinary related topics. He was a great supporter and enthusiast of the new London Veterinary School. Alexander Monro (1733–1817), Professor of Anatomy in University of Edinburgh, became recognised for his comparative anatomical work and as a physiologist, with many of his studies being made with the cow, horse and dog. Erasmus Darwin (1731–1802) FRS was an English physician and grandfather of Charles Darwin. He was a notable thinker in the evolution field along similar lines to J-B Lamarck. His book *Zoonomia, or the Laws of Organic Life* (1794–1796) was both an early attempt to classify pathology and a miscellaneous collection of observations on animals and their behaviour and ailments; many of these were later shown to be accurate. B Harwood FRS (n.d.) Professor of Anatomy at the University of Cambridge published *A System of Comparative Anatomy and Physiology* Vol. I, 1796. This is a detailed and well-illustrated study of the olfactory organs in animals, birds, fish and amphibia, described as 'a revelation of industry, sound anatomical knowledge and precise observation' (Smith 1976, pp. 226–227). No further volumes appeared.

T Champney (n.d.), a British surgeon who had studied the practice of what he termed the 'Healing Art' in European countries published *Medical and Surgical Reform Proposed . . .* 1783. A rather strange book, the author was keen on improving medical and veterinary education and suggested the two be taught together in every public hospital. He did not state who would teach students or how his scheme would be implemented. The London College already existed. Edward Jenner FRS (1799–1823), was a country physician, greatly influenced by John Hunter and who later made his name by proving and demonstrating the use of cowpox as an immunogen for smallpox prevention. Jenner was an observant investigator and explored cowpox and related conditions including horsepox which he probably confused with a now absent condition in horses termed 'grease'. There was some confusion over the calf lymph that was produced in immense quantity for smallpox vaccinations, was it the same material that Jenner had used? Animal welfare remained an ever present concern: progress was slow but aided by Thomas Young (n.d.), a Cambridge University academic and author of *Essay on Humanity to Animals* 1798. He covered a wide range of topics from cruelty in sports, hunting, farriery, slaughtering and even bees. It was abridged for a second edition in 1804, but was not widely read.

Continental Europe also showed similar advances, but with the earlier start in veterinary schools there was an earlier development of veterinary workers. One of the most important was Peter Christian Abildgaard (1740–1801), founder of The Royal

Veterinary School in Copenhagen, Denmark; he was a polymath who published zoological, botanical and geological studies, and also studied physics and physiology. Abildgaard had a particular interest in parasitism and described these in mammals, birds and fish as well as studying their complex indirect life-cycles; he made valuable observations on both fish and mammalian tapeworms. A biography details his life and work (Anderson 1985). Erik Viborg (1759–1822), a student of Abildgaard, published dissertations on rabies, glanders, foot-and-mouth disease and anthrax. Viborg became Rector of the Veterinary School in 1801, on the death of Abildgaard. He wrote *The Care and Management of the Pig* 1804, the first detailed text on the animal and its diseases, widely translated in Europe (Viborg 1804).

The Hungarian Veterinary College

Hungary commenced veterinary education by Imperial decree of the Austro-Hungarian empire, on 5th July 1787. A Chair for Animal Healing was created in the Faculty of Medicine in Pest. As this interest grew it was renamed the Royal Institute of Veterinary Medicine in 1851 and then again renamed the Royal College of Veterinary Medicine with the right to issue degrees. Further changes of venue and staff resulted in the College becoming the independent University of Veterinary Science in 1962. Restructuring in 2000 created the Faculty of Veterinary Science, Szent Istvan (Saint Esteban) University. In 2016 it became the University of Veterinary Medicine, Budapest, overseen by the Hungarian Accreditation Board.

The history is described as being divided into four periods – the classical era, the golden epoch, education in the socialist time and the modern period. Hungary became a leader in veterinary discovery and pathology with outstanding research during the period of the later 19th century and early 20th century with Professors Hutyra, Marek, Manninger, Mocsy and Aujesky. When they were originally founded, the teaching courses were strongly influenced by the German education system, now modified by English-American teaching and French methods. Teaching is now undertaken in Hungarian, German and English: if any examination is twice failed, no further attempts are allowed. While there have been many changes of name the College has remained in the same buildings for many years. These were built to the design of Imre Steindl (1839–1902), the architect of the magnificent Danube-side Hungarian Parliament building. The veterinary school does not have the exuberant exterior of the Parliament but does have many fine (and preserved) features.

Veterinary Education in Russia

Russia has a complex (and confusing) veterinary education history covering three main periods – the Russian empire, Soviet Russia and modern Russia. The first teaching began in Warsaw, Poland in the mid-1800s, it endured Russification in 1865 and became the College of Veterinary Medicine in 1889. During this period, several hundred veterinarians graduated, mostly Polish. Some veterinary teaching also started at Vilna (now Vilnius, capital of Lithuania) when this was part of Poland, this was probably between 1823 and 1832 when it closed due to the Polish uprising against the Russian occupiers. It restarted later but closed again in 1843 and its equipment was sent to Dorpat (now Tartu, Estonia). This appears to have been planned by the Imperial government in St. Petersburg. In 1848 the Dorpat Veterinary Institute was founded as a part of Dorpat University: both the teaching and research were good.

In Russia, the first veterinary actions happened in 1805 when a Chair of Cattle Medicine was created in the Moscow Medico-Chirurgical Academy of Moscow University. In 1810 it was renamed Chair of Veterinary Medicine and occupied by Theobald Renner (1779–1850) a German veterinarian. He left in 1812, the chair was abolished but a department was created with several teachers; graduates were produced between 1806–1842. The department was then closed and no veterinary education was available in Moscow until 1919.

Education also began in St. Petersburg in 1806 in the veterinary division of the Military Medical Academy which had a reputation for high quality work and teaching. The post of Professor was first offered to Delabere Blaine an English veterinarian. He refused the offer and the post was instead given to Professor I D Knigin, followed by Joseph Ippolitovitch Ravich (1822–1875) who became a leader in veterinary pathology and also founded *Arkhiv Veterinarnykh Nauk* in 1871 which became the most widely read Russian veterinary journal until its demise in the 1917 revolution. Kazan University had a Chair of Veterinary Medicine from 1841–1848 with some teaching. In 1873 the Kazan Veterinary Institute (Veterinary School) was created and opened with German Professors Constantine and Blumberg. Additionally in the Ukraine in 1851 the Department for Animal Treatment was created which became established in Kharkov University in 1873 as the Kharkov Veterinary Institute, and now is the Kharkiv State Zooveterinary Academy (KhGZVA). In the early days of Russian veterinary medicine the strongest influence was from Germany, where teachers were provided and Russian students were trained at the developing centres. The early work at Dorpat was excellent. In 1917, at the time of the revolution, there were five veterinary schools but only two actually in Russia – St. Petersburg, Kazan, Kharkov (Ukraine), Dorpat (Estonia) and Warsaw (as the German Army advanced in 1915 the Warsaw school was moved to Moscow and then on to Novocherkassk).

In 1919 the Soviet government decided to commence veterinary education in Moscow and Omsk, at the Siberian Veterinary Institute, which was a school for training feldshers, veterinary assistants. In 1926 the Moscow School was forced to close for a period due to the shortage of buildings in Moscow (Saunders 1980). Currently there are 37 State Universities with undergraduate veterinary courses and a total of 100 institutions providing courses on veterinary topics. The leading College is the Moscow State Academy of Veterinary Medicine and Biotechnology. Two interesting papers on veterinary schools and institutions following the 1917 Soviet revolution are by Podgaez (1922, pp. 304–314) and Hobday (1930).

Veterinary Education in Turkey

Turkey has a long history of animal healing which can be traced back to the Islamic/Arabic designation of *al-baytar* for a veterinarian. Training was given under the Ottomans in the 14th and 15th centuries, as described in the veterinary books (*baitarnume*) of that period. Advancement was halted by the *madrasas*, the schools of education and study of the Islamic religion with their fundamentalist and obstructionist attitude.

In the 18th–19th centuries the Ottomans tried to follow Western Europe teaching recognising the need for a veterinary school as there was much epidemic disease in the army horses. The madrasa tradition was breached in the late 1700s, when the army established engineering colleges. Finally in 1842 Brigade-Rossartz von Godlewsky, a Prussian military veterinarian opened the first veterinary school in Istanbul, for training army personnel. The class of 12 students graduated in 1845 and in 1849 the course was increased to four years. In 1888 to meet a civilian need, a second school was opened with teachers from France, Belgium and Germany – the tuition was based on the French course. In 1890 students were sent to the Alfort school in France and on their return in 1895 joined the teaching staff in Istanbul. The two schools were merged in 1920 as the *Baytar Mekteb-i Alisi* (Veterinary High School).

Following the 1923 creation of the Turkish Republic, an institute for the study of agriculture and animal breeding was established in 1927. In 1933 the *Yüksek Ziraat Enstitüsü* (Higher Agricultural Institution) was formed merging all agricultural interests including the Veterinary School. In 1946 this was moved to Ankara and in 1948 the Veterinary Faculty became a part of Ankara University. A second school opened at Elazig in 1970 and became part of Firat University in 1976. Currently there are 19 veterinary schools in Turkey, all are part of state universities and regulated by the Higher Educational Law No.2547. Of interest the first book on the history of Turkish veterinary medicine (*Nevsal-i Baytari*) was published in 1918. The history of veterinary medicine has been taught to veterinary students since 1933 and has been a compulsory subject since the late 1980s.

References

Anderson, S. (1985) *P.C. Abildgaard, Biography & Bibliography*. Copenhagen: Royal Danish Veterinary and Agricultural University

Cotchin, E. (1990) *The Royal Veterinary College London: A Bicentenary History*. Buckingham: Barracuda Books

Hobday, F. (1930) A Visit to Some of the Veterinary Colleges and Veterinary Research Institutes of the United Socialist Soviet Republic. *The Veterinary Record* **10**

Podgaez, H. (1922) The Past, Present and Future of Veterinary Education and of the Profession in Russia. *The Veterinary Journal* **78**

Pugh, L.P. (1962) *From Farriery to Veterinary Medicine*. Cambridge: Heffer & Sons

Saunders, L.Z. (1980) *Veterinary Pathology in Russia 1860–1930*. Ithaca, NY: Cornell University Press

Smith, F. (1976) *The Early History of Veterinary Literature*, Vol. II London: J A Allen (reprint)

Viborg, E (1804) *The Care and Management of the Pig*. Copenhagen: C.G. Prost (reprint)

CHAPTER 15

Veterinary Medicine Arrives in North America and Advances

The first colonists in North America were surprised by the absence of domestic animals, but within a few years all the European species of livestock had also crossed the Atlantic (see Chapter 9). Colonisation moved rapidly, the Spanish soon controlled Central America south to Panama, as well as Florida, and an advance into the west and California. The 13 British colonies occupied the east coast plain and the French occupied the Mississippi river system north from New Orleans. In Canada, the British and French competed for sovereignty.

As the population grew, pioneers crossed the Appalachian Mountains and found the Ohio river valley, a tributary of the Mississippi – this was farming land and there was a steady westward flow of hopeful farmers. Then the French in 1803 sold their interests to the young United States of America (USA), who also acquired Florida and later California from the Spanish. The USA was almost formed. Final treaties with Britain in 1818 and 1846 established the northern border and the Texas annexation of 1845 created the southern border with Mexico. The Great Plains of America were open for agricultural exploitation. At first the farmers only raised cattle for their own needs, but when the railroad was built across to Ohio in the 19th century the great western livestock industry began. By the time of the Civil War (1861–1865) Cincinnati had developed as the first meatpacking centre (Merillat and Campbell 1935, pp. 54–55). There was also an enormous horse breeding industry for riding and transport to and from the railways and riverboat steamers. The livestock were mixed breed cattle, coarse-woolled sheep and low-grade, but prolific, pigs.

In 1869 the railroad reached Omaha, and from this grew an immense cattle and sheep breeding industry from Texas to the Great Plains, sheep production started in the mountain states and the dairy industry followed on from the growth in population. After the Civil War, a pig (hog) industry evolved and in the 20th century the need for the horse rapidly declined.

One of the great stories of this period was that of the cattle drives, mostly from Texas, along defined routes with memorable names – the Shawnee, Chisholm and Goodnight-Loving Trails, as well as routes to the North such as the Western Trail. This boom however only lasted for about 20 years; as the railroads spread, the need for these drives evaporated. These drives included 500–2000 cattle and many millions moved along these trails. Between 1867 and 1881 more than four million walked from Texas to the railheads. The trail drives have become an attractive Western legend but in fact they were hard for both the cattle and the men. They are of particular interest for USA veterinary history as in 1766 the Colony of North Carolina passed laws to control these drives due to a reported disease occurring in local cattle – an action that resulted in Dr James Mease (1771–1846) being the first to suggest its infectious nature and to study it – later called Texas fever. This was the beginning of veterinary medicine in the USA.

A Need for Veterinary Medicine

Initially any health care needed for livestock was provided by the farmers, and was later supplemented by farriers or cow-leeches, usually unfortunately both as ignorant as each other. A man named William Carter in Virginia was described as 'an expert veterinarian or cow doctor who lived in James City in 1625' (Smithcors 1975, pp. 22–23), but the colonies had to wait two hundred years for graduate veterinarians. The first of these appears to be John Haslam of Baltimore who graduated from the London Veterinary College in 1799, to next appear in New York in 1803. Also listed is an R H Haslam of Baltimore who graduated from London in 1829. Another is Charles Clark, nephew of Bracey Clark one of the earliest British graduates. Charles is believed to have graduated in France, gone into practice in New York but returned to Britain in 1817 to join his ailing uncle's practice (Jones 2014, pp. 314–315; Smith 1976a, p. 37).

In 1827 a Mr Saunders arrived in Boston from England, and obtained a position as veterinarian with the Old Eastern Stagecoach Company in Massachusetts, which he held until his death. No record exists of him at the London College, but he is known later, as veterinary graduates began to organise, as the father of William Saunders, a prominent veterinarian. In the same year that Saunders arrived, there is also a record of John Rose, a Prussian graduate (possibly not a German national), building up a successful practice in New York (Liautard 1877, pp. 5–19).

There was then an increasing rate of immigrant European graduates, mostly of British origin: demonstrating both a perceived need and an opportunity. In the later 1820s, G C Grice arrived in New York, shortly followed by R H Curtis, A Lockhart and C Pilgrim. These London graduates were the pioneers of the New York Society of Veterinary Medicine. In 1831 R H Budd arrived in New York, to become known as a reliable author; shortly after A S Copeman arrived and set up practice in Utica, New York State, and in 1840 W H Lillyman arrived: all three of these came from London (Arbura 1934, pp. 11–38). There was then a regular trickle of graduates arriving from Europe. By 1847 there were believed to be 15 veterinarians in the USA, mostly of British origin (Smithcors 1959, pp. 330–341). 60 years later, in 1910 it was reported that there were 11,500 veterinarians, mostly United States (US) citizens and working mainly with horses in New York, Boston and Chicago. A number of students from the USA came to the British veterinary schools in the mid-1800s. One of these, William Miles, is known because he was a ringleader in student troubles at the London College in 1836, however on qualifying he appears to have remained in Britain (Smith 1976b, p. 23). Edinburgh produced their first US graduate, William Frater, in 1830 (Pringle 1869).

As the need for veterinary services grew, more 'practitioners' appeared. The backgrounds of these people and in fact most of their names are not known, but one man, Ezra Michener (1794–1887) a physician, developed a practice in Pennsylvania around 1830 (Bierer 1955, p. 33). He was well regarded, supported the 1854 formation of the American Veterinary Association in Philadelphia, served as Professor of Theory and Practice of Medicine on the faculty of the early Pennsylvania College of Veterinary Surgeons, and was father of C B Michener, an early US graduate who later became President of the US (now American) Veterinary Medical Association. Pennsylvania had a significant German immigrant agricultural community who used reprinted translated German veterinary texts, which influenced the regional practices. As times changed the community became known as the Pennsylvania Dutch.

George H Dadd, an Englishman who arrived in Boston around 1847, played a significant early role, but now usually downgraded; he established a veterinary practice and was involved in other veterinary activities. Another early player was Alexandre Liautard, a physician and graduate of Toulouse Veterinary College, France; he played a significant role in the development of veterinary education, the founding of the national association and journal in the USA, but retired back to France.

The Idea of American Veterinary Education

As in Britain the establishment of a veterinary education system was slow and difficult. The evolving US government administration had many, to them, more important issues to resolve in the rapidly expanding country. The education core of the few universities, themselves having to adapt to their environment, remained tied to their traditional subjects of theology, law and medicine. Philadelphia University was founded in 1749 and in 1765 added a Medical Department with a three-year course. Medical needs however had increasing demands and private schools began to open in the USA in the late 1700s.

There was recognition of a need to attend to animal diseases. This was usually expressed by physicians (as in Britain), with reports of several interventions and studies. With a growing interest in scientific farming in 1785 the Philadelphia Society for Promoting Agriculture was formed, followed by similar organisations in South Carolina and Massachusetts. The members of the Philadelphia Society included George Washington, Benjamin Franklin, Benjamin Rush, James Mease and Judge Richard Peters. The memoirs published by the Society indicate that they saw veterinary schools as the only way to solve the animal disease problems. Noteworthy was Dr Benjamin Rush (1745–1813), founder (1765) and head of the Medical Department of the University of Philadelphia. Visiting Europe in 1806 he saw the progress made in the veterinary colleges and in 1807 lectured Philadelphia medical students on, 'The Duty and Advantages of Studying the Diseases of Domestic Animals and the Remedies proper to remove them'.

He sent a letter to the Agricultural Society of Philadelphia urging the importance for the University of Philadelphia to establish a Veterinary Department: this was discussed but it was to be more than forty years before any further action was taken, and eighty years before the school finally opened.

Another public figure proposing the establishment of a veterinary profession was Dr James Mease (1771–1846), Lazaretto (quarantine) physician at State Island, Pa. Visiting Lancaster County in 1796, he found his hosts greatly concerned with the loss of cattle that had occupied a pasture which recently held a herd being driven from South Carolina overnight. Mease became interested and traced the epidemic spread including making autopsies; he continued his studies, eventually making them public in 1814 in a lecture to the Philadelphia Society for Promoting Agriculture. This was the first account of what became known as Texas fever. There was however still no apparent enthusiasm to create a veterinary school (Arbura 1934, pp. 11–38). Texas fever was responsible for the first animal disease legislation in North America, passed in 1766 by North Carolina State legislature introducing controls on driving cattle herds across the state.

Two events precipitated positive action for establishing veterinary schools. First, the horrific treatment of equines during the Civil War (1861–1865): an estimated one million horses and mules died from trauma, starvation or disease with minimal health or safety attention; with the average equine life in service being only about five months (Smith 2010a, pp. 317–327). Secondly, the economy started to expand after the war, the horse emerged as the essential means of transportation of people and goods in the rapidly increasing urban centres, and in the fast growing rural economy.

While there was a growing recognition of the need to improve animal health care, there was no recognised professional body of knowledge, no obvious patronage, and no students waiting. Religious denominational colleges occupied a position of primary importance in higher education, but after the Civil War the situation changed when these were replaced in importance by Land-Grant agricultural colleges (Miller 1988, pp. 4–50). Public support for veterinary schools could only develop when it became appreciated that there was a body of veterinary knowledge that could be obtained and utilised.

The Printed Word, and then Associations

Initially veterinary books and journals arrived from Europe, mostly from Britain. As printing and publishing became established in the USA, reprints were made of perceived marketable and valuable texts. The first of these appears to have been James Clark's *Treatise on the Prevention of Diseases incidental to Horses*, published in Edinburgh in 1788 and reprinted in Philadelphia in 1791. This was a good choice for a foundation book, as it represented the best of British knowledge and probably the best in Europe (Campbell 1934, pp. 48–52). It is believed that Dr Rush read this book: it would have stimulated his ideas on veterinary education. The publishing of this book, and such books were not cheap, indicated that there was a perceived readership able and willing to both purchase and utilise its contents. In 1798, a reprint of *Farriery Improved* by William Bracken appeared. It was a compilation of Bracken's texts plus those of other older British authors, put together by Matthew Carey. Most of the advice was very poor and the book did little to add to knowledge.

At that time books were expensive; literacy was not of a high level and the medical sciences were at a very early stage. At the beginning of the Revolutionary War (1776) there were estimated to be more than 3500 physicians within the colonies, but only about 400, at most, held degrees from regular medical colleges. In Britain in 1801, there were only 37 veterinary graduates. The idea of veterinary medicine was still in embryo.

The next book was *The Citizen and Countryman's Experienced Farrier* 1803, by J Markham, G Jefferies and Experienced Indians. Described as, 'a compilation of absurdities already 240 years old' (Campbell 1934, pp. 96–100), it was intended for livestock owners and listed almost unimaginable cruelties in animal treatment handed down since medieval times. Most of the text is from Gervase Markham written in 1610, of which much was copied from Blundeville (1560). It was worthless: the Jefferies name was probably an invention and the 'experienced Indians' presumably included as an indication of native folk medicine.

In 1812 William Taplin's *The Gentlemen's Stable Directory* was published in Philadelphia, it was a more useful contribution to knowledge. In 1813, *The Complete Cow Doctor: being a Treatise on the Disorders Incident to Horned Cattle . . .*, was published in Philadelphia by Anthony Finley: this was a much plagiarised English work possibly dating back to 1787 (Clewlow 2012, pp. 188–190). There were more books, but the most valuable of these was written by William Youatt, already popular and well regarded in Britain. His first book, *The Horse*, was reprinted in 1834 as *Youatt on the Horse* and edited by John Skinner (1788–1851) who was the editor of *American Farmer* and interested in veterinary progress. It sold 23,000 copies (and that on cattle 10,000) and was still to be found in use up to the end of the century.

The earliest American veterinary literature, that can be traced, is found in pioneer medical journals. The first appears to be by F.B. Sayre, in *Medical Repository* (New York) in 1800, entitled *Observations on the Disease commonly called Yellow Water in Horses*. There then were regular, but not a large number of publications in the US medical press. The first scientific paper on veterinary pathology in North America was written in 1870 by Jos Woodward, medical officer at the Army Medical Museum in Washington DC, describing the histopathology of contagious bovine pleuro-pneumonia (Saunders 1987, pp. 1–26). The first American authored book discussing veterinary medicine was *Husbandman's Guide*, written by an anonymous author and published in Boston in 1710 (Smithcors 1975, p. 36). In 1801 James Mease published *The Bite of Dogs*. At that time rabies was regarded as a medical, and not a veterinary problem.

The first known American authored book specifically dealing with animal disease was *The New England Farrier* (1795), by Paul Jewett of Newburyport, Massachusetts. Directing his book at the farmer, Jewett discussed horses, cattle, sheep and pigs; he had no training but had a large veterinary practice so the book was of some value. This was followed by William Carver, a farrier, who wrote *The Practical Horse Farrier* (Philadelphia, 1818), and was experienced and sensible in his advice, and humanity.

James Carver Member of the College of Veterinary Surgeons (MRCVS) (London 1815), unrelated to William, was described as 'veterinary surgeon, corresponding member of the London Veterinary Medical Society and the College of India'. James published *The Farriers Magazine or Archives of Veterinary Science* (Philadelphia 1818), apart from the grand title, it was an advertisement for his practice. Only two issues appeared, but the author did make a plea for the establishment of a veterinary school. In New York in 1831 R H Budd MRCVS published *A Practical Treatise on Diseases of the Foot of the Horse*. A second edition later appeared: it was well received and remained in print for many years. In New York in 1847 an interesting, but relatively short at only 227 pages, book was published titled *Illustrated Treatise on Domestic Animals*. The book was written by R L Allen, a well-known agricultural writer who tried to provide veterinary guidance for the owners of horse, mule, cattle, sheep, swine, poultry and dogs. The book's content is of extremely mixed quality but it illustrates the more common practices and medications of the period. From this date veterinary literature appeared regularly: there was a growing market. Veterinary books were printed in Pennsylvania for the large German farming population. The *Horse-Doctor Book* was reprinted several times up to 1822 (in German).

G H Dadd wrote ten veterinary books between 1846–1866 of which *The Modern Horse Doctor* 1854 sold no less than 20,000 copies (Liautard 1877, pp. 5–19). This was, for the time, a good book and better than his *American Cattle Doctor* published in 1850. He started the *American Veterinary Journal* in 1851, but struggled to collect enough subscribers. The journal finally ceased publication in 1859 when Dadd wrote the 'Report of the Transactions of the Veterinary School at Alfort' for the *New England Farmer*, including a plea for an US veterinary school. In 1862, he became the veterinary editor of *The Prairie Farmer*, a widely read magazine that gave generally sound advice to livestock farmers for many years. In his time Dadd was an influential veterinary journalist.

Veterinary medicine had begun to be recognised as a science and a particular discipline. Its participants now wanted to enforce standards and over two days on the 9th and 10th June 1863 a group, mostly with a European veterinary qualification, met at the Astor House in New York, and formed the United States Veterinary Medical Association (USVMA). J H Stickney of Massachusetts, an 1859 London graduate and a physician, was elected President. In 1898 it was renamed to the American Veterinary Medical Association (AVMA). Of the other officers, two were London graduates including R H Curtis who was elected Vice-President, W Saunders and Alexandre Liautard, a Toulouse graduate, as Secretary. The USVMA had partially grown out of the less successful, American Veterinary Association, founded in Philadelphia in 1854 (Jennings 1884, pp. 12–42). As the new Association grew, in January 1877, it launched the first successful US veterinary journal: named the *American Veterinary Review* it later became the *Journal of the American Veterinary Medical Association*. The founding Editor was Alexandre Liautard MD, VS with A Lockhart MRCVS as Assistant Editor. The first issue starts with a fourteen page article by Liautard titled History and Progress of Veterinary Medicine, an informative description of the evolution of the US profession (Liautard 1877, pp. 5–19).

US Veterinary Schools Open

As neither the government, nor initially the foundation universities, showed any inclination to fund the establishment of veterinary schools the process was left to individual entrepreneurs or interested groups. The first of these was established in Philadelphia, probably arising from the 1806 plea by Benjamin Rush for such educational establishments. In 1852, $40,000 was raised and a charter obtained from the State Legislature for a veterinary college with a planned opening in 1853: the venture failed due to a lack of students. The prime mover was R Jennings (who used the post-nominal of 'VS', but had no formal veterinary education). In 1854 the same group reformed as the American Veterinary Association, with President, T J Corbyn VS. A further effort was made in 1855, premises were rented and a dissecting room built. An architect was commissioned to draft plans for a new building, but the directors became discouraged and abandoned their building plans (Jennings 1884, pp. 12–42).

An unsigned letter, possibly written by Jennings, appeared in a June 1858 New York newspaper headed *Progress of Veterinary Science in Philadelphia*. The letter extolled the premises and work undertaken in 1855, stressing the dissecting room and museum with its anatomical and pathological specimens which had won an award from the Pennsylvania State Agricultural Society in 1854. The comment was made, 'we were struck by the grand and extensive field here presented for the study of human anatomy and pathology' (Anon 1858).

The 'one medicine' concept flourished well in the USA at that time. A new start in 1859 resulted in two students attending but this effort was dogged by troubles and finally suspended in 1866. Another attempt was made later that year, as the Pennsylvania College of Veterinary Surgeons, but this closed in 1870. Eventually in 1884 a viable veterinary school was established and later integrated as a faculty of the University of Philadelphia.

George H Dadd, born in England in 1813 but nothing else known of his early life, arrived in Boston in 1846 or 1847 as a ship's surgeon. He claimed to have studied both human and veterinary medicine and used the post-nominals MD and VS; he certainly had medical training but it is not believed that he had reached graduate status. He soon established himself in veterinary practice and from 1848 produced in rapid succession a series of veterinary books and voluminous writings in the agricultural press – described earlier in this chapter.

In 1855 Dadd founded the Boston Veterinary Institute as a veterinary school, but his ideas seemed to be too new. The establishment ran a desultory course until it closed in 1859, but it was noteworthy in that at least three members of his faculty became president of the USVMA (later the AVMA). He then ran the enterprise as the Boston Veterinary School, with students also attending classes at the Harvard University Medical School, but this also closed after a year. His efforts resulted in the graduation of at least 12 veterinary students, who were judged to be of good quality. In 1861 he moved to Cincinnati and advertised the Academy of Veterinary Medicine and Surgery but there is no record of its opening. By 1863 he had moved to Chicago, he was veterinary editor for the national *Prairie Farmer* and announced the Veterinary Institute of Chicago: this again appeared to have no uptake, the public was not ready. After 1865 his activities become something of an enigma, he died in Baltimore in 1868. While Dadd is not remembered as a father figure – mostly because he upset his colleagues by his active promotion of his own remedies and his rather dubious qualifications – he did make a valuable early contribution and instilled a spirit of medicine into veterinary medicine (Smithcors 1960, pp. 129–131). Dadd also should be remembered as a somewhat pivotal figure on the American veterinary scene – he advocated humane and rational treatment, he was against bleeding, blistering, 'calomelising', narcotising and so on: observations that alienated him from many of his colleagues. He was the first to use general anaesthesia in veterinary practice in the USA (first recorded in 1852, but he had been using it before then).

1855 was an important year: the Philadelphia group were trying to create a faculty, Dadd opened his first Boston School, and Captain John C Ralston MRCVS obtained a charter to open the Veterinary College Institute of New York. Ralston raised $40,000, built a school and hospital with accommodation for 50 patients, but had to abandon the project two years later. This was followed by the New York College of Veterinary Surgeons, chartered by John Busteed MD in 1857; a building was secured on Lexington Avenue and equipped, but had a chequered career due to internal strife until 1899. Alexandre Liautard was not only associated with the New York College of Veterinary Surgeons but he worked for high standards. Named the American Veterinary College between 1875–1899 and then the New York-American Veterinary College until 1922, it can be seen as the progenitor of US veterinary education. The New York schools produced some 815 graduates, mostly of acceptable quality, at a time when the USA needed them.

The Scottish Graduates and the Canadian Schools

The first viable and lasting veterinary school in North America opened in 1862 in Toronto, Canada because the agricultural population were concerned by the plagues devastating cattle in Europe. Cattle values were rising and farmers had little protection should these diseases spread to North America. The Board of Agriculture sent the lecturer in Agricultural Science at Toronto University to Scotland to speak to Professor Dick at his Edinburgh College. Following his advice, Andrew Smith MRCVS, an 1861 graduate, was selected to lecture on veterinary science. He relocated to Toronto, was appointed Veterinary Surgeon to the Board of Agriculture, and started lectures in October 1862. This date is usually given as the founding of the veterinary college, it was, however, only the start of veterinary lectures to the agriculture students which later developed into a veterinary course.

The Canadian government soon realised that the lectures alone were not enough and that much more was needed. In the characteristically parsimonious British way the government declined to fund this, but in 1864 they granted a private charter to Andrew Smith for the founding of a veterinary school. It was left to Smith to determine the entrance requirements and the course of instruction. While this avoided any expense by the government, it meant that Smith had to depend on tuition fees for the creation and maintenance of his school. To induce sufficient numbers of students to attend he had to accept low entrance requirements and a not too rigorous course. There was no governing body and no process to ensure ethical standards among the graduates: the result was almost a repetition of what had happened in England in the late 1700s. In spite of these problems many useful, and some eminent, men were graduates. However, the lack of any means of professional cohesion and adoption of ethical standards was felt to have cast a shadow on the early development of the profession in Canada (Mitchell 1938, pp. 91–95).

The first class of three men entered in 1864 and graduated in 1866. Gradually the college grew and standards were raised. College premises were built, and enlarged, until almost 200 students were graduating annually. Having trained over 3000 veterinarians, Smith passed his charter back to the Ontario Government in 1908 and the School was integrated into Ontario University as the Faculty of Veterinary Medicine. Smith had created and overseen the first successful veterinary school in North America and, with his upgraded teaching standards, made a major contribution to establishing a North American veterinary profession. One of his 1877 graduates, M H McKillip, went on to establish a private veterinary college in Chicago which in turn produced more than 1200 graduates of good quality, including one of the first two US women veterinarians in 1910, before it closed in 1920 (Smith 2010b pp. 90–91).

Andrew Smith had called upon a fellow Edinburgh graduate, Duncan McNab McEachran MRCVS who had moved to Canada in 1862, to aid in the instruction of the students. However, they parted company in 1863 after three months as they could not agree on either Smith's entrance requirements or the course structure. McEachran moved to Montreal in 1865, and in 1866 opened the Montreal Veterinary College (MVC), with the assistance of Sir William Dawson, Principal of McGill University and Dr George Campbell, Dean of the Faculty of Medicine. This was McEachran's opportunity to put forward his views on veterinary education. The MVC was initially affiliated to the university and in 1875 he built, at his own expense, the college buildings where the clinical side of veterinary medicine was taught; other teaching was coordinated with the Medical Faculty. He became associated with Dr William Osler, destined to become North America's leading medical teacher and to play an early important role in the first scientific investigations of animal disease in North America. The two men shared similar views in their approach to education and in 1889 were successful in having the college integrated into McGill University as the Faculty of Comparative Medicine and Veterinary Science. This functioned until 1903 when it was forced to close due to lack of financial support, resulting from competition from commercial (for profit) schools in the USA that charged lower fees and offered quicker graduation. Between 1866–1902 approximately 315 veterinarians graduated from the MVC.

McEachran had lofty aspirations for the veterinary profession. Together with Osler they believed that medicine was one field and both believed in rigid training in the common fundamentals of medicine. McEachran raised veterinary education standards (Mitchell 1939, pp. 255–258), he insisted on high quality matriculation requirements together with a three-year course – no other Anglo-Saxon country college had such ideals. He has to be recognised as a veterinary education pioneer and leader.

The McEachran and Osler relationship was incredibly productive; Osler had already applied the Virchow methods of autopsy technique and scientific enquiry to his teaching of pathology at McGill. By the time the US Bureau of Animal Industry was founded in May 1884, and Theobald Smith was hired as the first pathologist, Osler had already conducted research on hog cholera (swine fever) (1878), verminous bronchitis of dogs (1877) and Pictou cattle disease (1883) among others. Osler and McEachran created an enduring legacy, they produced high quality graduates and established the discipline of pathology as the cornerstone of veterinary education – where the basic science subjects meet the clinical subjects, and give the latter meaning (Saunders 1987, pp. 1–26). McEachran and Osler formed a formidable team for medical science, (Eby 1960, pp. 273–276). When Osler departed for Philadelphia it was a great loss. Several MVC graduates went on to make distinctive reputations including: A W Clement who wrote *Veterinary Post-mortem Examinations* 1891, the first book in English on the subject, and W L Williams, born in Illinois, reaching the peak of his career at Cornell University as Professor of Surgery, Obstetrics and Ethics.

McEachran was influential in livestock disease control (glanders, hog cholera, bovine tuberculosis) in Canada. He was aware of the risk of importation of disease and warned the Dominion Ministry of Agriculture; in 1875 he was appointed Executive Director (1876–1902) to oversee the livestock quarantine station established on Point Levis, Quebec. This was the first in the Western Hemisphere and kept Canada free from the plagues that decimated cattle in Europe (Mitchell 1939, pp. 255–258). In 1881 he had helped found the Cochrane Ranche in Alberta. When the MVC closed in 1903 he remained active in cattle ranching until 1909 when he retired to import and breed Clydesdale horses on his model stock farm at Ormstown, Quebec, dying there in 1924 (Vokaty 1979, pp. 149–156).

Veterinary Education Is Established in the USA

In 1870 the USA had an estimated 124 graduate veterinarians, about 50% came from England and Scotland, 30% from Canada and 20% from the New York City Colleges. By 1884 the total number had grown to about 500, of which 46% were from US colleges, 42% from Canada and 12% from England, Scotland, France and Germany (Miller 1981, pp. 583–593). In spite of the problems experienced by the succession of private colleges in New York they effectively halted the dependence on foreign migrants and diminished the importance of the Canadian schools.

The 26 privately owned colleges greatly aided the creation of the US profession. From the establishment of the first, the Veterinary College of Philadelphia in 1852, to the closure of the last, the United States College of Veterinary Surgeons, Washington, DC in 1927, an estimated 9388 veterinarians were graduated. Of these 58.3% came from three institutions – the Chicago Veterinary College 24.7%, the Kansas City (Mo) Veterinary College 19.8% and the McKillip Veterinary College,

Chicago 13.8%. In 1862 the Morrill Land-Grant Agricultural College Act was passed and veterinarians began to head up veterinary science departments. By the early 1880s 22 of the Land-Grant agricultural colleges had a veterinary science professor (Miller 1981, pp. 583–593).

The Scottish Graduates and the United States Schools

The Chicago Veterinary College, one of the most successful private schools with the largest share of total graduates, was founded in 1883 by Joseph Hughes MRCVS, an 1882 Glasgow Veterinary School graduate. The College produced 2397 graduates, including A D Melvin, Bureau of Animal Industry (BAI) Head 1906–1918, before its closure in 1920 (Smithcors 1975, p. 134). The McKillip Veterinary College (1892–1920) also in Chicago founded by A McKillip, a graduate of Andrew Smith in Ontario, produced 1212 graduates – almost 40% of the private school graduates received a Scottish based education.

The Land-Grant colleges, led by Iowa State Agricultural College in 1879, became the main providers of veterinary education. Cornell University, (Ithaca, New York) started as the New York State Land-Grant college in 1865, introducing veterinary lectures in 1868. Ezra Cornell instructed Dickson White, the Principal, to visit Europe in 1868 to hire a 'horse doctor'. In Scotland he met John Gamgee who recommended James Law, an 1857 Edinburgh graduate. Law returned to Cornell with him and started teaching: the veterinary faculty was formed in 1896. He enforced high admission standards for students and instituted, unique at that time, a four-year course. Only four students met his standards before 1896, these included D E Salmon and F L Kilborne. Later graduates included Cooper Curtice, Leonard Pearson and Theobald Smith, who all went on to become leaders in the profession. James Law was the most influential veterinarian in the USA in the late 19th and early 20th centuries. His inspirational approach to both comparative medicine and public health was responsible for establishing Cornell's reputation as one of the world's leading veterinary colleges. Law published *The Farmers' Veterinary Advisor* in 1876.

Harvard University, Boston, the oldest US University, also established a veterinary degree course and hired Charles Parker Lyman MRCVS in 1882, a graduate of the New Edinburgh Veterinary College (John Gamgee's school). He established a high quality standard of education, soon becoming recognised as one of the best. However, the Veterinary Department closed in 1902, the principle reason was the burgeoning of the 26 low-cost, low-fee proprietary veterinary schools which attracted students (these also affected the MVC). The closure was described as,

> *an ugly blot on the escutcheon of veterinary medicine in America for such a school to close when so many illegitimate institutions remain open and prosper. (Miller 1981, pp. 583–593).*

The 1914–1918 war affected student enrolment and the depression years of the 1920s–1930s finally ended the private proprietary schools; the later post-1939–1945 war expansion was in the Land-Grant colleges, thus separating human and veterinary medicine centres. Most US veterinary schools are in rural locations unlike Europe where the main colleges have maintained an urban, and close to human medical, connection.

National Disease Control and Eradication

As the livestock population increased and a meat packing industry developed, railroad transport links grew, and the deficiencies in disease control became obvious, but solutions only appeared to a limited degree, in certain States. The definitive moment came in 1884 when the BAI was created with D E Salmon in charge – the BAI was responsible for saving the livestock industry from disaster. There were five major problems.

Bovine Pleuro-pneumonia

Introduced from Europe in 1843 and again in 1847 and was soon widespread. Massachusetts State created a Cattle Commission in 1860, instituted slaughter and disease stamped out by 1864, but it still existed in other States. John Gamgee from England was asked to investigate in 1871, but James Law stated that national legislation and slaughter of infected animals was the only solution. The BAI had limited funds and staff, but in March 1887 extra funds were granted, this enabled the purchase and destruction of infected cattle in a major Illinois outbreak. Slowly other States acted and total eradication was achieved by 1892.

Texas Fever

This disease had long been recognised but not understood. The North Carolina Laws in 1766 were the first legislation introduced to control cattle movement. James Mease reported his extensive study in 1826 but could not identify the cause of the disease. More controls on cattle drives were serious for the stockmen who had commented on the cattle tick burden from about 1830. It was F L Kilborne, directed by Salmon, who proved that the tick was the cause, followed by Theobald Smith at BAI who found the blood-borne protozoan. Next Cooper Curtice worked out the life-cycle and proposed control measures. Dip usage began in 1895, then Mark Francis in Texas worked on improving dips and later, with J W Connaway, first specifically identified the *Boophilus bovis* tick as the transmitter and *Babesia spp.* as the parasite, and developed successful immunisation techniques. Gradually the problem of Tick Fever was controlled (Dethloff and Dyal 1991, pp. 22–37).

Hog Cholera (Swine Fever)

This was first noted in 1833, then as the railroad network grew the increased movement of pigs spread the disease rapidly. There was much confusion and debate as to the cause. It was thought to be bacterial until the viral agent was identified by E A Schweinitz and Marion Dorset working at BAI. Soon an effective antiserum was available and later vaccines. The disease was finally eradicated in 1932.

Foot-and-Mouth Disease

This disease occurred sporadically when introduced from Europe in both cattle and pigs. There were serious outbreaks in 1870, 1880, 1884 and the early 1900s. Under guidance to the States from the BAI the disease was eradicated in 1932. In the 1940s the disease became active in Mexico: joint US/Mexico cooperation controlled the outbreak and the southern US border was fenced to prevent cattle movements.

Bovine tuberculosis

This disease had a long history and little control until in 1895 when Theobald Smith and Salmon at BAI proved the infectiveness of the bovine bacteria to man. Public health considerations became prominent and a BAI Tuberculosis Eradication Division was set up in 1917, with final eradication of the disease occurring by 1940. However, sporadic cases still occur in some States.

Salmon had made the BAI a leading veterinary research organisation, he left in 1905 after 21 years and was succeeded by A D Melvin until 1918, and J H Mohler until 1943. In that year, the BAI was absorbed into the United States Department of Agriculture (USDA) as the Agricultural Research Service; it had had a remarkably successful 59-year record and had also worked on rabies, dourine, glanders and equine influenza. The voluminous BAI annual reports from 1885 to 1911 demonstrate a record of progress. The USDA issued Special Reports on animal diseases in 1881, 1890 and 1904, these were probably the first US reliable and authoritative textbooks.

The Early Spanish School in Mexico

The conquest by Spain of the territory now known as Mexico was followed by extensive granting of large areas of land, known as *haciendas,* by the Spanish Crown and the Church to reward certain individuals. These haciendas were invariably enormous in extent and in the control they provided for their owners. The land barons had little interest in animal health, horses were their main interest. Spain did have a veterinary culture with practitioners termed *albeytars*, following the tradition of their Moorish predecessors. They had acceptable expertise in horse medicine and farriery.

In 1853, by presidential decree a veterinary school was established near Mexico City attached to the agricultural school. A four-year course of 19 subjects was created including riding instruction and teaching in English and German, as there were no suitable Spanish textbooks. The total emphasis was on horses, mules and donkeys: Mexico had few railways and very poor roads; the equine was essential for transport and for the army. There were 330 graduates recorded between 1862–1934, these were state employees and either joined the army or the public hygiene service in slaughterhouses and dairies. There were few private practitioners, and the hacienda owners had few concerns (López et al. 2003, p. 87).

The political and economic climate was disruptive with war in 1911–1915 and a social revolution in 1934: following this the hacienda land was distributed to the local population. The veterinary school struggled through these years. In 1955 it was moved into the University City structure and in 1965 began an educational update aided by Food and Agricultural Organisation (FAO) (United Nations) funding.

References

Anon (1858) Progress in Veterinary Science in Philadelphia. *Porter's Spirit of the Times* New York, issue of 15th June

Arbura, J.M. (1934) History of Veterinary Medicine in the United States. *Journal American Veterinary Association* **38**

Bierer, J. (1955) The Validity of Psychiatric Diagnostics: A Suggestion for a New Approach. *International Journal of Social Psychiatry* 1 No. 1

Campbell, D.M. (1934) Development of Veterinary Medicine in North America, Parts I and II. *Veterinary Medicine* **29**

Clewlow, J (2012) An Unrecorded Treatise on the Disorders of Horned Cattle. *Veterinary History* **16**

Dethloff, H.C. and Dyal, D.H. (1991) *A Special Kind of Doctor*. College Station, TX: Texas A & M Press

Eby, C.H. (1960) Sir William Osler and Veterinary Medicine. *Journal of Small Animal Practice* **1**

Jennings, R (1884) The Early History of Veterinary Medicine and Surgery in the United States. *Journal of Comparative Medicine and Surgery* **5**

Jones, B.V. (2014) First Qualified Veterinarians to Practice in the United States of America. *Veterinary History* **17** No.3

Liautard, A. (1877) History and Progress of Veterinary Medicine. *American Veterinary Review* **1**

López, G.G., Alvarez, R.M. and Abarca, F.A. (2003) President A.L. de Santa Ana Decree, Establishing a Veterinary School added to the Agriculture School on August 17, 1853, in *Proceedings of the 34th International Congress of Veterinary Medicine*. Mexico City: División Educación

Merillat, L.A. and Campbell, D.M. (1935) *Veterinary Military History of the United States: with a Brief Record of the Development of Veterinary Education, Practice, Organization and Legislation.* Chicago, IL: Veterinary Magazine Corp.

Miller, E.B. (1981) Private Veterinary Colleges in the United States, 1852–1927. *Journal American Veterinary Medical Association* **178**

Miller, E.B. (1988) 19th Century Origins of the American Veterinary Medical Association, with Special Reference to Education. *Veterinary Heritage* **11**

Mitchell, C.A. (1938) A Note on the Early History of Veterinary Science in Canada. *Canadian Journal of Comparative Medicine* **2**

Mitchell, C.A. (1939) A Note on the Early History of Veterinary Science in Canada: Duncan McEachran. *Canadian Journal of Comparative Medicine* **3**

Pringle, R.O. (1869) *Veterinary Papers by Professor Dick.* Edinburgh: Blackwood

Saunders, L.Z. (1987) From Osler to Olafson. The Evolution of Veterinary Pathology in North America. *Canadian Veterinary Journal* **51**

Smith, D.F. (2010a) 150th Anniversary of Veterinary Education and the Veterinary Profession in North America. *Journal of Veterinary Medical Education* **37**

Smith, D.F. (2010b) 150th Anniversary of Veterinary Education and the Veterinary Profession: Part 2. *Journal of Veterinary Medical Education* **38**

Smith, F. (1976a) *The Early History of Veterinary Literature*, Vol. 3. London: J.A. Allen

Smith, F. (1976b) *The Early History of Veterinary Literature*, Vol 4. London: J.A. Allen

Smithcors, J.F. (1959) Medical Men and the beginnings of Veterinary Medicine in America. *Bulletin History of Medicine* **33**

Smithcors, J.F. (1960) Retrospect on some Anglo-American Relationships in Veterinary Medicine. *British Veterinary Journal* **112**

Smithcors, J.F. (1975) *The Veterinarian in America 1625–1975.* Santa Barbara, CA: American Veterinary Publications

Vokaty, S. (1979) The Adventures of Dr Duncan McNab McEachran in Western Canada. *Canadian Veterinary Journal* **20**

CHAPTER 16

From the 19th to the 21st Centuries

The establishment of education was the cardinal factor in the evolution of veterinary medicine. It produced dedicated colleges which graduated students who had acquired knowledge, and the ability to add to this. It also created the basis of a profession to utilise that discipline. Part III should be read for greater details on many of the developments cited in this overview chapter.

The 19th Century

Veterinary medicine was now in a position to build a science base and to define itself as a distinct medical discipline. Europe had many veterinary schools and they were also developing in North America. Both clinicians and teachers were now able to examine cases of disease, study causation, describe pathology and gain understanding. The quality and number of students was growing and a veterinary press was starting: journals appearing in many countries. To this date the main role of clinicians was to find a treatment, medicament advertising invariably promised a 'cure'. This was the century that human smallpox inoculation became acceptable and widely used. It was copied, with some success to control sheep pox, and was tried unsuccessfully for many other diseases. It was not until 1879 that the main veterinary event of the 19th century occurred – Louis Pasteur and vaccines.

Louis Pasteur (1822–1895) the French chemist and biologist discovered the methods of microbial fermentation, pasteurisation and vaccination. His studies disproved the belief in spontaneous generation and supported the germ theory of disease. At the same time Ferdinand Cohn (1828–1898) botanist and bacteriologist, and Robert Koch (1843–1910) bacteriologist were working. These three men established the discipline of bacteriology, and Pasteur that of immunology. His first experiments in 1879 produced a fowl cholera vaccine, followed by vaccines for anthrax and swine erysipelas and in 1885 a rabies vaccination method for humans. This work was to dramatically improve the capability of veterinary medicine – in the next 100 years many diseases were brought under control through vaccination programmes and immunology research becomes a most productive science.

The opening of the London College near the end of the 18th century was to be of importance not only in Britain, but also in the introduction of veterinary medicine to

North America, Australasia, India and much of Africa (Pattison 1984). Some of the more important British personalities involved in this expansion are identified below. (See also Smith (1976) for further detail.)

William Moorcroft (1767–1825) was an English surgeon who went to the Lyon School in 1790 and became the first British veterinarian. He built a successful London practice, rejected the Professor post at the London College after Sainbel's death, went to India to work and was later killed during exploration in the Himalayas.

Edward Coleman (1765–1839) was an English surgeon who was appointed Professor at the London College following Sainbel's death. He had no veterinary knowledge, yet at the age of 28 years he had charge of the only veterinary school in Britain, a post he held until his death 45 years later. He had also acquired the position as advisor to the military and therefore controlled the army veterinary intake. He did not leave a good legacy, education in his years was both of poor quality and solely devoted to the horse.

Delabere Pritchett Blaine (1770–1845) was born in London, the son of a clergyman. He was apprenticed to a surgeon working in hospitals and then in 1792 was appointed as assistant to Sainbel at the London College, probably had a disagreement with Sainbel and left. He set up his own country veterinary practice, joined the army as Assistant-Surgeon and later left for medical practice. After several more changes he started a London veterinary practice in 1802 and also promoted his publishing programme which included the books: *The Anatomy of the Horse* (?1796); *Domestic Treatise on the Diseases of Horses and Dogs* 1800; *A Concise Description of the Distemper in Dogs* 1800; *The Outlines of the Veterinary Art* 1802. Not every book was an advance, some of the early editions contained errors but others were commendable, in particular his work on distemper in dogs. His practice grew, he met William Youatt and they became partners, operating from their two separate practices. Blaine was guilty of promoting his medicines (and sales agents) and he was ostracised by the Veterinary College. When he retired in 1817 he was seeing up to 3000 dogs a year, had a lucrative horse practice, and significant wealth. *Canine Pathology* was published after retirement and has been recognised as a 'masterly study'. Blaine also wrote on other subjects: he was a gifted writer.

William Dick (1793–1866) was a Scottish farrier's son and a student at the London College. He graduated in 1818 with a very poor opinion of Professor Coleman and the knowledge that he could teach a better course. After some trials he built his own veterinary school in Edinburgh in 1833. He received local encouragement and the venture was successful with its own certification of graduates. He was a hard worker, a good teacher and was loved by his students, but he also developed enemies, whom he rarely forgave. While his clinical work was excellent some of his views, in particular those on epizootic diseases, were surprisingly ignorant. His graduates went on to become many of the leaders for the veterinary schools in North America, Australia and New Zealand; he had many publications, mainly in veterinary periodicals.

William Youatt (1776–1847) was the son of an English surgeon, educated for the ministry. Any reasons for why he left the Church and commenced veterinary studies are unknown. Youatt studied under Blaine who encouraged him to enrol as a student at the London College. He did this in 1813 while still working with Blaine, but Coleman, knowing of his friendship with Blaine drove him out of the College and he never graduated. Youatt went on to set up his own practice, near Blaine, and the two entered into partnership until Blaine retired in 1817. The practice mostly treated dogs and horses with a little cattle work (London had some 12,000 cattle in its dairies). He was much involved with rabies control. Youatt was interested in all livestock and their diseases, and continually regretted that the College did not teach the subject. When the Royal Agricultural Society was formed in 1838 he joined, was placed on the Council and pressed for more livestock tuition of veterinary students, until eventually a lecturer was appointed. In 1828 Youatt opened his own school to lecture, it was a success but in 1834 it closed due to his ill health. In 1828 the first English veterinary periodical, *The Veterinarian*, commenced and Youatt began a friendship with William Percivall, the founder. He contributed articles and soon began to share the editorship. In 1830 Youatt commenced the monumental task of writing a series of books on the history, breeds, management and diseases of animals. He produced five books: *The Horse* in 1831, *Cattle* in 1834, *The Sheep* in 1837, *The Dog* in 1845 and *The Pig* in 1847. The first was by far the most successful with many editions in Britain and the United States of America (USA), and in wide use up to the end of the century. This is the briefest of summaries of a complex life but Youatt's contribution to the British veterinary profession was enormous and his international influence significant. He was much criticised, but was usually proved to be right.

William Percivall (1792–1854) was the son of the Senior Veterinary Surgeon to the Ordnance at Woolwich, London. He entered the London College and graduated in 1811. In 1812 he also joined the army until 1816, when he took a medical qualification. In 1823 Percivall published the first volume of his *Series of Elementary Lectures on the Veterinary Art*. In 1828 he launched *The Veterinarian* periodical; the objective was to update and modernise veterinary work and the College. Further books appeared always in a well-written educational manner; they were widely read in the United Kingdom (UK) and North America. He built a good friendship with Youatt, they wanted the College to reform, but Coleman was unhelpful. Percivall received no recognition or honour for his work but has to be remembered for his efforts to continue the education of the profession after they had graduated.

William Haycock (1818–1872) was an Edinburgh 1842 graduate from Dick's Edinburgh College. He became known for the accurate observation of his patients and his frequent contributions to *The Veterinarian*, as well as several books. In one, titled *Elements of Veterinary Homeopathy* and published in 1852, Haycock was unusual in that he discussed this practice rather than condemning it, as most medical authorities had done. His interest was in the requirement of the careful clinical examination of the patient, he believed the homeopathic remedies would probably do no good, but importantly they would do no harm, unlike so many treatments then in use. He deplored the amount of bleeding undertaken and urged the use of more humane and gentle methods of treatment.

Edward Mayhew (d.1868), a member of the Mayhew brothers (one was the first editor of the celebrated *Punch* magazine). Initially in the theatrical profession, he enrolled at the London College and was an excellent student graduating in 1845. He wrote well and published frequently. His most important contributions were the introduction of the use of the nasally introduced stomach tube to administer fluids to the horse, and instructions on how to pass the catheter in the dog; he also wrote some of the earliest reports on the use of ether as an anaesthetic in 1847 and on the use of ether and chloroform as an anodyne in 1848. His illustrated study, *The Horse's Mouth, showing the Age by the Teeth* published in 1849, was probably his most important work. Mayhew also wrote in 1857 a condemnation of the sale of meat from diseased animals, and the existence of London dairies. He was a brilliant artist and has left many examples of his work. He also wrote several plays which were performed on the London stage; he was a versatile and talented man.

John Gamgee (1881–1894) was a member of a remarkable family. His father Joseph was an 1823 London graduate with a great thirst for knowledge who established a practice in Florence, Italy. Joseph prospered and educated his eight children: one son became a leading surgeon, another a physiological chemist and John a veterinary surgeon in 1852. After visiting the continental veterinary schools he was offered the Chair of Anatomy and Physiology at Dick's Edinburgh College. The relationship did not work and he left in 1857 and founded The New Veterinary College, in opposition to Dick. He also began, with his brother, a campaign against the sale of diseased meat. In 1865 he moved his College to London renaming it The Albert Veterinary College Ltd. In the same year, the most catastrophic outbreak of rinderpest struck Britain. The College failed in 1868 and Gamgee moved to the USA where the government employed him for a short while as a consultant for one project. He then began to work to develop low temperature technology used for ice skating rinks and for refrigerated meat transportation but died before the work was completed. Gamgee's importance to veterinary medicine was his interest in epizootic animal diseases and his efforts to try to introduce methods of control to combat them. The British authorities ignored his arguments and from 1838 had allowed the ports to freely trade in livestock. He had warned of the potential risk of rinderpest importation but the authorities did not listen. He wrote many books and published *The Edinburgh Veterinary Review* between 1858–1864 in which he campaigned against the sale of diseased meat. Many aspects of his work are now forgotten but he led the way in veterinary progress. Gamgee believed in high standards of education. He was responsible for James Law being selected to start the Cornell Veterinary School and also influenced Duncan McEachran in Montreal. His lasting legacy is that he organised and founded the first International Veterinary Congress at Hamburg in 1863 – which became the World Veterinary Association.

The 19th century in continental Europe was one of positive progress. Pasteur and Koch had opened the bacteriological era, the germ theory was disproved, hygiene better understood and epizootic disease control recognised (Blancou 2003). There was a gradual movement towards improved livestock care but no significant advance in therapeutics. As infection became better understood, not only bacteria but other organisms were also recognised and classified (spirochaetes, protozoa, fungi), and pure cultures produced allowing for closer study. The basic sciences were developing.

Central Europe – Germany and Hungary – became major centres of veterinary research with many notable leaders: R Virchow (1821–1902) pathology and cytopathology; F Loeffler (1852–1915) who discovered the first mammalian pathogenic virus causing foot-and-mouth disease (FMD); P Ehrlich (1854–1915) chemotherapy with Salvarsan; E von Behring (1854–1917) serotherapy and antitoxins; F Hutyra (1860–1934) and J Marek (1868–1952) leading the important Hungarian school of research (Karasszon 1988).

Following the discovery of the FMD virus in 1897 research soon also isolated those causing: rinderpest in 1899; African Horse Sickness, fowl pox and sheep pox in 1900; fowl pest in 1902; swine fever in 1903 and rabies in 1905. In 1893 the first really effective syringe, the Record syringe with a glass cylinder and metal pistol, was invented in Berlin and in 1865 the hygiene field advanced when Joseph Lister (1827–1912) introduced phenol to produce antisepsis in the operating theatre.

The 20th Century

Veterinary medicine had increased its knowledge and science base, but at the start of the 20th century it was still an essentially equine occupation. There was a gradual broadening of species involvement and narrowing by specialty interest, as private schools closed and the state and universities took over the role of veterinary education.

The integrated schools and also state-funded institutions provided an environment for the performance of veterinary research. This produced increased investment by developed countries, in particular to aid eradication of the main livestock plagues: rinderpest, bovine pleuro-pneumonia, FMD, glanders, anthrax, sheep pox, swine fever. All of these were eradicated or brought under a measure of control in the 20th century, first in Europe and North America followed by Australia and New Zealand and by many programmes in colonial territories, as these moved to independence in the later 1900s.

Due to the 1914–1918 war, the depression years and the 1939–1945 war, the real growth occurred from the middle of the century. A veterinary need was seen globally; in the developed world this also saw the practice interest move to companion animals and the student gender to female. In the less developed regions of the world the veterinary need was to control epizootic diseases in livestock, and then to aid healthy food production. The establishment of the United Nations in 1945 led to the creation of its FAO whose veterinary section was vitally important in progressing this work.

These radical transformations in veterinary education, research and practice happened against a continually moving background of social, economic and political change. Steam, motorised and jet transport, shifting demands and fortunes in agriculture and rising disposable income all resulted in a changing emphasis in species care. Another transformation was in the role of the army: in 1900 it was an important outlet for veterinary work for the maintenance of both cavalry and transport horses. This rose to its zenith with a peak of demand in the 1914–1918 war with the horrendous loss of some eight million equines, not in their traditional cavalry role, most of these were lost in providing backup to trench warfare. The 1939–1945 war saw the army service active again, mainly with mules. By 2000 the veterinary military focus was changing to the use of dogs for defence, tracking and detection, and food inspection as well as chemical, nuclear and biological warfare interests. Additionally the ranks now included female veterinary officers.

As a direct result of veterinary intervention, disease control was the major factor in the growth of the dairy, pig and poultry industries (these latter two becoming the main meat sources). Beef and, to a lesser degree, sheep output also showed significant improvements. As equine practice declined, the profession gained a more extensive role in the previously small livestock sector. This trend advanced in the 1930s, but it was the war of 1939–1945 and the post-war years that highlighted the need for improved national livestock production. This demonstrated the important role that, aided by new technical resources, veterinary clinical and research inputs could play. Veterinary expertise developed swiftly with the recognition of biosecurity needs: specialist farm units expanded both in size and intensive production output. In developed countries this changed practice operations, while practitioner numbers fell in the livestock sector, the specialisation level leapt ahead with a consequent ability to understand and control herd and flock health. Veterinary practice changed to meet the demand for small animal care.

Public and state services expanded during the first two-thirds of the century: major diseases were controlled, specific vaccines produced and effective prevention procedures devised. An enlarged veterinary role grew in meat hygiene and public health activities as well as increasing numbers employed in welfare societies, caring for dogs, cats, horses and other species. A new area of practice also developed in wildlife conservation, in Africa in particular. The veterinary role continued to expand in many directions.

Before 1935, in specific medication terms, the veterinary profession (as in human medicine) could do relatively little for many of their patients. Surgery was limited to mostly external procedures in livestock and horses with some internal operations in dogs and cats; anaesthesia (usually chloroform or ether) was a risky procedure – apart from morphine and these early anaesthetics there was little else one could do except to treat symptoms. Apart from calcium borogluconate injection for milk fever there were virtually no specific medications, none for the serious bacterial infections or normal disorders and few effective parasiticides.

A transformational change in treatment of bacterial infections began with the introduction of the sulphonamides in the 1930s and then penicillin in the late 1940s. These antibacterials and antibiotics revolutionised the treatment of many conditions in all species; wound treatments, mastitis in dairy cattle and systemic bacterial diseases were all treatable and curable. These were followed by a stream of discoveries from pharmaceutical innovators with corticosteroids, hormones, anaesthetic agents, endo and ectoparasiticides. Later behaviour-modifying, geriatric specifics and cancer control agents were introduced together with enhanced nutritional understanding being gained in all species and the development of specific dietary foods for dogs and cats.

The use of biological products developed early in the century: state veterinary departments produced biologicals to control epizootics then moved to brucellosis, swine erysipelas, swine fever and sheep vaccines, together with tuberculin and mallein diagnostics. From the early 1960s targets expanded rapidly in viruses, rickettsia and even parasites. Innovation and extension continued at an incredible rate, boosted by advances in biotechnology, in particular in the last quarter of the century. In this period genetic knowledge was also expanded by unravelling the genome of the major species and the infective agents, with the promise of a multiformity of advances.

With this expansion in pharmaceuticals and medications came a similar increase of surgical techniques, imaging procedures, diagnostic and other technologies, mostly derived from advances in human medicine. Advances in surgery in all species – in particular with dogs, cats and horses – and the associated aftercare and intensive care came to dominate the public perception of veterinary activity. It appeared that any procedure that could be performed on the human, with the most advanced methods, could be duplicated in animals and was expected; cost became almost the only limiting factor.

The evolution of the veterinary hospital started in the USA with purpose-built premises for all species, but mostly for dogs, cats and equines. By the 1990s, however, it had become the characteristic of clinical practice in the developed countries. Management of the veterinary practice developed as a business, operated with financial expertise to control cash flow and dealing with increasing regulatory controls. Pet insurance became important and could be said to have helped in the development of expensive procedures and technologies. House calls were a rarity by the end of the century. Animal ambulances were becoming common: the well-equipped hospital with available specialist referral centres became the norm. However, the growth of corporate owned veterinary practice chains had already become significant in North America and Europe by the end of the century, hinting of important changes in financing and ownership of veterinary practice in the future. A useful review and documentation of the British veterinary scene 1791–1948 has been written by Pattison (1984).

The 21st Century

The 20th century was when the veterinary art fully emerged as a science. It now entered the new century having made incredible advances but also facing many issues. The veterinary practitioner in 1800 or 1900, in both cases usually a single-handed man with his work keyed around the horse and the forge, would have been unable to comprehend practice in 2000. In the developed world this was small animal work in a well-equipped hospital with facilities, staff, proficient referral services and in many cases business management targets. In fact this had not been a gradual evolution, the same could be said for the 1950s graduate. It was in the last 30–40 years of the 20th century that the change came, and the 21st century seems to be developing with as many changes ahead. For the history records, an important event was the total eradication of rinderpest, declared in 2011. Notable as only the second disease to be so controlled (smallpox being the first) but a demonstration of what can be achieved with technological advance and global cooperation.

This is a history book, not a fortune-tellers guide, however events cast shadows that can often aid prediction of the future. The 21st century has opened with a recognition that antibiotic usage must be restricted due to the emergence of multi-resistant bacteria and a lack of new effective antibacterials. A greater emphasis has to be given to preventive measures to control infectious disease by employing enhanced hygiene and biosecurity. The previous century's rapid development of new pharmaceuticals has slowed, much of this due to the ever-rising cost of research (and the need to satisfy regulatory requirements). Genetic and genome studies could indicate the use of more effective vaccines, and possibly 'engineered' livestock to reduce the claimed polluting effect of ruminants. In these early years of the century it is not easy to see the outcome of the climate change threat. The possible global spread of African Swine Fever could also be a harbinger of what is to come.

Clinical practice remains the main role of the veterinarian, but with the female gender now, in many major countries, representing some 80% of student intake heralding a change in practice ownership: women prefer to have a more flexible life pattern and so practices become increasingly owned by corporate entities. Will this change the client/veterinarian relationship, and what service or services the practice will offer?

Education becomes increasingly sophisticated, and costly. Now that the majority of practitioners in the increasingly urban world deal with companion animals, will the state consider it is still their role to finance their training? Livestock production increasingly moves into larger corporate structures with highly evolved units for producing pig and poultry meat, milk and in some countries beef. Intensive livestock production brings many concerns, not just health, but also animal welfare. This topic will grow in importance, for the farming units and also for livestock shipment, and certain slaughter practices. Animal understanding and welfare will advance as a veterinary interest and will gain more public support. Increasing concerns about the welfare and slaughter of livestock, processing meats and a desire for 'naturally produced foods' together with vegetarian and vegan beliefs may have an effect on production – and the need for veterinary support. In the less developed regions of Africa, Latin America and Asia there remains a veterinary challenge in controlling and eradicating disease, as well as improving the health of livestock.

Two lessons can be learned from the history of veterinary medicine. The first is the 'wild card' effect – disease is frequently totally unpredictable and can produce catastrophic effects requiring an urgent response. The second is the one sure factor that veterinary medicine needs and practices in the future will not be the same as today.

References

Blancou, J. (2003) *History of the Surveillance and Control of Transmissible Animal Diseases.* Paris: Office International des Épizooties

Karasszon, D. (1988) *A Concise History of Veterinary Medicine.* Budapest: Akademiai Kiado

Pattison, I. (1984) *The British Veterinary Profession 1791–1948.* London: J A Allen

Smith, F. (1976) *The Early History of Veterinary Literature, Vol III.* London: J A Allen

PART III

Domestication, Utilisation and Disease Histories

CHAPTER 17

Equine: Horse, Donkey and Mule

Following considerable discussion on nomenclature, it has now been accepted that the horse is a member of the *Equidae* taxonomic family, genus *Equus*. The domesticated horse is named *Equus ferus caballus*, one of the two extant subspecies of *Equus ferus*, the other being *Equus ferus przewalskii* the only true wild horse, still surviving in a small number in Mongolia, and also in zoological collections.

Of the six other members of the genus only one is domesticated, the ass or donkey, *Equus asinus*. The others are three varieties of the zebra, the kiang (wild ass of Tibet) and the onager or hemione (Asiatic wild ass now only found in arid areas of Iran and central Asia). All members of the genus can interbreed and this ability has been used by humans to create the mule, a cross between a male donkey (a jack) and a mare, or rarely a cross between a stallion and a female donkey (a jenny) to produce a hinny. These hybrids are usually sterile.

Domestication of the horse was achieved after the other species, all of which served a purpose for their guard or herding abilities or for the provision of hides and wool. It is not known when riding was first attempted, but domestication for draught work commenced around or before 3500 BC in central Asia. The horse was soon placed in a different category to livestock. An animal–human relationship developed, but not in the same way as with the dog who became a home companion.

The derivation of the word 'horse' is not very clear. The Old English was *hors*, from the Old Frisian *hors*, *hars* or *hers*; the Old Saxon *hros* or *hers*; Old German *rus*, *ors* or *ross*; Old Norse *hross* and Proto-Germanic *hrussa* or *hrass*. In current languages the North European words are German *pferd*, Dutch *paard* and Swedish *häst*. South European words are French *cheval*, Spanish *caballo* and Italian *cavallo*. Derivation of other horse-related words is much clearer from the Latin *equus* and Greek *hippos*.

Horses are given a variety of names depending on their age: males and females under one-year-old are foals and between one and two years they are yearlings. A male under four-years-old is a colt and a female a filly. A female over four-years-old is a mare. An uncastrated male over four-years-old is a stallion and a castrated male is a gelding. These terms may vary in the racing world in some countries.

Natural History and Biology

Belonging to the order Perissodactyla, the horse is described as a solid-hoofed perissodactyl ungulate mammal. The hoof is a modified claw covering the original third toe, the others have disappeared but a vestigial form of the second and third toes is sometimes observed. The top of the toe is surrounded by cartilage and the interior walls by highly vascular laminae. The keratin cover of the hoof grows continually and needs to be trimmed; if shod the shoes need to be reset at regular intervals.

The equine skeleton follows the basic mammalian structure except that it does not possess an equivalent to the human collarbone: the forelimbs are attached to the spinal column by strong muscles and ligaments. The feet and limbs are the most important and defining characteristics of equine anatomy: their structure enables the speed of movement. The horse is a prey animal that has developed a rapid response ability to move quickly and outrun predators: they have a good sense of balance. Four basic types of motion are used: walk, trot, canter and gallop, each entails a different sequence and speed of leg movements. Horses are herbivores with teeth adapted for grazing, with 12 incisors, and 24 premolars and molars. The interdental space between incisors and molars is where the bit is placed, enabling pressure to be put on the gums and tongue. The alimentary tract has a one-chambered stomach and an enlarged caecum for the fermentation of cellulose. This is inferior to the ruminant and makes feeding a horse more expensive (Bokonyi 1984, p. 163).

Lifespan is determined by several factors but can reach 40 years. Gestation period is between 11 and 11.5 months, twin foals are rare. The oestrus cycle of the mare is about 21 days from spring to autumn and lasts three to seven days. Foals are capable of standing and running shortly after birth and are usually weaned from the mare at about six months of age. Sexual maturity in domestic horses is reached in about three years. This is the usual time to commence breeding domesticated animals, but the ability to breed might occur earlier. The horse has a chromosome diploid number of 64 (the ass has 62 chromosomes). The genome was mapped in 2007 and shown to comprise 2.7 billion base pairs (linked nucleobases): this is smaller than that of the human or bovine, but larger than the dog.

Species Domesticated

The two domesticated species are the common horse *Equus ferus caballus* and the ass or donkey *Equus asinus* together with their crosses, the mule and hinny. The domesticated horse spread to many regions of Asia, Europe and Africa but only reached the Americas and Australasia following European colonisation. The ass was probably domesticated in north-east Africa, in the Nile valley then spreading to Mesopotamia and Asia, and later to Europe.

Horses have been subjected to more training (taming) discipline than any other animal. It is difficult therefore to evaluate their inborne intelligence. It has been remarked that the intelligence of any individual horse reflects the intelligence of the trainer. As a species they are naturally curious and are able to resolve problems and learn. As animals of habit they react well to regular routines and regimentation and as herd animals they are hierarchical and recognise a leader, more usually a mare.

Domestication and utilisation of the horse as identified from archaeological evidence has been dated to around 3500 BC in both the southern Ukraine and on the central Asian steppes in Kazakhstan and Turkmenistan. These first animals were small, compared with the present-day breeds. Complete domestication is estimated to have been achieved by 3000 BC and widespread distribution in Europe by 2000 BC. Many different breeds developed depending on locality, but there are two major types – riding and draught animals. These two types have then each diversified into many specific breeds: the riding type are selected for speed, for both personal transport or pleasure and are of a lighter weight and form; the draught animals became heavier and slower and usually with a much quieter temperament. One of the most important developments in equine use was when the Hittites developed a lightweight, spoke-wheeled chariot to be drawn by one or two horses – these revolutionised warfare. The horse grew in importance in its evolution starting from the Eurasian steppes, moving to Mesopotamia, then to the Near East and also into mainland Europe. With its utilisation in chariots and then the development of cavalry by Alexander the Great, the horse became an important weapon of war.

A characteristic and significant feature of the horse is the variation in hair colour, there is no standard colour for most breeds. The genetics of colour and the early history of the horse and ass are discussed by Mason (1984, pp. 162–184) and Zeuner (1963, pp. 299–337 and 367–383).

DOMESTICATED HORSES AND CULTURAL GROUPS

A study of nearly 5000 of the earliest animal images, painted in caves in France and Spain, has dated these from between 30,000 to about 12,000 years ago. Bison, mammoths, ibex and wild ox all feature but a special place was given to the horse, whose images were placed in high and visible locations as if to symbolically signify that the horse was the leader.

The earliest domesticated animals were small, about pony size, but with the conformation of a horse. They were the last main species to be domesticated probably with first use for draught, as they were faster than oxen, and later riding. Archaeological evidence of broken bones and opened skulls suggest that they were also eaten (a practice that lasted until Roman times, ending in most of Europe with the end of the empire). The first deliberate horse selection and breeding appears to have begun in the broad region of Anatolia, north Iraq, Iran and into the steppes.

Ancient Times

Domesticated horses are known by bas-relief sculptures in Mesopotamia from the 3rd millennium BC. Just before the 2nd millennium, horse drawn spoke-wheeled chariots were in use for war in the Near East (and 18th Dynasty Egypt). The introduction of the spoked-wheeled chariot gave armies strategic mobility, and improved wagons which helped trade. Chariots then appear in Mycenaean art but mounted men are rarely observed in either Mycenaean or Egyptian art. Cavalry begin to be seen in later Assyrian depictions (Hornblower and Spawforth 2003, p. 728).

In the Iron Age the final wave of the Asian horses from Southern Russia reached Europe. It is believed that the Scythians, possibly the first to ride horses, invented the saddle and had sturdy, reliable horses. These horses were related to the breeds from Persia, where in the 1st millennium BC many types of horse evolved, they were larger and could carry heavier loads. The horse reached cult status in the Persian culture. At roughly the same time a West European breed type, the Celtic horse, was developed. These horses were smaller but were the beginning of the European equestrian tradition. The horse was soon held in esteem and found a place in mythology, with veneration for Epona (Celtic *epos* horse, *ona* on) who was the patron goddess of mares and foals in the Gallo-Roman lands. She protected all equines, as well as being goddess of fertility, and was worshipped in Rome from the 1st to 3rd centuries AD.

Greece

The Homeric epics suggest that chariots were used until the 8th century BC, but mainly for the transportation of fighting men. This changed over the years and horses increasingly became ridden for warfare, hunting and racing. The main use in the Greek world became riding and light draught work. There were two notable early Greek writers on the horse. Xenophon (431–354 BC), his instructions for horse management, hygiene and care are still valid today, he praised Simon of Athens, who predeceased him, for his work. Aristotle (384–322 BC) is remembered as the first veterinary scientist. He wrote extensively on the horse, not only on the gait and movement of the limbs, but also on the ailments. The Greek equine knowledge continued to dominate under the Roman Empire and survived into the Byzantine Empire. In the early years they had recognised horse 'doctors' or *hippiatroi*, a specialist who was not duplicated in the Roman world (see Chapter 2).

Roman Empire

Equines were important animals for the Romans: they aided the growth of their empire. Varro (116–27 BC), a very early author, classified their uses: in war, for transport, for breeding and production of mules, and for chariot racing. Vegetius (c.AD 400–450) emphasised the place of the mule, in his time this was the most important animal in warfare, in the drawing of the wagon train of supplies. Later the army learned the use of cavalry and from this developed the equestrian 'art', much favoured by the upper echelons of Roman society. Horse breeding became a major industry with some regions and countries becoming renowned for their bloodstock. Riding horses were frequently equipped with elaborate saddles, bridle bits and adorned harnesses. Several magnificent bronze equestrian statues have survived, the best known being that of Marcus Aurelius on the Capitoline Hill in Rome (Toynbee 2013, pp. 172–173).

Hunting became popular, both of fierce and dangerous animals such as lions, bears and bulls as well as more timid creatures like deer or foxes. All these exploits were portrayed in mosaic, frequently alongside fish and birds in similar panels. Mules were widely used for draught work in both private commerce, on farms and in the army; special facilities were constructed for their accommodation in the rest stations of the public and imperial *cursus* on the road system. Both horses and mules were sometimes utilised in the gladiatorial shows in the circus. Chariot racing was probably the most widely watched sport and invariably one of fatality for both horses and men. Donkeys were domesticated but were generally poorly treated. Epona was the goddess and patroness of equines and their keeper: she was worshipped in Italy in particular, but also in other lands of the Mediterranean basin. Good husbandry and care was generally practised, but veterinary knowledge was not as good as it was in the Greek world (see Chapters 4 and 5).

EUROPE: FROM MEDIEVAL HORSES TO RACING AND EVENTING

Europe reformed following the Roman years and the horse came to be a dominant influence in society. Its ability to carry a human determined the limits of personal land transport until the introduction of the steam-engine railway in the 1830s. The use of the horse in transport was only effectively replaced when the automobile came into general use in the 20th century: first called the 'horseless' carriage, and always classified by 'horsepower' (Francis 2015, p. 210). From the medieval to the early modern times humans lived in a horse driven society. The horse has always been able to maintain a place in human life, and affection; it has a recognised and respected stately image of beautiful conformation, graceful behaviour and sometimes temperamental.

The Medieval Years

The major factor in the feudal structure were the manors with big houses. These varied in size with the importance of the owner, but a prosperous English household in the 13th century with an annual income of £1000, would have 30–70 horses and 20–30 grooms and valets. This represented the largest department of the house, known as the Marshalsea, which comprised stables, staff and horses. The marshal was in charge and was responsible for household discipline (the name was derived from the French *mareschal* (farrier)) and for organising any events and travel and transport arrangements. Grooms were sometimes called *garciones*. Horses were most important in the Royal households, who would have many animals, each with one groom. In medieval Britain, a bodyguard was known as a 'Horse-thegn'. The warden of the King's horses was known as a 'Horseweard' and he was responsible for both the care of the horses and of the stud – a 'herd' of horses was one of 50 mares. The title changed to Chief Keeper under King John, to King's Farrier for Henry III, and later to Marshal.

An important member of the Marshalsea was the Clerk of the Avenary, he was the purchaser of oats; this was a major household cost. When the household travelled, oats had to be purchased along the route (similar to a petrol station refill). Feeding for the horses was costly and based on oats and hay, except for June and July when fresh mown grass was fed. Beans or bran might be added and for particular occasions horse bread would be baked. There were a variety of breads depending on the needs of the horse – training, pregnancy, or bread for travelling to be carried by the rider: the injunction was always 'water the horse before feeding bread.'

For major households travelling was a frequent event. The Marshal was in charge and led the procession of coaches, wagons and horses. The coaches would include elaborately decorated, four-wheeled conveyances particularly for the ladies. They were usually drawn by four or five dexter horses (who walked and trotted well). These expeditions were to other big houses or to, or with the Royal court.

Veterinary needs were the responsibility of the Marshal (later to become part of the farrier's work). Account books of the time list regular purchases of grease or tallow fat (the common treatment for limb ailments), wort (unfermented ale), lard, garlic, olive oil and plasters. Special breads would be made, often including herbal medications. Honey and butter was purchased for treatment of the palfreys (a more upper-class horse).

By 1066 shoeing had come into general use in much of Europe, but its application varied by the work of the horse, and the cost. It created the role of the farrier. The cost of owning horses grew as saddle and harness makers evolved, and in turn enlarged the leather industry. Similarly the loriners, the makers of stirrups, bits and bells for pack horses in both iron and bronze, became a large trade.

The Role of the Horse

As the years passed and affluence expanded so did the role of the horse, the species became classified into many types. From previously a rough grouping of riding, war and draught animals, a horse for almost every purpose developed: *courser* ideal parade animal; *ambler* a smooth easy gait, by lifting each foot individually; *pacer* a natural gait, later harness racers; *trotter* trained to trot; *hackney* medium-sized, light compact harness horse; *dexter* popular medium size ride; *palfrey* early term for ambler; *hobbies* small size, ponies; *runceys* lower grade riding horses; *nag* small riding horses; *sumpter* pack horse used to carry goods for upper classes; *pack* for movement of goods, in particular bales of cloth or with panniers, coal, bread, or dung; *mail* and *bag* the post horses for mail delivery; *coach* good looking strong horses; *cart* for general haulage, and *great* or *war* horses, big massive animals to carry armour and armoured rider. In turn this produced the 'sport' tournaments and jousting; the competition of two armoured men charging at each other with lances which was popular, but dangerous for both horse and rider.

From these groups evolved the *hunters*, chosen by the riders depending on type of hunt, and later the highly specialised *racehorses*. Horses varied by size, shape, colour and utilisation, there was almost a type for every job: agriculture, transport, building, mining, anywhere where their energy could be utilised by treadmills or pumps. Frequently these animals were badly treated and poorly fed. It was a stratified society from the nobility to the serf, where a person's position determined the 'quality' of their animal (Macgregor 2012, p. 21).

Horse breeding became a major industry – initially the 11th century monasteries were involved – to satisfy an ever growing market which reached its apex in the Victorian age. Colts not selected for breeding were castrated, between the ages of nine days and two years. Horses were mainly sold at the regular horse fairs and markets. Mules and donkeys were generally not considered to be important animals in northern Europe; the donkeys in particular were much used in the Mediterranean world. Ireland was an exception for a while when the English purchased all the horses, then the ecclesiastical community tended to use them more as a gesture to humility. Mules, however, were good as pack animals as used in mule trains.

Equestrianism and the Manège

Horse riding or 'horsemanship' became both a distinguishing feature for the upper classes and an entertaining sport. Following the school started by Federigo Grisone in Naples in 1532 (see Chapter 12) the interest was aroused in England in the time of Henry VIII, and followed by Elizabeth I his daughter, whose Master of the Horse invited Claudio Corte to come to England. The art of virtuoso horsemanship became a popular pursuit. A leader was William Cavendish, Duke of Newcastle (1592–1676) who wrote his influential book *A New Method and Extraordinary Invention to Dress Horses* in 1667. He also constructed a remarkable riding school at Bolsover Castle, which is still perfectly preserved. This practice and pursuit is well described by Edwards (2007, pp. 82–87). The art of the manège, but at a very advanced sophisticated level, is preserved by the Lipizzaner horses in the Spanish Riding School in Vienna, Austria. The breed, originally from Spain in 1700, are bred at the Lipica Stud Farm, Slovenia which was established in 1580.

Horses and Hunting

By AD 1000 hunting had become an exclusive sport for the upper classes in most of Europe, and elsewhere. To hunt required horses, clothes and money. Large tracts of forest were declared Royal or private and used to hunt boar, deer and sometimes wolves, using hounds, nets and men. The first English book on hunting, *The Boke of Seynt Albans* by Dame Juliana Berners published in 1486, is a collection of essays, one on hunting, but with little original content. This was followed by a book attributed to

George Turberville titled *The Noble Art of Venerie* 1575, much of this was based on the classic work by Gaston Phoebus, the *Livre de Chasse* (see Chapter 12).

Racing and Polo

Racing originally began as a two horse contest but by the mid-1500s had acquired the characteristics of modern horseracing, essentially a sprint race for young thoroughbreds with small jockeys. Caliph Mahdi of Baghdad in the 8th century AD is reputed to have laid out the first racetrack for racing (not with chariots) with ten horses in a race. By 1600 Britain had become a leading nation for the breeding of racehorses, and by the early 1700s the sport had become organised (apart from a period under Oliver Cromwell's rule when it was banned). The Jockey Club, formed in 1750, formalised racing procedures in Britain and Newmarket became a racehorse centre. James Weatherby produced his *Introduction to a General Stud Book* in 1791, which became the *General Stud Book* published by Weatherby's since 1793. All pedigree British horses are registered in the Stud Book, based on three Arab horses: the Byerley Turk, the Godolphin Arabian and the Darley Arabian.

Polo is probably almost as old as racing. The game originally started in Persia and came to Britain via army officers from India, with rules formalised in 1875 by the Hurlingham Club. The early game is believed to have been played from 500 BC with a leather ball and long-handled wooden mallets. It was popular in Asia and spread to Byzantium by AD 1100 and to China by the 8th century, where local nobility had specially bred horses (James and Thorpe 1995, p. 556). Recent archaeological evidence also indicates that the game was played by Tang dynasty Chinese noblewomen riding on donkeys.

Horses for Transport

Horses were first used to pull wagons and carry goods. There was always a certain competition between the horse and the ox for draught work. While the horse lacked the pulling power of the ox, it did move faster; however, they cost more to feed, shoe and harness. Ploughing was more suited for horses, with a big animal and an iron plough. In Europe horses first pulled carts, then in about 1560–1570 wagons began to be used to convey passengers. By the 1600s coaches evolved to provide a more comfortable journey. 'Posts', a reliable system of horses to move mail first appeared in France (partly designed on the Roman *cursus publicus* system). Next the Holy Roman Empire in about 1491 introduced a network to carry mail, followed by Britain under Henry VIII in the early 1500s. In Britain, the Postage Act of 1657 made the postal service a government monopoly and by 1835 the service had about 700 mail coaches, said to have been the envy of other countries. Coaches were improved, and regular passenger services introduced when road surfaces enabled faster travel: these created a new industry with coaching inns, and ostlers to handle the horses, including changing them for the fast services.

A dramatic development was the horse bus, or omnibus, first built in Paris by an Englishman, George Shilliber, and then introduced to London in 1829; 25 years later there were 1000 buses on the streets. In the 1860s the first horse trams, used on iron tracks to reduce friction, started in Birkenhead, England, soon to be followed by most other major cities, worldwide. By the death of Queen Victoria in 1901, the largest London bus company had some 1400 omnibuses with about 10,000 horses. Used in shifts, these animals had short working lives, seldom above five years. Horse cabs also became popular, epitomised by the London Hackney cabs. Horse numbers increased when in the later 1800s steam trains operated widely and required horse transport to take people and goods to and from the train stations. This was the peak of the horse era, by the early 1900s motorcars had arrived. The 1914–1918 war is remembered for the years of static trench fighting with the struggle to keep the frontlines supplied. It was horses and mules that provided this resource, and resulted in an appalling loss of equine life, not so much by bullets and bombs but by sheer exhaustion. The war also stimulated the use of motor transport, the use of equines in later wars was much reduced and is now negligible.

Recognition of Equine Diseases

The earliest evidence of equine disease comes from fragments of 7th century BC cuneiform clay tablets found in Assyria: mention is made of horse medications (see Chapter 1). This was followed by tablets excavated at Ugarit in the Levant, dated to c.1500–1300 BC: the fragments detailing the medication of horses by nasal application.

The Years of Antiquity to AD 400

The first known written text on the horse, in Greek by Xenophon (430–354 BC) is *Peri Hippikon*, dealing with horsemanship with an emphasis on management and hygiene. The book is not a veterinary text but does deal with foot care as well as stressing a humane approach to the animal, 'never act with anger towards a horse' (see Chapter 2).

Aristotle (384–322 BC) was the first veterinary scientist. He made many original observations on the gait of the horse, ageing by the teeth and was the first to notice the absence of a gall bladder. In *Historia Animalium* he discusses foot problems, a syndrome termed *ileus* in stabled horses, laminitis, broken wind and *melis*, from his description almost certainly glanders (see Chapter 2).

In his text titled *Universal History* which provides a history of Rome and the Roman world, Polybius (c.200–117 BC) mentions that the horses of Hannibal's army were affected by a disease, while in the forests of Etruria, Italy, that caused the loss of their hoofs. Virgil (70–19 BC) in his poem the *Georgics* describes diseases of horses, in one of which 'the nostrils run black blood', possibly referring to anthrax. Equine medicine in the Roman Empire was essentially derived from Greek authors whose work was pragmatically used by Romans to advance their livestock industries. While these were very important, economically the status of veterinary medicine never reached the level of human medicine. The horse and mule were most important for the army, initially more for the mules who pulled the wagon trains, but later in the cavalry when they learned horse warfare tactics.

Animal disease was the subject of a series of compilation books, by Pelagonius (4th–5th century AD), Chiron (4th century AD), Vegetius (c.AD 450–AD 500) and in the *Hippiakrica* by an unknown author in the 10th century AD. Individual authors of significance were Varro (116–27 BC) and most important Columella (AD 4–70). These two men gave good practical advice and sensible hygiene recommendations. The books and authors are discussed in Chapters 4 and 5. Apsyrtus (3rd–4th century AD) was a Greco-Roman soldier in the Roman Army and is recognised as the most important early contributor to the advance of veterinary medicine. All ancient authors are discussed in the Introduction.

A wide range of equine ailments were recognised and described. In the earlier days of the empire the horse was mainly used for personal riding, draught work was by oxen on farms and general haulage, and mules were used by the army. Lameness and foot problems were significant issues for army animals as were the treatment of injuries, in particular puncture wounds from arrows and javelins, yoke and saddle sores and skin diseases (mange). Colic, tetanus, internal parasites were all known. Glanders, strangles, epizootic and ulcerative lymphangitis were all described and the serious nature of the diseases recognised. Many medications, mostly herbal, were used as well as bleeding and cautery. Horseshoes were only being developed towards the end of the empire.

The practical economics of the Romans and the veterinary expertise of the Greeks enabled a reasonably effective system of equine disease control, except for epizootic problems, but the application of hygiene and good management was appreciated and some sensible treatment procedures were used. As the empire declined, so did the recognition of these principles, with magic, incantations and spells becoming a significant part of diagnosis and therapy.

The Period of Natural Observation, AD 400–AD 1699

There are very few records of disease in horses in the early chronicles, this only means that other matters were deemed to be of more importance, or that these records no longer exist. The first reference that has been found dates from AD 581 and refers to an 'epizooty' in horses in Bordelais, France, 'which would not cease its ravages until vows were made to St. Martin and the solipeds had their heads branded with a red-hot key from the church door' (cited in Fleming 1871, p. 40).

Most of the cases cited in the following list are derived from the Fleming books of 1871 and 1882 (see Introduction) where source references are given, but frequently incomplete. Records of equine diseases occur from a broad geographic spread, but mainly England, France, Germany, Hungary, Ireland, Italy, Spain,

Switzerland with Iceland, Syria and Yemen. There is little or no indication of precise symptoms.

1252 *England and France* experience horse disease outbreaks (probably anthrax).

1320 *England* report of 'ffarsine' in horses (farcy/glanders).

1328–1615 *Europe* only nine reports of equine disease.

1640 *Spain* death reported of 500 horses, probably glanders.

1648 *Germany* a disease, probably influenza, reported by Sollysel in French army horses.

1686 *Germany* a description of probable farcy in horses.

1688 *Europe* England, Germany, Ireland, influenza described.

1693 *Europe* outbreak of ergotism in all species including horses, recognised to be caused by 'diseased' wheat.

1699 *Europe* England, France, Ireland an outbreak described of catarrh in horses, much coughing.
America outbreak of influenza in people and horses.

The Development of Biological Observations, 1700–1799

Diseases of the horse now become a regular item of record; this was the age of the equitation art with many competent horse masters. Disease became of greater interest as individual horses achieved significant value as elite animals; at the same time army cavalry units were growing in importance. Medical science was developing and epizootic diseases were getting increased attention from physicians and surgeons. In 1762 Claude Bourgelat opened the first veterinary school at Lyon, France. This was rapidly copied across Europe and more intense study of animal diseases commenced.

The most frequent ailment reported, as an epizootic or epidemic, was termed either influenza or catarrh. These were followed by reports of anthrax and glanders. Many cases of *glossanthrax* were noted, a disease characterised by carbuncles on the lips, mouth and tongue of the horse, and which was probably anthrax. Most disease reports were from England, Germany and France, followed by North America, Russia, Siberia and the West Indies. These indicate countries where records have survived, as well as the growth of colonisation.

1704 *Europe* Germany, Alsace, Belgium, Netherlands and Poland. Horses died in great numbers. Equine imports to Britain banned.

1705 *Europe* Epizootic still raging in horses in Poland, Germany, France and Switzerland, probably influenza.

1712 *Europe* France, Germany, Hungary, equine epizootic said to be anthrax.

1718 *Germany* A horse disease *pferdstaupe* raged in Silesia, believed to be glossanthrax.

1720   *Europe* Poland, Russia and Courland (Latvia) epizootic of *glossanthrax* in horses and cattle.

1721   *Europe* In central region of Silesia (part Germany, Poland and Czech Republic) ergotism seen in horses and pigs. King of Prussia banned use of rye tainted with ergot.

1725   *Europe* Bavaria, an outbreak of *impetigo erysipelatodes* also called grease in horses. Over 400 were affected on the feet and skin. They could not walk and healed slowly.

1727–1750   *Europe* Outbreaks of equine influenza reported in most countries, intensity varied by year.

1751–1755   *Europe* An epidemic of catarrh seen in horses in Ireland, Austria and elsewhere. Also called 'malignant fever' or 'distemper'. Possibly a chronic influenza with complications.

1758–1768   *Europe* Equine influenza reported most years, and some anthrax cases. In 1776 an epidemic of influenza reported affecting humans, horses and dogs.
America Equine influenza reported in 1766 and 1768.

1775   *Europe* Equine influenza and anthrax recorded.

1775–1776   *Europe* Glanders reported by La Fosse in southern France, in 1776 'glanders continued to rage in epizootic form in France'.

1777–1782   *Europe* Italy, Germany, France, England, Denmark all reported influenza, and some anthrax.

1783   *Europe* France and Italy, severe glanders outbreak in army horses and in Paris.

1794   *Europe* Southern France, horses and mules affected with mange, and scabies reported in men.

1795–1796   *Europe* Germany, glanders reported in Bavaria and Rhine provinces.

1798   *Europe* England, Bavaria and Prussia all report influenza outbreaks. In Piedmont (France/Italy border) glanders occurred.

Science Evolves With a Developing Veterinary Discipline, 1800–1900

In preparing this listing the basic information has been taken from Fleming's *Animal Plagues: Their History, Nature and Prevention*, Vol 2, 1882. Fleming was head of the British Army Veterinary Department; he knew horses and their diseases and was writing about the time of significant veterinary advances. Study of his book reveals pages of disease descriptions, post-mortem results and discussions. By 1850 veterinary schools were well established in Europe and producing many clinical observations, but the cause of most conditions was not yet understood – this was the way to that knowledge. Many of the reports identified are from France, which by 1825 had three veterinary schools, and Germany which was fast developing its position as the leader in pathology. Of interest, the occurrence of the skin condition in horses termed 'grease' which was a well-recognised condition (investigated by Dr Jenner in his smallpox-related studies), but now apparently not seen.

1800   *Europe* In Spain a 'malignant yellow fever' was observed which affected birds, dogs, cats and horses who had 'marble-like coldness of the extremities or general convulsions'. Outbreak of glanders in horses in British Army transport ships to Egypt.

1802–1830   *Europe* Equine influenza regularly reported across the continent. Glanders also reported in France 1807, Russia 1812 and England 1827. An outbreak of equine ophthalmia in France in 1827. Anthrax reported in horses in Germany and France 1818, and Russia 1826.

1830   *Europe* A 'mysterious' disease of horses seen in the Somme, France: no symptoms, sudden death and little seen post-mortem except 'little colour in blood with packets of fibrin'. In Germany, a widespread attack of *mauke* or grease, affected animals developed pustules and fever.

1831   *Europe* An outbreak of 'cholera' in horses in Poland, and in Prussia cases of *brust-seuche*, influenza.

1832   *Europe* Influenza reported in many countries, glanders in the Netherlands and 'cholera' in England and Scotland.

1833–1836   *Europe* Influenza in many countries, glanders in Germany.

1837   *Europe* Influenza in England, France, Switzerland and Germany where the epidemic was serious, called *pferdseuche* or horse-plague.
     Africa Cape Town reported serious mortality due to Horse Sickness.

1838   *Germany* An epizootic venereal disease of horses described with genital lesions; only seen in stallions and mares, not geldings.
     South America In Los Llanos the grasslands east of the Andes in Colombia and Venezuela a disease described as a *peste*, plague of horses. Seen first in crocodiles, wild animals then horses, not in donkeys or cattle. Main symptoms coughing and vomiting 'black' blood, then death.

1834–1841   *Europe* Influenza appeared in a greater part of Europe, described as 'a very universal fever'. In France in 1839 an outbreak of abortion in mares, also outbreaks of anthrax.
     Algeria Serious glanders outbreak in army horses, 1900 out of 2400 horses died in 1840 and a further 2000 in 1841.

1841–1843   *Europe* Influenza, most serious in France and Germany.
     India Calcutta, glanders and farcy very prevalent in army horses.

By the middle of the 19th century there was a clear recognition that glanders (and farcy) were the most serious condition affecting horses. Influenza also was a frequently occurring diagnosis but strangles was seemingly rather rare. All these conditions are of a respiratory or nasal character, at a time when diagnostic procedures were in their infancy there was obviously much confusion.

Glanders

Glanders, now known to be caused by *Burkholderia mallei*, was the major problem. The disease was first recognised by Aristotle (384–322 BC). It manifested in both rhinitis/respiratory form and cutaneous form (known as farcy) and was the major cause of death in equines for centuries. A true understanding of the disease only began when Abildgaard and Viborg in Denmark recognised that the pulmonary and cutaneous forms had the same origin. In 1797 Viborg stated the disease, in both forms, was contagious and indicated the expected incubation period. The major advance was made in 1882 with the isolation of the causative bacterium almost simultaneously occurring in France by Bouchard, Capitan and Charrin, and Löffler and Schuetz in Germany. This was followed by Helman who in 1890 in St. Petersburg prepared mallein, which was then used by Kalning at Dorpat (now Tartu, Estonia), as an intradermal diagnostic test. This is now used as an intrapalpebral injection or eye drop test, which produces reliable results.

Many treatments for glanders were tried in the past and it is now known that this can be achieved by sulphonamide medication. The disease has been eradicated in many areas of the world but still exists as a problem; slaughter and safe disposal of the whole carcase is recommended. A further difficulty was one of differential diagnosis between farcy and epizootic lymphangitis (sometimes called African glanders). In 1883 Rivolta and Miallone discovered the causal agent of epizootic lymphangitis to be *Cryptococcus farciminosus*, which is unrelated to the causal agent of glanders. A very full and excellent review of the history of glanders is given by Blancou (2003, pp. 107–131).

Strangles

Strangles has been known as a disease for many centuries but the early equine specialists frequently confused it with other catarrhal and respiratory diseases. This confusion was recognised and noted by Ruffus in 1251. Strangles was first transmitted experimentally by Viborg in 1802 and the causal bacterium *Streptococcus equi* was isolated by Schuetz in 1888. Vaccines are now available but have a variable preventive capacity. Antibiotic therapy is used for the treatment but the disease remains a worldwide equine problem.

Epizootic Lymphangitis

This disease originally was confused with the farcy form of glanders, a problem that was not resolved until the causal agent, *Cryptococcus farciminosus* was isolated in 1883. It is a notifiable disease in many countries, but now only found in Africa and Asia. Effective control is by slaughter, sometimes surgical excision of the localised nodules and ulcers is undertaken.

Equine Influenza

This disease has a long history in horses, and was frequently confused with glanders and strangles in earlier days. While the mortality rate is usually low there is always a long period of recovery. An outbreak in earlier years would disrupt the use of horses in the many capacities they held, in particular in transport. A serious epizootic in horses in North America in 1872, as well as in mules and donkeys in Canada, the United States of America (USA) and Mexico caused enormous disruption for about six months: in New York, some 7000 of the 10,000 horses in the city were affected. Another outbreak in 2003 also appears to have infected dogs. Globally the virus strains have to be checked to allow effective vaccines to be produced, currently the H3N8 strains are the common causal agent. Without vaccination an infection rate of up to 100% is seen across equine populations. The main equine sector affected in the developed world is the racehorse industry. A common sequel to influenza is a secondary bacterial infection, usually requiring antibiotic therapy.

Parasitic infestation

Equine parasitic infestation is a common problem being caused by helminths, mange mites and other ectoparasites and requiring treatment. Lice were reported by the Greek *hippiatroi* and by other authors, and mange (*Sarcoptes spp*) was recognised from the earliest times, identified by the Moors in Spain and then again in 1657. The use of many medications produced rather poor results until in the late 1700s a decoction of tobacco leaves began to be used. Endoparasites were recognised and many early authors from the ancient Greeks (Aristotle) recognised round worms in the horse as did the Roman authors, with Borgognoni in the 13th century describing equine *strongyles*.

Anthrax, tuberculosis and tetanus in the horse were all described by early authors. African horse sickness was recognised in the Islamic lands in the 13th or 14th century, probably first in the Yemen. It was reported in Southern Africa in the 18th and 19th centuries, and was a serious cause of horse deaths during the Boer War. The virus was identified by J McFadyean in Britain in 1900, and later there was an understanding of the role of insect vectors in spreading the disease. Apart from infectious diseases and wounds the main health issue, throughout equine history has been lameness, with many causes and many treatments. The most effective treatment for many cases is rest and a good diet.

The horse has played a pivotal role in animal–human relationships enabling transport, warfare and sport – the latter in many forms ranging from riding for pleasure to many team and individual competitions. In all of these the important factor is animal–human communication. That this has been developed so well has earned the horse an elite status in most societies and cultures.

Many civilisations and religions feature the horse, sometimes with wings or additional limbs. The characterisations may range from mythological references and beliefs to religious representations or worship. The horse is generally well regarded in all societies, the other equids are not so fortunate: the donkey is seldom admired and much abused, and the mule is more seen as just a work animal.

Equines and Public Health

In developed countries there are only minor human health concerns related to horse diseases, but in some regions glanders still exists and presents a serious hazard. Influenza does exist as a potential risk should a virus strain develop in horses which has a level of communicability to humans. Ringworm can be a problem in certain situations: mostly in the racing world where horse blankets are transferred between animals by humans (to avoid public scrutiny the disease is given colloquial names such as 'Newmarket itch').

Horse meat is only eaten in a limited number of countries, but with horses in some areas of the world infected or dying from diseases such as anthrax and glanders, such meat would be highly dangerous for human handling or consumption.

An Equine Epilogue

The horse, its relationship to humans and their efforts for advancement and for pleasure, has demonstrated its very close involvement with almost all human activity, and their recognition of its diseases. This was brilliantly illustrated by William Shakespeare (1564–1616) in *The Taming of the Shrew*, when Biondello described the rather decrepit horse that took Petruchio to Padua to marry Kate:

> . . . *his horse hipped with an old mothy saddle, and stirrups of no kindred; besides possessed of the glanders and like to mose in the chine; troubled with the lampass, infected with the fashions, full of windgalls, sped with spavins, rayed with the yellows, past cure of the fives, stark spoiled with the staggers, begnawn with the bots, swayed in the back and shoulder shotten . . . (Act III, Scene 2)*

This catalogue of ailments, headed by glanders, would indicate that the general population would recognise the names and understand the diseases – and the condition of the indispensable horse. Most of the vernacular terms will still be recognised except perhaps 'mose in the chine', this is more usually written as 'mourning of the chine' and described chronic nasal discharge (a main diagnostic sign of glanders). An early belief was that this discharge came from the spinal marrow and was described in French as *mort-du-chine* or death of the chain (the vertebrae), which was then anglicised! The terminology was used for several centuries.

References

Blancou, J. (2003) *History of the Surveillance and Control of Transmissible Animal Diseases.* Paris: Office International Des Épizooties

Bokonyi, S. (1984) in *Evolution of Domesticated Animals* (Ed. I.L. Mason). London: Longman

Edwards, P. (2007) *Horse and Man in Early Modern England.* London: Continuum Books

Fleming, G. (1871) *Animal Plagues: Their History, Nature and Prevention.* London: Chapman and Hall

Francis, R.C. (2015) *Domesticated: Evolution in a Man-Made World.* New York: Norton

Hornblower, S. and Spawforth, A. (Eds.) (2003) *The Oxford Classical Dictionary.* New York: Oxford University Press

James, P. and Thorpe, N. (1995) *Ancient Inventions.* London: Michael O'Mara Books

Macgregor, A. (2012) *Animal Encounters.* London: Reaktion Books

Mason, I.L. (Ed.) (1984) *Evolution of Domesticated Animals.* London: Longman

Toynbee, J.M.C. (2013) *Animals in Roman Life and Art.* Barnsley: Pen & Sword

Zeuner, F.E. (1963) *A History of Domesticated Animals.* New York: Harper & Row

CHAPTER 18

Bovine: Cattle, Buffalo, Yak and Others

Cattle belong to the Artiodactyla order of even-toed (hoofed) ungulates, of the family Bovidae, sub-family Bovinae and genus *Bos*. They are separated sub generically from the so-called 'wild cattle' (yak, gayal, banteng, water buffalo and bison) but they can interbreed to produce hybrids, which are usually sterile. Bovids possess either two or four toes and keratinised hoofs.

The original wild cattle of Europe were called *urus* in Latin, *auroch* or *auer* in Old German, and *thur* in Polish; all words related to the Latin *taurus* and Greek *tauros*. The auroch is named as *Bos primigenius* with the nomenclature of *Bos taurus* for European or 'taurine' cattle and *Bos taurus indicus* for the Zebu or Indian cattle, including the Sanga cattle, also termed *Bos taurus africanus*.

The words and names associated with bovines demonstrate their importance to humans, and the role that they have played in our culture and social structure. The word cattle is derived from the Middle English *catel*, which itself was probably derived from old Norman French, from the French *chatel* property, or wealth. In English chattels also mean property or goods, related to the Latin word *cattallum*, meaning property or moveable goods.

Bovine, a word used to describe cattle is derived from the Latin *Bos* meaning an ox; *bovarius* was a term used for a tenant who looked after the plough and oxen of the manor in medieval times. A *bovate* was the amount of land (10–20 acres) which notionally supplied one ox to a team of eight oxen (as seen in Domesday Book 1086). The word pecuniary, meaning related to, or consisting of, money is derived from the Latin word *pecunia* meaning money. The term *pecu* cattle, literally meant 'rich in cattle' as cattle were a trading commodity and property was valued in terms of cattle.

The word 'capital' has the same root as 'cattle', both are derived from the Latin *caput* (head). A Roman who could call many heads his own – someone who owned many cattle – was truly a capitalist. The earlier Old English word *feoh*, meaning cattle or property, and the Old German word *feo* referred to *vieh* (cattle), a meaning that exists in English as 'fee' (Werner 2011, pp. 14–15). The relationship of cattle to money remains strong in our symbolism and language, the figure of a bull represents a strong stock market and 'cash-cow' terminology indicates a nice little earner. The Medieval English word *bugle* meant an ox horn from the Latin *bucalum*. The horns were used by early hunters and soldiers for sending signals, later the horn was developed as a brass instrument.

Adult males are called bulls, sometimes termed 'intact' to differentiate them from castrated males called steers. Males that are one or two-years old may be called yearlings or stirks. Adult females are called cows once they have produced calves, the name of all young stock up to weaning. A female before calving is called a heifer. A female twin to a bull calf is infertile and known as a freemartin. There are innumerable words for varying ages and types of cattle in the different regions of the world: in the United States of America (USA) and Canada an unbranded bovine is called a maverick.

An old English word for horned cattle was neat, from the Old Frisian *nat* or *naet* from a Germanic base *nait*. Boiled hoofs of these cattle were used to extract neatsfoot oil, widely used to dress leather, in particular harnesses.

Natural History and Biology

Cattle are ruminant herbivores, typically they will graze for eight hours a day and will then rest while ruminating. The dental pad replaces upper incisor teeth aiding grazing and chewing. The multichambered stomach system of rumen, reticulum, omasum and abomasum, plus regurgitation of the cud and multiple chewing, together with the bacterial rumen population provides an efficient mechanism to digest and utilise cellulose. Cattle have a double-pulley system of leg tendons which restricts rotation but aids forward movement and long distance travel.

The gestation period is about nine months long. Oestrus (bulling) lasts for about 15–18 hours with the cycle averaging about 21 days. Cows remain fertile for 10–12 years (depending on species and nutrition) and may live for 22–24 years. Both *Bos taurus* and *Bos indicus* have the same chromosome number 60, and readily interbreed. A 2009 study by the United States (US) Department of Agriculture mapped the bovine genome and found some 22,000 genes: this has enabled increased study of meat quality and milk yields in the different breeds. Full background on bovine history, domestication and breeds is available in Porter (2007), Mason (1984) and Zeuner (1963).

Species Domesticated

All domesticated cattle are derived from the ancient auroch, *Bos primigenius*, now extinct since the last individual died in 1627. The aurochs existed over a vast range of the Eurasian continent from the Pacific to Europe, India and North Africa. It is suggested that the aurochs first evolved in India and then spread to Asia, North Africa and Europe. Illustrations of the wild animal exist from cave paintings in many locations and in wall paintings in early Egypt (c.2700 BC).

Domestication probably began in the Near East, upper Tigris region, Iran and Anatolia. Dating is imprecise but the earliest is suggested in about 8000 BC–7000 BC in southern Anatolia. An increasing number of bovine bones and teeth specified as Longhorn cattle have been found in later dating excavation sites across the Middle and Near East and in Europe, commencing from the Ukraine region and northern Greece dating from 7000 BC–6000 BC. It is possible that this domestication stream was separate from that originating in the Near East. Cattle arrived in Europe by two routes, the population spread and growth around the Mediterranean basin and by movement along the Danube river to populate northern Europe.

Shorthorn cattle, possessing a different conformation of the cranium and horn length and shape, appear to have been domesticated first in Mesopotamia about 3000 BC and have developed from the beginning as a milking variety. They became common across Europe by 2000 BC. Both the longhorn and shorthorn cattle are *Bos taurus*, the taurine type.

Zebu, or humped cattle (*Bos indicus*), became domesticated in the Indus valley (now Pakistan). They have a prominent hump of muscle and connective tissue and a well-developed dewlap. As a breed they have an ability to cope with high temperatures and sunlight, and a greater resistance to rinderpest, ticks and intestinal parasites. The Sanga cattle of East Africa and Ethiopia have long horns but reduced humps. The development of African cattle, along with the movement of the humpless shorthorns and longhorns with zebu and Sanga cattle both around the continent and into Europe, have been the subject of much discussion (Epstein and Mason 1984, pp. 12–16). The important African cattle regions are in a band from the West to East Coast, along the East Coast and into Southern Africa; the dwarf trypanotolerant breed that provided milk for the indigenous peoples are found in West Africa.

Other Domesticated Bovidae

There are four species of *Bubalus bubalis*, the water buffalo, but only one is domesticated, with river and swamp types. It is a wallowing animal, and does not tolerate heat so in hot climates it must have access to shade, wallow or spray of water. The species does well on poor quality feed, will produce about ten calves and yield milk for 18–20 years, or work in yoke for up to 30 years. The gestation period lasts between 308–320 days. The water buffalo was first domesticated in Mesopotamia or the Indus valley before 2500 BC as a draught animal. They are easily trained with a placid temperament and can be used for field work, road haulage, pack or riding. The water buffalo is a good milking animal, and is widely used in India. Its main populations are now found in India, Pakistan, China and Indonesia (Ross Cockrill 1984, pp. 52–63).

Bos grunniens, the Yak, is a species adapted to live outside at high altitude in dry and very cold climates on poor feed. It was probably domesticated following the capture of wild calves seeking salt, which is deficient on the Tibetan plateaus. Yaks are sturdy animals with shortish legs and very dense, dark, long fur. Hybrids are frequently bred, mostly with cattle to produce the male *dzo* or female *dzomo*. Utilisation of yaks or hybrids is mainly as pack animals or milk producers: the milk is high in fat and used to make butter and cheese. Little yak meat is eaten in Buddhist Tibet but it is popular in Mongolia and other regions. The yak features in Tibetan mythology and certain body parts or products are used in traditional Tibetan medicine. The yak was known in Roman times, for its tail. This was highly prized as a fly whisk or duster, and was also used by the old Turks fixed to a staff as an emblem of nobility. The tail is also used in some Indian religious ceremonies and also when dyed red by the Chinese to decorate headgear (Bonnemaire 1984, pp. 39–45).

Bos (Bibos) gaurus, the gayal or mithan sometimes termed *Bos frontalis*, is a domesticated bovine found in the hilly regions of East India, Bangladesh and Myanmar. It is said that domestication began because the native wild animal had a craving for salt. The primary purpose of domestication is to have a supply of sacrificial victims. The religions of the indigenous peoples have a need for many sacrifices for a variety of reasons; the flesh is always eaten. Following the end of colonisation in these countries there was a move to try to identify an economic reason to justify the species (Simoons 1984, pp. 34–39).

Bos javanicus, the banteng or Bali cattle, are domesticated wild Javan banteng. Domestication probably occurred around 3500 BC. The animal is timid and docile, can be used for ploughing rice paddies but are mainly bred for meat production, they only provide limited milk. They are traditionally kept by peasant farmers on smallholdings and are primarily distributed across the Indonesian islands, Malaysia and Australia.

Bison, the American bison, has not been domesticated but has been crossed with cattle to produce the 'cattalo' and the 'beefalo', although many claims have been made that neither hybrid has made a major impact on the beef meat market.

Bison bonasus, the European bison also called the wisent, has never been domesticated, but is of interest as the heaviest wild mammal surviving in Europe. It is probably unrelated to the extinct auroch. Currently the largest population of European bison is conserved in the Białowieża Primeval Forest in Poland.

DOMESTICATED CATTLE AND CULTURAL GROUPS

Cattle have played an instrumental role in civilisation: for early humans they provided the power to do work in pulling, ploughing, carrying and producing calves and milk – and when dead provided meat, hides, bones, ligaments and tallow. Cattle were also a great aid in colonisation when taken to the Americas, Australia and New Zealand. Cattle became a major influence on society when it was realised that cattle meant wealth, a factor that had a significant cultural influence in both Europe and Africa. An animal of such importance soon began to play a role in many religions, rituals and forms of entertainment in different cultures. Cattle health was soon recognised as an important part of livestock ownership and epidemic disease has played a role in many society structures. Cattle, by being host to cowpox, were the key to the eradication of smallpox in humans, the first disease to be so controlled, and the fact that rinderpest has been the first animal disease to be eradicated illustrates the importance of cattle to human society and civilisation.

Cattle in Europe

Aurochs (*Urus*) were known to the Romans, Julius Caesar commented on their strength and speed of movement (as did Pliny). Domestication of cattle had happened many centuries earlier. As the Roman civilisation developed it copied many of the rituals and practices of the Greeks, one was to incorporate the bull in their myths and bulls featured in wall paintings and mosaics. They were often seen in the arenas in combat with gladiators or with elephants, to produce a bloodthirsty spectacle. One Roman arena sport involved a bull-fighter approaching a bull (already made tired), jumping onto its back, seizing the horns and twisting the neck, bringing the bull to the ground and frequently breaking its neck.

Cattle served as draught animals for farms and general transport. The army used some for draught work but they were also used as a source of food for the soldiers. Beef was also eaten by the civilian population but was second to pork, mainly due to price. A more important use was for ritual sacrifice in the state religions; the main annual festival was the *suovetaurilia*, where a great sacrifice of premium beasts – a bull, a ram and a boar – was made to the god Mars to bless and purify the land. The ceremony was also used for other purposes with the livers being used for divination and the flesh being cooked and eaten by the onlookers (Toynbee 2013, pp. 151–152).

Cow's milk was seldom drunk as the animals were used for work in pulling ploughs, carts, wagons and river barges. The most important breeds were the large white cattle from Umbria and some small Alpine types. Breeding was carefully managed, mostly in ranches in southern Italy with great care being taken on the breaking-in for work.

Cattle in Post-Roman Europe

In the early years after the Roman Empire and into the Middle Ages most cattle were working oxen on peasant holdings in the large feudal system. There were few identified breeds, the stock was mainly Roman-derived, later there were introductions of long-horned Steppe cattle into south-east Europe then moving to Italy, south France, Spain and Portugal. Various wars and conflicts resulted in cattle movements and by the 1500s many had migrated from the Netherlands and Norway to England, Denmark, Sweden and the Baltic coasts. Swiss Alpine cattle spread to France, Italy, Germany, Austria, Hungary, the Balkans and southern Russia (French 1966, pp. 5–26).

The basis of cattle utilisation was transport and traction, peasant oxen in particular were used for ploughing. As excess stock could not be kept over winter due to feed shortages, they were slaughtered in the autumn. In Britain in the early 1500s there was a growing interest in the consumption of beef, which began with the butcher-grazier in market towns with strong links to the expanding yeoman farmer class. By the 1600s the large landowners also became involved to profit from the growing market. This is reflected in the publication of such works as *The Boke of Husbandry* 1523, attributed to Sir Anthony Fitzherbert, *A Hundred Good Pointes of Husbandry* 1557, by Thomas Tusser, and author Leonard Mascall in the late 1500s and Gervase Markham in the 1600s (these books are discussed in Chapter 12).

Britain was in advance of much of Europe by the end of the Middle Ages in the consumption of beef, but the main role of cattle was still in traction power with most animals yoked to a cart or plough, in teams of up to 20 oxen. Milk was mostly used to make butter and cheese, until in the 17th century milk consumption became a worthwhile market. There was still no significant selection or breeding plans for cattle and endemic disease was a constant problem, as waves of rinderpest and other diseases ravaged the continental herds. Since the 13th century people had tried to build herds but with difficulty due to constant disease epidemics, and wolves in many areas – frequently the cowherd would sleep out at night with his stock. Only a few animals would be selected to overwinter, others would be gelded or spayed (frequently by the cowherd) or slaughtered (Macgregor 2012, pp. 441–444).

Cattle breeds did not really exist throughout the Middle Ages, but a growing urban need for milk, and the import of Friesian stock crossed with local shorthorn cattle, resulted in the development of a dairy industry, probably more rapidly in Britain than in other countries. In the 18th century, British cattle, mostly of the shorthorn type were exported to Europe influencing the Dutch and German lowland breeds, and some French, with much genetic interchange.

In the 18th century the British Agricultural Revolution began led by Jethro Tull (1674–1741) an early agronomist, Charles Townshend (1725–1760) the developer of crop rotation, Thomas Coke (1754–1842) an agricultural reformer and Robert Bakewell (1725–1795) notable as the implementer of systemic breeding of cattle. Bakewell crossed a shorthorn heifer with good sturdy bull and began to produce quality beef cattle. He knew what he was doing, using 'in-and-in' breeding to fix particular characteristics; he sought 'a natural propensity to acquire a state of fatness at an early age'. Until the 18th century the role of cattle in Europe was not important, except for draught work, which could be undertaken by horses. By the 19th century this changed, the place of cattle grew in importance, exemplified by cooperation between countries to control epidemic disease. Slowly rinderpest, the main problem, was controlled allowing the dairy and beef industries to develop, and cattle types to become recognised regional breeds.

Cattle in India

India has traditionally regarded cattle as important. The original Vedic literature mentions them more than any other species, they clearly represented agricultural value and wealth, they provided draught strength and meat, milk, and useful dung. They played a key role in Vedic religious ritual as the principle sacrifice victims (the cooked flesh was afterwards eaten by the priests). The Vedic texts contain many metaphysical references to cattle in natural phenomena such as rainfall, streams, the dawn, fecundity and maternity. The cow was a mother-goddess and the bull represented virility – a belief system and ritual that has lasted for at least 5000 years (Porter 2007, pp. 240–241).

The *Ahimsa* doctrine – avoiding harm to living things – evolved in the later Vedic years. By the 5th–6th centuries BC, Buddhism and Jainism emerged together and the concept of the sanctity of the cow was developed by the Brahman Vedic scholars. This did not happen quickly and it was not until about the 4th century AD that it began to be adopted in the Hindu culture. At the same time zebu cattle breeds were developed for work, strength and milk provision. Over the centuries *Ahimsa* (Sanskrit, compassion) has become a key virtue in the beliefs of Buddhism, Hinduism and Jainism and was entered into the *Yoga Sutras*, the moral imperatives, as one of the *yamas* (observances) that you should follow. See also Chapter 8, for a fuller description of these beliefs.

Cattle in Africa

In Africa cattle obtained a role in the developing cultures that was of greater importance and influence than in any other part of the world. Over the continent a diversity of breeds evolved and the value of the animal as a provider of meat, milk and leather was recognised, together with its major role in ceremonial and rituals. Above all, cattle represented wealth, the more cows a man owned, the wealthier he was. The tradition of 'bridewealth' (*lobola*) is not a payment but an expression of an act of faith between families. The cattle are held in trust for her to be a good wife (by having children), if she fails then the husband can demand the cattle back, and not any cattle, the actual animals that were given in the first place (Porter 2007, p. 195).

The Hamitic tribes in the northern half of the continent are mainly nomadic pastoralists, such as the Fulani in West and the Masai in East Africa, who move their herds according to season and water supply. South of the tropics the indigenous peoples are more sedentary and tend to be settled, possibly with shared grazing lands. The relationship with their animals is good, they understand 'milk let-down' and use the tethered calf, or the milkmaid will sing and produce a tranquil cow (some also have found that 'cow blowing', forcing air into the anus or vagina will produce the same effect).

Much of the early ceremonial and ritual is now lost but the extent and importance of cattle is increasingly revealed by archaeological excavation. In the old kingdom of Nubia (north Sudan) rock carvings dating back to 7000 BC illustrate the role of cattle in the culture. At the base of a mound in the necropolis, partial excavation has revealed more than 5000 bucrania (cattle skulls) 'row upon row of cow horns and eye sockets'. These were sacrificial victims and the origin of the cattle culture across Africa (Casely-Hayford 2012, p. 24).

Modern cultural and agricultural changes are quite rapidly replacing ancient beliefs, but the *kambala*, a much loved traditional dance and masquerade, continues with wearing the treasured cattle masks. In Uganda, the herders still move their long-horned Ankole cattle south, a traditional trade route. Traces of the old Bunyoro kingdom of northern Uganda can still be seen and judged by the size of their dung mounds and heaps of cattle bones – the kingdom had salt and the wealth produced was shown in cattle herds. The Masai people in the Kenyan Rift Valley still keep their cattle for bloodletting and a little milk (both for food), but now mainly as currency. In the south the Zulu people in Natal always had big herds for meat, milk and hides to make their shields. Traditionally they would barter women for cattle: the women looked after the crops and the men the cattle. The focus of a Zulu homestead is the cattle pen, only men are allowed to enter. Sacrifice of cattle was the way to commune with the departed ancestors – such practices slowly ended with the occupation by Europeans. The background to the African cattle culture has been explored and discussed by Casely-Hayford (2012).

Cattle and Religion

The cow has been, and still is, seen as a mother figure in both religion and mythology. A symbiotic relationship with humans has developed over the centuries. The cow has played a leading role in many cultures: most of all in the Hindu belief. The ancient Egyptians also held the cow to be sacred and believed that the heavens were really the womb of a gigantic divine cow and that the sun god Ra rode on the back of Apis, a bull. The Sumerians worshipped Enlil and Ninlil, the former depicted with hoofs and horns as the Bull God of Heaven: when they mated the Euphrates and Tigris would flood, and make the land fertile.

Cattle veneration in Europe began with bulls; depictions from Catalhöyük, Turkey dated to about 9400–8000 BP near the start of domestication, focus on the auroch and stress the masculinity in the skull and horns. This image was much used for the deities – Apis in Egypt, Moloch and Baal (associated with child sacrifice in ancient Canaan) and Minotaur in Crete. Bulls were prominently sacrificed to Yahweh, Zeus (Jupiter) and to Mithras. Bull-leaping was a ritual well-known from the wall painting in Minoan Crete, but it was also found in India with Jallikattu bulls and elsewhere in West Asia and possibly ancient Egypt (Francis 2015, pp. 130–131). Cattle also feature in many African tribal belief systems.

Cattle are not a major feature of Christian theology (but some old religious practices from the Roman times have survived). In the early years of Christian doctrine cows, bulls and calves were not well regarded in the Judeo-Christian world as they were revered by some of the polytheistic religions. They were seen to be in competition with the monotheistic belief of the followers of the Bible. It is recorded that in the proceedings of one of the early 5th century AD meetings of the Council of Toledo, a description of the devil was published, who was given the physique of a horned bull. The Christian Church sought to compare the devil incarnate as the god of its adversary: at that time, the bull was the central feature of the Mithras cult, a religious competitor in the later years of the Roman Empire (Werner 2011, pp. 168–169).

Cattle and Sport

In some countries in Asia cattle are used for racing, not like horse racing, more as an event at festivals. Bull fighting is a sport still active in Spain, this style, which results in the death of the bull is also practised in southern France and Mexico, Colombia, Venezuela, Ecuador and Peru. A variant form of bull fighting is employed in Portugal where a horseman first jabs *bandeiras* into the bull's back before an interplay with a group of men in the arena: the bull, if he performs well, may be healed and used again but is usually killed by a butcher following the 'show'.

In southern France there are two indigenous bull 'sports': the *course camarguaise* which involves young men endeavouring to take a rosette from a bull's head and the *course landaise* in which a team annoys a cow, usually with large horns, while someone jumps over its back. In the same region, the 'running of the bulls' through the local town is also practised. In neither exercise are the bulls killed, but it is dangerous for the participants. Other countries enjoy the spectacle of a man wrestling with a bull, to get subjugation. The USA rodeo shows often include a bloodless bull-fighting session. The ritual with Jallikattu bulls in Tamil Nadu was mentioned under the Cattle and Religion heading: the bulls are unharmed, they are praised.

In both England and Ireland a popular entertainment was bull baiting, confronting a bull (already agitated with pepper blown in his nose) with a trained dog or dogs who had to fasten their teeth into the bull's nose. The practice was finally banned in Britain in 1835 and in Ireland under a similar 1835 Act. In Mexico, under colonial Spanish rule, a popular pastime was watching bull and bear fights.

Recognition of Cattle Diseases

Each animal species has at least one major epizootic disease, these can be traced back to antiquity, but the early records seldom provide enough information for a precise diagnosis. In cattle the problem is made more difficult because of the confusion between signs, symptoms and names. The most frequent early English word for a livestock epizootic is *murrain* derived from the Greek *maraino* and Latin *moril*; this is also known in French as *murie*, Italian as *moria*, German as *mar*, Celtic as *muire* and Sanskrit as *mr*.

Over the centuries three epizootic diseases have dominated cattle husbandry – rinderpest, contagious bovine pleuro-pneumonia (CBPP) and foot-and-mouth disease (FMD), additionally anthrax in varying forms has frequently appeared. These have occurred as a series of disease episodes, either of a single disease or in coincidental timing with others.

The earliest evidence of these diseases is difficult to interpret. The el-Lahun Egyptian papyrus fragments (c.1900 BC–1800 BC) describe disease in a bull, one of the suggested causes is rinderpest. In the Bible there are mentions of animal plagues, specifically the sixth plague in the time of Moses (c.1750 BC) which can be attributed to carbuncular anthrax (see Chapter 1). Aristotle (384 BC–322 BC) stated that cattle suffered from two epidemic diseases, *podagra* the foot sickness and *craurus*. From his descriptions the former was probably FMD and the latter CBPP (see Chapter 2).

Possibly the earliest European record, derived from oral folk history, is found in the *Irish Annals of the Four Masters* (vol. 1), compiled between 1632 and 1636. Dated as AM 5001 (this was the *Anno Mundi* calendar based on the biblical account of the creation of the world in 5199 BC; a difficult chronology to understand), the item is from the *Annals of Clonmacnoise*, 'There was a great mortality of kine (cattle) in Ireland in Breasal's reign . . . there was such a moreen of cows in the land, as there were no more left alive but one bull and one heifer in the whole kingdom . . . in a place called Gleam-Saunasge'.

The event is remembered in the name Glensawisk (the Glen of the Heifer) in County Tyrone. It is the first record of a cattle epizootic in Ireland, probably mythology possibly based on fact.

The Years of Antiquity to AD 500

Rinderpest (cattle plague)

This proved to be the most persistent and dangerous cattle epizootic with its earliest (possible) recognition occurring some 4000 years ago in Egypt. Later disease descriptions by Columella (AD 4–AD 70) and Virgil (70 BC–90 BC) in the *Georgics* can be attributed to rinderpest. Vegetius in the 5th century AD discusses a *malleus* of cattle which was probably rinderpest and St. Ambrose, Archbishop of Milan (AD d.397) wrote of a *pestilencia* of cattle.

Contagious Bovine Pleuro-pneumonia (CBPP)

This disease was possibly described by Aristotle's term *craurus*. Virgil's later vivid description of cattle disease in the *Georgics* also could have been CBPP. It does not appear, from surviving records, to have been either a major or constant problem until significant epizootic outbreaks from the 16th century onwards in Europe, and also in the 19th century in the USA. The disease was characterised by J Scheuchzer's description in Switzerland in 1732.

Foot-and-Mouth Disease (FMD)

Although the history of this disease is difficult to trace, Aristotle mentioned symptoms which could indicate he recognised the infection, and Columella gave names to differing ailments with symptoms very similar to those seen in FMD – *fluidum salivas os*, hypersalivation; *febricitanti bovi*, cattle fever; and mentigo for a similar syndrome in lamb and goats. It was not until Girolamo Fracastro wrote his classic description of the epidemic diseases in 1546 that it could be distinguished from other epizootics.

344 • *Part III: Domestication, Utilisation and Disease Histories*

Anthrax

Anthrax is one of the most well recognised diseases, common in most species in the early years but now rare in developed countries. The sixth plague in Egypt as described in the Bible (c.1750 BC) was probably anthrax, Virgil described symptoms in cattle resembling anthrax and Vegetius (c.5th century AD) gave the disease the name *morbus alienates*.

The problems with epizootic livestock disease were well recognised in the early days of the Roman Empire. Little can be learned of the actual diseases because of incomplete, or confused descriptions. In the Tarention War a 'most desolating pestilence' was recorded in 278 BC, known as the *Abortus epidemicus*, it was particularly fatal to pregnant women and cows in Rome. Livy (59 BC–AD 17) the Roman historian, added to the records and confusion when he wrote of a disease in 175 BC that began in cattle 'and then attacked mankind'.

In 200 BC Cato the Elder wrote, 'If there be reason to fear the presence of an epizootic disease it is most essential to give the cattle a mixture of salt, laurel leaves, onions, cloves of garlic, incense, powdered rue and burning charcoal, made up with a little wine'.

Onions and garlic continued to feature in most treatments for rinderpest up to the AD 1865 epizootic in Europe.

The Period of Natural Observation, AD 500–AD 1699

The early records are confusing but do indicate that serious diseases of cattle were frequent occurrences. In the 4th century the poet Sanctus Severus described a serious cattle disease that commenced in Hungary and then spread.

For many hundreds of years, while there were many records of epizootics, and other cattle diseases, there was no effort to try to classify or categorise them. The writers were not diagnosticians but reporters, initially from the monasteries or religious houses. As seen in a sampling of the records for this first period.

> 547 *Britain and Ireland* Several reports of a pestilence affecting 'men, beasts and reptiles'; called the 'yellow pestilence' when cattle were affected.
>
> 569–570 *Italy and France* A great disease 'and neat cattle especially perished in these countries'.
>
> 580–581 *France* A great epizootic in cattle, 'a dreadful plague of dysenteric nature and great loss of cattle'.
>
> 582–584 *Europe* Reports from France, Italy and Ireland of a cattle plague.
>
> 591 *France, Belgium* 'A grievous plague among cattle and oxen and stags in the forest'; thought to be anthrax. From 600, there were numerous reports from almost every country of Western Europe of cattle

disease, cattle plague, epizootics and pestilence. The few words of description would indicate that the cause was probably rinderpest but also many outbreaks of anthrax (*milzbrand* in German).

1223–1225 *Germany, Spain* Further seminal disease outbreaks termed *bovum pestilens, bovina mortalitas, crabra.*

1514 *Italy* An epidemic disease of cattle in northern Italy, spread to France and then England. In 1546 Girolamo Fracastro wrote a treatise on the animal plagues and gave the first detailed description of symptoms. The 1514 plague he termed *fièvre pestilentielle exanthematique* which would appear to be FMD (also called *stomatitis aphthosa* by others). Fracastro also described the other diseases and named the rinderpest syndrome *phlogoso-gangréneuse*. Other names for the disease were *cachexia, diathése varioleuse* and *contagious typhus*. Anthrax was generally recognised as a specific syndrome called *ignea peste* or *milzbrand*. Fracastro provided the first reliable differentiation of these diseases.

1599 *France, Italy* A cattle epizootic killed more than 13,000 animals, mostly in northern Italy. Ramazzini (see later) regarded this as a rinderpest outbreak.

1625 *Hungary, Italy* Disease, probably rinderpest spread from southern Russia into Western Europe. Serious losses.

1693 *Germany* In Hesse, report of a 'pulmonic affection' in cattle. Possibly the first report of CBPP.

1694 *Italy* Outbreak of ergotism in cattle and other livestock.

1695 *Germany* Outbreak of *aphthous fever*, probably FMD.

1697 *Sweden* Outbreak of *glossanthrax* recorded.

The Development of Biological Observations, 1700–1799

A gradual distinction was being made of the mix of epizootic diseases, with an increasing awareness of the continent-wide threat of rinderpest, now seen as the main killer of cattle. By the end of the century veterinary schools had been established throughout Western Europe, driven by the need to control rinderpest. Some of the more important outbreaks are identified.

1709–1710 *Russia, Ukraine, Romania* The spread of rinderpest into Europe appeared to start in Asia or Tartary and spread across southern Russia into Europe, to Austria, Hungary and Italy. Study written by Kanold (*Jahreshistorié*).

1711 *Europe* Rinderpest recognised in Poland, Hungary, Austria, Germany, Bavaria, Dalmatia and Italy. Also raged across Russian lands (fully described in Fleming Vol 1, pages 179–227).

Italy 27th August 1711, rinderpest found in imported Hungarian cattle, close to Padua in northern Italy. Investigated by Lancisi and then Ramazzini resulting in Papal Edict and first effective control measures (see Chapter 13).

1720   *Europe* Poland, Prussia and Latvia *glossanthrax* in cattle and horses; also rinderpest with pneumonias (?CBPP).

1726   *Europe* Poland, Silesia and Saxony: many outbreaks of carbuncular fever (anthrax) and pleuro-pneumonia. In 1726–1727 'epizootic pleuro-pneumonia (bovine) spread everywhere in Switzerland and to neighbouring countries'.

1743   *Switzerland, South Germany* CBPP prevalent (Wirth, *Seucheulehre),* also rinderpest.

1745–1771   *Europe* Severe rinderpest outbreaks in almost every country of northern and central Europe. Very significant losses of cattle throughout the continent, including England, Scotland and Ireland.

The second half of the century recorded an almost continuous listing of cattle epizootics in the European countries. Cattle disease reports were also found from Turkey, St. Domingo, Guadeloupe, the USA and Iceland: these were a miscellaneous collection, the one reported in the USA being a strange problem called 'horn disease' or 'distemper'.

Of the almost annual reporting of cattle epizootic disease a total of 63 were identified by a diagnostic name. Of these, 20 outbreaks were listed as anthrax (of which three were *glossanthrax*, possibly FMD); 19 named as rinderpest; 11 as FMD; seven as CBPP and six undetermined epizootics being named by major symptoms as abortion (3), ophthalmia (2) and gangrenous sore-throat (1). What was clear is that anthrax and rinderpest were major problems, followed by FMD and CBPP.

Science Evolves with a Developing Veterinary Discipline, 1800–1900

Analysis of descriptions of disease at this time show that there was much confusion between rinderpest and anthrax (Spinage 2003, pp. 85–86). In the 19th century most years in Europe were much the same for epizootic cattle disease, except some were worse than others: an outline of some examples illustrates the situation.

1800   *Europe* With Italy recording a complex of diagnoses – *cancro maligno* (malignant anthrax), *flusso dissenterico* (dysentery) and 'epizootic pneumonia'.

1801   *Europe* Cattle plague recorded in France, Switzerland, Germany and Ireland.

1802   *Europe* Ireland recorded 'a bloody murrain'; Russia, Poland and Italy – cattle plague and Bavaria, anthrax.

1805   *England* Cattle plague.

1813   *Europe* Switzerland, Hungary and Rhineland reports of cattle plague, CBPP and anthrax.

1814 *Europe* Many army movements between countries created transfer of affected cattle with cattle plague reports from France, Italy,
Switzerland, Austria and Silesia.

1817 *France* A complex cattle disease observed, probably FMD.

1820–1822 *Russia* Cattle plague prevalent in Siberia.

1824 *Europe* Cattle plague reports from France, Italy, Germany and Russia.
Southern Russia reported an 'ekzematous fever'.

1827 *Europe* Italy, Austria, Germany reported FMD outbreaks; France
reported CBPP and Russia and Danube region, cattle plague.

1828 *Belgium* At a time when cattle plague was widespread across the
European continent an outbreak of what was initially termed 'exu-
dative pleuro-pneumonia' was seen in cattle in Belgium and the
Netherlands. This was traced to a shipment of animals from Italy, the
losses were devastating. The true nature of the disease and a control
method was described by Dr Louis Willems.

1831 *Europe* Cattle plague introduced by Russian troops to Poland and
then to Germany. France experienced the spread of CBPP lasting
until 1839.

1836 *Europe* Outbreaks of cattle plague, CBPP and anthrax reported from
Germany, Belgium, Austria and Italy.

1837 *Europe* CBPP reported from France, Holland and Lithuania. Cattle
plague and anthrax reported in Austria, Italy (Naples), Danube
region and Turkey.

1839 *England* The first appearances of FMD.

1840 *France* Report from Lyon Veterinary School of a disease (probably
FMD) widespread in France affecting cattle, pigs and sheep.

1841–1845 *Europe* There was pandemic disease across the continent including
Britain and Ireland, most records indicate cattle plague, and CBPP
particularly serious in Holland as the main issue. Cattle plague
reported in Russia, Bessarabia, Turkey and Egypt. At the same time
there was an influenza plague in humans, also reported in horses (and
in cattle in France).

The growing seriousness of cattle diseases and the enormous loss of animals had at
last begun to awaken governments to the need for action. The calling of the meeting
in Hamburg of veterinary leaders from all the veterinary schools, by John Gamgee
in 1863, opened the way for inter-governmental cooperation (the meeting resulted in
the creation of the World Veterinary Association).

Veterinary schools, now present in most European countries, assisted veterinary
specialists to develop and enabled the establishment of veterinary journals to publish
and exchange information. In the second half of the 19th century those in governments and veterinary medicine began to understand and start to control the epizootic cattle diseases.

Major Cattle Diseases

Rinderpest

It was not until the work of Lancisi in 1711 and Ramazzini in 1713 that an understanding of the disease began to develop. It has been estimated that between 1711 and 1769 nearly 10,000 animals in Europe died each day from rinderpest. Control could only be achieved by study and cooperation. Methods to reproduce the disease were studied and descriptions of the post-mortem lesions were written (Blancou 2003, pp. 164–167). Many treatments were advocated, sold and used for rinderpest medication over the centuries: none were effective. Many immunisation methods were investigated, in particular from the later 1700s, none were effective and several were dangerous. In South Africa in 1897 Koch used an injection of bile from an infected animal; this was soon replaced by using serum from a recovered animal and then again by a serum virus method. The Koch method was tried in India but soon dropped due to the necessity of killing a cow to obtain bile – unacceptable in a Hindu country. The virus was finally isolated in 1902 (Nicolle and Adil-Bey 1902, pp. 50–67). J T Edwards working at the Indian Mukteswar laboratory developed a goat spleen vaccine based on the attenuated virus. This breakthrough led to further improvements until the Plowright vaccine which was used to obtain final eradication in June 2011.

Britain suffered from rinderpest with imports of cattle from continental Europe. It was recognised that the disease could be controlled by radical slaughter of infected cattle, which was used on three occasions, together with a ban on cattle imports. This ban was lifted in 1842. At that time European controls were effective and no problems arose, but Professor John Gamgee (the founder and organiser of the 1863 European congress) warned of the risk; he was ignored. When a rinderpest outbreak happened in 1865, he proposed eradication by slaughter and prohibition of stock movements; this was rejected. By 1866 the situation had become alarming and legislation was introduced to implement control. The country was declared free of rinderpest in September 1867, after 420,000 cattle had died. The creation of a Veterinary Department in the Board of Agriculture represents the start of the British government veterinary service (Hall 1966, pp. 259–264).

Rinderpest was first mentioned in early epizootics in Europe, usually commencing in Asia. Successive waves of infection, frequently caused by invading troops, were experienced from the early 1700s and for almost 200 years wave after wave of infection swept across Europe. In Asia reports of the disease exist in Korea, spreading to Japan. In Africa, a catastrophic epizootic was started by importation of infected cattle to Egypt in 1890 and then Ethiopia and across the continent, mostly to the east and south. The pandemic caused the death of some 97% of cattle and decimated large numbers of wild African ruminants including gazelle, buffalo, wildebeest, kudu and giraffe. Full and detailed histories of the 1890–1902 pandemic are written by Spinage (2003) and Blancou (2003).

Contagious Bovine Pleuro-pneumonia (CBPP)

CBPP was described and characterised by J Scheuchzer in Switzerland in 1732, becoming a defined disease in the later 1700s, primarily as a result of work by Bourgelat and the Lyon Veterinary School. The signs of the disease were described with a final summation by P Chabert in 1791. The determination of quarantine times was finally resolved with a maximum of 180 days. An immunisation procedure was developed by L Willems by 1852 and, following testing by several national investigations and trials, was widely used. Control was slow and difficult because the actual causative agent of the disease was not isolated until 1898 by E Nocard and E Leclainche in France. They had discovered a previously unknown organism, the genus was later named *Mycoplasma* and the causal agent of CBPP, *Mycoplasma mycoides*. The disease was one of the most serious animal plagues as not all infected cattle develop clinical signs, but can still act as carriers. With a variable and sometimes very long incubation period control is difficult and mortality can reach 90% in some outbreaks. A full historical review is available by Blancou (2003).

A unique aspect of CBPP is the immunisation procedure that was used in Africa. It is unknown when the use of this began, but the subcutaneous insertion of a piece of diseased lung tissue on the bridge of the nose, or subcutaneous insertion of infective pneumonia lymph – either alone or on a saturated thread into the skin – was found to produce an immunity. Either method invariably produced a severe reaction, local or general, and sometimes death. When first observed the animals with a growth on their noses prompted the belief that these were three-horned cattle (De Rochebrune 1880, pp. 304–306) . First seen in West Africa, the procedure was found to be used in East and South Africa, and was still in use in recent times. This is well discussed by Blancou (2003, pp. 146–148).

Foot-and-Mouth Disease (FMD)

The cattle epidemic at Fruili, Italy in 1514, and the resulting classic treatise of Girolamo Fracastoro in 1546, is accepted by most scholars as being the first reliable description of FMD; a disease classed as 'among the contagious diseases whose origins will remain forever obscure' (Blancou 2003, pp. 53–54). There were many studies and descriptions as the disease was recognised in every region of Europe, now seen as probably the most infectious disease known to veterinary medicine. F Toggio in describing an 1810 outbreak was first to use *febbre aftosa* as a name. The early stages of the disease are characterised by fever and mouth lesions, after about 72 hours developing to the classical vesicles in the mouth, tongue and around the coronary band and interdigital space. The timing may vary between cattle, pigs and sheep. The saliva is highly virulent.

The virus aetiology of the disease was first demonstrated by F Löffler and P Frosch in 1897 and confirmed by Hecker in 1899; it was the first virus to be isolated in animals. In 1922 Vallée and Carré discovered two antigenic variants (types O and A) of the virus. Investigations of possible vaccination methods began in the early 1800s but progress was slow until Vallée, Carré and Rinjord in France (1925) developed a vaccine utilising a purified, formalinised virus. Following this development, the application and use of vaccines have enabled FMD to be eradicated from most developed countries, but it still remains a problem in the less developed world. The first appearance of FMD in Britain was in 1839, and in 1869 it was declared a notifiable disease allowing for a progressive series of regulations for restriction of movement, quarantine and slaughter. In 1880 Austria introduced official legislation, followed by France in 1881 and then other European countries. A full historical review is available (Blancou 2003, pp. 53–78).

Anthrax

The outbreak of anthrax in cattle would appear to have been more frequent in earlier years, it now seems that there was much confusion in the diagnosis with the anthrax name being applied to other conditions, partly because the so-called *glossanthrax* was confused with FMD. Additionally, anthrax as a disease is now not as frequent, its occurrence in multiple species was much more common in the earlier years of record keeping. The P Chabert treatise in 1788 succeeded in providing a clear description of symptoms and differentiation from blackleg (*Clostridium chauvoei*) infection, to be used by Bourgelat in teaching. The isolation of the causative organism, *Bacillus anthracis*, by C Davaine and P Rayer in 1850 was followed by the development of an effective attenuated vaccine for use in sheep by Pasteur in 1881 (however, Pasteur had used an attenuation method devised by J J G Toussaint in Toulouse). Today antibiotics are highly effective for treatment if administered in time, an anti-serum is sometimes used for protection or treatment.

Tuberculosis

Of other cattle diseases of significance, tuberculosis is the most important. The disease was recognised in humans from the very earliest of times and records exist of its description in elephants in South Asia, in Aristotle's writings and in the Roman literature. In earlier years, the disease did not appear to be a major problem in cattle. There were many reports, and much confusion, regarding the relationship between the disease seen in humans and that in cattle. A difficulty in diagnosis and control is that the incubation period can be prolonged and the disease many appear to be non-contagious in less-intensive farming. It was not until Koch discovered the causal bacterium (*Mycobacterium tuberculosis*) in 1882 that the situation began to be resolved, and that the one organism could be the cause of tuberculosis in both cattle and humans. Efforts to produce an effective vaccine have not been successful but in 1921 an attenuated bacterium grown on potato slices was developed by Calmette and Guerin, known as BCG vaccine. It has value for use in humans and is also used in cattle and other species, but with unproved effectiveness. No satisfactory treatment has been found and a control programme based on diagnostic testing and slaughter of reactors is the only reliable control method. Diagnosis has been based on skin testing with tuberculin (the supernatant of a tubercle culture) developed by Koch, but more sophisticated tests are now being investigated. Tuberculosis transmission from cattle to humans via meat or milk is a major public health hazard and controlled in developed economies, but eradication is difficult.

Cattle disease is related to the husbandry practice used. In intensive farming, such as dairy production, the main problems have been mastitis; infertility and reproductive issues; and foot care. In extensive husbandry, blackleg, helminths, liver fluke and fly parasites (*Hypoderma* spp.) need control: these are all problems identified from the early Roman literature. Other recognised herd disease issues include bovine viral diarrhoea, infectious bovine rhinitis, Johne's disease, leptospirosis and neospora infection (parasitic). Johne's disease is a progressive wasting condition characterised by diarrhoea and has been found to be caused by *Mycobacterium avium* subspecies paratuberculosis.

Recognition and control of cattle diseases has been a major challenge to livestock farmers across all continents. In 2011 rinderpest was the first animal disease to be eradicated, a major advance for both veterinary medicine and animal welfare.

Cattle and Public Health

The historical record indicates that while several cattle diseases were recognised from the earliest times, generally the relationship to human disease was not perceived. The early Mosaic Laws of the Jews had an emphasis on hygiene and health and their instructions for allowing meat of slaughtered animals to be consumed recognised lesions now attributed to tuberculosis infection. These early injunctions contributed to the basis for eventual public health and post-slaughter meat inspection being adopted worldwide.

Other diseases such as anthrax also need to be controlled at meat inspection but generally in developed economies these are rare.

References

Blancou, J. (2003) History of the Surveillance and Control of Transmissible Animal Diseases. Paris: Office International des Épizooties

Bonnemaire, J. (1984) Yak, in *Evolution of Domesticated Animals* (Ed. I.L. Mason). London: Longman

Casely-Hayford, G. (2012) *The Lost Kingdoms of Africa*. London: Transworld

Epstein, H. and Mason, I.L. (1984) Cattle, in *Evolution of Domesticated Animals* (Ed. I.L. Mason). London: Longman

Francis, R.C. (2015) Domesticated: Evolution in a Man-Made World. New York: Norton

French, M.H. (1966) *European Breeds of Cattle*. Rome: Food & Agricultural Organization of the United Nations

Hall, S.A. (1966) The Great Cattle Plague of 1865. *British Veterinary Journal* **122**

Macgregor, A. (2012) *Animal Encounters*. London: Reaktion Books

Mason, I.L. (Ed.) (1984) *Evolution of Domesticated Animals*. London: Longman

Nicolle, Ch. and Adil-Bey (1902) Etude sur la peste bovine. *Annales de l'Institut Pasteur* **16**

Porter, V. (2007) Cattle – A Handbook to the Breeds of the World. London: Black

De Rochebrune, A.T. (1880) Formation de races nouvelles, Recherches d'ostéologie comparée sur une race de boefs domestiques observée en Senegambil. *C.r. hebd. Acad. Sci* **91**

Ross Cockrill, W. (1984) Water Buffalo, in *Evolution in Domesticated Animals* (Ed. I.L. Mason). London: Longman

Simoons, F.J. (1984) Gayal or Mithan, in *Evolution in Domesticated Animals* (Ed. I.L. Mason). London: Longman

Spinage, C.A. (2003) *Cattle Plague: A History*. New York: Springer

Toynbee, J.M.C. (2013) *Animals in Roman Life & Art*. Barnsley: Pen & Sword

Werner, F. (2011) *Cow: A Bovine Biography*. Vancouver: Greystone

Zeuner, F. (1963) *A History of Domesticated Animals*. New York: Harper & Row

CHAPTER 19

Ovine: Sheep

The sheep is a member of the Bovidae family (sub-family Caprinae) of the order Artiodactyla – the even-toed ungulates. Other members of the Caprinae are the goat, *Capra*, and two closely related genera: the Barbary sheep of the Sahara and the Blue sheep of the Himalayas. The name for the domestic sheep is *Ovis aries*.

The original wild sheep, the argali (*Ovis ammon*), were distributed in the mountain ranges of Central Asia, from there the mouflon type (*Ovis orientalis*) moved into Europe, followed by the urial type *(Ovis vignei)* which also moved south towards India. The argali type migrated across eastern Asia and into North America as the bighorn *(Ovis canadensis)*. Of these four main types of sheep only the bighorn has not played a role in creating the current domestic breeds. The wild mouflon has probably been the main antecedent of the sheep breeds of Europe and also of Asia. See also Zeuner (1963, pp. 153–165) and Ryder (1984, pp. 65–68).

The word sheep originated in Middle English, derived from the Old English *scep*, in turn derived from the Old English West Saxon *sceap* and related to Old Frisian *skep*, Old Saxon *scap*, Dutch *schaap* and Old High German *scaf*.

Adult males are called ram or tup, and wethers when castrated. Adult females are ewes and the young, lambs. Meat from adult sheep is termed mutton and from the young, lamb. Today the primary produce are wool and meat plus milk, utilised for yoghurt and cheese. Collections of sheep are known as flocks, herds or mobs.

Natural History and Biology

Sheep are ruminant herbivores requiring some 10–11 hours of daily grassland grazing, followed by just a slightly shorter night-time period of rumination. With cloven hoofs they are well adapted for walking on both soft grassland and also more rugged stony hills.

Their cleft upper lip allows grazing closer to the ground than cattle, but their nibbling action has detrimental effects on land unless a sufficient area is available. The front teeth bite on a hard toothless pad on the upper jaw. The presence of the front teeth is essential for them to feed adequately. Tooth loss ('broken mouth') starts from about four years in domestic sheep and then the animal has a progressive declining value. The adult will live to about 10–12 years.

Sheep have scent glands on the rim of their eyes and between the claws of the hoof: the exact function is unclear and may be related to reproduction behaviour. Their sense of smell and hearing is excellent. As prey animals their all-round (peripheral) vision is good but forward vision is poor except for a small area directly in front of them.

Breeding season varies between North and South hemispheres and between temperate and tropical breeds. In the Northern hemisphere the usual season is between September and November. Except for certain breeds, such as the Dorset Horn, breeding is dependent on declining day length, thereby resulting in melatonin release. Ewes are seasonally polyoestrous during the breeding season; the ewe has only one pair of nipples (the cow has two pairs). The length of gestation varies significantly both within and between breeds – overall an average of 152 days but ranging from 143–159 days in the Merino, to about 144 days in the Southdown and Dorset Horn breeds. Sheep have 54 chromosomes and goats 60. The Barbary sheep has 58 chromosomes but the number of chromosomes in the Himalayan Blue depend on the population group, usually between 54 and 56.

A wide range of natural fleece colours are found, but domestic sheep have been selected for the white fleece which allows for easy dyeing. There are also several variations in fleece characteristics ranging from a dense, highly crimped wool to a wool type almost indistinguishable from hair.

Species Domesticated

Sheep were domesticated in the prehistoric period by people of the late Mesolithic age. There has been debate whether the goat or sheep was domesticated first. This is unlikely to be resolved as species differentiation from the fragmentary boney remains can be difficult to determine. As the early crop farmers would have had to clear scrub and woodland the goat would have been initially more useful.

The species *Ovis aries*, mainly derived from the wild mouflon, is well established but all sheep types will interbreed. The wild varieties (according to some authors) can be divided into two groups: the first group including the mouflon *Ovis orientalis*, argali *Ovis ammon* and urial *Ovis vignei*. Evidence suggests that urial were the first domesticated in southwest Asia, that the mouflon was the source of the European breeds, and the argali provided the Asian breeds. The second group, in North America, have never been subjected to domestication: the bighorn *Ovis canadensis*, snow sheep *Ovis nivicola*, and the thin-horn *Ovis dalli* only found in Alaska.

The first substantiated evidence of domesticated sheep has been found at Zawi Chemi Shanidar in Iraq dating from c.8500 BC (Leonard 1981, p. 77). Later remains have been found across the early Fertile Crescent region of grass-sloped hills in an arc, Palestine–Syria–Turkey–Iraq–Iran. Rock paintings at Tassili, in the Sahara, dating from 5000 BC–4000 BC show sheep.

The process of sheep domestication is of considerable interest to both anthropologists and zoologists. It is suggested that the initial flock creation could have been in the Neolithic period (c.6000 BC) when a hunter would return home with a newborn lamb to be suckled by his wife as wet-nurse. This imprinting would achieve bonding to the woman, enabling easy handling. There are also indications of castration of males at this time, demonstrating an understanding of selection. They developed a breeding programme and worked to build an animal type that met their needs – docile with particular characteristics: improved milk yield, development of the fleece quantity and selection of fleece type.

The domestication process could have progressed through three stages: the initial ties to humans, followed by confining groups and breeding from them, to the third stage of selective breeding. It is suggested that by 3000 BC recognisable breeds with chosen characteristics had been developed in the Middle East region. Four main types evolved: fat-tailed, fat-rumped, haired and thin-tailed fleece sheep. This has been well explained by Zeuner (1963, pp. 170–198) and Ryder (1984, p. 67).

Domestication of sheep has been fundamental to the development of many civilisations; they have played a major role in economic and social success. There was little evidence of positive breed selection in the Middle Ages in Europe, the more primitive breeds remained significant in the southern regions, while a greater interest in development occurred in the north where more hardy breeds were kept. This was particularly obvious in the British Isles and in later years in Australia, New Zealand and the southern countries of South America. Many breeds have developed; using rather broad categories, the Food and Agricultural Organisation of the United Nations (FAO) identified some 1300 different breeds (FAO 2007). Of this total maybe some 150–200 breeds have a true economic value, while in practice the number of principal breeds in use in the major sheep economies is comparatively small.

DOMESTICATED SHEEP AND CULTURAL GROUPS

The domestication of sheep has been complex and diverse, it was one of the first livestock farming ventures, achieved with the aid of the dog, who played an essential role in their management.

Ancient Times

Middle East

Sheep became important because of wool and milk production. This is demonstrated in the clay tablet records, in wall sculpture, and other art forms: those with corkscrew horns were frequently featured. Ancient Babylonian records list flocks numbering thousands of animals. Fat-tailed sheep were particularly important as a useful food and tallow source.

The Bible records the sheep flocks of the early Hebrew tribes, not a reliable historical document but a description of ancient lifestyles. Abel the son of Adam and Eve, a shepherd, offered one of his first lambs as a religious sacrifice. Later Abraham is said to have owned flocks and that his second son Isaac followed him as a shepherd, and that his son Jacob cared for the flocks of his relative, Laban, for fourteen years before he owned his own. The interesting Biblical (*Genesis* 30:32) story of Jacob and his ability to breed spotted lambs shows that he had learned to recognise which of his flock carried the recessive gene for this characteristic. The ram's horn, suitably fashioned, was used as a trumpet in Biblical wars and entered Jewish ritual as the *shofar*, to be blown at certain times in religious services.

Egypt

The arrival of sheep in the Nile valley in about 5000 BC resulted in the animal being depicted in tomb paintings and in carvings by 2500 BC – with corkscrew horns and hair coat. After 2000 BC the depictions were of a sheep with normal horns and a fat tail, it was not until after 1000 BC that they are shown with a fleece. Herodotus (c.484 BC–425 BC) wrote that generally sheep were regarded as sacred animals and were not used for sacrifice, except at the sanctuary of Mendes (a goat-like god) while worshipping Isis and Osiris. As livestock, sheep were of low importance to the Egyptian economy, probably the initial interest was for milk and meat. The production of high quality wool only developed slowly. Herodotus also wrote that Arabia had two kinds of sheep, one type had long tails, the other had broad tails, and that shepherds would use little carts attached to the tail to prevent injury.

The Hellenic World

In the early Neolithic period small mixed ovicaprine flocks were kept, mainly for meat. These were kept on little more than large gardens/smallholdings, the animals grazed on the fallow or scrub land and were also valued for their manure. In the Bronze Age the interest shifted and wool become important, with large-scale production on both Minoan and Mycenaean palace properties. Greek agriculture became based in sheep, olives and wheat. Evidence from Minoan clay tablets and wall paintings, about 1500 BC, show the national wealth was based in wool, with a similar development in the mainland Mycenaean culture. As the Hellenes established their colonies around the Mediterranean Sea, the Black Sea region and Asia Minor, they took sheep with them.

Later arable farming became the dominant activity until, under Roman occupation, the flocks grew again as the demand for sheep and goat produce (wool and cheese) increased. In this period transhumance developed making maximum use of available pastures. Religious and social functions provided important dates, creating an expanded sacrificial calendar, which required quality finished animals to a specific schedule.

Roman Empire

Sheep were an important livestock species. Pastoralism was recognised to be a profitable livestock system and if well conducted could be a lucrative venture.

Cato (234 BC–149 BC) gave practical advice on building a flock and outlining the established terms of a sale. The purpose was wool production and he discusses shearing methods, emphasising the need for skin health care.

Varro (116 BC–27 BC) again detailed the stock to buy: not too young nor too old, full-bodied, abundant fleece, short legs and long tail. He emphasised pasture provision, attention to feet, providing a fold (shelter) for weather protection, ensuring available water and a warning of skin disease, scab. Varro also wrote of the value of transhumance, he sent his sheep from Apulia to Abruzzo, and stressed the importance of informing the tax collector of the movements. Breeding is discussed at length. Castration of lambs at five months was advised. If the animals had valuable fleeces the use of hide jackets was recommended, and keeping the fold and housing clean. Farmers who preferred to pluck the wool were advised to starve the sheep for three days prior: to weaken the attachment of the wool. The owner should ensure the herdsman knew remedies for diseases and had them available, as well as having their uses written in a book that he should carry with him.

Columella (AD 4–AD 70) wrote, 'the sheep is of primary account if one has regard to the extent of its usefulness' identifying wool production as well as cheese and milk, both for 'country folk and people of taste'. Much emphasis was given to choosing good stock for the locality and suggesting that 'coated', that is, fine-woolled sheep should be kept in meadows on flat land. Columella discusses cross breeding for differing wool types and colours; while recommending white wool he wrote of the values of brown, black or red (*erytheon* sheep from Asia) wool. As a practical landowner and farmer he writes in detail on ram selection, and ensuring that the palate and tongue are not black or spotted, as these will produce coloured lambs. He suggested that ewes be mated on April 18th, which was termed *Parilia*, the feast of Pales the tutelary goddess, who watches over sheep and the shepherd. This date was to enable the lamb to get good autumn nutrition to see it through the winter. He also stressed that the flock owner replenish his stock all the time by rejecting older animals and always entering the winter with good strong sheep.

Columella emphasised that the owner of the flock should be knowledgeable on veterinary matters and in particular with lambing. If a breech presentation occurs and the lamb cannot be delivered, an embryotomy procedure was described, as one practised by the Greeks. The advice, also given by Varro, that the new-born lamb should not be allowed the 'beastings' or colostrum is repeated. [No reason is given for this potentially dangerous practice: today it is regarded as an essential aid to the immune protection of the new-born].

Sensible humane advice is given, that flock masters should always be 'observant and vigilant', be quiet and never shout at or hit their animals. They should also always stand as the guardian of the flock and watch over their care, grazing and provision of shade when needed. Shearing and treatment to control scab was also detailed. Columella advised care in preventing snakes entering the sheep houses, it was suggested regular fumigation either by burning various substances such as cedar wood, *galburnum* (a gum resin from *Ferula galbaniflua* grown in the Middle East), woman's hair or stag horns.

Palladius, writing in the 4th–5th century AD, produced a compilation book utilising many of Columella's suggestions. Feeding of Greek sheep, described as Asiatic and Tarantine breeds, in sheds is recorded. Snake control, copied from Columella, indicates that this was a problem in certain areas. Overall the emphasis is on wool production and the utilisation, and value of the dung.

The *Geoponika* anthology, dating from about AD 900, indicates the extent of knowledge at the end of the Roman Empire: Varro and Columella are still quoted, indicating their value. The emphasis on wool production with careful selection of breeding stock and on the value of dung for vine cultivation remains. There is also a content of folklore/magic, such as: if the sheep skip, a storm is coming; if the ewes want to repeatedly mate it indicates a long winter; and the interesting suggestion for a reliable fish bait – a baked ram's penis.

During the years of the Roman Empire sheep flock management and wool production reached a sophistication that was to be lost as their civilisation vanished. Within Italy sheep were important, particularly in Apulia and the Po plain, but the system needed teams of slave herdsmen. After the Roman times sheep survived well in Europe, but mainly due to the peasant class who had small flocks to provide clothing, milk, cheese and manure.

Medieval Europe

Over generations each region within Europe developed 'breeds' suitable for their locality. The Balkans and Greece produced varieties related to Turkish and Near Eastern types. Italy and its islands developed predominantly milking breeds while the plains of northern Europe produced hardier wool producers. Spain concentrated on high quality woolled sheep (Merino). By the Middle Ages Spain and Britain competed as the two major producers of fine wool. Eventually Britain became the principal supplier of cloth (mainly worsted) to Europe and sheep and wool became the cornerstone of the British economy. The development and evolution of the major sheep breeds, and in particular the European varieties, has been well researched and reviewed by Ryder (1984, pp. 76–83).

Post-Roman sheep initially had major importance as milking animals. In the English Domesday Survey, 1086, it was shown that sheep were the most numerous livestock animal: five ewes could produce as much milk as a dairy cow, but with a shorter lactation period. When wool production began to gain importance milk still remained significant. Additionally the manure was highly valued.

The Liber Bestarium (MS Bodley 764), a monastic book produced in the mid-13th century, contains a significant section related to sheep. It is recognised as an important provider of wool and that they 'eat voraciously' before the onset of winter before the frost stops the growth of grass. The ram is seen as the powerful male animal, the wether is also noted [but politely not mentioning castrating]; the male is recognised for strength and its habit of headbutting. The comment is made that 'he has worms in his head which cause such itching' [possibly a recognition of gid: parasitic infestation]. Imprinting is recognised allowing dam and lamb to find and recognise each other. These observations were written by someone who had observed sheep [the monasteries usually had large flocks]. The species provided opportunity for allegorical texts – the gentle sheep, the pugnacious rams and the baby lamb. All feature in the Bible with many attributions and available quotations. The illustrations in the *Liber Bestarium* all show horned sheep, the animals grazing and the dam caring for the lamb.

By the Middle Ages big flocks were common in Northern Europe, held by the monasteries and feudal lords. Most peasants had small groups of sheep grazed as a flock on common land under the care of one shepherd. Shepherding became a major occupation with flock masters holding important positions in rural society. The shepherd was truly the guardian of his flock, he and his dog would sleep in the fold and he had to be continually on watch, in particular for disease. It was customary for the shepherd to receive a daily bowl of whey all summer and ewe's milk on Sunday, a lamb at weaning and a fleece at shearing. These men would never leave their flock unattended (Macgregor 2012, pp. 426–430 and 456–475).

There was a gradual shift to wool production (in particular in Britain) with shearing a major local event. Sheep had to be first washed in a lake or river: clean wool fetched a higher price. The shearers always had a pot of tar or salve available for dressing wounds and cuts. Equally important was the castration, or gelding, of lambs, well described by Henry Best (*Rural Economy in Yorkshire in 1641, being the Farming and Account Books of Henry Best*). He wrote that a competent man could geld 100 lambs in three hours by slitting their scrotum with a knife, biting off the 'stones' and then dressing with tansy-butter to ward off flies and 'to keep healthy'. But this was a dangerous process and lambs were frequently lost due to infection. The origin of this particular practice dates back many years, but was still remembered in the 20th century. Disease was always a hazard, with sheep scab first recorded in Britain in 1275 and sheep pox in the 1300s.

The correct management of the flock was recognised as the essential factor in producing a profit. One of the earliest writers on English agriculture was Walter of Henley who wrote, in French in c.1280, a book of management of a large agricultural enterprise. Titled *Le Dite de Hosbandrie*, this book is usually presented with two similar publications – *Seneschaucie* by an unknown author, and the *Book of Robert Grosseteste*: together these lay down sensible management instructions. The Seneschal was the title of the senior manager of a property, responsible to the owner. The books were widely read, and highly regarded up to the 1700s. It was recommended that the flock be inspected three times a year: after Easter during May, to look for scab; before Lammas (celebrated between 1st August and 1st September) to sort and remove old or poorly animals; and at Michaelmas (29th September) to cull any poor stock before winter. The advice was, 'see that your shepherd be not hasty, for by an angry man some may be badly overdriven': the stress on flock welfare was sound, but it is not known how well it was observed.

The importance of the wool industry was demonstrated by the publication in 1353 of the Ordinance of the Staple, which described wool as 'the sovereign merchandise and jewel of this realm of England'. The monasteries, with big flocks developed a wool industry; they started spinning, used marketplaces and merchants, and their woven textiles moved to the export markets. In the later Middle Ages their influence declined and the main producers became the larger farmers. The 15th century saw a great improvement in waterpower, used for fulling mills and also the manufacture of cheaper grades of cloth. The export of fleeces to Europe declined and gradually England came to dominate the European cloth trade.

From the 17th century, meat production became more important than wool but sheep maintained their place as the most important part of the livestock industry. In certain regions the production of sheep cheese and butter was important: this was seen on the Essex marshes (east of London) which became the main supplier of lamb meat, and cheese and butter to the city. Butter was important as a much used salve (healing ointment) used on both sheep and humans. The marshes, however, were seriously infested with liver fluke which accounted for significant losses. By the 19th century this Essex trade had declined and soon vanished (Trow-Smith 1957, p. 131 and pp. 241–250).

Arable farms were anxious to have sheep graze stubble fields to acquire the valuable dung. This resulted in a complex system of renting, or loaning flocks in return for their manure. Elaborate systems of 'folding' developed, with hurdles that were moved to confine the sheep to a new area every day. It was estimated that at least 400 sheep were needed for the system to work well, overnight penning ensured the dung was deposited on the correct selected areas.

Europe: Agricultural Revolution 18th–19th Centuries

The sheep industry reached prominence by the middle of the 18th century with improved feeding methods and, by selective breeding, had developed many local breeds. A prominent figure was Robert Bakewell (1725–1795) of Dishley Grange, Loughborough, Leicestershire; now recognised as one of the most important contributors to the British Agricultural Revolution. Apart from his sheep breeding work he made successful improvements with beef cattle, some with horses, and was a leader in grassland improvement. With careful selective breeding Bakewell improved the Lincoln Longwool breed and used it to develop the New (or Dishley) Leicester breed. This was highly successful and sheep were widely exported to Australia and North America. This work was continued by Thomas Coke (1754–1842), later Lord Leicester, of Holkham, Norfolk. Among his other agricultural achievements he promoted and advanced the English Leicester Sheep, noted for fast-maturing, and thriving on a diet of turnips. The best surviving English breed from this early work was the English (or Leicester) Longwool.

While British sheep and cloth production was dominant in Europe there was a recognition that Spanish Merino sheep produced a particularly fine wool. The Spanish authorities were concerned to keep control, the export of the merino breed was banned. However, this did not prevent animals being smuggled out. The Napoleonic Wars disrupted Spanish regulations and the French were the first to break the export ban. Jean-Louis-Marie Daubenton (1716–1799), a leading French breeder, built a flock to attempt to break the British monopoly on quality wool. He headed a state-financed scheme and with good selective breeding was able, after a few years, to produce a fleece almost as good as that grown in Spain.

King George III of England (1738–1820), was interested in agriculture and was dubbed 'Farmer George'; the British Agricultural Revolution reached its peak during his reign. He had a flock of English sheep and tried to build a flock of Merino sheep. He purchased some and Daubenton also sent him some but it was not a success. Merino sheep were bred for, and were used to, a transhumance life – even temperatures, a good diet, plus they needed care and selection to thrive outside of Spain. Animals also reached Germany and Austria but with limited success. The first Merinos were shipped to Australia around 1793 and some wool shipments to England arrived in 1807, but it was to be another 35 years before Australia could ship more Merino wool to Britain than the Spaniards.

By the 19th century there were some 20 well recognised principal sheep breeds in Britain and these went on to provide the leading bloodlines for the global sheep industry; New Zealand in particular has made notable further improvements.

Mid-Near East, Africa, Asia

The main influence on sheep development and use was the rapid spread of Islam and the creation of a caliphate that at its maximum reached from Spain, North and East Africa, the Near and Middle East, Arabia and extending into present-day Russia and Pakistan. There, is however, little illustrative or written literature to aid the identification of breeds or management practices. Sheep not only were valuable to nomadic tribes, contributing to their ovicaprine flocks, but also became essential to provide sacrificial animals for the religious practices. Ovine milk products aided a staple diet and the flocks provided hides and fleeces which contributed to Islamic leather and woven products.

In the Middle/Near Eastern countries sheep were the basis of much of the existing nomadic and transhumance culture. The fat-tailed sheep were popular and sheep food products, leather and wool and use for religious sacrifice formed the basis of an economy spread across an enormous region of the world. In later years, the sheep provided the basis for an important carpet trade. Both fat-rumped and thin-tailed breeds also had local importance. The Karakul, for production of woolled lamb skins, evolved as a specific localised breed.

Central and Southern Africa

The breeds that developed in this region were almost all haired sheep, including the fat-tailed Somali breed. In 1652 the Dutch settled in Southern Africa with imported sheep which they bred with local fat-tailed sheep. Spanish Merino stock arrived in 1789 and a government Merino stud was founded in 1804 and the breed became of major importance. Other breeds such as the Blackheaded Persian were also introduced and became popular in Rhodesia (now Zimbabwe).

Asia

Most sheep were located in the mountainous ranges of the Himalayas, Tibet and China together with the steppe plains of Siberia (Russia). A major feature of their management was the transhumance nomadic lifestyle of the pastoral peoples. Sheep in the northern regions of the Indian subcontinent were used to carry salt over the mountain passes; pack flocks were much employed, with each animal carrying a 35–40 lb load. These were the Hunia breed, developed from the Urial type. In central India carpet-woolled breeds are found but in southern India there are mainly haired breeds. The sheep of Tibet are mostly thin-tailed with hairy fleeces while those of China are fat-tailed and many also fat-rumped.

The Americas and Australasia

In these continents the sheep have all been introduced, almost all with the European breeds and in particular those from Britain. Sheep proved to be an ideal colonisation animal that could be utilised in areas of poor pasture, and not only provided meat, but wool – essential for early colonists to spin and weave for home-spun cloth, but also a product that could be shipped and traded. Sheep in North America were mainly of British stock from the mid-1600s. In the 1800s sheep farming moved westwards. Central America received its first sheep in the late 1400s, Chile in 1540 and Merinos arrived in the Argentine in 1812. Mexico had Merinos in 1521.

Australia received British sheep in 1788, with the first settlement. Imports, mainly of British stock, rapidly increased when the inland expansion between 1840–1870 took place, at which time Australia had an estimated 50 million sheep. A Captain McArthur purchased three Merino rams from King George III flocks in 1793 and, with 30 ewes and some additional Spanish and Irish stock, started the breeding of Merino sheep.

New Zealand colonisation began in the 1840s and Merino and British breeds became established, first in the South Island and later in the North Island. Extensive pasture improvement and intensive selection, to provide either meat or wool for the changing market opportunities, have characterised the highly successful New Zealand industry.

Recognition of Sheep Diseases

Study of the literature from the past produces a confused record, in particular in the early years, because of the frequent incidence of epizootic diseases common to sheep, cattle, goats and pigs. The use of the word 'plague' is frequent. Care must be taken in interpretation of much of the early citations, the reporters were frequently concerned with occult, magical or religious causes of disease, which affected their clarity of observation. The sources quoted here are multiple and many are drawn from the listings included in Fleming's *Animal Plagues* Volume 1 (1871) and Volume 2 (1882).

The Years of Antiquity to AD 800

Examination of ancient and pre-history sources do not reveal any major health problems with sheep (Biblical references are dealt with separately). The first definitive information is found in the Roman agricultural treatises. Cato (234 BC–149 BC) only mentions one disease – 'scab' – it was the major recognised flock disease. Ticks were also recognised as being undesirable, but probably not directly related to any disease.

Treatment for scab was recommended for the flock after shearing by smearing the whole body for three days with a mixture of equal parts *amurca* (the watery residue left after oil drained from crushed olives), boiled lupin water and the dregs of 'good' wine. Then the sheep were to be washed in the sea or in brine water. The claim was made that it would prevent scab, produce better wool and also ward off ticks. A somewhat similar flock procedure was still being described in 1728, without any evidence of its value.

Sheep were also a part of most important Roman religious sacrificial rituals. At *suovetaurilia*, the most significant major public sacrifice, three species had to be offered – a bull, a ram and a boar. Cato describes a *suovetaurilia* sacrifice to be held on the farm, describing it as an important ritual to be undertaken, 'to purify the farm and the land', together with wine to be offered to Janus and Jupiter with cakes (described as like fingers joined together). Among the prayers to be said were the words, '. . . thou keep away, ward off, and remove sickness, seen and unseen . . . preserve in health my shepherd and my flocks . . .'.

It was also stated, presumably to reduce costs, that on the farm the sacrifice could be a calf, a lamb and a piglet.

Varro (116–27 BC), writing some 150 years later, discussed the state of knowledge on the causation of disease, 'In general, sickness is caused by the fact that the animals are suffering from heat or cold, or else from excessive work, or, on the other hand from lack of exercise . . .'. Varro also echoed Cato's writing with '. . . in the matter of health there are many rules; but as I said, the head shepherd keeps these written down in a book, and carries with him the remedies he may need'.

Presumably such literate and knowledgeable staff were available. Varro's instructions indicate that the knowledge of the time understood cleanliness, there is emphasis that sheep folds be kept clean and that the milking stalls have hard surfaces to drain away urine. Other rules were not explained, such as during the breeding period the ewes should always drink from the same source, 'as a change causes the wool to spot and is injurious to the womb'.

The two health problems that are mentioned are scab, obviously the main worry, and foot rot: '. . . the moisture of the ground injures not only the fleece but their hoofs as well and causes them to become scabby. . .'. [This is not explained but possibly indicates that both Psoroptic as well as Chorioptic mites were involved; the foot lesions could also be a sign of of virus infection, but lip lesions are not mentioned.] Much attention was directed towards examining each animal for scabs or sores, which had to be treated before shearing. All freshly shorn animals were to be rubbed down with a salve made of wine and oil with white chalk and hog lard. If the animal usually wore a hide jacket then this was to be greased inside with the salve before replacement. If any sheep were cut during shearing the advice was, '. . . smear with soft pitch' [to become a shepherd's staple for many centuries].

Columella (AD 4–70), the most practical and pragmatic of the Roman agricultural authors, wrote that while sheep are generally healthy one must choose a breed suitable to the type of farm that you have, and in particular to the type of land you own. He stated it was essential to provide a warm fold in winter and the availability of shade in summer. The folds should be kept dry underfoot and the sheep should be well fed. Ensuring sufficient feed was essential, but it could be made more attractive if troughs of salt were available, to act as seasoning to encourage feeding.

Columella advised that in general sheep can be treated as cattle with the same medications. However, if the whole flock were unwell the advice was to move them out of the heat or wind if it is present. This movement should be made slowly, some exercise would be valuable, but enfeebled animals should not be hurried. The most serious disease of sheep was seen to be 'scab', Columella wrote that it usually occurred when it was cold or frosty, or after sheep have been shorn. He advised that scab could be prevented if sheep were washed and anointed (as previously described). Diagnosis was made when sheep were seen to be rubbing against walls or trees; shepherds were advised to part the wool when they would see rough skin with a crust. When found, treatment had to be commenced at once. Several remedies were suggested but before treatment the crust was to be scraped away and then the medication applied with vigorous rubbing. A favoured treatment was a mixture of equal portions of crushed white hellebore with lees of wine, dregs of oil and the juice of boiled lupins.

For sheep with a fever it was recommended to bleed, either from the hoof or pastern, or between the eyes, or ears. Lameness was said to be due either to fouling of the division between the claws of the hoof or to an interdigital tumour containing a worm, which had to be carefully removed. Treatment was by anointing with liquid pitch (tar) or pitch with alum, sulphur and vinegar added. For lung disease it was suggested that a leaf of lungwort (*Pulmonaria officinalis*) be inserted through the ear of the affected animal. The disease named erysipelas, or by shepherds *pusula*, was deemed to be incurable [this was possibly sheep pox]. Columella stated that unless caught on the first infected sheep it will affect the whole flock, he noted that it could be eased by fomentation with goats' milk, but that this was not a cure.

Remedies for other diseases are suggested, such as for a sheep with catarrh (in translation written as 'rheum'), the stalks of wild mint should be inserted into the nostrils, or sour vinegar poured down the left nostril. Broken legs were to 'be treated as humans': wrap the limb in wool soaked in wine and oil and then bound with splints. A fatal disease of lambs called *ostigo* or lamb scab is mentioned, characterised by 'eruptions around the mouth and lips with filthy sores'. Having been described as fatal a cure is proposed by using hyssop and salt crushed together and rubbed all over the mouth, followed by a vinegar wash and finally anointed with liquid pitch and lard. [While this disease could be identified as orf, caused by a pox virus, its transmission to human handlers, a well-recognised hazard, is not mentioned.]

The observations of sheep diseases provided by Columella were to remain the basis of sheep health care for the remainder of the Roman Empire. While the methods of treatment and medications were in most cases of little efficacy, the overall guidance on management and flock care was both sensible and of value to the owner.

Palladius (4–5th century AD) provided an anthology of advice on agriculture and farming practices. He gives some importance, when discussing sheep scab, in quoting the lines from the *Georgics* by Virgil (70–19 BC). The words of particular interest relate to treatment where cutting open the scab is recommended as 'the malady lives and thrives by hiding', this could indicate an awareness of the presence of the parasitic cause, but not actually understanding the observation.

Palladius noted that cedar resin was used in Arabia for camel scab [sarcoptic mange remains a major camel disease problem]. Cedar resin was also recommended for tick control. Many other herbal concoctions were proposed for a variety of disease problems, additionally herbal mixtures or decoctions are suggested for dosing of all sheep in both spring and autumn to maintain health. Overall Palladius presents a compilation of knowledge that shows no significant advances from Columella.

The *Geoponika* anthology, compiled in Byzantium in the 10th century, was an agricultural reference guide. The diseases of sheep feature, Varro is quite extensively quoted and also, briefly, Virgil. Much of the disease related texts can be seen to follow the advice and precepts of Columella.

Of other authors cited, Florentinus is the most extensively quoted on sheep providing sensible advice on housing, feeding and care, but the only health advice appears to be to always have an odd number in the flock as it has 'some natural influence on their survival and safety'. Africanus, offered the wisdom that to make sheep follow you – block their ears with wool. Democritus gave the advice to keep lambs healthy, give them ivy as a food for seven days. Didymus was more rational and discussed the treatments for scab and ticks: all previously noted by Columella and Palladius. *The Quintilli* were concerned by an unidentified plague termed *loimike nosos*: the recommended treatment was to emulsify a stork's intestines in water and give each sheep a spoonful by mouth. Leonitus also wrote of this unidentified plague and proposed its control by dosing the flock with an herbal mixture every spring and autumn. Finally, Anatolius is quoted, mostly with his repeats of older knowledge and ideas together with advice on preventing wolves from attacking the flock: this was to fasten the squill plant around the neck of each sheep. The *Geoponika*, as far as veterinary care and medications are concerned, would suggest that no significant advances had been made over the previous 800 years.

The Period of Natural Observation, AD 800–1699

Many of the early references to disease in sheep are coupled with other species and without any diagnostic features. Where possible these are grouped to avoid repetition. This was a period when epizootic diseases were common. There was no real understanding of disease, and relatively little appreciation of prevention methods.

829 *Greece, Thrace and Bulgaria* A plague and with an 'epizooty among sheep'. (*Frari Della Peste* vol. ii, p. 211)

886 This year 'a pestilence in animals throughout the whole world'. (*Eulogium Historiarum*)

887 *France* A very severe and tedious winter, also a 'plague' among oxen and sheep extended beyond measure in France, so that scarcely any of these animals were left. (*Annal. Fuldens.*)

994 *Continental Europe* 'A terrible plague broke out among men, pigs and sheep . . . a grievous famine in Saxony'. (*Annals. Quedlinburgens* Pertz M. p. 72)

994 *Wales* During the reign of King Hywel Dda (r.AD 942–AD 950) the laws of the country were codified, and then known as the Laws of Wales. This was a very progressive move almost unique at the time. When animals were sold they had to be warranted by the seller against certain diseases, for sheep these included scab (mange), redwater (probably haemoglobinuria) and rot (liver fluke). In the latter it was stated the warranty was for 'three dew falls' until the 1st May (but no other date appears to be given), when 'she shall have satisfied herself three times with new herbage'. It would appear that the relationship of fluke infestation, and snails and wet herbage was recognised.

1086 *England* A year of bad weather, 'a severe season, and a swinkful [toil and labour] and sorrowful year . . . sheep as well as cattle suffered from the great intemperature of the air'. (Walter Hemingsford *Chronicles*)

1088 *Ireland* Recorded that a, 'great snow in this year and great mortality of oxen, and sheep and pigs. . .'. (*Annals of Innisfallen*)

1124 *England* An eclipse of the sun occurred on 3rd August, 'which was followed by a great pestilence among oxen, sheep, pigs and bees'. (*Cosmae Prag. Chronic.* Book III)

1149 *Belgium* '. . . by some death-bringing contagion a pestilence, sheep, oxen and all kinds of cattle were hurried away by death'. (*Acta Sanctor. Bolland* Jan 2, p. 318)

1171 *Germany* Disease in cattle, sheep and men throughout the country. (Hoffman *Annal. Bamberg*)

1201 *England* Continual rain and great floods. 'A great dearth of animals followed, but chiefly of sheep, possibly from dropsy or rot'. (T Short *A General Chronological History of the Air* London 1749)

France and Spain Disease in man, also 'for birds, cattle and sheep become sterile and brought forth no young'. (Villalbo *Epidemiologia Espanola* vol. i, p. 54)

1223 *England* A great death of sheep. (T Short *ibid* vol. i, p. 139)

1254 *England* After a severe winter there was, 'a great murrain, and death of sheep and deer, so that of whole flocks and herds scarce the half escaped'.

Later after more tempestuous weather there was, 'such a deadly disease among sheep and wild beasts, that the sheep folds were void of sheep, and the forests of wild beasts; indeed, in large flocks scarcely one-half survived'. (Matthew of Paris *Chronica Majora*)

1258 *England* A severe winter with wind, frost and snow, 'it seemed as if a general plague was raging among the sheep and lambs'. (Matthew of Paris *ibid*)

1274 *England* The first reports of a 'deadly disease' of sheep, called *Lues ovium*, it was to be reported for the next 25 or 28 years and was said to have nearly destroyed all the flocks in England. (Thomas Walsingham *Historia Anglicana*)

1275 *England* Commenting on the Walsingham report, that this was the first recorded observation of the disease later known as sheep pox. (Henry de Knyghton *The Events of England*)

Following the report by Thomas Walsingham it was also recorded that, 'A rich man of France brought into Northumberland a Spanish ewe as big as a calf of two years, which ewe being rotten, infected so the country that it spread all over the realm. This plague of murrain continued for twenty-eight years ere it ended and was the first rot that ever was in England.' [While the nature of the disease is unclear it is probably a plagiarism of the 1274 report, however it could also be the first record of a Merino sheep introduction to Britain.] (Stow *The Annals or General Chronicle of England* London 1614, p. 200)

1314 *England* A year of famine and great shortage of all foodstuffs 'No flesh could be had . . . sheep died of the rot, swine were out of the way. . .'. (Stow *ibid* pp. 217–218)

1333 *England* There were major losses of all classes of livestock, due to the general 'murrain'. For sheep this was reported as, at Maldon 'more than half his sheep and lambs', at Leatherhead 'little more than the same rate', at Farley 'more than twenty-five percent', at Woolford and Basingstoke 'about thirty-four percent', at Wolford 'a little less than fourteen' and 'at Cuxham about eleven'. (Rogers *Hist. Agricult.* vol. i, p. 53)

1338 *Ireland* A year of tempestuous weather and a common 'complaint' of oxen, cows and sheep. The latter were 'almost destroyed', said to be the first recorded ovine epizooty in Ireland (Clyn *Annals*)

1385 *England* In the accounts of Alton Barnes an entry reads, 'Great mortality among sheep – 15 per cent, 55 of lambs died'. (Rogers *ibid*)

1389 *England* The accounts of Alton Barnes have following entry 'Scab and sickness very prevalent among sheep'. A similar report was from Leatherhead. (Rogers *op. cit*)

1443 *Ireland* 'A rainy tempestuous year ... it much hurted bees and sheep. The second epizooty of sheep reported in Ireland'. (Mac Firbis *Annals of Ireland*)

1513 *Europe* In this, and the following year, there were reports of epizootic disease in animals and plague in humans from many parts of Europe, 'the plague did sweep away the wretched cattle, but also nearly the whole of the unhappy flocks of sheep'. (Fracastor *Tract. De Contagiosis Morbis* vol. i, cap. 12)

1515 *France* A disease of sheep, previously seen infrequently became contagious and pestilential. It was named *Febris pestifera* or *Vari nigri* or commonly 'Tac'. This can be traced back to Conrad Gesner who mentions the disease as scabies and a treatment called *huile de tac*. Tac oil was widely used by the peasantry of Gaul. The oil was derived from juniper oil, and the word 'Tac' from the recognition that it was spread by simple contact. (Paulet *Recherches sur Maladies Epizootiques* Paris, 1775 vol. 1, p. 88)

1523 *England. Boke of Husbandrie* by John Fitzherbert. Directs the shepherd to never be without his 'tar box', a mixture of tar plus oil or grease was in general use as a salve for skin disease (scabies and lice), wounds and fly control. Also written that sheep were 'the most profitabilest cattle any man can have' and also 'white snails be ill for sheep in pasture and in fallows'. [Fluke (rot) causation was recognised but not understood.]

1567 *Europe* Widespread smallpox outbreaks and similar outbreaks in sheep: attributed by many to be same disease. In Montpellier, France the sheep affection was named *picota* or *picotte* (the French term for *variola ovina* or sheep pox). In some areas a great loss of sheep, the thousands, was reported. (Joubert *De Peste Libellas* 1567 and Spangenberg *Mansfeld. Chronic.* book i, p. 402)

1591 *Sicily* A hot and damp year, forage blighted and cattle and sheep became emaciated. (Marcellus Capra *De Morbo. Pandemonio* Folio II)

1628 *Italy* In the states of Venice, Rot (assumed to be liver fluke infestation) was widespread. Locally also named *pourriture, biatta, marciume.* (Bottani, Vol ii, p. 37)

1649 *Italy* A skin disease of sheep was reported in the Padua region. Local diagnosis of smallpox [but no record of the disease in man], probably sheep pox.

1656 *Italy* Much epizootic disease in humans in many regions. Additionally, 'a cruel epizootic disease aggravated the pestilence by attacking and destroying the greater part of the oxen and sheep'.

From the report this was probably in the Ecclesiastical States, no details given. (Frari. Vol ii, p. 484)

1663 *England, Germany* and other countries. Rot of sheep was particularly observed, 'and even wild animals were said to suffer from this affection'. In Germany, the disease is called *egeln, egelichte or lebern.* The description states that 'the livers of stags were full of *vermium*' translated as 'hydatids'. The causes of the disease outbreak which lasted for two years 'were alleged to have been frequent inundations, the honey-dew and rust of herbage and corrupt water'. (Frohmann *Miscell. Nat. Cur.* p. 245)

Italy In the Venetian territories, 'this year and the following, the livers of all sheep, oxen, deer, hares and so on, were only bags of worms, like leeches, and often the lungs also . . . only old bullocks and sheep survived'. (Bonet *Sepulcr. Anatomic*)

England Sheep-masters called this the 'Rotten Year' as most of all of the great flocks died. (T. Short *op. cit.*). A German chronicler wrote,'the year was a very damp one in England, so that the cattle and sheep suffered severely from fluke-worms (*egelwümen*)'. (Schnurrer *Chronik. der Seuchen*)

1673   *Ireland. The Herdsman's Mate* by Michael Harwood. The first book published in Ireland with veterinary content. The author recognises the fluke as the cause of 'rot' and associates it with wet pasture, but not with snails.

1689   *England* Written that 'In mankind, spotted fever, small-pox and others, then followed by murrain of sheep' (but no details). (T. Forster *Atmospherical Origin of Epidemic Disorders of Health*)

1690   *Italy* In Lombardy the spring weather was without rain, crops were affected with rust, smut and other blights. Then insect pests arrived followed by heavy rains then very dry with great heat. 'Animals of every species (were) dying in great numbers, sheep were first affected, after a few days, variolous eruptions appeared on their heads and necks and generally caused blindness . . . died from hunger . . . and either whole flocks died suddenly, or were seized with smallpox. . .'. (Ramazzini *Const. Epid. Op.* Geneva, pp. 120–141)

   Another chronicler ascribed the losses in cattle, sheep and other animals to anthrax. (Wirth *Lehrbuch der Seuchen und Ansteckenden Krankheiten der Hausthiere* Zurich, 1846, p. 85)

1694   *Europe* Probably Italy. Reports of, 'a supposed epidemy and epizooty of ergotism . . . sheep, cattle, pigs, horses and geese were not free from the contagion'. Some wheat 'was so plainly diseased, that it was dangerous for man to eat of it'. (Brunner *Ephem. Nat. Curios.* Dec. 1694)

The Development of Biological Observations, 1700–1800

With the start of the 18th century the medical sciences were becoming more defined and specific disciplines were evolving. As these developed a greater interest in animal disease was seen, in particular where this involved epizootic disease with a zoonotic character. Most important, in 1761 the first veterinary school was established at Lyon, France – soon copied in other European countries.

   1708   *England. The Whole Art of Husbandry* by J. Mortimer, a Fellow of the Royal Society (FRS), published in London. The book is a comprehensive guide to agriculture and all types of farming. The observations on sheep are of interest as shown by the statement that they are a 'very useful creature, but very profitable too'. The breeds of that time and their wool types are discussed; the section on choice of stock reads much like Columella's advice. The management guidance is sound. Shearing is outlined with the emphasis on washing the sheep first, care in shearing so no cuts occur and watching for blow flies in the tail region.

Disease problems are described as, 'The great inconvenience which attends sheep is their being subject to the Rot; which is very hard to prevent, if the year prove very wet especially in May and June . . . the Rot, Red-Water and most of the Distempers that sheep are subject to, proceed from too much moisture of the land they feed on . . . keep on dry land in wet seasons and give fine hay, oats and bran with salt mixed in as the best preventive.' There is no mention of Scab or skin disease, other than blow fly strike. A series of plant/herbal based remedies are suggested. As earlier observers had also written Mortimer adds, of sheep faeces 'this is the best of all Dung' and advocates the practice of folding sheep on arable land after harvest.

1708 *Ireland* After bad weather there was 'another great Rot among the sheep here (Dublin)'. (Rutty *Registry*)

1710 *England* A 'fever' of sheep on the South Downs raged epidemically, the shepherds called it smallpox. It 'began with a burning heat and broke out in fiery pustules all the body over. These pustules maturated, and, if death had not happened first, dried up into scabs about the twelfth day . . . when it came it swept away whole flocks . . . it never affected mankind'. (Thomas Fuller MD *Exanthematologia, or an Account of Eruptive Fevers, especially Measles and Smallpox*, London, 1730)

1714 *Europe* 'In Alsace, cattle, fowls, hogs, geese, sheep and horses perished', but no details are given. (Kanold *Jahres hist.* pp. 119–206)

In many parts of *Germany*, the dropsy or rot had prevailed among cows, sheep and goats from spring until autumn. This disease also appeared in Paris region, and the following year, 'when so many sheep died, that an ordinance was issued to kill all pigeons and other birds that might diffuse the contagion'. The same disease was common in Italy (Kanold *ibid* p. 177)

France In a further report on the Paris outbreak a detailed description was given by the Faculty of Geneva: this covered the appearance and maturation of the pustules up to scab formation and skin cicatrices, 'very similar to those produced on man after the small-pox'. Two sheep were examined in detail together with the clinical signs as noted by the shepherd. The local French name is *claviliere*. This description follows the account by Fuller of the 1710 outbreak in England. Two medical authorities give the first good description of sheep pox. (*Reflexions, and so on* Geneva p. 130)

1716 *Ireland* 'A general Rot among the sheep ... after the great frost ... that destroyed the sheep even on the best lands'. (Rutty *op.cit*)

1718 *Germany* A year in which most species suffered from some form of epizootic, variously attributed to either anthrax or foot-and-mouth disease. In the autumn it was reported that the sheep 'in many places began to cough badly' – but no other details. (*Breslauer Sammlung* vol. vi, p. 1711)

1719 *Italy* An epizooty of *Variola ovina* was seen in the Vatican States. (Bottani *Delle Malattie Contagiose ed Epizoötiche* Rome, 1817)
Bohemia 'a disease resembling the small-pox of sheep, *schafblattern*' was seen. (*Breslauer Samml.* vol. x, p. 460)

1720 *Germany* An outbreak of 'smallpox' in sheep was reported from Saxony. (*Breslauer Samml.* vol. xiii, p. 622)

1724 *Italy* A report of 'a deadly epizooty of ovine small-pox in the Venetian States, lasting from August to December'. (Bottani *op.cit* p. 202)
France A paper by M. Astruc mentions the prevalence of sheep small-pox, noting it to be highly contagious in sheep. He stated it could be transferred to other animals, in particular rabbits who acted as the vectors to other flocks; he recorded that the shepherds of the Languedoc and the Cévennes were well aware of this and tried to eliminate rabbits in those areas. In the Cévennes the shepherds were aware to the pox problem and had a belief that if they passed by an infected flock they would immediately stop their own flock and remain there until the next day – the belief was that the cold of night together with any dew might destroy the potential particles which would communicate the disease. (M. Austrac *Dissertation sur la Contagion de la Peste* chap vi, Toulouse, 1724)
Europe In the years 1723–1724 'immense' numbers of sheep were said to have died from the 'rot' in Silesia, Poland and Prussia. (*Breslaur Samml.* vol. xxviii, p. 398)

1726 *Germany* Sheep smallpox was reported to be 'very destructive' in Eichsfeld and Thuringia (*Breslauer Samml.* vol. xxxvii, p. 57)

1729 *England. The Gentleman and Farmer's Guide for the Increase and Improvement of Cattle* by R Bradley Fellow of the Royal Society (FRS). Published in London. Bradley was Professor of Botany at Cambridge University; his book covers all livestock species including horses, and discusses management and their 'respective distempers, and the most approved medicines for the cure of them'. There are also special mentions of 'the benefits' of wool and the 'great advantages arising from Hides, Tallow etc'.
Chapter 1 is titled '*Of Sheep, and the several ways of* ordering them for Profit'. The importance of sheep at that time is illustrated by the opening sentence, 'The sheep being a Creature of extraordinary Profit to Britain, from the Riches which proceed from its wool, and the great convenience arising to the generality from its nourishing Flesh, its

Tallow, and its Skin, I think it proper to give it the Preference in this Treatise'. Bradley makes his point.

Following a sensible and mostly rational discussion of sheep types, feeding, pasture and management: mentioning only one disease – the Rot – liver fluke infestation. Rottenness is then discussed in detail with both external signs and post-mortem findings including, 'if we cut open the Liver . . . we find small Worms of the Shape of Flounders, that sheep is rotten'. He also states that 'wherever the Speerwort or the Flamula grows, which for the most part is found in wet Grounds, there the Sheep rott'.

There is quite a long comment on choice of pasture and, 'in some Pastures there are great Numbers of Snails and Sluggs, which while they are small, the Sheep will take in with the Grass, and are distempered by them . . . in dry Weather, Sheep are not in danger of the Rot by these Creatures'. Bradley demonstrates that while the causation of fluke infestation and the actual fluke had been recognised the relationship between the two remained unknown. This knowledge, however, enabled sound advice to be given on pasture selection and preventive grazing, feeding, management, selection of rams, raising and suckling lambs and the best time for castration of lambs. In writing about washing of sheep prior to shearing Bradley quotes from John Fitzherbert 1523 (see above) noting that he was the English writer of husbandry 'of any note'. He also cites the ancient Roman writers on agriculture. There is also a long and detailed dissertation on the wool, weaving and cloth trade, demonstrating its importance in the English economy.

In discussing sheep diseases Bradley emphasises that first every shepherd must have a salve for topical treatment of the Scab or Ray [Ray was a term used to describe the skin inflammation and fly strike area around the tail, derived from the Old French *raié* meaning a stripe or streak in 16–17C. English. The word was used for diarrhoea in sheep and cattle, also for smear or bespattering]. He stated that these were the 'most common Distempers Sheep are subject to', but added 'both proceed from poor Food'. However, he then wrote of Scab that 'one has good Reason to judge it infectious'.

A salve was a mixture of tar [now termed Stockholm tar] with the Grease or fat of poultry, geese or pigs or unsalted butter. Also recommended was a 'Broom Salve' as this was a cheaper ingredient than tar. The recipe was 20 gallons of spring water from a gravel soil (preferred) to which was added about ten gallons of Broom tops, stalks, leaves, flowers all shredded and boiled to the consistency of a jelly. Then two quarts of stale human urine was added with the same volume of strong salted beef or pork brine plus two pounds of melted mutton suet. Stir together, strain and store for use. This salve was also claimed to destroy ticks and sheep lice.

Other remedies, all plant based are listed. Juniper berries are used as a 'regular medicine' with the observation that where the Juniper grows sheep are never subject to Rot. A tick remedy based on a decoction of 'tobacco stalks' was cited as a 'sovereign Remedy against Ticks' [a recognition of the antiparasitic activity of nicotine]. The 'worm in the foot' as a disease is discussed with a long quotation from John Fitzherbert, *The Boke of Husbandry* 1523; a myth that can be traced back to Columella.

Many other diseases and remedies are listed but recognition of the actual condition is not easy to determine. The two most serious ovine problems in Bradley's estimation were the Rot and the Scab.

1735 *England* A report of the 'most noted sheep rot of 1735', it was said to have been observed in deer, sheep, lambs, hares and rabbits that were on wetlands. Very severe in the Vale of Aylesbury. (*The Shepherd's Sure Guide*, London 1749)

 Ireland It was recorded that notwithstanding the excessive rainfall that no 'general rot' appeared in the sheep. (Rutty *op.cit*)

1740 *Europe* A rainy summer resulted in sheep rot in the low countries. (T Short *op.cit* p. 254)

 Ireland Mentions of sheep dying from rot and redwater, also rabbits. (Rutty *op.cit*)

1741 *England* A severe winter and horses, cattle and sheep all died from starvation. (Huxham *Observations on the Air and Epidemical Diseases* London, 1758)

 Ireland 'Horses, cows, sheep, pigs and poultry, all were struck by the plague and perished'. It was known as *Bliadhain an air* (the year of the slaughter). (*Famine in Ireland in 1740, 1741*, a pamphlet)

1743 *France* 'The whole of the sheep in the territory of Arles, died from rot'(*pourriture*). (Hurtrel d'Arboval *Dict. de Méd. Vét* vol. i, p. 249)

1746 *France* 'Sheep small-pox did great mischief among the flock', in Beauvais. (Barbaret *Maladies Epizootiques* p. 16, also Paulet *op.cit* vol. i, p. 267)

1747 *England* Rot in sheep after a wet spring, in particular in Vale of Aylesbury and in Middlesex. (*Shepherd's Sure Guide*, London, 1749)

1750 *France* Sheep attacked in January, February, April and November by *Picotte (variola ovina)*, many in particular those affected in January died [sheep pox]. (Marcorelle *Mém. de l'Acad. des Sciences* vol. ii, p. 622)

1753 *Ireland* Following very wet weather this was reported as the cause of 'great destruction of sheep throughout the island'. (Rutty, *op.cit*)

1754 *Germany* During the winter sheep, pigs, ducks and geese were attacked by, 'glossanthrax, or a form of gangrenous sore-throat presented itself as an epizooty among animals in Hanover . . . the sheep and swine and also the geese and ducks were attacked'. [The term glossanthrax is sometimes interpreted as foot-and-mouth disease, if so the perceived avian infection, possibly avian influenza, would have been unrelated]. (*Hannov. Gen. Anzeig* 1754 also Fischer *Lieflandisches Landwirthschaftsbach* p. 625)

1755 *Germany* From May to September *ekzema epizootica* or aphthous fever affected all domestic animals in Franconia and also in Bamberg and Nuremberg: 'the feet of affected animals became swollen and the hoofs sloughed off'. This affected cattle, horses, swine and sheep. 'The same appearances were observed in the mouth, both sides being covered with vesicles which became confluent. . .'. 'Turkeys also had their feet so diseased that they could not walk. . .'. [While this outbreak can be suggested to be foot-and-mouth disease the report of signs in horses and turkeys has to be questioned, the mild disease has been seen in fowl and other birds but is generally not recognised in the horse]. (*Frankische Samml.* vol. i, p. 349)

Switzerland Sheep smallpox was reported in the Basel region. A report suggested that inoculation such as that used for human smallpox could prevent the disease in sheep. (Zuinger *Acta Helvetica* vol. iii, p. 301)

1756 *Germany* Sheep smallpox was prevalent in Saxony. One infected flock was quarantined in a garden containing pepper plants (*Capsicum Indicum*), the sheep fed on these and were reported as, 'all recovered'. (J Wolf *Geschichte. u. Beschreib. der Stadt Duderstadt* p. 207)

1757 *Germany* In this and the two following years ovine smallpox was very common, and fatal, eye lesions and lip gangrene were frequent concomitants. (Fink *Pockenkrankheit d. Schafe* p. 1)

England Observations on Husbandry by E. Lisle, 1757, published in London. The most important sheep disease was 'the rot'; a problem that could halve a flock kept on heavy clay and undrained sodden soils. Management was recognised as important and herbal remedies were used. The other problem was skin disease, but the renewed use of mercury preparations was seen to be useful for treating scab. Tar was the panacea for skin wounds and for prevention of fly strike. The shepherd's teeth were still seen as the handiest tools for castrating the ram lamb, 'he has his two hands at liberty to hold back the strings of the stones that are not all drawn away'.

1761 *France* Heavy winter and spring rainfalls were seen as the cause of rot (*pourriture*) in sheep in the Boulonnais region, 'lambs were fewer, feebler and smaller than in ordinary years'. The outbreak became widespread except where the land was elevated, dry or sandy. The sheep died showing extensive dropsy beneath the lower jaw; the livers were filled 'with flat worms which the country people called *dogues*'. Affected sheep continued to eat well until death. (Desmars *Mem. sur la Mortalité des Moutons en Boulonnais. Epidémiques d'Hippocrate* Paris, 1767 p. 289)

In some districts of France ovine smallpox was seen (Heusinger *op. cit.* p. 237)

1762 *France* Sheep smallpox widespread in Beauvais and other provinces, also glossanthrax in sheep in Lorraine. (Paulet *op. cit* vol. i, p. 248 and Schnurrer *Chronik. der Seachen* Part II p. 325)

1763 *Europe* A year of moist and sultry weather, poor harvests for both cereals and olives. Many human epidemics were recorded and similar epizootics in animals, all species appear to have been affected with differing signs in most countries.

'Malignant Anthrax' was reported across *France* including sheep; glossanthrax also in many regions affecting sheep (and cattle and pigs). An 'anthracoid' disease also reported in sheep in *France* with the best animals the first to die. An epidemic of apthous fever (*eczema epizootica*) recorded in cattle and sheep in *Moravia* [includes a reasonably reliable description of foot-and-mouth disease and symptoms]. Nearly all sheep affected cast their hoofs, goats were also affected. A possibly similar disease was reported from northern Europe in the Hulstein and Nordhausen regions. (Duhamel *Mem. de l'Acad. des Sciences* 1764; Barbaret *Mémoire sur les Maladies Epidémiques des Bestiaux* Paris 1765; Sagar *De Morbo Sing. Ovium Vinob* 1765; Paulet *op. cit* vol. i, p. 397)

1764 *Europe* Apthous disease in sheep in The Netherlands, northern Germany, the Rhine provinces and elsewhere in central Europe. (Paulet *op. cit* vol. i, p. 397; *Frankische Sammlung* vii, p. 544)

1765 *Europe* In Moravia a great many sheep died, 'may have been either rot or malignant catarrh'. (Sagar *op. cit.*)

1766 *England* Rot in sheep 'experienced all over England . . . when whole flocks perished'. (Mills *Treatise on Cattle* 1766)

1771 *Russia* Ovine smallpox reported to be prevalent in Siberia. (Pallas *Voyages dans Plusieurs Provinces* vol. iv., p. 19)

1775 *France* Smallpox in sheep reported to be 'making great ravages' in Aix vicinity, and also smallpox in man. (Darluc *Hist. de la Soc. Roy. de Médecine* vol. i, p. 250)

1776–1782 During this period cattle plague dominated all animal disease reports throughout Europe.

1783 *Iceland* Severe earthquakes and volcanic eruptions in Iceland. Over 190,000 sheep perished (also humans, horses, cattle). The losses continued into 1784 and post-mortem examinations of sheep revealed multiple lesions in body organs and severe bone loss: attributed to inhalation of volcanic dust.

1786 *Germany* An infectious disease initially called anthrax was observed in cattle, the main signs related to the tongue with a 'ropy mucus flowing from the mouth . . . in bad cases . . . a painful tumour under the jaw'.

The infection spread across the German States in cattle, horses, sheep and pigs. Later it spread to Italy and diagnoses included Cattle Plague and 'the glossanthrax' (foot-and-mouth disease); other variations were termed gangrenous erysipelas, malignant anthrax and there was a claim that it spread to mules and humans. Rot was also seen in sheep in Bavaria. (Will *Kurzer Unterricht uber den jetz herrschenden Zungenkrebs* Munich, 1786; Plank *Veterinar-topographie von Baiern*, p. 137)

1787   *Italy* and *Germany* The epidemics of the previous year continued. In Bavaria, an epizootic of sheep pox broke out with stated 'deadly' consequences. The report added that the disease has continued in the region since that time. (Laubender *Seuchengeschichte der Landwirthschaftlichen Hausthier* Munich, 1810)

     Ireland A very wet year 'disorder among the sheep – particularly the murrain'. This was characterised by blisters on the mouth, the comment is made that this might be the mild form of glossanthrax that was prevalent on the Continent. (*Dublin Chronicle*)

1790   *France* Smallpox in sheep was 'rife' in Normandy. (Chabert *Instructions, Etc.* vol. i, p. 399)

     Germany Haematuria was observed in sheep, supposed to be caused by the larvae of *curculio pisi* (?). (Laubender *op. cit* vol. i, p. 399)

1791   *France* A contagious foot rot of sheep was said to have crossed the Pyrenees from Spain, termed *pedero*. It became prevalent on the area of the river Gironde and the Lower Medoc. (Chabert *op. cit*)

1792   *England. The Shepherd's Guide* by James Hogg, published in London. James Hogg (1770–1835) was born at Ettrick, a small village in the Borders area of Scotland, 17 miles from Selkirk. While as a young man Hogg worked as a farmhand and shepherd, for the majority of his life he was known as a poet, novelist and essayist – and termed the 'Ettrick Shepherd'. *The Shepherd's Guide* was written in 1792, when Hogg would have been aged 22. While Ettrick was in the heart of the sheep region and there would have been good local knowledge, possibly some caution should be taken in his judgements and attitudes. This book tries to deal with diseases of the sheep in a logical and 'scientific' manner. Clearly laid out, it is an attempt to bring order to a complicated picture. The author appears knowledgeable on his subject. In the Introduction the two diseases which he declares are the most serious are 'the Rot' and 'the Braxy'. The liver fluke issue had been well recognised as a problem for many years but 'the Braxy' is not the clostridial infection to which the term is now usually applied to sheep in Britain.

    The opening chapters deal with the diseases of lambs and young sheep, the latter termed 'Hoggs'; castration of lambs by 'incisoring' is recommended, followed by pulling the tail sharply a couple of times! This is followed by a long and essentially incomprehensible section on the four types of Braxy and methods of cure and prevention – 36 pages of a 188 page book. A similar number of pages are devoted to the rot, however, in spite of the numerous prior publications relating the disease to wet conditions and snails on the grass Hogg writes,

'I hold it as an incontrovertible fact, that *a sudden fall in condition* is the sole cause of the rot'. Scab is discussed in six pages, giving stress to it being highly contagious, the advice that treatment by topical application of mercury compounds was a useful advance in therapeutics, but with a potential toxicity.

Apart from a rather gruesome description of Hogg's 'operation' for gid (hydatid cysts) by inserting a wire up the nostrils into the brain the book has an interesting listing of old names for sheep diseases, many of which are not easily recognisable. Of particular interest however are the three appendices: two by Daubenton, the notable French veterinary writer, one on methods of bleeding sheep and the other on ovine diets. The third is by Vitet, another recognised French author, on sheep pox in France. **Note:** the above has been written using a facsimile copy of Hogg's book, dated 17 July 1792. Two other reports have been seen both of which give a publication date of 1807.

1795   *France* 'Smallpox committed great ravages among sheep'. (F.H. Gilbert *Recherches sur les Causes des Maladies Charbonneuses dans les Animaux* Paris, 1795)

1797   *Germany* During this year (and next) 'smallpox was very fatal in sheep'. Efforts at vaccination were made. (Fink *Beschreibung der Pockenkrankheit*, p. 22)

1799   *Italy* In the Venetian States and in Lombardy 'sheep suffered much from smallpox'. (Faggiani *Topografia di Padova*, p. 111)

Science Evolves with a Developing Veterinary Medicine Discipline, 1800–1900

With the establishment of the first veterinary school at Lyon, France in 1761 a central point was created for specific studies. This was important for sheep diseases in France in particular with the serious sheep pox problem.

1801   *France* Sheep in the Haut-Pyrénées [region] were 'decimated by *variola ovina*'. (*Ann. de l'Agriculture Francais* vol. xii, p. 69)

1802   *France* In Crease region, '*variola ovina* was very destructive among the flocks'. (no reference)

1803   *France* In the Rhone Department 'ovine smallpox caused much destruction among the sheep'. (Gohier *Mém. sur l'Epizootie de Trannois* Lyons, 1804)

1804   *Germany* Rabies in foxes was widespread in Wurtemberg and Baden who attacked both humans and animals including sheep. The outbreak spread to several cantons of Switzerland (*Sammlung d.d. Veterinärpolisei in Würtumb. betreffenden Verordnungen* p. 218)

1805   *Europe* The 'Spanish foot rot', described as a contagious disease of sheep appeared in Switzerland, Piedmont and other countries; previously recorded in 1791 (see above). (Heusinger *Recherches de Pathologie Comparée* Cassel, 1853)

Switzerland 'An epizooty of rot accompanied by flukes in the liver, among ruminant animals in Zurich Canton, in this and the next year'. (Wirth *op. cit*, p. 123)

1807 *France* In the Departments of Aube and Gers, 'the sheep flocks were nearly exterminated by sheep pox'. (no reference)

1809 *France* A skin disease in dogs, diagnosed as *variola canina*, or canine smallpox, was observed in kennels at the Lyon Veterinary School. Attempts were made to inoculate both sheep and dogs: sheep showed a slight eruption of pustules around the inoculation site, but nowhere else. (Hurtrel d'Arboval *Diction. de Méd. Vétérinaire*)

France and *Germany* Rot (here termed *cachexia aquosa*) was reported to be prevalent in both countries. (Sander *Vermischte Beitrage zur Praktischen und Gerichtlichen Thierheilkunde* Berlin, 1810)

England. A Treatise on the Diseases and Management of Sheep by Sir George Mackenzie, Edinburgh, 1809. A rather strange mixture of contents: Part I deals with the anatomy of the sheep written by a surgeon, James Wardrop and Part II is surgical, mostly where the author describes the use of a trocar and cannula that he had devised for draining hydatid cysts (cases of 'gid' or 'sturdy'). He has based the technique on the 'Hogg operation', and states that the procedure is frequently fatal. The rest of the text is copied from other authors and is of little value.

England. A Practical Treatise on the Merino and Anglo-Merino Sheep by C.H, Hunt, London, 1809. Mainly an opinion of regret on the lack of knowledge on sheep diseases and an appeal for greater action to understand the problems.

England. Facts and Observations Relative to Sheep, Wool, Ploughs and Oxen by John Lord Somerville, London 1809. While this is a most attractive and well-presented book, no doubt due to the eminence of its author, it is not really a text on sheep disease. Of the 256 pages in the book, 107 are devoted to sheep, 53 to cattle and farming generally and 96 to farm accounts and shows. It does demonstrate the continuing importance of sheep and wool production to British farming at the start of the 19th century and in particular the arrival of the practical application of new technologies (in ploughing, grassland, water supplies and so on). The author defines himself as not just a sheep man but a British sheep man – 'I am resolved never again to wear superfine cloth, or Kerseymere' [a coarse cloth woven from short-stapled wool]. There is an explicit well written discussion of British sheep and farming and the end products required in wool, meat and tallow. Merino sheep and the signs of health are sensibly reviewed (he refers to Columella, showing the continuing influence of the ancient texts). The incidence of foot rot in Merino sheep is noted and treatment sensibly discussed. Construction of sheep folds is covered in detail with attention to both shelter and ventilation. Nutrition is discussed based on the use of salt, either as a supplement or in a lick made from saturated salt solution and ground chalk in 'cakes' following drying. The work of Daubenton, France, is quoted here – 'Salt gives them appetite and strength . . . promotes digestion. . . .'. The practice was apparently widespread in France, Sweden, Saxony (Germany) and Silesia.

As the 19th century advanced there was a gradual evolution of a scientific method, the recognition of specific diseases and the factors related to their cause. Rational treatments were (slowly) being introduced and some ideas of prevention were becoming proven. In continental Europe sheep pox had become a major disease problem, liver fluke disease (rot) was a universal disease and mange (scab) was broadly spread. The two main sheep countries were Britain and France, followed by Spain with their traditional transhumance practice and Merino sheep. In Britain sheep and the wool trade was the major economic activity of the country.

Rot was known to be related to flukes in the liver and to wet seasons and grass, and possibly to small snails seen on such pasture, but there was no understanding of the life cycle. Vermifuges of such substances as nitre with ginger, vitriol and salt were in common use, but no value. Scab was coming under a measure of control with improved salves, blends with tobacco juice, aged human urine, gunpowder or turpentine all helped. The reintroduction of the old medieval treatment based on mercury was efficacious if used well. Ewe milk butter salve was considered the best. There were no sheep dips.

Sheep foot rot was known but was seldom perceived as a major problem. Braxy as a disease entity was becoming recognised, mainly in Britain, it was seen in flocks in the western counties and was rapidly fatal. Mainly occurring in store lambs with a full bladder and when there was a heavy frost; keeping the sheep moving was found to be a preventive. Hydatid cysts in the brain (causing gid or sturdy) was a variable problem, shepherds drained the cysts by various methods, often fatally. The disease that is now known as scrapie was probably first recognised in 1732 in Cambridgeshire, England (Trow-Smith 1959, pp. 199–201 and pp. 212–213). Occurring initially mainly in the Cheviot and Suffolk breeds it is now known to be one of the transmissible spongiform encephalopathies, caused by prions.

Recorded disease in European sheep to the end of the 19th century, shows regular reports of rot, frequently with dropsy (liver fluke disease) in Britain, France and Germany; in France sometimes with huge losses (1812). Foot rot was commonly reported across Europe but seldom serious until in 1815 an outbreak of what was termed *contagious ovine paronychia* in France, Germany, Piedmont (Italy) and Switzerland: many local names were used – *pedero, pietin, limace, fourchet, crapaud contagieuse, cuidite, pustuleuse, Franzosiche Klauenseuche* and others. The most serious and important sheep disease in Europe was sheep pox. The losses in France were particularly high, there was a particularly bad outbreak in Germany and the Haute-Marne in France from 1822–1834. Italy and almost all other countries also reported outbreaks.

A book by M. Gasparin, *Des Maladies Contagieuses des Bêtes á Laine* published in 1821 in Paris, discusses methods of prevention of sheep pox. In the Languedoc region, 'from time immemorial to prevent epizooties' every autumn the shepherds, when the weather was becoming colder, would hang the skin of a sheep that had died of pox in the sheep fold. All the lambs, six to eight months old, would acquire the disease 'and the health of the flock is ensured'. No details of losses due to this deliberate infection are given. Gasparin reviews the value of various inoculation techniques (termed *ovination*) that had been employed by both veterinary and medical men in the 18th and early 19th centuries. The procedure was known to work in certain circumstances but had never been properly investigated. When human smallpox vaccination came into general use the technique was investigated again with much work in the early years of the 19th century. The conclusion was that inoculation was an unreliable prophylactic. It was also recognised that some breeds of sheep had a very low, or no incidence of the disease. This publication by Gasparin was an important landmark in the understanding of sheep pox as there was an attempt to provide a scientific analysis.

Early reports of sheep pox in Britain are unclear; it was said to have been known in the 9th century but there is no convincing documentary evidence. Another reported introduction of skin disease in 1275 could have been pox, it was said to have persisted for 25 years. There was always an awareness of the disease because of the known regular outbreaks in continental Europe. The first recorded case of sheep pox in Britain was in 1847, described by J B Simonds, lecturer in cattle diseases at the Royal Veterinary College, London. A flock of 56 Merino ewes had been imported from Tonningen (Tonning, Germany) and sold at Smithfield Market (London). There was then a rapid spread of the disease and heavy losses of up to 50% of flocks. A year after the introduction, two Acts of Parliament were introduced to prohibit imports and provide orders to control any spread: by 1850 the disease had disappeared.

The disease was reintroduced in 1862 with the loss of some 400 sheep from a flock of 1700 animals. Simonds discussed the situation with human smallpox specialists and tried *ovination* using lymph from mild cases, but with limited success. Stringent movement controls and 'stamping out' eradicated the outbreaks. There were three further introductions to Britain and these were soon eliminated by strict controls; since then all imported cargoes have been checked on arrival and any infected animals slaughtered at the port (Ministry of Agriculture 1965, pp. 162–164). An interesting observation was made during the sheep pox outbreaks in Britain. A trial was made with a child who was inoculated with the 'matter' from a poxed sheep. It was recorded that it produced, 'a disorder corresponding with the cow pox' (Spooner 1878, p. 273).

Reports of sheep diseases began to appear from other countries. An 1829 serious rot outbreak was described in sheep and cattle in Egypt, as the Nile river water level fell in the Delta following the annual floods. Dropsy was an important sign, described as 'a bag of water under the jaw and neck', losses were high. Sheep pox was reported from Russia in 1829.

Reports began to appear of undiagnosed diseases in sheep: a 'catarrhal fever or influenza' in England, 1838; an illness termed *Raphania*, but undescribed, in Germany in 1834; reports also of a 'trembling disease' in France, Germany and Scotland in 1839. In Scotland it was called 'leaping ill' [now termed 'louping ill' and recognised as a viral encephalomyelitis spread by ticks]; good early descriptions are by W Matthewson, *Edinburgh Veterinary Review* May 1892 and J Fair, *The Veterinarian* vol. xii, p. 162. There is an excellent description of a disease in lambs and ewes, 'their mouths presented a mass of disease being one complete ulcer . . . I found a large fungus issuing from all around the lower gum . . . the lamb communicates it to the ewes udder . . .'

The description is totally characteristic of contagious ecthyma or 'orf', now recognised to be caused by a pox virus related to bovine papular stomatitis virus; this first description was by Rawlings in *The Veterinarian* (1838) vol. x, p. 205. As specific diseases were described some clarity was developing for the recognition of sheep ailments.

The publication of a book by Spooner (1878) a veterinary surgeon and teacher at the Royal Veterinary College, on the diseases and management of sheep provided a text that advanced the understanding of sheep diseases. As was the way in the Victorian era education was broad-based, the text is in three parts: 1 History and Breeds; 2 Anatomy and Economy; and 3 Diseases and Treatment. While the understanding of many of the diseases lacks the later knowledge, it is an intelligible and rational book. In the section on liver fluke infestation (the rot) there is recognition of *Fasciola hepatica* as being the cause of the disease, but no knowledge of the complex life cycle that results in the clinical signs. It was known that cercaria develop in water snails and that sheep close-crop the grass; the fourth edition of the book (1878) comes very close to an understanding of the life cycle of the liver fluke.

Two discoveries in sheep diseases happened towards the end of the century. J B Simonds published the results of his investigations on the sheep lungworm, *Dictyocaulus filaria,* and enabled an advance in pasture management (Simonds 1874, p. 265). This started a more detailed examination and interest in the gut helminths of sheep. Of more importance was the final elucidation of the life cycle of the liver fluke by A P Thomas (1883, pp. 99–133) an Oxford zoologist, following a particularly serious outbreak in 1879. After so many years the cause of 'the rot' was understood, this provided a boost to better pasture management. The study of sheep diseases had now moved into the hands of scientists.

Ovine Disease and Welfare

Sheep are often regarded as one of the 'lesser' livestock species, cattle usually dominate the picture. However, an historical assessment shows they have been an important, and for certain communities vital, part of the economy. Being one of the very earliest domesticated animals, sheep have possibly been of more value to evolving human civilisation and societies than any other animal. Initially they provided fat, previously only obtained from wild animals (while this was later replaced by vegetable fats in the West, in the East it remains an essential part of their culinary practices). Having a sheep flock assured a permanent source of meat as well as a constant supply of milk, cheese and hides. As religious practices evolved it also provided a convenient and reliable source of suitable animals for ritual sacrifice.

Later wool was seen to be of value, probably first by felting wool plucked from moulting animals (still practised in some Asian regions) and next by spinning and weaving to produce cloth. The latter appears to have first happened in more northern climates. Felting, spinning and weaving are among the first technologies devised by humans and date back to the earliest times. Spinning and weaving were initially developed for flax to produce linen, suitable for hot climates. Wool provided a better cloth for the colder regions and when finer wools were available more woollen cloth moved south. Wool remains a unique and valuable product.

Wool not only created the cloth trade, it also revolutionised clothing and built trade and wealth. These properties enabled colonisation with the sheep being the major economic driver in Australia, New Zealand, South Africa, areas of Latin America and North America, as well as providing early settlers with the material for their home-spun clothes. The economic value to both Europe and their colonial expansion was particularly important for Britain, who became an initial leader in developing and selecting for new breeds of sheep for wool and meat production. The Merino sheep was developed in Spain with unique husbandry practices: a breed that has been significant in global development. Additionally, sheep have played a very important role in French agriculture, and in Germany.

Throughout this long history disease has been recorded as a factor in sheep farming. Some interpretations of the Bible consider that Moses, himself a shepherd, remarked on what could be scab in sheep. From the early Roman agricultural treatises it is scab (psoroptic mange) that is specifically recorded. In the greater than two thousand years overviewed in this study four diseases are seen to be significant: scab, rot (liver fluke infestation), sheep pox and foot rot.

Sheep scab was recognised and diagnosed by early shepherds. In the late 1800s the nature and life cycle of the invasive acarine parasite became understood. The disease still exists globally: it can be eradicated but is now regarded as a problem to be kept under 'control' as the economics of sheep farming are not as flourishing as in previous years. Liver fluke disease was a major cause of loss by both death and poor condition for centuries: it was clearly recognised as early as in the late 10th century, but it was not until 1883 that the life cycle of the parasite was finally understood. The disease remains a problem unless strict pasture management methods are followed.

Sheep pox was for many years the most serious flock problem in mainland Europe, in particular in France. There is much of interest in the French literature of the 1800s on the disease and its possible relationship with human smallpox and other pox diseases. Now, sheep pox is eradicated from all major sheep markets but occurs elsewhere; a vaccine is available. Foot rot was recorded from quite early times, frequently as an epizootic, this remains unclear and may have been associated with outbreaks of mild FMD, which were recorded in continental Europe. The disease is now better understood and regular hoof care can play a major role in its control.

The now well recognised group of sheep diseases caused by the anaerobic *Clostridium* spp. bacteria were not understood until the early 1900s. The signs and deaths described in the early literature can be recognised in some cases. *Clostridium perfringens* was first described in 1892, but the actions of the complex toxins have taken many years to understand. The most widespread of these diseases are enterotoxaemia in lambs: *Cl. perfringens* type B, causing lamb dysentery and *Cl. perfringens* type D causing pulpy kidney. *Cl. perfringens* type C is the cause of the rarer enterotoxaemia in sheep at pasture, usually called struck.

Other clostridial diseases, all of which were known by colloquial and often dialect names before the cause was identified, include braxy (*Cl. septicum*), typically in spring lambs; redwater (*Cl. haemolyticum*) also termed bacillary haemoglobinuria; bighead (*Cl. novyi*) usually seen in rams, and rarely blackleg (*Cl. chauvoei*) where cases are usually found dead. Tetanus (*Cl. tetani*) and botulisum (*Cl. botulinum*) are very rarely seen. While the cause was unknown the colloquial names have generally survived and give an indication of the length of time over which these diseases have been recognised. As with all livestock disease the incidence and frequency changes with the husbandry method. More intensive practices usually result in higher disease incidence, or where there is more buying-in of animals.

In the later 1800s, as the parasitology discipline developed so did the recognition of the number of helminths found in the alimentary and respiratory tracts of sheep: early studies aided pasture management. In the 1900s developments in therapeutic and prophylactic products for use in sheep was significant. Now effective parasiticides for both endo- and ectoparasites are available, as well as vaccines for most of the recognised problems.

The welfare of sheep probably features more in their history than in that of other livestock. Sheep are recognised to be timid animals (actually based on their lack of binocular eyesight). Since Roman times it has been recognised that good management demands care in their movement between pastures and provision of shade, water and shelter, depending on the season and at lambing to ensure that time and space is allowed for the essential ewe/lamb imprinting process. While such good welfare practices have not always been followed throughout history there has always been an awareness of such requirements, and usually followed by the more progressive farmers.

Sheep and Public Health

The disease hazards listed below, while individually serious, have a low frequency in developed countries with veterinary and public health controls. Many of these problems have not been identified in the historical record. While they undoubtedly existed they were not seen to be of sufficient significance to be mentioned in the available records.

Meat inspection for transmissible diseases must be undertaken for, in particular tuberculosis (very rare in sheep), and anthrax (equally rare with none in developed countries). Other transmissible diseases are orf (the skin lesions can affect handlers) and anthrax from spores in wool, originally called 'woolsorter's disease'. Enzootic abortion in sheep due to *Chlamydophila abortus* presents a hazard to pregnant women and can cause severe illness. The danger is associated with aborted lambs and placentae.

An indirect hazard to humans is infection with *Echinococcus granulosus*. This tapeworm has dogs, foxes and wolves as the definitive hosts and sheep, goats, cattle and pigs as intermediate hosts – and also humans when they have accidentally consumed the embryonated eggs. The resultant hydatid cysts, if located in the brain, can be fatal.

References

FAO (2007) *State of the World's Animal Genetic Sources for Food and Agriculture* Rome: FAO

Fleming, G. (1871 and 1882) *Animal Plagues, Vols 1 and 2*. London: Baillière, Tindall & Cox

Leonard, J.N. (1981) *The First Farmers*. Netherlands: Time Life

Macgregor, A. (2012) *Animal Encounters*. London: Reaktion Books

Ministry of Agriculture (1965) *Animal Health: A Centenary 1865–1965*. London: HMSO

Ryder, M.L. (1984) in *Evolution of Domesticated Animals* (Ed. Mason, I.L.). New York: Longman

Simonds, J.B. (1874) On the Parasitic Lung Disease of Lambs. *Jnl. Royal Ag. Soc.* **X** No.ii

Spooner, W.C. (1878) *The History, Structure, Economy and Diseases of Sheep*. London: Crosby Lockwood

Thomas, A.P. (1883) The Life History of the Liver Fluke (Fasciola hepatica). *Quart. J. Microscop. Soc.* **23**

Trow-Smith, R. (1957) *A History of British Livestock Husbandry to 1700*. London: Routledge and Kegan Paul

Trow-Smith, R. (1959) *A History of British Livestock Husbandry 1700–1900*. London: Routledge and Kegan Paul

Zeuner, F.E. (1963) *A History of Domesticated Animals*. New York: Harper & Row

CHAPTER 20

Caprine: Goat

Taxonomically the goat is a member of the Bovidae family (subfamily Caprinae) of the order Artiodactyla – the even-toed ungulates. The other members of the Caprinae are the sheep (*Ovis*), and two closely related genera: the Barbary sheep of the Sahara and the blue sheep of the Himalayas.

The genus *Capra* has nine recognised species, of which the most significant are *Capra aegagrus* the bezoar or wild goat, generally accepted as the ancestor of the domesticated subspecies *Capra aegagrus hircus*; and *Capra ibex* and *Capra pyrenaica,* the Alpine and Spanish varieties found in Europe, the others are in Asia and the Near East.

The word 'goat' is derived from the Old English *gat,* and Old Saxon *get,* Old High German *geiz,* Old Norse *geit*; from the Germanic base *gaitaz.*

Male goats are called bucks (from Old English *bucca*) or billies (introduced in the 19th century). Female goats are called does or nannies (introduced in the 18th century). They are often simply termed he-goat (from 12th century *hegote* or *hegoote*) and she-goat. Juveniles are called kids. Goat meat has a variety of local names, often the adult meat is termed mutton (as is sheep meat).

Goats acquired an unjustified reputation in the past. The Biblical reference (*Matthew* 25:32–33) to separating the sheep from the goats, with the sheep being 'on his right, but the goats on his left' led to the interpretation that Christians were the sheep and that the 'goats i.e. non-Christians were not good people. Goats came to represent evil and became incorporated into the symbolism of Satanism. The shape of the head of the goat was found to fit into a drawing of an inverted pentagram. The figure of Baphomet, which displayed the head and legs of a goat, was said to be worshipped by the Knights Templar, and subsequently was used in occult and Sabbatic traditions.

The goat is also represented in Greek mythology by Pan, 'the God of the wild', part human and part goat. Goats are also known in other Greek mythology fantasies, and in Capricornus, the sea-goat, one of the oldest recognised group of star constellations. Capricorn is included as one of the twelve signs of the Zodiac, a concept that originated in Babylonian astrology.

Natural History and Biology

While goats and sheep are both members of the Caprinae subfamily, there are important differences in their ecological requirements and in the raw materials that they provide for their owners. The goat is a browser not a grazer and prefers shrubs to grass. They are hardy animals, well adapted to many climates; in particular both mountainous and arid regions which have small shrubs, and frequently aromatic herbs that other ruminants leave. Goats can survive in harsh desert-like conditions with poor quality feed.

Goats can be found all over the world, but are common in the warmer, drier regions. As they produce meat they are an important species in Muslim countries. They are good milk producers and are sources of hides for water and wine carriage, fibres and manure. They can be used for transportation of minor loads. These characteristics of the goat make it an ideal animal for people living at subsistence levels, rather than suppliers of export quality produce (Zeuner 1963, pp. 129–130).

Goats differ from sheep by possessing a beard and in the male having cornual scent glands situated at the base of the horns (usually in an anterio-medial position). The most obvious distinguishing feature is the tail – held erect in the goat, except in the Nubian breed, and pendant in the sheep. Many goat breeds also have wattles, one on each side of the neck. Sheep have suborbital tear glands and foot glands, and the latter are sometimes seen in goats. Most goats have horns with differing shapes and sizes depending on the breed. The skull shape shows significant differences compared with that of the sheep, who have both a greater thickness of skull (they head butt with considerable force) and also have thicker and more twisted horns than those of the goat.

The goat is polyoestrous, in warmer climates they will breed throughout the year, in temperate regions most breed in the autumn season. Kidding age is usually between 15 and 18 months. Pregnancy varies by breed and averages 150–152 days, but only about 145 days in tropical breeds. Life expectancy can be up to 18 years depending on the husbandry system and forage source. Goats have 60 chromosomes (sheep have 54).

Species Domesticated

Current evidence indicates that the goat was the earliest livestock animal to be domesticated, and in many regions of the world it was the first domesticated farm animal. There are some 300 recognised breeds, but the precise origin of the domesticated animal is unclear, because of the difficulty in distinguishing between the early domesticated and wild goats. Another difficulty in using the osteological evidence is determining differentiation in bone fragments between those of sheep and goats.

Neolithic farmers in south-west Asia were probably the first to domesticate the goat. DNA studies from bone remains found in the Zagros Mountains, on the borders of present-day Iraq and Iran, indicate that the domestication date was about

8000 BC. Other osteological evidence from 7000 BC–6000 BC has been found in sites at Jericho. Bones identified in Tepe ali Kosh, Iran date from before 7000 BC; since this site is well away from the natural habitat of *Capra aegagrus*, the recognised progenitor, it is suggested these were from a domesticated animal.

Capra aegagrus the originator species, is colloquially known as the bezoar. The name is a modification of the Persian (Farsi) *pád-zahr* meaning counter poison (*pád* = protecting (from) *zahr* = poison). The word in English dates from the late 16th century, used to refer to a concretion found in the stomach of ruminants (and presumably more common in wild goats due to their habitat and feed). These bodies were believed to act as poison antidotes, when ground up and administered to the patient. The word can be traced back to the Arabic *bádizahr* or *bázahr*. The mountain goat in Persian is *pázan* (the two words have a similar root).

DOMESTICATED GOATS AND CULTURAL GROUPS

The utilisation of goats shows enormous variations by both geographic region and by culture. Initially in ancient times goats were kept in herds that roamed on hilly or available grazing areas and were valuable in helping to clear scrub and woodland for arable farming. Goatherds, frequently children, are still a feature of the husbandry in many areas of the world. Only two breeds, the Angora and Cashmere, have been developed for wool production.

Ancient Times

Middle East

Reliable evidence provided by osteological remains (cited previously) indicate that the first domesticated goats were existing in the present-day Kurdish lands of Turkey, Iraq and Iran about 8000 BC. Other sites examined on the Iranian plateau suggest a similar date. In a variety of sites in present-day Turkey, Iraq, Israel, Palestine and Jordan, goat bones have been identified with dates about 6000 BC. Goats are believed to have been present in association with human habitation before sheep.

Ancient images show a variety of goat horn shapes, all basically derived from the straight form, or the twisted or corkscrew type. In ancient times the horn type conveyed much significance. The horn has value for making spoons and other objects, as well as also being used, with the ram's horn, to make the *shofar*, a form of trumpet used in Jewish religious ceremonies, and also as a war trumpet in Biblical history. A more detailed study of the development of the goat as a domesticated animal in ancient times, and in particular the significance of horn shape is given in Mason (1984, pp. 87–91) and Zeuner (1963, pp. 131–138).

Egypt

Goats are illustrated in tomb wall paintings from 4000 BC but were present in the region from 5000 BC. Horn shape is well shown from the many illustrations, but in 1700 BC the spiral corkscrew horned type became dominant, having entered the region from about 3500 BC.

The goat became important, more than the sheep, in the Egyptian economy, as a provider of meat and milk, as well as a source of hides used to make containers to carry water. Goat skin was also used as a wrapping for the dead. That the animal was valued is recognised from remains found along the Nile valley into Nubia (now Sudan) and also westward into Libya; these had occurred by 2500 BC as the goat evolved to an obviously popular lop-eared, screw-horned type.

The Hellenic World

It appears that Crete and possibly some Aegean islands had *Capra aegagrus* wild goats, but elsewhere in Europe the wild species were probably all of the *Capra ibex* variety. It is suggested that the domesticated goat entered Europe with initial introductions into the Hellenic (Greek) area, in the Neolithic period. Goats with both scimitar and twisted horns are shown on ancient Greek coins. A particularly interesting seal impression from the Late Minoan period in Crete shows a chariot drawn by goats, but it is not known if they were used as draught animals to any extent. The goats illustrated on this impression have bezoar distinguishing sabre or scimitar shaped horns.

Roman Empire

Goats of the scimitar/bezoar type arrived in Europe prior to the Roman expansion. Remains have been identified in many sites, in particular in Germany and Switzerland, Hungary and Scandinavia. During the Roman period hornless goats were reported, these were probably dehorned when young, rather than bred. *Varro* (116 BC – 27 BC), one of the earliest writers on livestock farming, not only noted the presence of wild goats in Italy, but also recorded the value of the domesticated animal for milk production. He stressed that in creating a herd one should buy young goats of a strong and large physique, with a thick haired coat, wattles and a large udder. He recommended that males should be chosen as one of twins and preferably with white hair, and also proposed one buck to ten does, but said others had one buck to twenty does.

Goats were of value on farms as they preferred woody shrublands to grassy fields, however they were found to be difficult to manage as they frequently had wounds from thorny shrubs or from fighting. Varro emphasised that goats felt the cold and therefore their stalls should face the sunrise, and be floored with stone to keep them clean and enable dung removal.

Columella (AD 4–AD 70), described goats as one of the 'lesser' farm animals. His comments on grazing and stock selection were similar to those of Varro, except he recommended keeping black haired animals to be shorn, 'for use in camps and hapless sailors coats'. Breeding was advised in the autumn, before December, and again stressed the value of twins or triplets in selecting stock. Columella also stated that their housing should have a stone floor for cleanliness and that goats needed a lot of 'keeping in their place' as they are most inquisitive and energetic. Their primary value for milk production was identified, he described in detail the cheese making process, for a good marketable product.

Palladius (4th–5th century AD) repeated many of the previous observations, the value of the goat in milk production, and the value of goat dung, not only as a fertiliser, but also for its use in treating damaged vine roots. There are also references to the use of burned goat hoofs being used as a snake deterrent, the use of goat milk to promote the production of peach trees, and goat blood being used in the manufacture of copper hoes, which when used will 'cause grass to die'.

The *Geoponika* anthology of farming information provides an overview of the status of the goat in the years leading to the end of the Roman Empire. While not described as a major livestock species it was valued for milk and cheese, meat, leather and hair: the latter was particularly favoured for ropes and nautical equipment.

There was also much use of goat products as medications and for a variety of other purposes: goat blood and vinegar was used to smear on walls and so on to control bedbugs, and was also said to kill fleas. Goat dung was rated fourth in value as a fertiliser, after that from pigeon, human and donkey. Various authors cited its particular usefulness for fertilising vines, date palms, vegetables, and combined with human urine as an apple feed. When burned it was said to control rust in grain crops and would fumigate vines. Goat fat smeared on pruning knives was used to control vine parasites and burning goat fat was claimed to drive away scorpions and other insects. A mixture of ground up goat hoof with herbs was used to deter snakes. Goat horns, inserted in the ground around vines were used to aid the fruiting, together with varied uses for the blood, fat, horns, dung and hair. Goat parts and produce were included in many recipes for animal treatments. Practical advice to the consumers of alcohol was to bake and eat a goat lung before heavy drinking: the recipient was said to remain sober.

Medieval Europe

Post-Roman Europe goats spread to all countries as populations migrated, adopted and adapted farming practices. Three main breeds developed, all arising from Swiss antecedents: the *Saanen*, with the highest milk yield; the *Toggenburg*, with a good milk yield and the *Chamois Coloured*, with very distinctive colouring of stripes. One other important breed is the *Appenzell*, similar to, but smaller than the Saanen. All of these breeds are horned and attempts to breed polled varieties have failed due to the creation of genetic abnormalities. Spain developed breeds without introducing Swiss stock, they produced two good dairy types: the *Malaguena* and the *Murciana-Granadina*.

The goat has been poorly documented in Europe because it was not perceived as a major livestock species, but there was a widespread population, in small herds and groups, mainly kept by peasants.

The *Liber Bestiarum* (MS Bodley 764) an early Medieval bestiary book, produced in the mid-13th century, features the goat, unusually with four illustrations (more than any other species), with well-drawn figures showing animals of the bezoar type, non-lop-eared, with erect tail and in most images demonstrating the habit of browsing on trees. In the text there is little mention of natural history but much on the activities of the he-goat and the character of the kid, and the utilisation of these to illustrate the meanings of Biblical texts.

In *Cheape and Good Husbandry* published in London 1616, Gervase Markham wrote that the distribution of the goat population varied widely depending on the availability of woodland and hilly country such as 'wilde and barraine places'. The goats were kept in small herds, not exceeding 100 animals, and it was noted that they did not like weather that was too hot or too cold. The value of the goat was in milk production, 'an excellent restorative' and in the kids, as a source of tender venison.

Thomas Moffet, in *Healths Improvement* published in London 1655, suggested that he-goat flesh was improved by placing them under stress before slaughter. The nature of the stress was not specified. Thomas Pennant wrote in *British Zoology* (1768) that goats were mainly found in mountainous regions. He noted their preference for tree shoots and bark, which could result in their being a nuisance animal and a problem; comments that would apply elsewhere in Europe. A particular wool industry developed in the Ankara region of Turkey, with a high value fleece being obtained from the native Angora goats. Greek and Roman writers in the 5th century BC had mentioned goats with 'fine fleeces' in Cilicia and Phrygia (Turkey).

Overall during this period the goat was valued for its milk and cheese, together with its meat when the haunches were salted and dried like bacon; for its fat for use in candles; the skin for fine glove leather, and the hair for making the 'finest periwigs'. As other meats and products came to the market and fashions changed, the role of the goat became primarily one of a dairy producer, and for some meat production.

Other Countries

The distribution of goat breeds and types from the initial domestication focus of the Near and Middle East, apart from their introduction into Europe, is not described in detail here: the subject is well covered by Mason (1984, pp. 88–96) and Zeuner (1963, pp. 140–152).

The one Asian breed that has become internationally known and valuable is the *Pashmina*, also known as Cashmere, because it was first encountered by Europeans in Kashmir, India. The breed developed in the mountains of central Asia, in particular in Persia, Tibet, Kashmir, Kyrgyzstan, Mongolia and Xinjiang, China. The fine-woolled fleece was named Pashmina meaning fine wool from *Pashm*, Persian for wool.

Extensive utilisation of the goat developed in the Indian subcontinent (India and Pakistan), which now has the largest regional global goat population: the animal is of importance for milk, meat and also hair. Many breeds are involved. While goats were known in India by 100 BC, it took several centuries for the species to spread throughout South-East Asia, probably only reaching Indonesia in the 14th century.

Many breeds of goat have reached China, these tend to be of the smaller breeds with characteristically short legs. The goat did not reach the main islands of Japan until the late 19th century when the European breeds were introduced.

The first goats to reach the Americas appear to have been introduced by Spain in the early 16th century. Initially introduced to South America, these Spanish types have developed to a well-adapted, but low productive *criollo* race. Similarly in Brazil, breeds now termed *crioulo*, were introduced by the Portuguese colonists. Many types of goat were introduced to North America, probably commencing first in the south-west, by Spanish colonists – this admixture has resulted in milk producers, meat and Angora goats all being present.

Goats in Africa developed most strongly from the early Egyptian introductions and then along the countries of the northern coast, typically with those of the Middle/ Near East breeds. The Sudanese breed is much found in East Africa, the breeds south of the Sahara tend to be small or dwarf.

The introduction of goats to islands in the Pacific were by early sailor/explorers: knowing that the species reproduces well it was a custom to leave a few on isolated islands hoping they would breed and provide a food source for future travellers. Captain Cook left the first goats in New Zealand in 1772 and Hawaii in 1778. Captain Vancouver also visited Hawaii in 1792 and left goats, as did Admiral Perry on the Bonin Islands in 1853.

Recognition of Goat Diseases

The goat, probably the first livestock species to become domesticated also became regarded as a lowly animal, mainly kept by the peasantry. As a result, compared with other species, the diseases occurring have been poorly recorded. After observations made by Roman authors, very little appeared in the national records of the European countries to indicate any serious health problems. As the species has a reputation for hardiness this might also be a true reflection of the situation.

The Years of Antiquity, 200 BC–AD 1000

The first extant treatise on agriculture, by Cato (234 BC – 149 BC), makes no mention of goats (but does of sheep). In the next treatise Varro wrote, '. . . no man of sound mind guarantees that goats (which are never free of fever) are sound of body' and 'What can I say of the health of animals which are never healthy? I can only make one remark: that the head goatherds keep written directions as to the remedies to be used. . .'. He noted frequent flesh wounds due to their habit of fighting and using their horns, as well as thorn wounds from their grazing habits. Varro also recommended several herds, each of no more than 50 head, be kept rather than large herds, so that if an epidemic occurs the losses are reduced. The diseases are not described.

Columella (AD 4–70) noted that 'disease strikes suddenly on plump and lively animals', but does not qualify this observation. He wrote that their diseases should be treated in the same way as those of sheep.

Palladius (4–5th century AD) made quite extensive observations on the goat but followed Columella in stating that they will be well and then 'suddenly fail and be laid low'. He wrote that if a plague occurs and some of the herd are affected then the others should be bled at once and then shut up for four hours in the middle of the day. Without any descriptions he then states, 'if another type of ailment occurs medicate with a draft of roots of reed with whithorn and no other drink'. If this fails to cure he suggests to either sell or kill and salt down, and then only buy new stock 'after waiting a time'. Various remedies are noted including those for dropsy (without explaining the condition), post-parturient damage and retained placenta, but otherwise to treat as for sheep. In a description of medications Palladius gives some emphasis to the use of goat tallow as a pharmaceutical: uses include being dripped into an abscess cavity, or on to a cauterised area; also as an ointment base with ox marrow, pitch and old olive oil to massage into the swollen necks of yoked oxen.

Goats' milk was suggested as a remedy for erysipelas or pustule in sheep [possibly sheep pox or orf], and it was emphasised that it must be used as a matter of urgency otherwise the disease will spread through the flock. Goats' milk was also suggested as a cure for a fevered horse, 'as a result of work' and also a cure for equine haematuria, when mixed with eggs, meal and olive oil, administered as a drench.

In the *Geoponika* (c.9–10th century AD), while there are many entries related to the goat, none of these relate to diseases of the species, not even the concerns shown by the earlier Roman authors that they were prone to ill health. There is a considerable amount of comment on the value of the goat in its many productive capacities and also in the use of the blood as a counter to bed bugs and fleas, the use of goat fat (tallow) in treating lameness in the ass (a prescription noted by Apsyrtus), and also for treating ox foot wounds. The two remedies for equine 'fever' and haematuria listed by Palladius are repeated with the source being given as Apsyrtus. Finally a dubious remedy for a bull who fails to perform – burn the tail of a goat, pound, knead with wine and then use to anoint the penis and testicles: the bull will then mount.

The Period of Natural Observation, AD 1000–1699

Very few mentions of specific disease in goats are found in the old records, however this was a period when epizootic diseases (plagues) were common in livestock (and in humans). Although goats are not mentioned they would have been affected by the frequent disease outbreaks, probably due to rinderpest, foot-and-mouth disease (FMD) and anthrax, or combinations of these infections. The only specific mentions are:

1127 *Europe* A plague was reported in oxen, cows, pigs, bears, stags and goats. This heavy mortality appears to have continued for several years. (*Saxon Chronicle*, p. 229; Anselm Gemblac. *Chronic. Pistor.*)

1599 *Italy* A plague 'among cattle and goats . . . and by them communicated to other animals'. Other reports indicate that a similar epidemic affected cattle in most European countries. (Cole, quoted by T. Short *A General Chronological History of the Air* 1749, London p. 287)

The Development of Biological Observations, 1700–1800

1713 *Europe* In Naples kingdom some 50,000 sheep and pigs perished and in Poland, Prussia and Silesia sheep and goats were also hit by 'the disasterous epizooty' (Kanold *Histor. Relationen.* Chapter II)

1714 *Europe* Many reports of epidemic diseases in cattle, horses, pigs, sheep, poultry and 'in many parts of Germany dropsy or rot had prevailed among cattle, sheep and goats'. (Kanold *op. cit.* p. 177)

1764 *Europe* Reports of pestilence in most species of animals and humans. From Sweden a specific record of mortality among cattle, horses, sheep, goats and swine. No description of signs but one suggestion from Spain that the cause was 'old and corrupted corn'. (Rutty *The Weather and Seasons*)

1778 *Germany* In both Thuringia and other regions 'an epizooty of anthrax showed itself'. Cattle, horses, asses, goats, pigs and deer all died. An anthrax epizooty was also recorded in France. (Glaser *Von der Knotenkrankeit.* p. 3, p. 7 and p. 32)

The late 1700s into the 1800s appears to have been a particularly bleak period for the publication of observations on diseases of the goat.

One publication is of interest, containing an observation made around 1810–1812, specifically related to the Cashmere breed in either Kashmir or elsewhere in the Himalayan region. It was noted that there was a widespread 'and fatal epizooty' among the Cashmere breed, but no details of specific signs is made. The observation was made by William Moorcroft, the first British veterinarian (trained under Bourgelat in France). One of his expeditions into the mountains north of India was an effort to obtain Cashmere goats to ship to England to breed to start production of this valuable wool, used for manufacturing pashmina shawls. The term derived from the Persian *pashm shal*. Moorcroft also mentions that he diagnosed 'gid' (the intermediate stage of tapeworm infestation in goats, located in the brain); and also found adult tapeworms in the animals at post-mortem (Moorcroft and Trebeck *Travels in Cashmere and Thibet*, Vol. II, p. 167).

Two unrelated mentions in the literature concerning goat health are of interest: (1) in West Africa some breeds of goats were recognised to have developed a trypanotolerance (similar to that seen in cattle), a valuable evolutionary change; (2) the introduction of the Angora/Mohair goat to New Zealand, to start a new industry sector, failed due to a recurrent foot rot problem. Both of these are cited in Mason (1984, p. 97).

Caprine Disease and Welfare

The previous review illustrates the paucity of historical recorded goat disease data: presumed due to the perceived low value of the animal in the European livestock industry. However, it was, and remains, almost the mainstay of both milk and meat supply to peasantry worldwide.

It is difficult therefore to present a well-balanced appraisal of goat health over the past centuries. One has to be careful not to dismiss the comment by Varro that goats were never healthy. It is more likely a reflection of the fact that goats are in fact hardy animals used to mountain, scrub and woodland locations; the Roman farming habit, based on confined and housed stock for milk production did not provide a suitable environment. However, his advice that one should never have a group of more than 50 animals because of the risk of contagious disease was sound.

While not mentioned in the early literature it is now recognised that goats can acquire significant helminth infestations on pasture, they appear to have less natural resistance than sheep. Additionally coccidiosis can be a problem in housed goats unless good hygiene is maintained – and hygiene was recognised by the Romans to be an essential part of good husbandry.

We know that historically epizootic diseases were a major constraint on all species utilised in livestock farming: most of which would also affect sheep and goats. They were considerable hazards, which would have had a dire and rapid effect on an animal already in an unsuitable environment. Columella wrote that in goats disease strikes suddenly 'to plump and lively animals', unfortunately without any qualifying descriptions, an observation followed by Palladius. He also wrote of plagues affecting the herd. In spite of these problems it is obvious that the goat was a useful contributor to the Roman economy in terms of food, hide and hair, and in dung (valuable for vine cultivation, an essential feature of their Mediterranean agriculture).

In the post-Roman years in Europe the goat declined to become a peasant's sub-sistence animal, but with a specific value in milk and cheese production. From the Middle Ages up to the 19th century this situation persisted. There was not the same interest in the goat compared with other livestock.

The enormous areas of the Middle East (the original home of the domesticated goat), Asia, India and Africa have all continued with a traditional husbandry system based in herding groups, to graze in shrub and scrubland areas. Transhumance is still practised in many areas of the world, probably mimicking the natural treks of the wildlife. This is an important husbandry system used to ensure a feed supply year round. It is now also recognised as a significant method of disease spread in many regions.

The goat in fact is subject to a wide range of diseases, many of which are shared with sheep, and some with cattle. While there is no evidence to support the sugges-tion, it is possible that an important 'plague', that would have troubled the goat over the centuries in Africa and Asia is what is now known as Peste des Petits Ruminants (PPR). Caused by a rinderpest related virus, and infecting goats, sheep and some wild ruminants, it remains a serious problem in affected regions, with a mortality level of 20–90% in infected groups.

Another problem is goat pox, a highly contagious virus, antigenically related to sheep pox. Goat pox infection is more serious than sheep pox and the disease is now recognised as an important issue in both Asia and Africa, and also with a few foci in South East Europe. Parasites such as helminthiasis and liver fluke infection can be much more serious in the goat than in sheep, with life-threatening infestations. Moorcroft found tapeworms in wild goats sharing pasture with the domesticated animals in India.

Little if any, specific therapeutics or prophylactics had been either studied or developed in the period studied. Goat welfare is not a topic that appears to have been either practised (in a humane manner) or studied in past centuries.

Goats and Public Health

From the review of available literature there do not appear to be any significant diseases that are transmissible to humans specifically related to the consumption of goat milk or meat or as a result of contact with the animal. The goat, however, can transmit some zoonotic diseases, as can sheep and cattle, to humans: tuberculosis, brucellosis, anthrax and rabies being the most obvious.

References

Mason, I.L. (Ed.) (1984) *Evolution of Domesticated Animals*. London: Longman
Zeuner, F.E. (1963) *A History of Domesticated Animals*. New York: Harper & Row

CHAPTER 21

Porcine: Pigs and Peccaries

Taxonomically the pig belongs to the Artiodactyla order in the even-toed ungulate family Suidae (subfamily Suinae) in the genus *Sus*. The ancestor is the Eurasian wild boar *Sus scrofa* and the name used for the domestic (European type) pig is *Sus scrofa domesticus*.

There are a variety of words used to describe the species: the English word 'swine' is derived from the Latin *suinus,* as are *Schwein*, German and *Zwijn*, Dutch. The word 'pig' is derived from the early Middle English *pigge*, which has unknown etymology. 'Hog' is also of Middle English origin, today in Britain it refers to a castrated male pig to be reared for meat, while in North America it has a more general meaning for all pigs. Old English contributed both 'boar' from *bár*, an uncastrated male, and 'sow' from *sugu*. A 'gilt' is the term for a female until her first litter. There are in fact a multitude of words for the species, in particular the smallest piglets in a litter: pigling, critling, nisgul, creet, and so on (Henderson and Stratton 1963, p. 115).

Apart from the specific use of the words listed above, these same words moved into vernacular conversation in a wide variety of descriptive roles: in English usage in Britain a 'hog' was a term for a shilling coin in the 17th–20th centuries and a 'pig' was a sixpence coin in the 17th–19th centuries (both currency units now discontinued). Another word 'grunter', of obvious etymology, was in general use for pigs from the mid-16th–20th centuries. The same word was used for a suckling pig in the 17th century, and then used for a shilling coin in the late 18th century. It is also a derogatory term applied to British policemen from the 19th century. The number of pig derived words that have entered the English vernacular tongue is extensive, and generally applied in a rather uncomplimentary usage. An interesting listing of these words is found in Lutwyche (2010, pp. 12–32).

The pig-human relationship is interesting and differs significantly between cultures and civilisations. While the pig appears in many folklore and traditional legends, it tends to be regarded on a lower scale to that of other animals. In Europe it was represented in heraldry, with associations of bravery and boar hunting. One of the most long-lasting domestication and utilisation systems originated in China dating from about 8000 BC with many pig bones excavated from the Yang Shao period c.2900 BC. The pig is well regarded in Chinese culture and the wild boar/pig image is found in the Chinese zodiac symbols. However, in almost all other societies where the pig is accepted as useful as a food source it invariably also has negative connotations, as noted above in its usage in words; in spite of this, today pig meat is possibly the world's most consumed meat.

The pig is also an animal of religious significance, in as much as two world religions (Judaism and Islam) abhor both the consumption of pig meat and the presence of the animal. This particular relationship between pigs and humans is of uncertain origin but has a long history. It is discussed later in this chapter (see also Chapters 1 and 6).

Natural History and Biology

The farmed animal, *Sus scrofa domesticus*, has a large head with a long mobile snout, strengthened by a unique prenasal bone, and ending with a cartilaginous disc at the tip. This is both a sensitive sensory organ as well as a useful aid to digging in soil. Each foot (trotter) has four toes. The central two are the main weight bearers, but the outer two may also help on softer ground.

Wild pigs have a total of 44 teeth but this is reduced in some domesticated breeds. The rear teeth pulverise and grind the food. In the male the canine teeth become tusks and grow continually. The stomach is simple with two chambers: pigs are omnivorous and in the wild will eat acorns, roots, plant stems, chestnuts, insects, worms, reptiles, frogs, manure and cadavers. Their greatest activity period is at night when they will travel in groups in search of food; in daytime, if available they will wallow in mud for long periods. Adult males are more solitary and more widely roaming; European wild boar (single males) are reported to roam for long distances in a single night.

Given a good diet and being cared for in a suitable environment, the gestation period is about 116 days with a farrowing number of eight to twelve piglets, in some domesticated breeds the number of offspring can be higher. Reproduction rate is rapid: oestrus occurs about every 21 days, and lasts for two to three days. Modern breeds may achieve puberty in five to six months, possibly even younger in some of the Chinese breeds, for example, the Meishan. Lifespan, usually shorter in domesticated pigs bred for their meat, can easily be 16–20 years.

The pig is one of the most numerous domesticated animals with a global population of about one billion, dominated by China with about half the global total. Other major players are the United States of America (USA), Russia, Brazil, Germany and Poland. There are also significant numbers (about or over ten million) in Mexico, Canada, Denmark, France, Netherlands, Romania and Spain. In Africa, most pigs are held in South Africa. Of veterinary significance it has to be noted that bush pigs and warthogs, related species that are widespread in sub-Saharan Africa, can act as carriers of pig disease pathogens, such as African Swine Fever.

Species Domesticated

Based on osteoarchaeological evidence, domestication of the western type of pig probably started between 12,000–10,000 BC in the Tigris river basin, from this region they slowly spread into Europe and to Persia (Iran).

Domestication almost certainly only occurred after human settlement and farming commenced, and after sheep and goats. Pigs immediately found a place in meat production. Initially a herd would be kept wild in local woods and culled as needed (a practice still popular in some areas of Eastern Europe and the Caucasus and now responsible for the wild boar spreading African Swine Fever); later, to produce fatter animals, they were confined. They were seen as an animal of convenience – useful scavengers and consumers of food waste, cheap to fatten in small groups, and prolific suppliers of meat and fat for the pantry. They lagged behind other farmed species in veterinary care.

The domestic pig is derived from the species *Sus scrofa*, originally the wild boar listed by Linnaeus, 1758. This genus has about ten other members (and osteoarchaeology has identified at least 13 extinct species). The probable ancestor of the genus was *Sus strozzi* of the Pliocene period, in Europe and Asia, now extinct. The wild boar was a widely distributed species group spread from Europe to Asia with the representative species being *Sus scrofa* the wild pig for the west, and *Sus vittatus* the banded pig for the east. These two differ in head shape – the European being more elongated and the Asian being smaller, in body size and weight. There are several subspecies and transitional races derived from where the two regions connected, these progressively evolved as civilisations exchanged breeding stock. This is well described by Epstein (1984, pp. 145–162) who in particular details the several species, and Zeuner (1963, pp. 256–274). The European domestic pig is now commonly regarded as a full species and termed *Sus scrofa domesticus*.

Apart from the domestic pig reared for its meat and food products, there are several other varieties that are kept for specific or local reasons. The Vietnamese pot-bellied pig had a short period of popularity in Western countries as a pet – until it was realised that they grew to a significant size. Of some interest also is the *Kunekune*, a small domestic pig developed in New Zealand from imported Asian varieties in the early 1800s. It is a small hairy pig of various colours, often with wattles on its lower jaws. It is noted as a friendly, placid animal, often treated as a pet. A type of porcine found in the Coromandel region of New Zealand is known as a *Cooks* or *Cookers* pig. These small, black pigs are a wild breed that has evolved from animals left by Capt. Cook when he visited the country in 1769. The pigs were part of the stock bred for food on his ship, the *Endeavour*, and gifted to the resident Maori. Now they are mainly hunted, using dogs.

Mention has to be made of the *peccary*. This is also classified in the Artiodactyla order, suborder Suina but in the family Tayassuidae. While classified Suina, these are New World pigs, not to be confused with the Old World pigs described above. They are native to Central and South America. A domesticated variety is raised on farms by local communities, they cannot be said to be commercially exploited.

DOMESTICATED PIGS AND CULTURAL GROUPS

The pig is one of the most useful animals for humans, virtually all of the carcase can be utilised. The meat can be eaten fresh, but also salts and smokes well; the fat is valuable in cooking, apothecary formulations and perfume production; the skin makes good leather for saddles and book covers and the bristles for brushes; there are also recipes for pig ear pies. From the earliest times there have been significant differences in domestication practices between the West and the East. The Western approach was to keep pigs in groups or herds, while the Eastern method evolved from housed pigs and in particular a house-pig, as in China.

The history of the domesticated pig probably begins in China, where it has, for millennia, been regarded as a major, and much appreciated, food source. In the West, starting from the Middle East, the domesticated pig became a valued item of food throughout the Mediterranean region and Western world. In India, its acceptance has been slower, and almost negligible in the African continent.

Middle East

The earliest dated bones of domesticated pigs have been excavated in the region of southern Turkey and Iraq; pig bones comprise over 7% of domestic animal bones found at these sites. Pottery and carvings of pigs have been found in northern Mesopotamia dating from late 6000 BC and their bones discovered at major archaeological locations such as Ur (c.3000 BC). Pig bones at Ashnunnak (Tell Asmar) late 2000 BC, comprise almost 30% of total domestic animal bones. From this region the spread of the domesticated pig can be traced to Iran, Turkistan and possibly to the Indus valley.

The ancient Egyptians, Hebrews, Phoenicians and Carthaginians all considered the pig to be an impure animal, some groups even identified the wild boar with evil. The belief might have been introduced to Egypt by the Hyksos, who conquered early Upper Egypt, and are thought to have been Semitic Bedouins from Syria, who held the pig to be unclean. It would appear that pigs were attracted to early communities as scavengers, both of waste food and also human faeces. This habit, together with their enjoyment of carrion and even human flesh if a corpse was available, violated two taboos of virtually all civilisations.

Pigs were seen as 'unclean', their meat was the food of the poor segment of the population, it was not well regarded. Because of this the pig was not used in early sacrificial rituals (unlike cattle, sheep and goats). A Babylonian text reads, 'The pig is impure, it makes the streets stink . . . [and] besmirches the houses'; another stated, 'The pig is not fit for the temple . . . [it is] an offence to all the gods'. Pigs in the Middle East were mostly found in the poor regions of the early cities – they ate the waste and also provided a food source for the people. A Hittite text, written c.1300 BC, included the words 'neither pig nor dog is ever to cross the threshold' of a temple, and an Assyrian one, written c.670 BC, includes the curse 'may dogs and swine eat your flesh'. Around 1200 BC the Hebrew tribe settled in Canaan in Palestine, like their neighbours they did not eat pig meat. However, unlike their neighbours this tribe, to later become the Israelites or Jews, were to make this rejection a core part of their religious belief (Essig 2015, pp. 48–64).

While not followed by all Middle Eastern cultures the rejection of pig meat was a widespread practice until the Greeks conquered the Persian armies and introduced their cultural characteristics which included the consumption of pork. This cuisine was also followed by the Romans, who in turn had conquered the Greeks. The attitude towards pigs and pig meat changed across the region – until the Arab/Islamic conquest occurred with their belief, which followed the Judaism custom, and banned pigs and their meat.

Herodotus wrote that the Libyans (then located on the border between Libya and Tunisia), as the Egyptians, did not raise pigs or eat pork. He also recorded that the Scythians (Southern Ukraine region) were unwilling to raise pigs.

Egypt

Based on the dating of excavated bones the domesticated pig first occurs in Egypt in the later 5th century BC. Pigs thrived in the Nile Delta, using the moist soil and water holes as wallows. The pig does not appear in Upper Egypt until about the mid-4th century BC.

Herodotus recorded that the Egyptians considered the pig to be unclean, 'if anyone touches a pig he goes immediately to the river and submerges himself, clothes and all' (Strassler 2007, p. 138). They were used to tread seed into the earth after sowing, and also to thresh the grain harvest. All management and care of pigs was the work of swineherds, whom Herodotus said were not allowed to enter any Egyptian sanctuary. Because of their work they could only intermarry with the families of other swineherds: a particular caste was created. Pigs were only used in sacrifice to Isis and Osiris, and then only at a full moon. After the sacrificial ceremony to Isis, the tip of the tail was cut off, and together with the spleen and belly fat, was wrapped in the omentum and totally burned as a funeral offering. The rest of the meat was then cooked and eaten on that full moon night. On any other day people would refuse to even taste pig meat. At the Isis ceremony poor people would bake cakes shaped like pigs and sacrifice them on the altar fire. At the Osiris festival the custom was to slaughter a young pig at the entrance to the home and then give it to the swineherd who had sold it to the house-owner. Herodotus added that he was told the reason for the Egyptian aversion to pigs, 'but it would not be very proper for me to divulge here'!

Following the conquest of Egypt by Alexander the Great in 332 BC, and the establishment of the Ptolemaic Kingdom as an Hellenistic state, the aversion to the pig gradually died out. The Greeks ate pig meat and it became a popular Egyptian food.

The Hellenic World

By 6800 BC Greek farmers had domesticated pigs. This could have been related to their religious sacrificial practices. They were raised on small farms and mostly fed on kitchen waste and acorns. Excavated bones indicate that most animals were killed young, presumably with more tender meat. In certain regions, such as Aetolia, Demeter (goddess of the harvest) was admired as the 'sow mother', whose swineherd Eubulus helped her to find Persephone, her daughter. Also in mythology Eumaeus, Odysseus' swineherd, was an expert in foretelling the future, and was highly regarded. The religious use of pigs for sacrifice had an effect on management practices as only perfect animals were accepted by the priests. Also the more valuable the animal (that is, being perceived as a prime specimen), the more likely was the success of the sacrifice.

By the Archaic and Classical periods it appears that animal husbandry and sacrificial ritual had become closely related as most pigs were slaughtered as sacrifices. Priests would kill the pig and butcher the carcase, the fat and femur bones were burned on the altar as a gift to the gods, and the rest of the meat was distributed to the participants, a practice which was welcomed by the poor. Votive pig terracotta figures and pig-shaped rattles have been found in the sanctuaries of Demeter and Eleusinian Mysteries. The latter was the basis of a major cult (c.400 BC) and can be dated back to the Mycenaean period (c.1600–1100 BC). Demeter and Persephone were the central figures of the Eleusinian Mysteries that predated the Olympian Pantheon. Most of the practices have remained unknown but in the Lesser Mysteries the initiants would sacrifice a piglet to Demeter and Persephone and then ritually purify themselves in the river Ilisos.

The basis of the Greek agricultural economy was livestock, and extant writings indicate that they made significant advances in livestock improvement. The early Greeks would appear to have been the first Europeans to breed swine and consume pork. Notably Aristotle (384–322 BC) in *Historia Animalium* (Book VIII) wrote on the diseases of pigs.

Roman Empire

Pigs were a part of Roman agriculture. They were recognised for their roles in the food supply and as a sacrificial animal in religious rituals. It was customary to sacrifice a pig (a sow was preferred) to Ceres at the start of a harvest, and to Bacchus at the start of a vintage. There was a profitable market in providing sacrificial swine for slaughter in the state religion. The most solemn ceremonial offering was that termed *suovetaurilia* which involved the killing of a bull, pig and sheep. Many Roman artworks show boars and pigs in sculpture, bronzes and glass.

Almost every country of the Roman world had a wild boar population. Hunting was widely practised, both as a source of food for the poorer population and as a sport for the more affluent. Wild boars were also kept in the private parks (*vivaria*) of the gentry for both pleasure and food. The hunting of wild boar with dogs and spears was a favourite field sport of certain emperors, and also featured in killing spectacles in the arena. The animal features in many surviving marble statutory groups (there is a fine sculptured panel, now in the Roman Curia of a boar with a head dressing and a meander pattern embroidered body girth), and also on coins and medallions of Vespasian and Titus Antoninus Pius.

Several pig types were raised in the Roman world for both domestic consumption and breeding: larger pigs were mainly of the early turbary type and smaller pigs of the *scrofa* group. Both adults and sucking pigs were sold to pork butchers and either consumed as meat or preserved as ham or sausages. Fat was regarded as a useful by-product. Romans studied the art of breeding, rearing and fattening pigs (*porculatio*). The earliest extant writing on pig farming was by Varro (116–27 BC) who wrote 'every farmer raised pigs' and also stated that the Latin *sus* derived from the Greek, meaning to offer as a sacrifice. In the early days of the Empire there was a premium added to really fat pigs. Varro recounts that some were so fat they could not walk and required carts to move them. He noted that Gaul produced the best pigs (the Gauls gave the boar special sanctity and put the images atop their native standards). Strabo (65 BC–AD 23) the Roman historian, wrote that Gaul and Spain supplied Rome with gammons, hams and sausages.

Varro wrote on pig health and Pliny (AD 23–79) quoted much of his text, additionally stating that pigs were subject to many diseases, in particular *squinancie* (?quinsy). Pliny described the feeding procedures – giving dried figs and honeyed wine to produce a 'monstrous' liver, and the culinary practices of the affluent: a whole pig stuffed with delicacies bathed in wine and a rich gravy, being boiled on one side and roasted on the other. Columella (AD 4–70) writing after Varro, regarded the pig as the least important of farm livestock.

Europe: Medieval to Agricultural Revolution

In the Middle Ages, pig types were essentially local, there was little concept of breeding and most were farmed as a small entity in a general mix of livestock and arable. On some monastic farms large groups were kept, providing food for the community.

Before 1750 the pig was mostly kept for individual farms or houses as a cheap meat source: the animals were low value but the rapid breeding rate made them economical. There was little effort to keep breeding or ancestry records, those who kept them in quantity were deemed to be low status.

Medieval pigs were usually put out to 'pannage' (roaming the forests for food), they were lean, razor-backed but sturdy animals adapted to rooting in the soil for food. Woodlands provided acorns and beech mast. The practices varied across Europe but the derided swineherd would take groups of pigs into the woodlands. He collected, for a fee, small numbers of pigs from many households and could, by now lost training methods, weld the animals into controllable herds. This defined behaviour was controlled by the swineherd's horn in France and Britain, by a cow horn and whip in Germany and bagpipes in Calabria and Tuscany – a well-developed practice and culture that existed for some hundreds of years.

An indication of the value of pigs is found in early Welsh law, codified by King Hywel Dda (Hywel the Good) (c.AD 880–950):

The price of a little pig from the time it is borne, until it grows to burrow is one penny; when it ceases suckling, which is at the end of three months it is worth two pence; from that time it goes into the wood with the swine, and is considered as a swine its value is four pence . . . and from the Feast of St. John [24th June, Midsummer Day] its value shall be twenty-four pence, the same as its mother.

The value of a boar was stated to be equivalent to the value of three sows. The laws also provided for compensation to be paid for damage done by pigs (presumably to crops).

The Welsh laws also required the seller of a pig to, 'warrant a sow to be sound against quinsy for three days and nights after she is sold'. If the sow developed symptoms the seller had to return one-third of the sale price to the purchaser. Another disease is mentioned which translators have interpreted as 'strangles', but its exact nature is unclear. These definitions indicate a quite sophisticated society, unfortunately there does not appear to be reliable information on how well or widely they were applied.

The sections of a bestiary book, *Liber Bestarium* (MS Bodley 764) written in the mid-13th century, dealing with the pig are totally disparaging – 'the sow is a filthy beast', the boar 'is wild and rough'. Followed by a lengthy allegorical descriptive text, to be used by religious scholars for meditative thought. No mention is made of its food value, the illustrations show a bristly brown long-legged long nosed type, including a sow with piglets.

The monastic houses, however, recognised the economic value of the pig. In the early years of the 14th century the records of Peterborough Abbey, England, show an ownership of 1394 pigs in 18 manors, five of which had herds of 100 or more. This demanded a feed source of legumes and grains. The meat and products were all consumed by the Abbey and workshop staff.

As pannage access to the forests became more restrictive, and costly, pigs had to be contained in paddocks and housed. This in turn produced a demand for feed. Initially these were home-made, one was described by Gervase Markham, (c.1568–1637), never a reliable author, but in this case probably reasonably accurate, 'From the Husbandman he taketh Pulze, Chaffe, Borne-dust, Mans-ordure, Garbage and the Weeds of his Yard, and from the Huswife her Draffe [kitchen waste and refuse], Swillings, Whey, washing of Tubs, and such like'.

In other words there was little attempt to provide a logical, balanced ration. Until the improving livestock breeders in the 18th century the pig remained essentially a poor man's animal, mostly hidden away on farms, but in total in the main countries of Europe there was a very large population.

Many other factors were involved in the slow development of the pig industry. As urban populations grew there was a demand for cheap meat; this produced a demand for a specialist pig and this required a feed supply. At the same time other industries were developing, the dairies producing butter and cheese had whey to dispose of, the brewers had used grains, the starch makers wheat refuse and the distilleries, lees. These all provided a valuable feed stock and enabled large pig feeding units to be created. In turn, as the improved regular meat supply developed so did the opportunity to produce salted meat (of value to feed ships crews), ham and sausages.

Agricultural Revolution to 19th Century

Robert Bakewell, in England in the late 1700s, investigated and understood the method of fixing inherited characteristics to improve sheep and cattle. He turned his attention to pigs and by repeatedly inbreeding he found that he could fix characteristics: he aimed at a 'natural propensity to acquire a state of fatness, at an early age'. Both cattle and sheep ownership had a place in social status, however, pigs carried no such social standing and were only kept for profit; when it was seen that the new breeding methods, together with the prolific reproductive cycle could result in increased and rapid profit, success was assured.

Bakewell took the local varieties of British pigs – essentially short-legged, docile and prone to fatten (fat pork and bacon were popular foods) and introduced new stock. Chinese, Siamese and Neapolitan strains were imported and crossed with native pigs. These produced the Yorkshire pig, which farrowed five times in two years with six to eight piglets each time. The pace of improvement increased. Next the Black Berkshire pig was created, very fat and popular, even to the 1920s.

The new breeds of Wessex and Essex pigs in the United Kingdom (UK), and the Hampshire in the USA, became popular and moved away from the massive fat pig. In the 1800s the Wiltshire lean pig was developed and valued for its hams, and the Large White, a general pig, became a global breed. In Denmark similar lines were followed resulting in the development of the highly successful Landrace breed, also widely adopted. German breeders followed similar lines. Polish immigrants imported their native stock to the USA in 1830 and in Ohio created the Poland-China breed. The practice continues to the present time, now with very sophisticated genetic planning.

In *The Pig*, William Youatt (1847), the British author, describes not only the wild boar, but also details 20 local British breeds recognised in England, Scotland and Ireland, with illustrations, by county including the Yorkshire, Berkshire, Wiltshire and Essex – all as improved breeds (Chapter VI). Youatt discusses the Chinese pig, as well as pigs and pig farming in the USA, Canada, China, Japan, Germany, France, Russia, Hungary and Sweden (Chapter V). The book gives the first overall review of British pig diseases and their treatments, plus chapters on anatomy, breeding, feeding, housing and pig products: providing an insight into the industry in the 1800s (Chapters VII–XV).

The domestication and use of the pig as a significant source of human food came comparatively late to Western (Europe, Near and Middle East) civilisations. It was, however, adopted much earlier in the Eastern (Chinese) culture, as judged from a cookbook found in the tomb of Wu Yang (died 162 BC) which contained many meat recipes, mainly for pig meat, as well as details for butchering and cooking.

Recognition of Pig Diseases

There is a significant absence of any mention of pig diseases in the early ancient literature. Pigs violated two taboos by eating both human cadavers and faeces. This behaviour contributed to the lack of comment on pig diseases.

The Years of Antiquity to AD 400

The first known observations were by Aristotle (384–322 BC) in *Historia Animalium* (VIII Book) who noted a lethal disease of pigs [possibly anthrax] and another with high fever, diarrhoea and loss of condition. He recorded the occurrence of larval tapeworm cysts in the tongue, warned that the overfeeding of acorns could cause abortion in sows and observed dermal pustules and pimples. *Hippocrates* (c.460–370 BC) does refer to oxen, sheep and swine as being infested by 'hydatids' (*De internis Affect.*), but this is while discussing dropsy in humans, and suggesting a possible relationship.

Pigs were increasingly kept in the Roman Empire, they provided meat for the lower section of society and slaves, and were much appreciated for salting and smoke curing to produce speciality meats; pig fat was also seen to be a valuable by-product. The job of swineherd was very low in the social system. There is little surviving mention of disease problems, apart from that written by Columella and Palladius.

Columella (c.AD 4–70) regarded pigs as the least important farm livestock. He emphasises careful selection of the boar and attention to choosing breeding stock of the right conformation. Castration was recognised for male piglets, to be undertaken in spring and autumn: two methods are described. In the first method incisions were made in the scrotum over each testicle and then the testicles themselves squeezed out, or in the fascia and cut off. In the second method one mid-line cut was made in the scrotum and then the testicles were pulled out with a crooked finger and removed. He describes neutering of the sow: first give no food for two days, and then to spay, hang pig by the forelegs, make mid-line incision and remove the 'stones', 'they will then grow fat'. Also mentioned is spaying by a form of uterine intervention (not specified) to produce scarring and infertility.

Diseases are mentioned as a fever, or when they are 'scrofulous', with treatment by bleeding either from the tail or tongue together with various doubtful medications including fish-pickle and ivory dust. Columella emphasises the importance of hygiene, the separation of sick and healthy animals, and the provision of water and shade in the summer. While noting that pigs will exist on very poor food, he also recommends good pasture and feed to produce fat animals, keeping them in orchards with dropped fruit available is suggested. He advises that pig houses should not create overcrowding, which could indicate that he was aware of this as a means of disease spread. Many of the issues discussed by Columella are copied in Pliny's (AD 23–79) encyclopaedia *Naturalis Historia*.

During this period, the pig became well developed in the Chinese culture, there is little available literature (in translation) but the animal was seen as an essential food source. The Emperor Fo-Hi ordered his subjects to breed from Western pigs and to import stock. There was also much cross breeding with wild stock in the early days which accounts for the numerous different breeds. With typical Chinese ingenuity they developed the pig-privy (known from surviving earthenware models). A privy was placed above a pigsty into which the human waste fell, to be consumed by the pigs below. This was also an efficient method of parasite transfer.

The Period of Natural Observation, AD 400–1699

Palladius' treatise *Opus Agriculturae* (The Works of Farming) dates from late 4th to early 5th century AD (Fitch 2013). The section, covering pig diseases is almost a *verbatim* copy of the writings of Columella. This could suggest that the most significant disease issues were fever and 'quinsy', swollen glands (probably of the throat). [The term 'quinsy' as a disease description frequently occurs in the old literature, current expert opinion suggests that it refers to peritonsillar/lymph node abscessation, not currently seen as a common condition. Both classical swine fever (CSF) and Aujeszky's disease cause tonsillar erosion, as can PCV2, but are generally only seen at post-mortem examination as the relevant lymph nodes are well buried and not easy to observe].

Palladius included a long list of suggested medications, none of which would appear to have much logic, such as one which involved the boiling of a toad in water and then feeding it to pigs to, 'cure all their diseases'. The diagnoses offered are vague (that is, pull bristles out of pig's mane, if the ends are clean the pig is healthy, if bloody it is diseased) and if any prognosis is given it is always expressed in a positive manner. He suggested that should the whole herd sicken to the point of emaciation – induced vomition and purging was proposed as a cure. Another suggestion was: 'to prevent pigs falling sick, you will give them river crabs to eat'. The final words in the veterinary text are, 'For diarrhoea in any animal or in a horse: you write on a papyrus sheet the name *honore panassi* and fasten it on the top of the tail next to the excretory ring'. Little progress had been made in 500 years.

Many of the literature references below are derived from ancient chronicles, as listed by Fleming. Caution should be used in interpretation of these records; the absence of data does not indicate freedom from disease. In many years there were serious outbreaks of disease in both humans and animals and claims, probably unjustified, for transmission between species were made.

c.900 *Cyfraith Hywel* Welsh Law, as codified in the 9th century by King Hywel the Good, specified certain diseases against which animals could be warranted. For swine, the diseases were (as translated) 'quinsy' and 'strangles'.

c.936 *Geoponika* This Byzantine Greek farming manual is a compilation of Greek and Latin authors from the previous millennium. Almost all the pig management and disease observations are those included in Columella's treatise; however, the individual sources are cited (*Florentinus, Didymus, Praxamus* and *Democritus*) all of whom predate Columella, but whose writings are now lost. The Praxamus observation, 'neither hens nor pigs should approach the cow's manager because the dung of either if eaten will harm them . . .' might relate further back to the concept of the pig being 'unclean'. The recommendation of river crabs being fed to pigs to prevent disease appears to be derived from Didymus who prescribed precisely 'nine river crabs'.

994   *Germany* 'A terrible plague broke out among men, pigs and sheep', with a famine in Saxony, which lasted into the next year. The pestilence was named *Osterludi*, in many towns all the populations died. (*Annales Quedlinburgens*, M. Pertz)

1041   *Ireland* A mortality of cattle and swine. This appears to be the first epizootic specifically mentioned as affecting swine in Ireland. (*Annals of Innisfallen*)

1088   *Ireland* A great mortality of 'oxen, sheep and pigs', following very heavy snowfall. (*Annals of Innisfallen*)

1124   *England* An eclipse of the sun, followed by 'a great pestilence among oxen, sheep, pigs and bees'. (Cosmae. *Prag. Chronic.* book 3)

1125   *Italy. Anatomia Porci* (*The Anatomy of the Pig*), a book possibly authored by Kopho, of the Salerno Medical School. The pig was used as a dissection model. Some observations made on reproduction.

1129   *Europe* Plague reported in oxen, cows, pigs, bears, stags and goats. In Ireland, a 'murrain' killed most of the cows and the pigs. (Gale. *Annals de Margan.* Scrip, II, p. 6)

1131   *England* High mortality in domestic animals, 'the pig sties were emptied, and the stalls of oxen deserted'. William of Malmesbury wrote, 'entire herds of swine suddenly perished'. Another historian wrote that there was a great cattle plague that affected oxen and swine. (Gale. *Annals de Margan. ibid*)

1133   *Ireland* An epizootic outbreak which killed a majority of cows and pigs. (*Chronic. Scotorum*)
      Note: the available published records of the years from AD 1133 to 1504 contain no mention of the words pigs or swine, however other animal plagues are listed with regularity. The use of the word 'cattle' is frequent, in Medieval English the term was used for personal property as well as a generic word for all livestock including pigs. Many epizootics were recorded in this period and must have equally affected pigs.

1504   *Germany* A year of severe drought, crops failed, food was scarce, there was a great heat and 'pigs died in large numbers'. (Spangenberg, *Mansfield Chronic.* book i, p. 402)

1508   *Austria* An epizootic in cattle and hogs, named *lues intercus*, or 'dropsy under the skin'. (*Chronic. Mellic.*)

1529   *Germany* A significant epizootic reported in pigs at Augsburg and Thuringia during an outbreak 'of sweating sickness in mankind'. In Ceyca 600 pigs died. (Mencken *Scrip. rer. German.* i, p. 1992)

1534   *Germany.* 'Disease among pigs continued in Ceyca, and in the country around, to the great detriment of the poor people'. (Languis *Chronic. Nurembergens*)

1566   *England. The Fower Chiefyst Offices Belonging to Horsmanshippe* by Thomas

Blundeville published. This book states a relationship between pigs and anthrax outbreaks; urges that pigs be kept out of stables.

1601 *Italy. De Vocis Auditusque Organis Historia Anatomica* by Guilo Casserio (1552–1616), published 1601, illustrates the anatomy of the ear and vocal organs of the pig (and other animals).

1610 *Spain* 'Gangrenous sore-throat occurred in Old Castile and destroyed entire herds of horses, cattle and pigs', with a suggestion that this was anthrax. (Fontecha *De Angimis Disput. Compent.* 1611)

1612 *Germany* In Hesse and other regions a great 'pestilence' was observed in pigs and cattle.

1690 *Italy* Following dry years in 1689 heavy rains fell throughout the spring and summer. Rust (fungal disease of wheat) became widespread including beans and pulses. In 1690 rust appeared in June and spread to all crops. 'Pigs perished in droves from suffocation . . . arising in my opinion from the acid nature of the mildew'. (Ramazzini *Const. Epid. Op.*, ed. Geneva, pp. 120–141)

1694 *Italy* A supposed epizootic due to ingestion of ergot, humans and all species of livestock affected. (Brunner *Ephem. Nat. Curios.* Dec 1694) [*Claviceps purpurea* is now recognised as the cause of the infestation of in particular rye, and related plants. The alkaloid, ergotamine, has a range of biological actions, mainly effects on circulation and neurotransmission – the problem was well understood in the Middle Ages].

The Development of Biological Observations, 1700–1800

Diseases of pigs start to become seen as specific entities. An interest by medically qualified individuals helps to identify symptoms and suggest causes, frequently incorrect but an indication of progress.

1708 *Hungary*, and in Transylvania, a disease of a carbuncular nature among animals. A physician stated that, 'a black cloud obscured the sky and filled the air with a foul odour'; soon after this cattle, horses, pigs, dogs, wolves, hares and foxes died in great numbers. (Loigk *History of the Pest*, P. 358, p. 421 and p. 437)

1712 *Hungary* An 'extraordinary mortality' was seen in wild hogs, the epizootic was also seen in Augsburg (Germany), pigs, horses, cattle and poultry were affected. Symptoms were of 'hard tumours' on the breast and groin that quickly spread leading to rapid death. It was suggested that it was spread by hornets who had fed on corpses of animals affected and killed in the previous year. (Schroeckius *Constit. Epid. Nat. Curios.*, App 27) [John Gamgee (Britain), later commented on this carbuncular fever as a form of anthrax infection]

1714 *Germany* Recorded that in Alsace, cattle, pigs, sheep, horses and poultry died and also at Frankfurt; no reasons are given. (Kanold *Jahres hist*, pp. 119–206)

1715 *Germany* Many pigs died in the country around Cologne, but no symptoms or descriptions given.

1717 *England* Recorded that in October 'the weather was clear and air healthy . . . but a fatal month to oxen and swine'. (T Short *A General Chronological History of the Air* London, 1749, vol. ii, p. 20)

1718 *Germany* In Trebnitzschen pigs in the oak forests died, from a 'special malady'; in Medziborschen a disease also appeared in pigs – symptoms were 'a tumour on the throat, which threatened suffocation', when cut into many animals were saved. (*Breslauer Sammlung*, vol. iv, p. 1711)

1721 *Germany* In Silesia the weather induced epidemic ergotism, the problem became so serious that the King of Prussia issued an edict banning the feeding of rye tainted with ergot because of the effects on horses and pigs. (*Breslauer Sammlung*, vol. xvi, p. 436 and p. 556)

1729 *England* In his book *The Gentleman and Farmers Guide to the Increase and Improvement of Cattle*, Richard Bradley describes a disease of pigs called 'choler'. The symptoms described were intestinal plus loss of appetite and body weight together with lethargy. (The description resembles swine fever/hog cholera, but this was not officially recognised in Britain until 1862.)

1741 *Ireland* Following disease in both humans and horses and starvation in 1740 the next year was even worse. Horses, cows, sheep, pigs and poultry were all 'struck by the plague'. The year was always mentioned as *Bliadhain an air* (The year of the slaughter). (In pamphlet *Famine in Ireland in 1740, 1741*.)

1755 *Germany* An epizootic disease 'raged among cattle in Bamberg, Nuremberg and their neighbourhoods'. [The description indicates that it was foot-and-mouth disease (FMD)]. The 'inflammatory symptoms were more urgent than usual, pigs in particular suffering severely, and frequently losing their hoofs'. (Hoffman *Frankische Sammlungen*, vol. i, p. 384 and Reuss)

1757 *France* In Brie 'a very peculiar carbuncular epizootic appeared affecting pigs and all other species including fish as well as humans'. A description of symptoms is given: the suggestion is made that it could be associated with stagnant water. (A. de Chaignebrun *Relation d'une Maladie Epidemique et Contagieuse*, Paris, 1762)

1763 *Europe* A wet and sultry summer with poor harvests. Many maladies were reported in both humans and animals: much of this was attributed to anthrax. Sheep, horses and pigs were equally affected as were dogs who ate the carcases of dead cattle. In one outbreak in Moravia, cattle, sheep and pigs all shed their hoofs, in pigs these were the ones who survived. It was also recorded that men were affected and had great difficulty in swallowing. One expert attributed this epizootic to an eclipse of the sun, the red blight (rust) on plants and the 'intemperature' of the air. The disease was termed apthous fever. [From the descriptions some outbreaks were due to FMD]. (Hurtrel a'Arboval *Dict. Vet.*, I, p. 110 and Paulet *Recherches sur les Maladies Epizöotiques*, 1775)

1765 *Switzerland* and *Germany* Erysipelas reported in epidemic form and was fatal. (Wirth *Lehrbuch der Seuchen und ansteckenden Krankheiten der Hausthiere*, Zurich 1846, p. 110)

1770 *Germany* Erysipelas of pigs, described as a form of anthrax, was prevalent, and noted that this malady has repeatedly appeared in Switzerland during the last century. Also termed (in German) 'Brown disease of swine'. (Wirth, *ibid.*, p. 110)   1777   *Germany* 'A curious epizooty was noticed in Germany, cows and breeding sows aborted in large numbers'. (Chabert *Instructions* and so on)

1778 *Germany* There were widespread cases of anthrax reported in cattle, horses, asses, pigs and deer; these started in July and August and ceased in September. (Glaser *Von der Knotenkrankheit*, p. 3, p. 7 and p. 32)

1786 *Germany* Anthrax described as a serious problem. Moving across the states from Swabia and Franconia into Bavaria, attacking cattle, horses, sheep and pigs. Later was observed in Italy, Transylvania and Sweden with pigs affected. In Hanover 'gangrenous erysipelas', described as a variety of anthrax, with up to one-third of the pigs dying. (Lippische *Verordnung Beitr. z. Thierheilk*, vol. iv, p. 133; Will *Kurzer Unterricht uber den jetzt herrschenden Zungenkrebs*, Munich, 1786; Flormann *Neue Schwed. Abhandlung*, vol. viii, p. 209)

1788 *Germany* Anthrax appeared in many parts of the country and in Krandsberg 247 horses, 389 oxen and 201 pigs died before any assistance could be obtained. (Laubender *Seuchengeschichte der Landwirthschaftlichen Hausthiere*, Munich 1811, vol. i, p. 134)

Science Evolves with a Developing Veterinary Medicine Discipline, 1800–1900

With the commencement of veterinary education in the late 1700s, there was a rapid development of an appreciation of the value of veterinary science. While initially the horse received the most attention, there was also soon an increasing concern about understanding and control of epizootic diseases in all livestock species, including the pig.

1804 *Denmark* One of the most significant advances in understanding the pig was the printing of an illustrated book by Erik Viborg. The first publication that could claim to be a textbook on the use of the pig in animal production. Aimed at the farmer and educated estate managers, it created a significant impact, and was translated into French in 1805, German in 1806, Swedish in 1835 but not into English until 2006. However, English literature would suggest that the early translations had been read. Viborg, a veterinarian but better described as an animal scientist or agronomist, can be seen as the 'father' of the modern pig specialist. Viborg became Director of the first Danish Veterinary School, founded in 1773 by Peter Christian Abildgaard (1743–1801) his teacher and mentor. (E. Viborg *Veiledning til Svinets Behandling som Huusdyr*, 1804 Copenhagen) (Viborg 1804)

1805 *England* In *General Treatise on Cattle*, John Lawrence wrote that he had 'an infectious disease among his hogs' and that a skilful cow leech cut off half the tails of the fattest. As a result, 'they had to be bound up otherwise they would bleed to death'.

1805 *Italy* An outbreak of an unidentified epizootic disease was seen in pigs in the Panaro district. (Misley *Deser. Della Malattie Serp. su i Majali nel Departim. del Panaro* Modena, 1805)

1811 *France* A disease described as gangrenous erysipelas (*erysipelas carbunculosum*) was seen as an epizootic in the Allost district in this year, and again in 1821. There was a high mortality of up to 90% and an extreme course with death in eight to ten hours [possibly anthrax]. (*Nouveau Diction. de Méd. Vet.*, vol. vi, p. 320)

1817 *Germany* A disease of pigs termed epizootic gastritis (*magenseuche*) was observed. (Busch *Zeitschr. fur Thierheilkunde*, vol. ii)

1821 *France* During the summer heat 'an extensive and fatal epizooty manifested itself in many departments of France, but particularly in the north'. It was called pleuro-pneumonia by Saussol, but Wirth believed it to be the erysipelas (*rotlauf*) of swine. It affected all ages and sex of pigs within one region, Tarn, 'one-fifth of every 400 animals were affected'. Symptoms are described in detail [the disease was possibly swine fever]. (Saussol *Rec. Med. Vet.*, vol. xiv, p. 233)

1832 *Germany. Raphanial*(?) in pigs was witnessed by a Dr Helm: '. . . 12 pigs of various ages were fed with rye which contained much ergot. A few hours afterwards convulsions set in, with foaming at the mouth . . .' Symptoms and post-mortem details were presented. A skin disease termed smallpox (*blattern*) was also seen in pigs. (*Provinzial-Sanitatsbericht von Pommern*, 1832)

1835 *Germany* Swine were reported to have perished in large numbers from a 'rapid and deadly quinsy'. *Milzbrand* (anthrax) was also reported to be widespread in all species in Russia, Lithuania and Prussia. It was thought that the quinsy was also anthrax, as pigs were recorded developing symptoms after eating the cadavers of other dead animals. (*Rec. Med. Vet.*, 1834 and *Sanitatsbericht Konigsberger*, 1835)

1836 *Ireland* Disease in pigs was reported from Cavan county and other places: initially 'called cholera, on account of the black colour the animal assumed'. Also termed *morbus niger*, it was a febrile disease with inflammation of the bowels. One report stated that after the cholera epidemic, a malignant disease attacked the swine, and swept them off in immense numbers. (*The Limerick Standard*)

1837 *France* Near Brest 'after the damp heat of July epizootic erysipelas fever (*febris erysipelatosa maligna*) attacked pigs, and within a fortnight but few were left in the villages. . .'. The same disease, termed *rotlauf* was also seen in Switzerland. (Kazean *Ann. de la Soc. Vet. du Finisterre*, vol. ii, p. 20 and Pommer *Schweiz Zeitschrift*, vol. v, p. 352)

1838 *Ireland* The pig epizootic reported in 1836 continued with particularly fatal results in Munster. (*The Limerick Standard*)

1840 *Ireland* An epizootic disease in pigs, usually fatal, occurred in the north of the country, and also in Galway. It was seen as an 'eruptive fever, which in a short time assumed the appearance of measles in the human subject, and finally the whole skin became one universal patch of floridity'. (*The Irish Farmer's and Gardener's Journal*)

Germany In Hesse an outbreak of intestinal helminthiasis in pigs was reported. The parasite was named as *Echinorynchus gigas*, in several cases the intestinal wall was perforated. (Walch *Zeitschrift fur Theirheilkunde*, vol. viii, p. 149)

1841   *Germany* In the Treves district a pox disease was observed as an epizootic in young pigs. In the following year, the same symptoms were also seen in pigs at Kissiten, Prussia. (Leichter *Magazin fur Theirheilkunde*, vol. x, p. 112 and p. 98)

1847   *England* The reports of swine diseases from British sources (*The Veterinarian*), indicate a recognition of pigs as a valuable part of the livestock economy, and an appreciation of this by veterinarians. The first British book on the pig published: discussing history, management and diseases (Youatt 1847).

By the middle of the 19th century a pig industry was becoming established. Denmark and Britain had led the way in improving pig stocks, and knowledge of correct dietary needs and housing was developing. There was pressure from the agricultural community to control the now recognised disease problems. The publication of Youatt's book in 1847 was a result of this concern, its appearance, however, was not appreciated by many of the British practising veterinarians. Their position was difficult, many felt that any new knowledge should be kept within the profession, but Youatt felt everyone should benefit. More clinical papers appeared in professional journals and expertise increased: however, there were still no effective medications for the diseases, which were almost all of unexplained aetiology.

Pig farming was making progress, but the major problem was frequent outbreaks of epizootic disease, usually with catastrophic consequences. In retrospect, swine erysipelas, anthrax, FMD and various intestinal/respiratory diseases were taking a heavy toll – without any understanding of the actual causes.

Significant progress was made in 1881 when Friedrich Loeffler identified the bacterial cause of swine erysipelas. This widespread disease was known by several names – *rouget du porc* (France), *mal rossino* (Italy), *schweinerotlauf* (Germany), *vlekziekte* (Netherlands) and diamond-skin disease in England. Theobald Smith (1859–1934), working at the Bureau of Animal Industry, also described the organism in the USA in 1885.

Louis Pasteur had been asked by the French pig industry to try to find an answer to the problem in 1877, and in 1883 he developed a swine erysipelas vaccine utilising rabbit passage of the bacterium. About the same time Loeffler, with W. Schutz, also produced a vaccine. Additionally Loeffler and Schutz isolated *Pasteurella suisepticus*, which at the time was believed to be the cause of swine plague, and developed a vaccination method for the disease. Emmanuel Leclainche (1801–1953), working with E. Nocard (1850–1903), published definitive reports on swine erysipelas in France in 1895.

The background to the other major swine disease entity – swine fever/hog cholera – is unclear. The probable origin is related to the improvement of pig breeds and the introduction of new stocks from Asian and other markets, but this remains an hypothesis.

The disease became significant, and particularly important in the USA. The first recorded report details an outbreak in Ohio in 1833, thought to be related to the importation of Polish breeding stock, but the disease may, and probably did, exist earlier. The rapid development of the railroad system allowed for widespread dissemination, and recognition. An 1860 report by the Agricultural Division of the United States (US) Patent Office revealed the prevalence of the disease named 'hog cholera'; this led to the establishment of the US Department of Agriculture in 1862, and the introduction of regulatory veterinary medicine to the USA.

The disease was recognised in Britain in 1862 (but probably had existed for some time). It was first recorded in a paper by Professor Varnell of the Royal Veterinary College, published in *The Veterinarian* (1864). The first classical report of the disease in Britain and (possibly in Europe) was published by D W Budd in the *Journal of the Royal Agricultural Society of England* (1867): described as *Typhoid Fever in Pigs*. The author added that his investigation started as a result of Professor John Gamgee advising him of an outbreak of typhoid fever in pigs, in Edinburgh.

The spread of the disease in Britain led to the *Typhoid Fever of Swine Order* 1878, involving notification of an outbreak and obligatory slaughter. The disease proved to be very difficult to control and eradicate, the symptoms were frequently confusing, and diagnosis problematic. Before the recognition of swine fever/hog cholera veterinarians had paid little attention to pigs. Horses and cattle were the important species. In Europe it was the care of army horses and cattle rinderpest that dominated veterinary attention.

The disease became a major problem for the pig industry in Continental Europe, in particular in centrally located Germany and Austria, where it was named *schweinpest* (swine plague), and Hungary, where there was a devastating epizootic outbreak in 1895. This outbreak was studied by Jozsef Marek (1868–1952) and by Ferenc Hutyra (1860–1934), both of whom became leading veterinary pathologists. An immune serum was produced in Hungary by H Preisz (1860–1940) in 1897 which soon became important, and was used either alone, or with a live virus in a simultaneous vaccination procedure.

Finally the causation was proven by the work of Marion Dorset (1872–1935) and Alexander de Schweinwitz (1866–1904) who, whilst working at the US Department of Agriculture in a programme of work in 1903–1904, succeeded in isolating the swine fever/hog cholera virus. Dorset and Schweinwitz had been investigating the disease for several years but had been concentrating on *Bacillus cholerasuis*, originally believed to be the causative agent. Following the virus isolation there was much work in both the USA and Europe on the development of reliable vaccines. One of these was based on virus inactivated by crystal violet and was much used successfully in eradication schemes in the 20th century.

Also of importance in the study of pig diseases was the recognition of *Trichinella spiralis* as the cause of trichinosis in the human. The parasite was investigated in detail in 1861 by Albert von Zenker (1825–1898), who revealed the true danger of eating raw pork. The life cycle was then elaborated by Karl Leuckhart (1822–1898), to be followed by Rudolph Virchow (1821–1902) who studied the endemic disease in humans. This work resulted in the introduction of compulsory microscopic examination of pig meat before sale, first introduced in Berlin in 1865.

By the end of the 19th century, with the elucidation of the cause of swine fever and development of a vaccine, together with the introduction of swine erysipelas vaccination and trichinosis meat inspection, the importance of pig diseases was recognised and began to be controlled.

Porcine Disease and Welfare

It was not until the early 1800s that the pig began to be seen as an animal to be commercially exploited and therefore demanding of higher standards of care. The initial impetus came from Denmark in 1804 with the publication of Erik Viborg's book. This presented a clear case for proper management, feeding and care with a listing of diseases and suggested treatments (which were limited by the knowledge held at the time) but Viborg did present a logical approach to disease control. In 1847 a similar book by William Youatt, published in England together with a good circulation in North America, advanced this interest. Both Denmark and Britain, at the same time, led the way in improving pig stocks by introducing other varieties utilising successful selective breeding programmes.

In retrospect the defining issue in pig diseases and their control was swine fever/ hog cholera (now known as classical swine fever, CSF, to differentiate from African swine fever, ASF, which did not appear as a problem disease until its appearance in Portugal in 1957). There has to be a strong possibility that CSF was present long before it was definitely diagnosed in the USA in 1833. The significant research effort made following the continual epizootics have resulted in eradication from the USA in 1978, Canada in 1962 and the UK in 1966 (but with an outbreak occurring here in 2000). CSF is now also absent in Australia, New Zealand, Ireland, Scandinavia and much of Europe. The disease is troublesome and difficult to eradicate, with both acute and chronic infection forms and difficult differential diagnoses. The use of vaccines, both crystal violet and lapinised, together with a rigorous 'stamping out' slaughter policy with strict controls is required.

The result of swine fever elucidation and control have resulted in the establishment of very significant large scale pig operations in the USA, Denmark, Germany, Russia and China in particular, but to a degree in all developed economies. As a result swine disease problems, due to the close confinement of so many animals, have multiplied providing a constant pool of disease research entities to be studied, as well as an ongoing search for new vaccine types and therapeutics. Global pig production is currently threatened by the spread of ASF and at the time of writing no preventive vaccine is available.

By the end of the 19th century bacteriological and serological methods had been introduced to support clinical and post-mortem diagnoses. Laboratories in slaughterhouses began to drive public health aspects in meat inspection. In Hungary Joseph Marek joined Ferenc Hutyra to form an impressive team in investigative pathology

– in the view of many observers this was when the discipline of internal veterinary medicine began.

It is important to note the role that pigs are now recognised to play in the evolution of the Influenza A viruses as human, avian and pig pathogens. This is usually ascribed to rural housing conditions in China where people, pigs and ducks share the same home. While this has only been recognised within the last century, the conditions have existed for much longer and may well account for some of the 'plagues' described in the early literature.

Over the known history of the pig as a farmed animal, its welfare has seldom been a major concern, as confinement husbandry was never a significant factor. Once large production systems began to develop in the 20th century the situation gradually deteriorated. To a degree this has improved in the 21st century, but swine welfare issues have lagged behind the consideration of care given to other livestock.

An important part of pig production, recorded from the earliest times is the castration of male piglets, in the first week of life, and without anaesthesia. The procedure prevents 'boar taint' in the meat and reduces aggression towards other pigs, and caretakers. This is now recognised as a painful procedure and several strategies are introduced to overcome this welfare issue. The vast majority of male piglets are castrated surgically; the procedure has not been practised for many years in the UK and Ireland: to avoid taint, pigs are slaughtered before puberty. Since 1998 Australia and New Zealand have replaced surgery by immunocastration. Immunocastration, by the induction of antibodies to gonadatrophin releasing hormone (GnRH), requires two injections to produce a temporary form of castration. In the EU measures were introduced from 1 January 2018 to ban the surgical procedure.

Pigs and Public Health

Apart from possible bacterial diseases, such as anthrax (now very rare in developed countries) and occasionally erysipelas (a possible hazard to butchery workers) the main potential human health hazards are parasitic. The rarity of anthrax is unexplained as the spores are known to have a long viability in soil. The *kashrut* and *halal* dietary laws of Judaism and Islam prohibit pig meat consumption, eliminating risk for these two groups.

Trichinosis, caused by *Trichinella* spp. cysts (usually *T. spiralis)*, can be a human health issue unless precautions are taken. This helminth is spread by the consumption of undercooked or raw pig meat: fully cooking the meat kills the parasitic cysts. The disease is now rare in developed countries and controlled by public health ordinances – no feeding of garbage and food waste, rodent control, good hygiene, disposal of carcasses of dead pigs and rats (both possible carriers) and limiting wildlife contact. The introduction of microscopic examination of pig meat after slaughter effected control.

Taenia solium infestation can result in what is known as 'measly pork', the presence of the cysticercus stage of the adult tapeworm in pig muscles. Pigs, the intermediate host, contract the infestation by consumption of human faeces containing the embryonated eggs. These develop to larvae and ultimately the infective form of cysticerci, embedded in muscles. Humans consume the uncooked meat and develop the adult tapeworm in the gut. Infestation in humans is usually benign, however sometimes humans become accidentally infected with the oncospheres and become the intermediate host, with the larvae having a predilection for brain tissue and soft muscle, a serious condition in the former location. Distribution is global but is mainly found in Central and Latin America, and South-East Asia.

References

Epstein, H. (1984) *Evolution of Domesticated Animals* (Ed. I. L. Mason). New York: Longman

Essig, M. (2015) *Lesser Beasts.* New York: Basic Books

Fitch, J.G. (2013) *Palladius: The Work of Farming.* Totnes: Prospect Books

Henderson, G.N. and Stratton, J. (1963) *Baillières Veterinary Handbook.* London: Baillière, Tindall & Cox

Lutwyche, R. (2010) Higgledy Piggledy: The Ultimate Pig Miscellany. Shrewsbury: Quiller

Strassler, R.B. (Ed.) (2007) *Herodotus: The Histories.* New York: Anchor Books

Viborg, E (1804) *A Guide to the Care and Management of the Pig as a Domestic Animal.* Original publishers C.G. Prost, Copenhagen. English translation by Lorraine Steen Svendson (2006). Printed at Reproenheten Alnarp, Denmark

Youatt, W. (1847) *The Pig.* London: Cradock & Cox

Zeuner, F.E. (1963) *A History of Domesticated Animals.* New York: Harper & Row

CHAPTER 22

Canine: Dogs

The taxonomic classification of the dog places the species in the order Carnivora, family Canidae, and genus *Canis*, which includes the wolf, *Canis lupus*, the coyote and jackals. The original classification by Carl Linnaeus in 1758 listed the domestic dog as *Canis familiaris*, separate from the wolf as *Canis lupus*. There is discussion and controversy about the origin and definition of the species name but zoologists prefer the subspecies terminology of *Canis lupus familiaris*. For this discussion, the species and genus used is *Canis familiaris*, the name for the common domestic dog in its many breeds.

The dog is recognised as the first animal species to become domesticated, but that the original species was the wolf. Dates have been suggested for when this genetic divergence process started, probably around 40,000 to 20,000 years ago with domestication about 16,000 to 12,000 years ago. Complete sequencing of the dog genome has proposed a date of 27,000 years ago, based on nuclear DNA (Derr 2012, pp. 33–35). It is also suggested that the actual ancestor wolf from which the domesticated dog has evolved is now extinct. While the evidence is not fully proven it appears that domestication of the wolf had multiple origins, but all in the northern hemisphere.

The reason for domestication was probably one of mutual advantage; the dog acted as a guard, herder and companion and the human was a source of food, warmth and companionship. It is obvious that a very strong relationship developed and from this, selective breeding over thousands of years has produced canine types suited for herding, hunting, guarding or just as companions. The animal–human relationship has grown to be not only very pronounced, but has also made the dog an elite species.

The derivation of the words used for dog is complex. The English word is believed to be derived from *docga* a late Old English word that originally meant 'once', the origin is unknown. The word hound is derived from the word *hund* used in Old English, Old Frisian, Old Saxon and German; in Dutch the word used is *hond*. The French word *chien* has derived from the Latin term *cane/canis*. The Greek word *kokoni* for dog is derived from the word *kotona*, meaning daughter, reflecting its place in the household. Early Greeks used the word *kynikos* meaning doglike, from which the word 'cynic' evolved as well as *cynegeticus*, literally meaning 'about dogs', used as a title for poems.

Recognisable breeds of dogs have been discovered in many archaeological sites dating back to Mesolithic times (at least 10,000 years ago). It is obvious that humans soon began to adapt the species in ways that would be of benefit, sheep and hunting dog types have been found as well as miniature breeds of the Maltese type (Fiennes 1968, pp. 4–5). From the earliest illustrations of dogs in pottery and sculpture from Mesopotamia, Egypt and Greece it can be seen that the main breed varieties of dogs had already been evolved, and their importance in hunting, and demonstration of the owner's status, identified.

Natural History and Biology

Despite the great variety of sizes and shapes, the basic anatomy and physiology of the domestic species breeds remains essentially the same. The dog is a carnivore with a muzzled head (of variable length by breed), prominent ears and a tail, usually long. The body is adapted by breed for either fast running or endurance walking. The jaws are strong and developed for a basically meat diet. All senses of sight, hearing and smell are enhanced and in certain breeds have been selectively amplified (as is the case in sight and scent breeds). The dog is a strongly social animal with a clearly defined hierarchy within groups. Facial expression, vocalisation, body posture and tail wagging all serve to communicate with either dogs, other animals or humans.

The dental array is dominated by the large and pointed carnassial teeth, a strong resemblance to those of the wolf. Average lifespan is about 12 years but can extend to 15 years, except in very large breeds where the maximum is six to eight years; lifespan is related to breed type, mixed breeds invariably live longer. Gestation is about 63 days (the range is 58–68 days) and semi-annual oestrus cycles which are about 21 days in length. Puppies are blind for the first two weeks of life and are suckled for five to six weeks. Litter size varies with the breed. The male dog possesses a baculum or penis bone, and male and female will remain tied for about 30 minutes after copulation. The chromosome diploid number is 78. Most dogs become sexually mature by 12 months of age.

Species Domesticated

Canis familiaris is recognised as the common dog, probably evolved from the now extinct grey wolf. Two other variants are recognised, the Australian *dingo* and the New Guinea singing dog: the two are closely related. Both dogs live with local aboriginal peoples and are domesticated to the level of that relationship.

The domesticated dog is widely distributed globally, probably there was no single ancestor and no single original point of the dog-human relationship. As humankind evolved and migrated it appears that dogs accompanied them, probably also interbreeding with related species such as the jackal in these progressions. These are complex and not fully resolved topics, several authors have written at length on the early development of the domesticated dog, in particular Zeuner (1963), Clutton-Brock (1984) and Derr (2012).

Domestication of the canine species has been a process spread over several millennia with the aim of developing specific characteristics, in behaviour, conformation, size and appearance (colour and hair length). Recent work on genome comparisons between breeds of dog has revealed more than just genealogical information; it has shown that there are five types of genetic mutations or alterations in the dog (as in most species). This has been aided by genome mapping which has revealed the genetic basis for many specific physical traits which have been utilised by breeders. Such breeder activity has disrupted the normal process of canine evolution, frequently to create undesirable characteristics (Francis 2015, pp. 45–47). This inbreeding depression in several breeds has resulted in a decrease in litter size and an increase in the number of puppies which are stillborn or die prematurely.

The outstanding features of the dog, and the major contributors to the relationship with humans, are its perceived intelligence and the behaviour patterns related to this. Uniquely among animals, the dog has behavioural characteristics that are similar to those of humans, in many respects they are compatible. As a social animal with an hierarchical understanding, dogs are more receptive to training, which is actually the 'taming' of the animal. Two types of dogs had particular abilities to assist hunters, from which specialist breeds developed – the sight (or gaze) hounds and the scent hounds. The former are excellent runners and the latter more endurance walking animals. The sensory capabilities of the dog are still being understood: they are trainable to guide blind humans; have an ability to detect certain cancers; can be trained by scent to detect many specific substances or objects such as illegal drugs, foods or landmines; can be aware of pending epileptic attacks, and have been shown to be of comfort to hospitalised and psychiatric patients. In all of these roles a specific bond develops between the handler and the dog.

The recognition of these abilities meant that different types of dogs were bred from early times, probably as early as the 5th or 4th centuries BC. These separate varieties can be seen in early art works in bas-reliefs and wall paintings in Mesopotamia (Assyria and Babylonia) and Egypt. Large, well-built hunting dogs and greyhound types, as well as miniature breeds, can all be seen. A small dog, of the Pekinese type, has been known in China from about 2000 years ago.

DOMESTICATED DOGS AND CULTURAL GROUPS

The dog has played an important role in aiding the advance of human development. This has varied in different parts of the world but appears to have started around 10,000–12,000 years ago. The first utilisation was in hunting and then, as permanent settlements and farms began, in herding sheep in particular, and as guards. In remote Arctic regions the adaptation of the wolf to draw sledges enabled expansion of the lives of those peoples. One of the earliest archaeological findings of a wolf/dog skeleton was in Oberkassel, Germany, found with human remains in a habitation excavation, and dated to the later Upper Palaeolithic period, about 14,000 years ago (Nobis 1979, p. 610).

Many sites including bones with doglike characteristics have been found, one of the earliest claimed findings has been in China, dated earlier than 15,000 BC, indicating that domestication might have begun in the Far East. Others have appeared to be more in keeping with human developments, in the fertile crescent territory dated to 12,000 BC; Turkey 9500 BC; Idaho 9000 BC; Romania 5000–4000 BC; Assyria and the Nile Delta 4000 BC. Those regions that also had developed art forms in bas-relief and wall paintings are those that provide reliable evidence, these were in the Nile valley and Mesopotamia regions.

Ancient Times

From 5000–4000 BC good evidence is available of the canine types that were being bred. Assyria had evolved strong and well-built mastiff-type dogs, shown in many bas-reliefs of hunting scenes (and the associated dog-keepers) accompanying the royalty and nobility. The Assyrian cuneiform for dog was *kelb* with spoken sound of *ku*. Herodotus wrote that they used Indian dogs (which the Greeks termed mastiffs). The dogs used were scent hounds with broader heads, larger noses and loose lips. He also observed that certain villages were given the task of providing the food for the Royal Hounds, and that a form of taxation was imposed for the 'hound bread'. The saluki was also a much praised hunting dog in Assyria.

Egypt developed possibly the strongest early dog culture. The placing of most animals in their religious pantheon of gods resulted in at least 12 recognisable breeds and strong indications of a jackal ancestry, with a significant jackal input into the creation of *Anubis* the dog-headed god, who was the Lord of the Necropolis and patron divinity of Lykopolis, his cult city, now called Asyut. Anubis, represented as a dog-headed man, or a black jackal-like canine with exaggerated upright ears, had a pivotal role in funerary rites. There were several other canine gods, two of the more important were Khentiamentiu and Wepwawet. The word for dog in ancient Egyptian was *iw* which was transliterated as *oau-oau*. Rice (2006, p. 194) suggested that this term could sound like bow-wow. An excellent example of Anubis, in black and gold, was found in the Tutankhamun tomb. Herodotus recorded that if a dog died it was mourned by the family and buried with special rites; there are huge numbers of mummified dogs buried in the Anubeion at Saqqara.

Hunting with dogs was a highly developed sport much enjoyed by the Pharaohs. Egypt with its dry sandy soil was not a country for following a scent. Egyptians bred the Pharaoh Hound, a highly specialised sight hound for hunting with a golden coat, narrow head with a long nose, strong jaws and excellent vision. The Egyptians called these hounds *tjesm*. The dogs were very elegant and had a strong bond with the owner. Egypt was the first country to show an animal–human relationship. All types of dogs as well as the prized hunters were kept, and have been well described by Rice (2006) and Hancock (2012).

Greece

Dogs played a significant role in the Hellenic region. They were used for guarding both livestock and buildings and for hunting, and as pets. The only early Greek text to have survived on the hunting dog is the *Cynegetica* by Xenophon (430–355 BC), he valued the Laconian hound, as well as the Castorian and Vulpine (a claimed fox-cross). For boar hunting the Indian, Cretan or Locrian hounds were favoured (the word 'Indian' at that time indicated a country in Persia, possibly by the Caspian Sea, these dogs were possibly the same as the Molossian mastiff). Aristotle (389–322 BC) the notable naturalist and the first veterinary scientist also mentions the Molossian and a small breed, like a Maltese, as portrayed on Attic vases. Both Xenophon and Aristotle believed that some of the dog breeds were a result of crossing with the fox (Merlen 1971, p. 281). Xenophon and Aristotle and their works are fully discussed in Chapter 2.

Roman Empire

Animals of all species and breeds feature in any history of Rome, including the appalling cruelty and slaughter that occurred in their sporting arenas, and hunting. Yet at the same time, an almost cloying affection is shown to certain individual horses, and in particular to dogs. As a species, dogs were used as guards for livestock, buildings and army camps and they played a role in the army being used as the front row of attack. They were also sometimes used to pull small carts or chariots or as performers. But their main roles were in hunting and in the home as pets. These types are well illustrated in wall paintings and mosaics: a good example is the mosaic at the entrance of the house of Paquius Proculus in Pompeii showing a guard dog. While the many breeds are named they were also grouped as *canis venaticus*, the hunting dogs, *canis pastoralis*, the farm dogs, and *canis villatici* the guard or house dogs, with pet dogs called *catelli*.

Hunting became increasingly popular after the full subjugation of Greece in the 2nd century BC. Virgil (70–19 BC) in his poetry wrote of the use of the Umbrian breed in the stag chase. The sport was adopted by leading Romans such as Cato and Cicero, and by the 4th century AD it had become the principal pleasure of most of the emperors.

Pliny the Elder (AD 23–79) in *Natural History* wrote of the hunts and the Colophonius and Castabaleans who maintained squadrons of mastiffs for war service – they were in the front rank in battle. He recorded that Romans relished the meat of suckling whelps and also used dogs for sacrificial expiation (Fiennes 1968, p. 9). Martial (AD 39–103) wrote his well-known epigram relating to Issa a pet dog, which has been open to interpretation (Ferris 2018, p. 45).

Varro (116–27 BC) recommended the use of dogs to protect sheep and goats from attack by wolves. He stressed the best size and colour of dog to use, these were similar to today's Pyrenean Mountain dog.

Gratius Faliscus (63 BC–AD 14), a poet, wrote *Cynegeticus Liber* the first of the Roman hunting books. He recognised and described 22 breeds from all over the Roman Empire naming the Celtic and the British dogs as two of the best from north-west Europe.

Lucius Junius Columella (AD 4–70) in writing on agriculture, emphasises the value of dogs for guarding, but stresses they should have short names to get a quick response when called, suggesting 'Ferox', 'Celer' or 'Lupa'.

Flavius Arrianus (c.AD 86–160). Arrian wrote his *Cynegeticon* in prose, with much discussion of breeds, conformation and colour. He liked the Celtic (Irish Wolfhound) and Segusian hounds; laid down rules for kennel management; and recommended an annual sacrifice (of sheep, goat or calf) to the goddess of the hunt, Diana Venatrix.

Claudius Aelianus (AD 170–230) wrote *De Animalium Natura*. In this text he discussed the character and personality of the dog, and the devotion they showed for their master.

Oppian (2nd century AD). The *Cynegetica* attributed to him was probably written by another author with a similar name. It is presented as a poem and praises the Agasseus from Britain as an excellent tracker, but of unattractive appearance.

Olympius Nemesianus (c.AD 283). The last of the Roman Empire writers on the dog, only fragments of his *Cynegetica* have been found. He added more breeds from Spain and Italy and praised British dogs, 'the fleetest hounds, the best in the wide world over for the chase'.

Hunting was the main role for a Roman Empire dog. The Romans obtained the fastest coursing hounds from Britain and Gaul, and the best scent hounds from Germany, then a region of dense forests. The role of dogs as pets became important with many small breeds selected. They were also much represented in carved and bas-reliefs in funerary art, on sarcophagi and tombstones; they were used as a symbol of death, but in a comforting way. Dogs symbolised the 'healing' of the dead by rebirth into the afterlife (Toynbee 2013, p. 123). The many books named in the list of references provided in this volume contain an abundance of information and stories on dogs in the Roman world and are recommended reading. The role of the dog and the Romans who wrote about them are all discussed in Chapter 4.

Medieval Dogs

As the Roman Empire collapsed, the continent was split by factions and wars until a new structure of countries evolved. In all of these new entities, dogs formed an important part of the new societies. These all, mostly, had a similar social structure and feudal system: the land was divided into 'manors' with controlling lords. Dogs were found in four main groupings – hounds for the hunts, guard dogs, shepherd dogs and dogs as pets. From the beginning there was a constant awareness of the risks of rabies. Although the disease was regarded as a human problem – hydrophobia – it was recognised that the dog was the vector, the animal that carried and spread the disease. Rabies was described by the French surgeon Henri de Mondeville (c.1260–c.1320), but well-known to other authors and feared in every community (Walker-Meikle 2012, p. 47).

An appreciation of the role in society played by dogs can be seen from the illuminated manuscripts which were a feature of the medieval years: everyday scenes and characters were seen in the marginal figures. The *Lutteral Psalter*, an English work from around 1330–1345, has many drawings of dogs acting as guards (with belled collars), shepherding or performing tricks. In Folio 11V of the *Holkham Bible* (1328–1340), an illustrated holy book, the Virgin is shown rising from a chair on which sits a capped lapdog, an example of the extravagance of fashionable society. In Geoffrey Chaucer's *Prologue to the Canterbury Tales* (c.1380s) he writes of 'Nonne, a Prioresse' the owner, Of smale hounds had she, that she fedde with rosted flesh, or milk and wastel-breed'.

Dogs and Medieval Law

As the new country entities emerged in Europe their leaderships introduced legal codes. Those in the south of Europe tended to follow the previous Roman Law, in the north a Teutonic (or German) Law evolved, either used alone or blended with Roman codes. The dog featured in all of these, the reason being to put honour prices for the penalties imposed following either the damage or death of a person due to a dog's attack, or the damage or loss of a dog belonging to another person. The legal codes included the *Lex Alemannarum* and *Pactus Alemannarum* (German), and the *Salic Law* of the Franks. The legal systems, now extremely complex to understand, show that dogs had value, as shepherd dogs, guard dogs or hunters, and also that ownership carried a responsibility: the person who fed the dog was usually defined as the owner.

The Laws of Anglo-Saxon Britain list fines levied on the owners of dogs who attack people. Alfred the Great's laws valued a dog collar at one shilling. The Welsh laws of Hywel the Good in the 11–12th centuries classified three types of animals 'a beast, a dog and a bird' and then listed three kinds of 'higher dogs'. Hywel's laws even quoted the value of the chief huntsman's needle 'for sewing up torn hounds', at four pence. There were many similar laws both in Britain and continental countries, all mentioning the custom of the lesser nobility setting aside a portion of manorial land for the growing of crops to feed the dogs of the Kings or Lords as they travelled. Irish laws, some dating to the 5th century, listed fines related to dogs which were classified as hunting, guard or lap (household) dogs. These laws are discussed and explained by Merlen (1971, pp. 90–116).

Hunting and Guard Dogs

These two main types of dogs were to be found associated with the royal courts, nobles and big households. The hunting dogs were highly prized as seen in the superbly illustrated manuscript of the late 1330s by Comte Gaston de Foix (aka

Gaston Phébus), *Les Deduitz de la Chasse*, a notable sporting and hunting work. There are pages of illustrations of hounds, hunting and the management of dogs, executed with clarity and care, one of which shows eight dog 'valets' each with a different breed of dog receiving inspection, bandaging limbs, cutting claws, bathing feet and applying topical dressings. In the 15th century this was translated by Edward, Duke of York and formed the main content of his *Masters of Game* book.

Many other books followed with the first serious book on the dog in English, *De Canibus Britannicus*, published in 1570 by Dr John Caius. He attempted to produce a full classification of the species. While not acceptable today he identified 16 canine types, all except one, *Canis delicates* a pet dog, were working dogs. The emphasis, however, was on the sporting dogs with one of the best books being *The Noble Art of Venerie or Hunting* published in 1575 and attributed to George Turberville. It is based on a translation of *La Venerie* (1573) by Jacques de Fouilloux, and also on parts of *Les Deduitz de la Chasse* by Gaston Phébus. This book was important as it was the first English language work to discuss dog care and disease as well as dog types, rearing of hounds and kennel construction. The hunting library was enlarged with mostly similar books, with much plagiarism and one common factor: all mentioned the madness in dogs – rabies. Later typical works were *The Gentlemen's Recreations* 1686 by Richard Blou and *Essays on Hunting* 1781 by William Blane.

The country houses of the feudal lords and nobles in most countries of Europe all had dogs. These were used by the owner to accompany him on his hunting and fowling days. Sometimes, for the bigger households, there would be a pack of hounds, and often some smaller breeds for the ladies of the house. If guests visited it was expected that they would bring their dogs and all would receive hospitality. Most dogs were fed on specially prepared bread, for the hunters this would be a good ration of one or two loaves a day and sometimes a special black bread made with bran would be fed (Woolger 1999, pp. 193–194). Following a successful hunt the entrails of the butchered quarry would be cooked and fed to the hounds. In big households the fewster (the keeper of hounds) would have responsibility for the dogs, their kennels, feeding, daily exercise and health.

Hunting dogs were usually a mixture of breeds, greyhounds were popular as were alaunts (a large wolfhound), spaniels, mastiffs and 'hounds'. Their use varied by the quarry – boar, deer or hare. Good kennel buildings were constructed with a loft to aid cooling in summer and for holding heat in winter; heating was incorporated and floors were sloped with gutters for drainage. Those dogs allowed in the house were made to behave, they were not allowed in bedrooms (a rule frequently ignored by guests) and stroking at the dinner table was not acceptable! Dogs had many names – Jakke, Bo, Terri and Gerland are all recorded – with one 15th-century manuscript being said to list 1100 names of hunting dogs (Walker-Meikle 2013, p. 21).

Pet Dogs

The keeping of pet dogs was common in Roman times and continued in the medieval years. Dogs were the favourite medieval pet, they ranked higher than cats, monkeys or squirrels – they showed loyalty and faithfulness. As the society structure evolved, the majority of pet dogs were living in an indoor world with either women or clerics, mainly in religious houses. Secular men preferred animals that reflected the outdoor life with qualities they hoped to copy – strength, loyalty and fierceness. John Caius, in his 1570 classification of dogs, had identified the *Canis delicates*, which he described as, 'Of the delicate, neate, and pretty kind of dogges called the Spaniel gentle, or the comforter, in Latine *Meliteus* or *Fotor*'.

This indicates the supposed Melita or Maltese dog of ancient times. Caius noted that it was 'Little, pretty, proper and fyne' and a luxurious plaything for the gentler sex, they were 'play fellowes for minsing mistrisses to bear in their bosoms' in the bed chamber or when out driving. It was also believed they had a health benefit as, 'these little dogs are good to asswage the sickness of the stomake . . . or borne in the bosom of the diseased or weake person'. He also reported that the *Meliteus* was useful to 'bewray bawdery, and filthy abominable lewdnesse . . .'; he was apparently referring to adultery, but did not explain how. William Harrison in 1586 added to this general picture of the pet dog in the *Holinshed's Chronicles of England* writing that, 'dainte dames and wanton women . . . in their chambers, to succour with sleep in bed, to nourish with meat at board, to lie in their laps and lick their lips'. Pet dogs not only had collars and hats and cushions but were said to be fed on 'scraps and indulgences'.

Hildegard of Bingen in the 12th century commented on the loyalty of dogs and noted their ability to tell the future, by their posture. This was also a time when astrology was important for prediction, notice must have been taken of *Canis Major* and *Canis Minor* in the Orion constellation with Sirius the 'dog-star' located in the nose of *Canis Major*. It was, however, recognised that some dogs, in particular large ones, had disadvantages and King Henry VIII (r.1509–1547) decreed that the only dogs allowed in court were 'some few small spaniells for ladyes or others' so that 'the house may be sweet, wholesome and clean'. And so, through all the changes in society, by the 21st century dogs still retain a unique position in human homes throughout the world and have earned the title 'man's best friend'. Dogs have retained a role in shepherding sheep, as guards and also with a role in the police and army for detection of illegal drugs, explosives and people.

Dogs and Sport

Humans have found many ways to use dogs in competitive situations, usually with a financial prize or some benefit to the owner. Dog racing with specially trained greyhounds is popular in many countries, it can be the cause of injuries and damage to the limbs. Similarly sledding races are popular in northern climates, frequently involving long cross-country races. Competitive dog shows with judging for specific characteristics by breed and agility and related competitions are popular, but the activities of breeders in selecting specific characteristics to emphasise a breed have not always been to the advantage of the dogs. The ability and intelligence of dogs has enabled the creation of competitive sports, and also their use in circuses and other forms of entertainment.

Dogs and Religion

The mythology of many cultures includes dogs, beginning from early times with Anubis the dog-headed god in Egypt, and Ninisinna an ancient Babylonian goddess of healing who was frequently offered votive gifts of canine images. In many mythologies dogs guard the gates of the underworld. Most well-known is Cerberus, a three-headed dog who is the guardian of the gates of Hades, with similar representation in Norse, Welsh, Persian and Hindu folklore. China has a 12-year cyclical series of animals each representing a year, the dog is one of these (and seen as a good omen for that year).

Christians accept dogs and in their religion they are seen to represent faithfulness and loyalty, featuring in many stories of the saints. The Dominican order is said to have their name, *Dominicanus* derived from the Latin 'dogs of the lord', but this has been questioned. Dogs also feature as one of the animals in the medieval *Bestiary* books written by monks in England and France as aids to study of 'natural philosophy'. The dog sections have strong allegorical meanings to aid meditation. Church teaching was based on the works of St Augustine, producing a theology that taught that animals, including dogs, were without spiritual souls. This was expanded by Thomas Aquinas (1225–1274) who followed this belief. The idea was originally proposed by Aristotle (384–322 BC) who believed that animal souls disappear when they die. That this theology was not universally recognised was shown in the writings of Adelard of Bath in one of his dialogues in Platonic style *Quaestiones naturales*, where he argued that animals do have immortal souls since they have the power of judgement to desire or avoid things, and such a property can only exist in the soul and not just in the body. However, regardless of the theological teachings, both monks and nuns were regularly criticised by their bishops and others for keeping dogs and providing food for them, which properly in the teachings of the Church should have been given to the poor.

Muslims follow the word of the Prophet who did not like dogs, mainly it seems on hygienic grounds; Muslims practice ritual hygiene (*wudu*) five times a day at prayers. An exception appears to be made for the *Saluqi* (Saluki). Muslim laws only allow the consumption of meat from religiously slaughtered animals. However, to enable the consumption of hunted animals, when the dogs are released the words 'In the name of God' had to be said, which allows consumption later.

Jews generally were known to originally dislike dogs, possibly a result of their time in Egypt and knowing of the Anubis cult. This attitude is demonstrated by the words 'Give not that which is holy unto the dogs, neither cast ye your pearls before swine' (*Matthew* 7:6). It is unclear as to the actual relationship because their shepherds had dogs and their later kings engaged in hunting. As it was lawful to eat wild meat there must have been some exemption.

Dogs in Other Civilisations

Dogs were used in several capacities around the world, as guards, herders, as sledge teams in the Arctic and as draught animals for small carts. They featured in religious rituals in many countries, probably most significantly the Zoroastrian belief at the time of human death, and in pre-colonial west and central Mexico associated with the god Xolotl where they guided their masters into the underworld after death, a belief also held in ancient China. These uses lasted for many thousands of years and are still employed in many countries.

Another practice that has been widespread is the consumption of dog meat, it was known in Roman Europe, in the Middle Ages, in Africa, the East Indies, North America and in particular in China and some neighbouring countries, for example, Korea. The Chinese originally bred Chow dogs specifically for consumption (feeding them on vegetables before slaughter to improve the flavour) but later, and today, many breeds may be used. In Siberia, the Samoyed tribes also ate their dogs and prized their skins as fur coats. While the consumption of dog meat has markedly reduced, it still remains a recognised food in some far Eastern countries. The native Mesoamerican dog was a hairless creature. While being a household pet, it was principally raised as a foodstuff, and was often force-fed.

The barbarously cruel sports of bear and bull baiting by dogs has now ceased. Doubly cruel as bears were blinded and bulls tormented before the dogs attacked. These and other customs have been described by Fiennes (1968, pp. 99–111).

Recognition of Dog Diseases

The earliest record of canine disease was given by Aristotle (384–322 BC) who wrote that dogs suffered from three diseases: *lyssa* (rabies) which was spread by the bite; *quinsy* a throat condition and *podagra*, a foot ailment. He also stated that humans would not develop rabies if bitten (see also Chapter 2).

In the Roman era dog diseases were well recognised and are discussed in the works of Grattius, Arrianus and Nemesianus. Rabies, and its risk of transmission, was known of. The best described were the skin diseases of mange, fleas and ticks with the anti-parasitic activity of sulphur being used. Foot problems and coughs, diarrhoea and constipation were all treated.

The Period of Natural Observation, AD 400–1699

Canine disease was not a major feature of early records until the 17th century. The reports in this listing are derived from the 1871 and 1882 books compiled by Fleming (see Introduction). Literature citations have not been included but can be traced by the year of reporting. These observations must be read with caution. Disease causation was unknown and naming was undecided, except in the case of rabies where most reports were probably accurate but may not reflect the epizootic proportions of the outbreaks.

1028 *Europe* Bohemia, 'dense, foul smelling vapours' followed by 'an invasion of cicadae and caterpillars . . . swarms of butterflies . . . everything green was devoured', there was then 'a great mortality among men and animals, but especially dogs'. This then spread across Europe, including England.

1414 *Germany* A severe form of dysentery affected horses, cattle, dogs, cats and humans, reported by Saxo Grammaticus in *Gesta Danorum*.

1500 *Spain* Ravaged by 'rabies caninum', in Blaine, *Canine Pathology*.

1586 *Europe* Flanders, Hungary, Austria and Turkey, epizootics of both human plague and canine rabies.

1603 *England* A pestilence reported in humans, cattle and 'even dogs suffered greatly'.

1604 *France* A rabies epizootic in Paris.

1690 *Italy* An epidemic in dogs in Anda described as 'anginous' with a 'suffocating, oppressive pain', like quinsy (possibly anthrax).

1697 *Germany* Dogs died from an epidemic marked by a 'burning fever and black bile'.

The Development of Biological Observations, 1700–1799

Reports begin to show more study of clinical signs, the first reports of canine distemper and the recognition of a global rabies problem.

1708 *Europe* An epidemic in animals, including dogs, of 'carbuncular nodules'.

1710 *Germany* 'dogs driven to madness . . . gasping . . . marked on the body with carbuncles'.

1715 *Germany and France* An epizooty of gastrobronchitis in dogs (?distemper).

1719–1724 *Europe* Outbreaks of rabies, in particular in Silesia and France (up to 1721), in Silesia and Hungary to 1722 and also seen in wolves in 1725.

1734–1735 *England* Serious rabies epidemic, 'many mad dogs run up and down'.

1735 *South America* First report of 'the distemper in dogs' in Peru, but not seen in Paraguay.

1741 *Barbados* Outbreak of rabies.

1757 *France* A 'carbuncular epizooty' affecting cattle, deer, asses, pigs, dogs, fowl and fish (it was often reported that disease outbreaks affected almost all species, these were almost certainly incorrect, this was most likely an anthrax epizootic and the public fear would attribute it to all disease in all species).

1759 *Peru* An outbreak of disease in dogs, they could not stand, many suffered and a few died.

1760   *United States of America (USA)* Reports of a disease in dogs causing great mortality.

1761–1764   *Europe* A great epidemic of disease in dogs seen. Termed distemper (English), *maladie de chiens* (French) and *hundestaupe* (German). Rare or unknown symptoms, seen first in Spain where it spread across whole country only affecting dogs. Spread across continent reaching England (London) in 1760. 900 dogs died in Madrid in 1763 and in the same year the disease spread across France (well described) with many packs of hounds affected. In 1764 it spread across Ireland, Bohemia and Franconia (Germany).

1763   *Europe* Many epizootics in animals, also affecting dogs reported. In France anthrax outbreaks, also seen in dogs.

1766   *England* An inflammatory catarrhal disease called 'horse cold' observed in horses and dogs.
France Many dogs died of a malady, also in horses and sheep.

1766   *USA* Distemper reported in Louisiana, many dogs died.

1770–1771   *USA* Rabies outbreaks commenced in June.

1771   *Russia* Moscow, a disease reported as distemper described.
Romania, distemper in dogs reported in Wallachia.

1775   *England* Horses and dogs affected with a malady, called influenza.
France Dogs and fowls reported with 'catarrhal angina'.

1776   *West Indies* Rabies outbreak in French Antilles, many people died.

1779   *America* Rabies reported in Jamaica for first time. Also in Hispaniola (1783 – 84), many people died.

1782–1784   *France* A 'distemper' reported in dogs and also cats with a similar disease.

1785   *USA* Rabies, 'canine madness raging all over the Northern States' and into 1786 in the Southern States with 'much hydrophobia in men'.

1786   *France* In Southern Pezanus region a 'catarrhal fever or distemper in dogs'. Written that it had caused 'dreadful ravages among dogs' for 20 years.

1789   *Germany* A rabies epizootic in Westphalia.
USA Much rabies seen, including New York.

1797   *USA* Rabies reported on Rhode Island. Recorded that before an outbreak of yellow fever in humans it was observed that 'many dogs showed a sickness'.

1799   *France* Canine distemper outbreak in Paris and into 1800.
Italy In the northern region 'an epizooty which destroyed a great number of dogs'.

Science Evolves with a Developing Veterinary Discipline, 1800–1900

The Lyon, France veterinary school had opened in 1762, soon followed by similar schools across Western Europe including England and Scotland. While dogs were not a major species in the course taught, the schools soon developed clinics and began to treat cases. The problem of rabies and its control had become important throughout the world. The study of pathology was beginning.

1800   *Spain* A disease affected many species particularly dogs, in Cadiz and Seville: haemorrhages and 'black vomit' were observed.

1803   *Peru* Rabies seen for the first time in 1803/1804, many people died, dog extermination attempted in Lima. Outbreak spread across the country.

1805   *England* Distemper seen as an epizootic (in Blaine *Canine Pathology*).

1806   *England* Rabies cases very frequent up to 1808, then less prevalent (Blaine *Canine Pathology*).

1807   *Ireland* Rabies prevalent in the Spring.

1809   *France* Lyon Veterinary School reported variola or 'canine smallpox', it was easily cured and had been previously seen in the region.

1810   *USA* Rabies epizootic in Ohio, also seen in wolves and foxes.
        England An epizootic seen in dogs; the bladder was much inflamed.

1813   *Mauritius* Rabies reported for the first time.

1815   *Denmark* and *Norway* Rabies epizootic.
        Austria Rabies frequent outbreaks.

1818   *France* 'Malignant distemper' reported in Lyon region.

1820   *England* Rabies very common in dogs over a three to four year period (Blaine *Canine Pathology*).

1821   *Russia* First appearance of distemper in Northern Siberia, extensive epizootic and very serious for local population who depend on sledge dogs.

1822   *Holland* Rabies cases 'markedly common'.

1823   *Europe* Rabies in most countries and species: *England* in dogs and cats; *Norway*, *Denmark* and *Russia* also in wolves, and in reindeer in *Lapland*. In *Switzerland* and *Southern Germany* lasted to 1826–1827 in dogs, cats, goats, sheep, cattle, horse and humans, also in foxes.

1827   *Germany* An epizootic in dogs called 'Yellow Fever', well described jaundice and post-mortems, no diagnosis.

1829   *Germany* Rabies outbreak in Saxony from 1828–1830.

1832   *Germany* Rabies very common in Saxony, dogs biting cattle.

1833   *Barbados* Rabies 'prevailed to an alarming extent'.

1834   *Germany* In Saxony both rabies and distemper 'extremely widespread and fatal' also 'bilious fever' present in dogs.
        France A pulmonary catarrh in dogs and horses reported in Lyon region, 'not a simple infection'.

1835 *Luxembourg* Outbreak of 'yellow or bilious fever', described as similar to 1761 outbreak.
      Chile Rabies, very prevalent in North Chile, many people died.
1836 *France* Rabies very common in Paris for whole year.
      India, Afghanistan Rabies common in wolves.
      Mexico, Brazil, China, Ceylon Canine rabies in all countries.
1837 *Germany* Rabies in dogs, foxes also cats in Württemberg (1836–1837).
      Austria Many rabies reports.
      Lithuania Rabies outbreak.
1841 *Austria* Canine rabies. A study showed first report was in 1808.
      Germany Rabies in Württemberg and Baden, foxes probably involved.
      France Lyon reported that both rabies and distemper were prevalent in dogs 1839–1841. Rabies also reported in Aix, Rouen and Nimes in 1842.

By the mid-19th century veterinary medicine had become an established and recognised science. The numerous veterinary schools were developing their role in studying diseases. In the 1841 year, listed above, the Lyon College reported rabies had been the cause of death of 104 dogs that had been in their hospital in the years 1839–1841. They also reported that in the 30-year period,1811–1842, a total of 779 dogs died of rabies in the hospital, with most deaths occurring in June and fewest in December. The Vienna College also reported on dog diseases most frequently seen; rabies was the most common but occurred in cycles; on a regular basis rheumatism, arthritis and mange (*schäbe*) were the most frequent diagnoses.

The chronological list of canine diseases clearly shows the increasing incidence and importance of canine rabies and its progressive spread around the world. While the records show the canine importance, together with its occurrence in other species, the actual importance was the human form, hydrophobia. Rabies was regarded as a human disease; veterinary involvement only became of significance in the mid-1800s.

From 19th to 20th Century

The listing also shows the first report of canine distemper in Peru in 1735 (well described in 1746 by Ulloa in *Relación historica del viage a la América Meridional*), then its appearance in Europe in 1761 and epizootic spread. A condition described as anthrax is quoted as a problem in some years and also mentions 'bilious fever', an undetermined problem, but possibly related to undisclosed canine distemper. The progression of the understanding of canine diseases is outlined in the content of published books. A discussion of five of these books follows; the first two were probably unique in Europe.

A Dictionary of the Veterinary Art was written in 1805 by Thomas Boardman, a graduate of the London College. His entry for the dog is mainly concerned with hunting hounds. The emphasis is on the maintenance of health with clean kennels, regular changes of straw bedding to control fleas and regular attention to the coat at least twice a week to prevent 'greasy skin' and mange. The need for a clean water supply is stressed, along with a diet that is dominated by farinaceous foods, little meat (always to be boiled first) and baked sheep's feet. The main problems described are bites and wounds, mange, poisoning, worms, sore feet and 'coughs and colds'. Various medications, of doubtful value, and bleeding are recommended, except in the case of 'but if it be what is called the distemper' where no bleeding and a nutritious diet of meat broth is recommended instead. Rabies is included in a list of types of madness, five of which are said to be curable. A good description of rabies is followed by the advice 'you should immediately knock him on the head as the only cure'.

Canine Pathology 1824, written by Delabere Blaine, has the subtitle '*or A Description of the Diseases of Dogs with their Causes, Symptoms and Mode of Cure Drawn from Twenty Year's extensive Veterinary Practice*'. It also noted that it included a Treatise on Dog Breeding and a copious detail of the Rabid Malady; all preceded by a Critical Enquiry into the Origin of the Dog. Blaine had attempted to provide total cover! He stresses at the beginning of the text the maintenance of health by attention to the diet and regular exercise. The list of diseases is very similar to that met today with only two described of what we now know to be of viral origin – distemper and rabies. Of interest, on page 165, he describes 'excessive fatness' as the most common complaint among dogs and suggests it 'proves a source of numerous diseases'. Skin diseases are well covered, and obviously a problem, he includes the comment 'if I am not greatly mistaken the canine mange is capable of producing the human itch' (Blaine did not know that Avenzoar, a physician in 12th century Seville, had recognised a mite as the cause of human scabies, see Chapter 6). There is a good description of canine distemper including rebuttals of Dr Jenner's efforts and claims regarding smallpox vaccine as an effective preventive, and Dr Erasmus Darwin's views on distemper treatment. The rabies section is good and extensive (Blaine does not mention his outrageous claim, made some years before, of his 'efficacious' remedy). Overall this was a good book, valuable for its clinical descriptions and Blaine's stress on humanity in all work with animals. The treatments recommended would in most cases be of little value but also of little harm, which was progress, of a sort.

Dogs: Their Management was written in 1858, by Edward Mayhew MRCVS. He was a talented artist and the book is illustrated with woodcuts. Written for the public, the text is well presented. The rabies section (pp. 155–164) includes the observation 'Of the causes or treatment of this disease we know nothing'. In discussing canine distemper Mayhew observes (p. 33) 'Of all diseases to which the dog is subject this one is the most dreaded'. However, he then states that he treats the cases and cures them: one has to question his original diagnosis. The book does provide an overview of canine disease in the mid-19th century. The advice is generally good. There are few treatments but Mayhew stresses care and a humane approach.

The Management and Diseases of the Dog was written in 1881 by John Woodroffe Hill, MRCVS. By the end of the 19th century the dog and its care had become a part of urban family life. Hill commences with sound advice on nursing, feeding, exercise, washing and grooming: he emphasises a wholesome, nutritious diet but with not too much meat included. For house pets he suggests a meaty gravy or a bone, or bread or biscuit with milk, potatoes and vegetables twice a week. For sporting types, or those used as guard dogs, meat was to be fed with discretion – and checking for tapeworm cysts. Regular exercise is advocated to make life interesting for the dog. Rabies is well discussed with much use of the French literature and the observation that the 'true nature of rabies is still involved in mystery'. When a case is found the recommended method is destruction of the animal with a revolver. Distemper is reviewed with the statement that 'nature works her own cure in many instances' but adding numerous treatments 'produce mischief and result in death'. Hill quotes reports from the Lyon College, notes the occurrence of glanders in dogs, cites a case of a dog contracting measles from a human and records *variola canina* as a variant of smallpox. While much of these reports are of limited interest, or accuracy, they demonstrate the increasing study of canine disease, and the role of the veterinary schools and their clinics; both sarcoptic and demodectic mange were then known as parasitic infections, increased knowledge of canine helminths and cestodes was developing, but effective treatments still needed.

The Dog's Medical Dictionary, written in 1934 by A J Sewell and F W Cousens (veterinarians to the British royal family), had appeared in several editions since 1906. It provides good advice, in particular on nursing: the authors also state that obesity is a common complaint and give advice on feeding. Canine distemper is correctly described as a contagious febrile disease of viral origin with an incubation period of five to fifteen days; the occurrence of fits and chorea is recognised. The authors note that a vaccine had been developed at the National Institute for Medical Research (London) but was not yet on sale. Rabies is reported as of viral origin and that if diagnosed the dog should be shot. By this date, the disease had been eradicated in Britain and in developed countries it was under control. Mange treatment with sulphur-containing products was said to be successful but slow.

Canine Disease and Welfare

Over the centuries rabies was recognised as most serious and dangerous, but regarded as a human disease, although spread by dogs. The work of Geog G Zinke in 1804 established that the cause of the disease was an infectious agent, which was followed by Louis Pasteur and Emile Roux in 1881 who were able to immunise dogs with an attenuated vaccine, published in 1887. Pasteur used his vaccine method of treatment on his first patient in 1885. In 1931 Joseph Pawan noticed negri bodies in an infected bat brain. In the following years, a variety of vaccines have been produced first using diploid cells, then chicken cells and tissue culture on egg embryo vaccines both live and inactivated. These are now employed worldwide to hopefully eventually eradicate the disease.

Canine distemper was proven in 1905 by Henri Carré in France to have a viral origin. Many attempts at vaccine production were made until immunisation systems using serum and virus, or vaccine, were developed in the 1930s by J Laidlaw and H Dunkin in England. This provided effective, but costly, protection. In 1948 D A Haig in South Africa developed an egg-adapted vaccine strain which provided effective, low-cost protection, when introduced in the 1950s, including against a resistant 'hard-pad' form of distemper in Britain. Since then several improved vaccines have been developed.

In more recent years, a wide range of other viral infections (parvovirus, coronavirus) have been studied together with bacterial infections (those caused by rickettsial, babesia and coccidial bacteria). The development of antibacterials, antibiotics, parasiticides and endocrine products has now provided the veterinarian with a well-supplied pharmacy.

The dog has a unique animal-human relationship, it appears to be the longest such partnership and one that exists in most cultures and civilisations. The benefits are obviously mutual. In recent years, the highly developed canine senses have been trained to aid human health in various capacities, as well as tracking people and substances. The dog, however, also holds a special place in human affections for its value (and obvious enjoyment) in hunting; by nature a pack animal, it behaves well in the hunt environment. Many countries have national organisations (like the Kennel Club in Britain) devoted to canine care and management, and the preservation of the wide variety of breeds.

Canine veterinary practice has now become a major part of companion animal practice which, following the 1939–1945 war, has advanced with rapidity to serve the large dog and cat populations in developed countries, and in the increasing urban populations. Hospital and consultant services are generally available with high quality surgical procedures. The creation of the World Small Animal Veterinary Association in 1959 has encouraged similar global standards, now with affiliated groups in 133 countries and a membership of over 200,000 veterinarians (2020).

Dogs and Public Health

The historical record shows that from early ancient times the danger of rabies and its spread by a rabid dog has been known and feared. Of other diseases the human recognition has mainly been from ectoparasites, but as more of a nuisance. However, ringworm has sometimes been difficult to control. The human, usually children, can also act as a variant intermediate host for some canine nematodes, termed visceral larval migrans. Dogs can be infected with tuberculosis and in a companion animal, this can be a human threat. As most cultures do not consume dog meat, any hazards from this practice are not known.

References

Clutton-Brock, J. (1984) in *Evolution of Domesticated Animals* (Ed. I.L. Mason). New York: Longman

Derr, M. (2012) *How the Dog became the Dog*. London: Duckworth Overlook

Ferris, I. (2018) *Cave Canum: Animals and Roman Society*. Stroud: Amberley Publishing

Fiennes, A. and Fiennes, R. (1968) *The Natural History of the Dog*. London: Weidenfeld and Nicolson

Francis, R.C. (2015) *Domesticated: Evolution in a Man-Made World*. New York: Norton

Hancock, D. (2012) *Sighthounds: Their Form, Their Function and Their Future*. Marlborough: Crowood Press

Merlen, R.H.A. (1971) *De Canibus: Dog and Hound in Antiquity*. London: J A Allen

Nobis, G.J. (1979) Der alteste Haushund von 1400 Vahren. *Umschau* **79**

Rice, M. (2006) *Swifter Than the Arrow*. London: Taurus

Toynbee, J.M.C. (2013) *Animals in Roman Life and Art*. Barnsley: Pen & Sword

Walker-Meikle, K. (2012) *Medieval Pets*. Woodbridge: Boydell Press

Walker-Meikle, K. (2013) *Medieval Dogs*. London: British Library

Woolger, C.M. (1999) *The Great Household in Medieval England*. Cambridge, MA: Yale University Press

Zeuner, F. (1963) *A History of Domesticated Animals*. New York: Harper & Row

CHAPTER 23

Feline: Cats

Taxonomically the cat is a member of the Felidae family – of the order Carnivora, suborder Feliformia. There are two subfamilies: the Pantherinae – tigers, lions, jaguars, leopards; and the Felinae – all other non-pantherine cats including *Felis catus* the domestic cat.

The domestic cat is an extremely popular household pet, probably equalling or possibly exceeding the dog in total numbers. Its popularity is global, across all countries, climates and regions. It is kept as a domestic pet/companion, but is also seen as a useful economic animal in farmsteads and commercial premises, where it is recognised as having a value in controlling rodent (mice and rats) pests.

Most European languages have a word which derives from the Roman Latin *cattus*: French *chat*, German *katze*, Dutch *kat*, Anglo-Saxon English *catt*, current English *cat*. The word *cattus* appears to have been first used by Palladius in the 4th century AD and is obviously derived from one of the Arabic/Berber tongues from the word *quttah*, meaning cat. Also with Arabic roots is the word 'tabby' used for the typically striped fur pattern. This word was first seen in Medieval Latin as *attabi* from the Arabic *attabiya*, itself derived from *al-Attabiyya*, a quarter of Old Baghdad where a characteristic striped silk fabric cloth was woven in the 12th century. It is said that either the fabric or the district was named after the Umayyid Prince Attab. There is also a, probably apocryphal, story of the Prophet Mohammed who, finding that a cat had fallen asleep on the sleeve of his gown, cut off the sleeve when he wanted to move, rather than disturb the cat; another version states that Mohammed loved cats and that he would do without his cloak rather than disturb a cat sleeping on it. He was said to have had a favourite cat named 'Muezza'. While there are no specific animal species sacred to Islam, in general cats are revered by Muslims. There are obviously strong relationships between cats and Arabic peoples. A Turkish word *utabi* for a cat, shows a similar origin.

There is a strongly recognised connection between Egyptians and the cat; it has been suggested that the word 'puss' may be derived from the name of the Egyptian goddess Pasht, more usually translated as Bastet, but this is dubious because 'puss' is an ancient English word for a she-cat, later used for both sexes, and also in the 1600s was a term used for a hare. In some English texts of the late 1300s the word in Latin for cat was written as *musio*. The Egyptian connection between cats and humans is, however, very strong, in Ancient Egypt it was regarded as sacred, as many animals and birds were. An illustration of this affectionate relationship is seen in the trans-literation of the Egyptian hieroglyph for cat – *miw*, which was pronounced 'miaow'.

Natural History and Biology

The cat is an agile, flexible-bodied, light-footed, frequently nocturnal, quadruped mammal, with usually smooth fur and protractible and retractable claws. The species are obligate carnivores, meaning that they are adapted to eating meat and have difficulty with plant-derived foods: sources of the amino-acids taurine and arginine are essential to their diet. There are many species or subspecies of cats, together with a lack of clarity on the exact relationship of these varieties to the common domesticated animal.

Cats have quick reflexes, a powerful jaw and teeth designed for killing small prey. Senses of smell and hearing are very good, night vision competence is well developed, but colour vision is poor. Cats have a rather unique capability reflex to right the body in a fall. Its whiskers aid navigation and sensation detection. Cats have many vocalisations, while they are a social species they are solitary hunters. With a gestation period of about 64–67 days they have a high breeding rate: the female is facultatively polyoestrous and usually only ovulates following foreplay and coitus. In domestic environments a cat will usually live at least 15 years or more, aided by neutering.

It is currently recognised that the domestic cat (*Felis catus*) is derived from *Felis silvestris-libyca*, part of a mixture of a number of races of small wild cats originally found in Europe, North Africa and Southern Asia. Until recently it was believed that this was not a distinct species, but a complex with two principal subspecies: *Felis s. silvestris* (European wild cat) and *Felis s. libyca* (African wild cat). Both are very similar except that the latter has a more supple body, lighter coat colour and less well defined striped or mackerel tabby coat pattern.

Recent analysis of mitochondrial DNA from a sample of 209 cats that lived between 8000 BC and the 20th century AD has provided data that helps to illuminate, and confirm the domestication process. The DNA was extracted from bones, teeth, hair and skin of animals that were found at sites in the Near East, Africa and Europe. Phylogeographic analyses of the genetic material indicates that all domestic cats today descend from *Felis silvestris libyca*, the subspecies found in North Africa and the Near East.

The study showed that two distinct populations contributed to modern domesticated cats. One from the Middle East spread to Europe as early as 4400 BC; the other, a separate lineage, was initially common only to ancient Egyptian cats then spread to Europe and the Middle East from the 5th century AD onwards. Expansion patterns suggest that they followed maritime and land trade routes. A coat-colour variant was only found at high frequency after the Middle Ages, which suggested directed breeding of cats occurred much later than with most domesticated animals (Ottoni et al. 2017, p. 139).

Other species which are recognised, but are probably not involved in the genetics of the domestic cat, are *Felis margarita* (sand cat), *Felis manul* (Pallas's cat), *Felis temmincki*

(Temminck's cat), *Felis silvestris ornata* (steppe cat) and possibly *Felis chaus (jungle cat)*. This complex topic has been well studied by Robinson (1984, pp. 217–223).

Species Domesticated

The history of the domestication of the cat is unclear. Cats exploit their owners, unlike dogs: it is often claimed that dogs have masters and cats have servants. Their relationship with humans has caused far less changes to their physical form than that seen in dogs; they have had relatively little genetic manipulation (until some recent interventions), compared with other species.

The cat is probably the most recently domesticated species, but possibly 'domesticated' is not the correct word, 'semi-domesticated' may be a better description. While the cat satisfies, in broad terms the four characteristics of domestication, it is not dependent on a human relationship. The cat will leave human habitation, breed and will thrive. A reversion to the feral state is seldom satisfactory for other species, invariably they are either unable to survive on available food sources, or are targeted by predators.

Felis catus (F. domesticus): the first name is due to Linnaeus, who used it to designate the tabby variant of the wild cat. *Felis* is in fact a much earlier word which originally meant a yellowish coloured carnivore. The domestic cat is closely related to the common wild cat *F.s. silvestris*. This is extinct in many areas of the world but is still found in some parts of Scotland and possibly elsewhere. In Scotland, the total population of wildcats still existing outside captivity was estimated in 2016 to be no more than 100.

Domestication developed (from archaeological evidence) in the Near East at the time of the rapidly expanding early civilisations. Agriculture created a need for grain stores, which were soon populated by mice (and rats), in turn to be followed by the cat seeking a food source. Arising from this close human contact the domestic cat appears to have evolved as it was seen to have an economic value in pest control. At the same time the Egyptian civilisation, with its interest in all forms of animal life, was becoming a dominant power. The cat became easily adopted into Egyptian society, where it was highly regarded. The domestication process based on archaeological evidence has been studied by Zeuner (1963, pp. 387–391).

Breeds of cats appeared relatively late in their domestication, the idea started in the Middle Ages in Europe and then developed in Britain from about 1850. The standards, based on head shape, body structure and fur type and quality are well covered by the cat breed societies. One of the first breeds to be recognised was the Manx cat, with its lack of a tail, due to a dominant gene. The breed did not arise in the Isle of Man: such cats are found in many regions of the world. In 1884 the first imports of the now called 'Siamese' mutant arrived in Europe and created a demand for totally different standards to be defined, due to the different body (more sinuous) structure. The geographic origin of the Siamese is questionable, however due to the skull shape it is almost certainly of Eastern origin. These have been followed by an ever growing selection of breeds, such as the initially termed Persian (now

Long-hair), the Burmese, the Abyssinian and Egyptian variants. There are some 100 cat breeds and many cat associations, anxious to define standards for their particular designated feline type.

The story of the cat in society is one in which the animal has been tolerated, respected, despised, associated with witchcraft, or cruelly treated for various purposes. This alteration in attitude is also reflected in the use of its names, usually associated with women. In everyday English language 'puss', 'pussycat', 'tabby' and 'tabby cat' are usual homely speech. In England in the early 1600s 'puss' was seen as a term of contempt, but now it is a term of endearment used for girls or women. In the mid-1700s 'tabby' denoted an elderly spinster in a derogatory manner, but by the early 1900s it was used to describe an attractive young woman.

DOMESTICATED CATS AND CULTURAL GROUPS

The early relationship of the cat with humans, and its subsequent domestication, is complex and is still a subject of both study and contention. Different civilisations and societies have reacted with a diversity of attitudes. The domestic cat possesses 'desert' characteristics inherited from its Near East and North African antecedents – it can tolerate quite high temperatures; cats generally lack the circadian rhythms seen in dogs; they have a strong nocturnal instinct (often seen in desert species as cooler nights are more suitable for hunting) and, if on their natural meat diet, they can live on a minimal water intake.

Egypt

The Nile valley is generally recognised as the region where the cat first gained significance, due to the preservation of both written and illustrative images and archaeological research. There is real evidence that the Egyptians were the first to domesticate cats, but this was a society that regarded many animals (including birds) as being sacred. The first record of the cat in a domestic context is seen in a wall painting in the Middle Egyptian tomb of Baket III at Beni Hasan, dated around 1950 BC. In this painting a cat is illustrated confronting a rat in a bakehouse, confirming its recognised utility value. The cat is well portrayed in tomb paintings and sketches from 1550 BC onwards: there are frequent pictures of cats joining the hunt for wild fowl, catching mice or playing under the chair of the owner.

The main focus of interest in the cat was the cult of the cat goddess, Bastet, shown as a cat headed woman, or as a cat. Bastet was originally regarded as an aspect of Sekhmet (the lioness goddess, known as 'The Powerful One', a guardian of the Pharaoh), but then took the form of a domestic cat. The cult was based in Bubastis (House of Bastet), a royal city from the 22nd Dynasty. This was a great sanctuary and held a major cat cemetery, there were many others but those at Bubastis and Saqqara were the largest. An annual Bastet festival was held and the city flourished, in particular in the 26th Dynasty. Herodotus, who visited in the 5th century BC, recorded that some 700,000 people attended from all over Egypt and that it was ranked at the top of all great Egyptian religious gatherings. He also noted that it was characterised by being a drunken, ribald occasion (women 'ritually' exposed their breasts to much jollity). It was also the time when huge numbers of mummified cats were offered as tribute to the deity. For a long period in Egyptian history a dead cat was embalmed, elegantly wrapped and cased before being taken to a feline specific cemetery.

In the late 1800s an entrepreneur brought a shipload of cat mummies to England in the hope they could be sold as fertiliser. His venture failed, but as a result a significant number of mummified cats are now in British museum collections. In recent years x-ray imaging of these has shown that many either contain kittens, part of a cat or in some cases no trace of a cat. Obviously, the demand at festival time was high, and unscrupulous dealers provided the pilgrims with the offering they had to have. It also indicates a cat breeding industry to meet the demand.

The cat cult was very popular in the Late Period, many bronze statues of both cats and Bastet were produced (Bastet statues and images at this time often include kittens, to show her benevolent nature). Apart from the Bastet cult the cat also had serious religious associations, as a manifestation of Ra (or Amun-Ra, the King of the gods) or battling with the serpent Apophis, or generally as a sacred animal with various deities. As the ancient Greeks began to explore the gods of Egyptian religion they related their two pantheons, Bastet was equated with Artemis.

Herodotus, who was much interested in animal–human relationships, incorrectly recorded that all were considered sacred in Egypt. He devoted time to describing the national practices, noting that every household had designated separate caretakers for the raising and feeding of each type of animal, and that their children would inherit these offices. People would take vows and offer regular prayers to the god to whom the animal belonged. The system was such that if someone killed an animal deliberately the penalty was death, if accidental the priest would assign a punishment. These practices and systems gave the priesthood domination over virtually every aspect of the life of the population.

Herodotus (bear in mind that in his time there were practically no cats in his home country, Greece) wrote that male cats always seek intercourse and, 'outsmart the females . . . by killing their offspring, although they do not eat them . . . the females, bereft of their babies, feel a desire to mate and so go back to the males. . .'. He also recorded that, 'whenever a fire breaks out, some divine seizure comes over the cats . . . if they fail to extinguish the fire . . . the cats rush into the flames'.

While many of the observations of Herodotus may seem to be those of a very gullible person, they must be viewed in the context of the time. There is, however, no truth in the above story concerning fire, and none in the following where he reported that when a cat dies the Egyptians are overcome by intense grief (probably true) but, 'All those who live in a household where a cat has died a natural death shave their eyebrows. For the death of a dog they shave the entire body and head', this was not true but he had a Greek audience who knew nothing of the cat (Strassler 2009, p. 146). The story is, however, much quoted.

Respect for and care of cats was important. Evidence from papyri is fragmentary, but there is one portion of a papyrus which discusses removing poison from cats stung by a scorpion – an indication of the concern for their health. The export of cats was not allowed and if Egyptian traders and sailors found cats outside of their country they would try to catch them and return them to 'home'. However, following the invasion and conquering of Egypt by Rome, and the later introduction of the Christian religion, the export ban was lifted. There was no overt restriction on the activities of the Bastet cult, it just gradually dissolved.

The ancient Egyptians were undoubtedly very fond of cats. Diodorus Siculus (c.60–30 BC) wrote of a Roman diplomat who, when visiting Egypt accidentally killed a cat. He was lynched, not because it was a cat, he would have had the same treatment if it had been an ibis – certain creatures held a very sacred place in the culture. Diodorus also recorded that the Egyptians would feed cats with bread in milk or raw cut up fish; also that they called cats with a special 'clucking' sound.

The Hellenic World

Knowledge of the cat was first available to the Hellenes from the writings of Herodotus. Obvious representations of cats appear on marble reliefs dating from c.500 BC and cats are shown on vase paintings from the 5th and 4th centuries BC; these were probably the first cat images to be seen in Italy, and appeared in the Greek colonies in the south of the country. The common representation was of a cat with women, playing with a ball of wool. It was not until later Roman times, when the cat became popular in the Greek world as a pet and a pest controller, that the economic value of the animal was appreciated.

Roman Empire

Cats began to be introduced to the Roman world following their conquest of Egypt, initially by ships which began to carry cats as a method of rodent control. Gradually specific imports were made as their vermin control capabilities became recognised. There are animal images in Etruscan tombs, the predecessors of the Romans, some claim that these are of cats, but the consensus view is that they are of small dogs.

Cats began to appear in Rome in small numbers from the Imperial period and by the Christian era they were fairly widely spread. A particularly well-known mosaic, found in the Pompeii excavations, features a tabby cat playing with a fowl (now in the Naples Archaeological Museum). In later years domesticated cats were found throughout the Roman world (as shown by osteoarchaeology). They were primarily utilised to control vermin; it would appear that they joined and then gradually replaced the ferret, proving to be a more easily managed animal pest control agent. Excavations in the English Roman town of Silchester have uncovered skeletal remains of cats and also cat footprints on roof tiles (made in the drying process). These would suggest that the cat was well integrated into Roman society.

Many Roman authors referred to cats. Strabo (63 BC–AD 23) wrote that wild cats from Libya were regularly imported to Spain to hunt nuisance rabbits. Pliny

(AD 24–79) observed the tactics of the cat, how it would walk silently, then creep, watch and pounce, and how they would bury their faeces to hide the smell which would reveal their presence. Seneca (4 BC–AD 65) noted that chickens were afraid of cats, but not dogs. The Romans, who admired their own culture, were rather dismissive of the ancient Egyptian civilisation, Juvenal (AD 47–127) in his writing poured scorn on people who worshipped cats and crocodiles.

As practical farmers both Columella (AD 4–70) and Varro (116–27 BC) advocated making smooth plastered walls around compounds where chickens, ducks and geese were held with their young, to prevent entry by cats. One of the first mentions of a cat by the word *cattus*, in extant Roman literature, is by Palladius (4th or 5th century AD). In his work *Opus Agriculturae*, he writes, 'Against moles it is useful to keep cats in the middle of cardoon (artichoke) beds. Many people keep tame ferrets', he does not say how either animal is kept in the middle of the beds.

Of European interest are the Norse myths (of indeterminate ancient origin), Freyja, the goddess of love, beauty and fertility, is depicted in a chariot drawn by two cats. It raises the question, was the wild cat domesticated in the Norse countries in ancient times? Today it would be strange to depict the goddess of love drawn by wild cats, but possibly relationships were different in early Norse times. In the study by Ottoni et al. (2017) genetic material was collected from Viking graveyards, which would suggest a relationship with the cat kept as a pet.

Medieval to Renaissance Europe

Cats enjoyed a very mixed reception, and domestic life, during the Middle Ages. They appear to have begun as economically useful creatures to control mice and as a result were introduced to many households and religious institutions. Laws in Wales, Switzerland, Saxony and elsewhere in Europe, all protected cats and imposed a heavy fine on cat killers. However, later in the period fortunes changed as superstitious beliefs developed and cats were associated with witchcraft and magic. The main involvement with humans was in the house, it would appear that the majority of homes had a cat, either in residence or on the property – in barns, stables and outbuildings. Overall they were valued as mousers, but in many houses they were just pets. While the keeping of such animals was frequent, in wealthy establishments this often went to extravagant extremes. Common household pets at the time also included caged birds, squirrels, monkeys and dogs (except those kept for hunting). In big households there were well defined rules of behaviour, 'courtesy manuals' were written to instruct the residents and guests. One rule was that cats (and dogs) should not be stroked at mealtimes; another rule was that cats should not be allowed in bedchambers, but the rules were frequently ignored.

From the beginning of the 14th century Middle Eastern cats were imported to Europe from Syria, via Italy. These were regarded as exotic creatures, they had a different coat: a brown tabby pattern with black stripes, termed herringbone. As these imports increased and the cats bred, the influence of the pet culture grew. There were many stories of ladies who had special cushions or beds made for their cats.

Sometimes cats were given jewelled collars with bells, and were generally spoiled. It was recorded that Eleanor de Montfort had a cat that almost certainly shared her bedchamber, records show she ordered milk to be provided for her cat and also for her dogs. While the cats were companions and pets, they had the freedom to wander and their hunting value was recognised.

The literature of the time also includes names given to cats: old Irish legal texts include *Méone* (Little Meow), *Cruibne* (Little Paws), *Bréone* (Little Flame) and an Irish monk and poet in the 8th–9th centuries AD wrote of his cat *Pangur Bán*. These names and their origins are discussed by Walker-Meikle (2011, pp. 4–5). A cat named Mite was recorded in Beaulieu Abbey, England in 1270. In the Middle Ages tom cats were generically called Gyb or Gibb (shortened form of Gilbert); in French this became *Tibers* or *Tibet*.

The monasteries and nunneries invariably had cats for vermin control, and some recorded the costs for food for the 'mousers'. The keeping of pet animals and birds in these establishments became something of a problem in the Middle Ages, and presiding bishops frequently had to instruct the houses that only cats were acceptable as pets, a ruling that was often flouted.

Cats featured in ancient laws: *Catślechtae*, a medieval Irish legal edict valued a cat as worth three cows if it could purr and catch mice (the circumstances of this ruling are not known and it would appear unlikely that it was enforced). Of more interest is King Hywel Dda (Hywel the Good) (c.AD 880–950) who was putative ruler of Wales (or most of the territory). He codified Welsh law, in one section 'The value of wild and tame' it is written that a kitten, from the night it was born until it opened its eyes was valued at one penny, from that time until it killed mice at two pence, and after it had killed it was valued at four pence.

Medieval literature has frequent mentions of cats, manuscripts in particular religious works are well illustrated with drawings and paintings. Usually the pictures are not related to the text, and typically in Psalters such as the massive British Luttrell Psalter, there are numerous pictures, drawings and sketches utilising animals. Cats, and mice, were frequent choices and their use in elaborate initial letters, marginalia and filling gaps in lines of text is extensive. While one reason for these illustrations may be to introduce a light-hearted tone to amuse the reader of a serious text, it is also suggested they were used as 'markers' by monks and others who would use the text for meditation, often a word or a line for a day. These images show that the cat was seen primarily as a mouse killer, but also an animal that would play with a mouse before its termination – it introduces a different aspect from the image of the cat beside the hearth.

In both the 13th and 14th centuries cats, or allusions to their characteristics, frequently appear in poems and verse. As the Middle Ages progressed there was a developing interest in natural history (in the early sense), much of this was based on the ancient authors (Pliny, Aelian and so on) but it was also gradually forming its own character. One of the first attempts was in the bestiary books. These were an interesting literary innovation common in the mid-12th–late 13th centuries. While composed in several European countries, the majority appear to be of English or French origin. The content described a mix of real, exotic and imaginary animals.

The pictures were often anatomically incorrect (but invariably beautifully presented). The intent was both to educate on natural history and convey a moral lesson: the illustration was used to demonstrate that the world was the word of God. The moral or allegorical interpretation of each animal used its behaviour as a symbolic language. These texts played a significant role in determining the use of animals in Western Christian art and literature.

One of these, the *Liber Bestiarum* (Bodleian Library, Oxford MS Bodley 764), probably written in the late 1300s, has an illustration of three cats: one sleeping, one opening a birdcage and reaching in, and the third carrying a mouse to what could be a fire. The text (Folio 51) translates, 'This creature is called a mouser because she kills mice. The common word is cat because she captures them. They have sharp sight that the brightness of their glance overcomes the darkness of light. 'Catus' is the Greek for cunning'. It is a message that does not totally portray a friendly animal, but one that could be a good subject for moral and religious interpretation and meditation.

During the later medieval years the cat encountered its most difficult relationship with humankind. This was a period in Europe when the Christian church was not just the dominant faith, it also dominated society in almost every function. There was a belief in angels, the devil, and witches. The cat became associated with witchcraft and was seen as a 'familiar' – extending the meaning of the word from friendly and intimate to a demon, in the form of a cat who attended a witch. Because of the habits of the cat – nocturnal, stealthy, killing, scratching while also purring – an unfavourable image was created. The first recorded English witch trial that involved a cat (white spotted and called Satan) and associated it with the Devil, was in 1556.

The stories grew: cats were associated with all forms of magic and heresy, both the Cathars (an heretical Christian sect) and the Knights Templar were alleged to worship a cat (usually black). Increasingly cats were used in ritual sacrifice: the intention was that this act would drive out the Devil (Zeuner 1963, p. 397). The Lent period became a particularly unpleasant time: cats were killed and buried in Oldenburg, Westphalia, Belgium, Switzerland and Bohemia; they were burned on Shrove Tuesday in the Vosges and in Alsace at Easter. On the first Sunday in Lent in many places, but in present-day Belgium in particular (from the records), they were thrown into bonfires or roasted on the ends of long poles. In Ypres, on the second Sunday in Lent, cats were thrown from a church tower and in Paris, on the eve of 24th June, St. John the Baptist's day, one or two dozen cats in bags were burned over a fire before a feast was held. There is a similar story of roasting black cats alive in Scotland, in the medieval period (Spence 1945, p. 97). These horrifying actions and stories were manifold. In a world that believed in magic, witchcraft and the Devil, and also held that 'brute creatures' had no souls, one can seek an explanation of the practices, but not an understanding of why both the Church and the legal system not only allowed these acts, but also participated.

An interesting side-light on medieval customs is revealed in the English Sumptuary Law of 1363 (such laws were common in Europe, lasting up to the 17th century, but with dwindling respect). The law defined who could wear what type of apparel and tried to regulate the colours, fabrics, trims and fur used. Cat fur was listed, it was seen as poor quality, below lamb, rabbit and fox, and allowed for use by lower grades of society. The laws were intended to restrain extravagance in clothes, food and luxury expenditure. Cat skinners were active in Britain, France, Germany, Italy and most European countries. 24 cat skins were estimated to be the number required for a topcoat. Cat skin was prized by glove makers, in particular for ladies wear.

Albertus Magnus (1193–1280), a man with polymathic knowledge including alchemy, zoology and physiology, wrote in *De Animalibus* of the cat's delight in being clean and liking warm places. He stated that cats can be kept at home if their ears are trimmed to prevent dew dripping into them. He also noted that the flesh of wild cats was good as a treatment for gout and that cat's bile was a valuable treatment for pain.

Geoffrey Chaucer (1343–1400), in *The Canterbury Tales*, frequently included a mention of cats. The Wife of Bath uses a cat allusion to one of her former husbands; in the Manciple's Tale a lustful wife is compared to the difficulty in controlling a wilful cat and in the Miller's Tale there is not only a description of a cat-hole in a door but also a reference to a man's desire for a woman in cat–and–mouse terms. In almost all cat references made across the literature of the period, and later, the human involved is female. Good descriptions of these literary sources are given by Walker-Meikle (2012, pp. 10–13). Even Desiderius Erasmus (1466–1536) the classical scholar, remarked that some men did not like cheese, as others did not like cats. The cat was able to attract the attention of all levels of society.

As the Middle Ages, or Medieval period, passed, the practices and rituals described above either died out or were banned, and the cat returned to its place as a mouse catcher and pet. However, another practice emerged, that of immuring or entombing cats in walls, under entrance steps or floorboards. These are discovered in the course of demolition or rebuilding works. Possibly some were accidental due to a cat's natural inquisitiveness, however several have been found that are seeming 'set pieces' of a cat and rat or bird (probably already dead when incorporated in the building). It has been presumed that the intent was to act as a rat or mouse-scare. Dates, when they can be estimated, run from the late 1500s up to one found in Sweden from a house built in 1920 (Zeuner 1963, p. 399).

Other Countries

Apart from Europe and the Near East there is little documented evidence on cats.

In **India** cat keeping and domestication has been known for more than 2000 years, possibly earlier if the remains of a cat, found in an Indus Valley excavation dating back to 2000 BC was domesticated. Indian feral cats mix and interbreed with the wild *Felis libyca ornata*. The cat-keeping custom may have reached India from either Egypt or Babylonia as early as 2000 BC.

Domestication of cats in **China** could date from about 3300 BC based on archaeological studies conducted in 2013 on village grain stores with bones of both cats and rodents.

In **Japan,** the *maneki neko* cat is a symbol of good fortune dating back many centuries. The typical image, with front paw raised is still widely sold and kept in the home. In ancient Japanese religion cats were held to be exalted souls, companions and guides for humans; they were all-knowing but mute, so could not influence human behaviour.

The native cats of **Burma**, **Siam** and **Malaysia**, of undated domestication dates have all proved to be popular breeds in the West.

Recognition of Cat Diseases

The earliest mention of cat health occurs in a fragment of an early Egyptian papyrus, c.1800 BC. This gives a formula for removing poison from a cat stung by a scorpion, (James and Thorpe 1994, pp. 439–440). That it was written is an indication of the regard for cats and their well-being that existed at that time. Study of other literature sources appear to have very few mentions of the species – except those by Herodotus and Palladius, quoted earlier – and no mention of disease or any health related conditions. The cat was absent from both Greek and Roman civilisations for the majority of this time.

The Period of Natural Observation, AD 400–1699

No reports of feline disease have been identified before 1414. Those listed from here on provide a series of mentions of feline epizootic diseases but little detail, many are derived from ancient chronicles as extracted by Fleming (1871 and 1882). Where possible literature citations are included. Particular care should be taken with many of these early observations, they do not give full representation of the cited situations, but in later observations do indicate serious epidemic problems.

> 1414 *Germany* A severe form of dysentery ravaged the country, affecting horses, cattle, dogs, man and cats. (*Saxo Grammaticus* is cited as the source, but since he probably died around 1220 this may refer to an outbreak at that time.)
>
> 1514 *England* An epizooty was observed in cats but no details of symptoms are given. (Forster, *Disorders of Health*, p. 153 and N. Webster)
>
> 1578 *France* An epizootic disease of cats and poultry reported in Paris. (Paulet, *Recherches sur les Maladies Epizootiques*, Vol. I, p. 56)
>
> 1613 *Turkey* An epidemic of human plague occurred in Constantinople. The local cats were transported to Scutari, as it was believed they were the cause of the epidemic, being themselves 'distempered'. (Forster, p. 157 also T. Short and Mignot)
>
> 1630 *Italy* Many reports of plant disease, famine also a bovine 'pest' and in Padua 'an epizooty among cats'. (Muratori *Govern. delle Peste*, p. 8)
>
> 1671–1672 *Germany* An 'extensive exanthematous epizooty' of cats was observed in Westphalia. It was reported as, 'The head was covered with scales, and at first the ears were inwardly crusted with scaly matter. The

eyes seemed as if they were covered with a film, although the animals could see until suppuration took place; after this period they died'. The affected cats were mostly inactive and sleepy and it was stated that the skin disease only affected the head and neck. Almost all houses with cats were affected, even if the cats were shut in; medicine (only the use of whale-fat was described) was of no help and only 'few survived'. (Wedlius. *Miscel. Nat. Curios.*, 1 December)

1679 *Austria* A great 'epidemy' was reported, particularly serious in Vienna. The summer was hot and damp, 'cats and birds died during the plague'. (Stegmann, *Ephem. Nat. Curios.*, Vol. II, p. 427)

The Development of Biological Observations, 1700–1800

Recognising and reporting of disease in cats start to identify symptoms and some cases are investigated by medical professionals.

1712 *Hungary* An 'epizooty' was reported to have 'raged' among cats in Kaskow county. It was said to have killed all cats in many villages, resulting in swarms of mice invading the houses. (Loigk, *Histor. Pestis.*, v.437)

1782 *France* In the region of Chartres during the period 1782–1784, a 'distemper in dogs prevailing as an epizooty'. There was a similar epidemic in cats, which was thought to be the same as that affecting dogs. Many farmers in the region lost all of their cats during the winters of the three years. (Barrier *Instructions et Observations sur les Maladies des Animaux Domestiques*, Paris 1813, Vol. I, p. 208)

1789 *Egypt* In Cairo during an outbreak of plague in humans, 'cats died in large numbers'. (Enrico di Volmar *Pest.*, p. 178)

1796 *Netherlands* 'The cats . . . had been attacked with a peculiar skin disease, which had the appearance of scabies'. They also had an acrid stinking discharge from the eyes, which eventually blinded them. It was observed that in the previous months . . . 'they were excessively lascivious and their night cries were particularly loud'. (Blumenbach *Voigt Magazine*)

     England Quotation from Dr Darwin of Derby: 'The *parotitis purans*, or mumps with irritated fever, is at times epidemic among cats, and may be called *parotitis felina*: as I have reason to believe, from the swellings under the jaws, which frequently supperate [*sic*], and are very fatal to those animals . . . I recollect being inclined to believe that the cats received the infection from mankind, though in all other contagious diseases, except the rabies canina can be so-called, no different genera of animals naturally communicate infection to each other; and I am informed, that vain efforts have been made to communicate the small-pox and measles to some quadrupeds by inoculation.' (Dr Darwin *Zoonomia* London, 1791, Vol. II, p. 229) [the author is Erasmus Darwin, grandfather of Charles. This report is discussed later].

1797   *United States of America (USA)* It was recorded that 'an extraordinary epizooty' among cats was seen in many countries and was believed to have started in the USA, at the same time as the epidemic of yellow fever [in humans] the previous year. It was noted that the disease was similar to that seen in the Netherlands the previous year. In Philadelphia, shortly before the commencement of the yellow fever outbreak there was 'a great disease among the rats and cats, from which many hundreds died'. This was reported in New York, and again in 1796. The cats lost their appetite, became thirsty, were sleepy, looked ill and soon became emaciated. Some died in a stupor and others 'towards the termination of the disease, become mad, vomited, and foamed at the mouth'. Many believed the disease generated spontaneously. Estimates were that 5000 cats perished in Philadelphia and 4000 in New York and then spread across the Northern States. (*New York Repository*, Vol. I)

England In March and April of the year in London and elsewhere a 'remarkable disease' appeared in cats: in three London Parishes, within two weeks, over 5000 cats died. It was likened to the epidemic disease in the USA and a similar outbreak reported from Bordeaux, France.

Ireland Another similar outbreak was reported and cats died in great numbers, 'for some of the skins of the cats . . . being dried and the hair taken off with lime, appeared full of small holes caused by numbers of worms or insects that thus penetrate . . . the poor animals appear to be in the greatest of agony'. (*Hibernian Magazine*)

Europe Many other reports indicate the widespread epidemic: 7000 cats died in Copenhagen; also seen in Stockholm, Netherlands, Germany, Italy and Austria (Vienna, 25,000 cats reported dead). In Lyon, France an eruption of itch (*gale*) destroyed almost all cats. A conclusion was that the epidemic spread across Europe from the north-west to the south-east, and followed a similar route to both yellow fever and distemper in dogs in 1761. The disease descriptions from the different countries were much alike. The most comprehensive outline of symptoms was by Buniva who quoted Dumas, professor of medicine at Montpellier, 'the symptoms of the disease are dullness, loathing, debility, rigidity of the members, drowsiness, frequent yawning, alteration of the voice and trembling of the head and extremities'.

It was also stated that in both succession and nature these symptoms may vary. Initially the cat will appear uneasy, will lose its vivacity and nimbleness, lose its appetite and its courage. As the disease advances it becomes, 'timid, melancholy, restless, and feeble . . . evades its master and drags itself along with slowness and difficulty; it withdraws itself to the most secret places in the house . . . *Valeriana marum* and *Nepeta cataria* no longer excite it. Then it has difficulty in walking, the ears hang flaccid and cold, the eye is sunken and tearful and pupil contracted; the tongue is dry and covered in yellow mucus and the mouth dribbles a white frothy saliva deepening to green. In the early stages there appears to be constipation, laboured breathing and an intense heat of the skin, the belly becomes tympanitic and there are ineffectual efforts to vomit.'

Other reports from both the USA and Europe refer to fetid yellow mucus and also a yellowish tinge to the body. Post-mortem findings frequently mention gangrenous patches in the viscera and elsewhere. The respiratory tract was usually full of a mucous matter, white, yellow and sometimes blood-coloured. Dead wild cats were also found in France showing similar signs. Both the Society of Agriculture and of Medicine in Paris reported on the outbreak and undertook investigations. (Buniva, Sedillot, *Recueil pér de la Société de Médicine*, Vol. VII, p. 273; Hundius, *Dissert. Morbi Epizootici Felibus an. 1797 fatalis historia.*, Viteberg 1800, p. 6; Brera, *Memoria Sul attuale Epidemia dei Gatti*, 1798 Pavia)

Science Evolves with a Developing Veterinary Medicine Discipline, 1800–1900

As recognition of the problem of animal disease grew, the first veterinary school had opened in Lyon, France 1762. Gradually investigation and study of animal disease evolves. The cat does not feature in this work but medical clinicians and pathologists begin to study specific issues.

1800 *Spain* A plague-like epidemic, similar to the outbreak described in the USA 1797, was seen in Cadiz and Seville. First birds died, then dogs were badly affected and then cats – they were said to be liable to haemorrhages, black vomit and dark-coloured fetid faeces; and later horses died. (Arejula *Succinta Exposicion de la Enfermedaden*, Malaga, 1804)

1803 *England* During an outbreak of influenza at Droitwich, many cows and sheep were also unhealthy, and many lambs died. 'Cats were also affected, and many perished'. (*Mem. Medical Soc. of London*, Vol. VI, p. 316)

Europe It was stated that the distemper of cats was general throughout Europe (no source given). Dogs and cats were affected, 'and each is capable of giving or receiving it from the other. . .'. The disease was said to have ravaged Europe and nearly one-half of the cats died. Symptoms were described as cough, sneezing, running from the nose and eyes, with great wasting and weakness, and sometimes purging. (Delabere Blaine, *Canine Pathology*, 1817, p. 170).

1804 *England* In one of the first veterinary dictionaries the cat is given a specific mention observing that it is 'a domestic animal, of known utility, but of whose diseases we have scarcely any knowledge'. It was noted that cats are subject to inflammatory infections, intestinal and glandular obstructions, epilepsy, tapeworm, internal hernia (a case of diaphragmatic hernia was described by a Mr Spry in the *Medical and Surgical Journal*), 'and to peculiar epidemic disease'. There is also a report of a hairball, believed to be the matted hair of a rat found on post-mortem. Also reported is, 'A female cat died in consequence of glandular obstruction, as was supposed from having stolen away, and eaten, a piece of the skin of a horse affected with the Farcy [glanders]. This portion of skin was studded with the buds or excrescences usual in that disease, and had been set apart for examination by a medical gentleman. The parotid glands were remarkably enlarged.' The work of Dr Valeriano Brera (1797) on the epidemic disease of cats in Europe is also cited. He had concluded it was a 'nervous fever' derived from the atmosphere, but advocated euthanasia of affected cats and deep burial and fumigation of their houses with vinegar. The comments on the cat close with Brera's work and the words, 'The purring tribe, which has already found a Homer in Mr Desherbier, has found an Esculapius in Dr Brera'. (*A Dictionary of the Veterinary Art*, 1805, Thomas Boardman, published by George Kearsley, London). [This report is discussed later in this chapter.]

1821 *Germany* A 'contagious epizooty' appeared in cats in Cleve, towards the end of the year. It spread rapidly and was very fatal in a short time. Initially the cats showed a loss of appetite, sought warmth, had muscular debility, then intense thirst, staring coat, watery eyes and bilious vomiting. The disease was highly contagious and all affected cats died within 24–48 hours. (Rust *Magazin.*, Vol. XIV, p. 109)

1823 *Norway*, *Denmark* and *Russia* Rabies was a frequent occurrence in dogs, cats and wolves. Also reported in England (*Hamburg Magazin. fur Ausl. Méd. Lit.*, Vol. VIII, p. 273)

1824 *Sweden* Rabies widespread in dogs, wolves, foxes and cats. Also generally reported in Northern Europe, England and Ireland. (*Svenska Lak. Selísk.*, arb. 1824)

1831 *Bohemia* (then in Austro-Hungarian Empire) Widespread disease seen in cattle, goats, dogs, hares and cats. Large number of cats affected, showed dullness, loss of appetite, great thirst, violent vomiting, slimy watery diarrhoea, usually died in convulsions. Post-mortem examination showed engorged brain blood vessels, mouth rigidly closed and full of viscid saliva, dry pleural membranes, with reddish spots, friable liver, distended gall bladder, slimy fluid in intestines, empty bladder. A similar picture was reported for cats in Austria. (*Oesterreich Med. Jahrbuch*, Vol. XVII, p. 442)

1832 *Syria* An epidemic disease of cats reported in Aleppo. Some 300 cats in the city died due to 'the plague' (Vere Monro, *A Summer Ramble in Syria*, London 1835, Vol. II p. 235)

An important and significant advance in the veterinary study of the cat in England occurred in 1841. The November issue of *The Veterinarian* (Vol 14) included on page 676 a paper titled 'On The Diseases of Cats', while no author's name is given it is attributed to W A Cartwright, a veterinarian practising in the town of Whitchurch. This is, as far as can be determined, the first feline related publication in an English-language veterinary periodical. The content is a listing and discussion of clinical cases (including an operation on a cat undertaken by a human surgeon). [The description of surgery on restrained, but non-anaesthetised animals, is particularly noteworthy, illustrating the problems for the surgeon and the suffering for the patient.] He comments on the great age of some cats, living from 18 to 25 years old; the death of cats in households of painters and those who deal in lead; describes tapeworm infection and undertakes post-mortem examinations, with a record of his findings.

By 1850 the veterinary discipline had become established. There were numerous Colleges throughout continental Europe, the London College (1791) was followed by others in Edinburgh (1823) and Glasgow (1862). None of the courses taught at these Colleges featured the diseases of the cat, except for the occasional mention when discussing the dog, which at that time itself only received cursory attention. But all these Colleges had clinics: cats were increasingly presented and required a diagnosis. Verge and Christoforoni (1928, p. 312), in France demonstrated that the cause of the epizootic disease now called feline infectious enteritis (FIE), and probably so frequently described in the above literature review, was due to a viral entity. Feline disease research was recognised and the current era had commenced.

Feline Disease and Welfare

The bond between the cat and human society is unique. From its earliest domestication, which mostly grew from a recognition of its economic value as a controller of vermin, the cat has had a complex relationship with humankind. Humans eat all the major, and most of the minor, species that they have domesticated. This includes the dog, although this is essentially limited to China and Korea. The cat, however, is the exception: it has never been either a primary or a ritual food. In times of deprivation, in towns undergoing siege or poverty, cats have been eaten (in the 1920–1930 depression years in Britain a feline-based dish called 'roof-rat pie' was eaten). In 2015 it was reported that an annual festival is held in La Quebrada, Peru which involves the skinning and eating of cats: described as a centuries-old tradition born out of an earlier time of a struggle for survival. The practice is, however, in decline.

For most of the known past, based on existing records, the health of cats has received practically no attention. From the late 1700s reports begin to appear with an attempt to characterise the symptoms. The first of these featured in the book *Zoonomia* written by Dr Erasmus Darwin (1794–1796) who was an English physician and is recognised as one of the key thinkers of the 'Midlands Enlightenment'. His description of *parotitis felina*, which he classifies with human mumps, is not readily recognisable as a common cat problem but he does comment on it spreading rapidly to neighbouring cats, which has some similarity to FIE. The Darwin report is confusing, until it is read in conjunction with the case history extract from Boardman's Dictionary (1805). This provides strong grounds for suspecting that cats can develop glanders, based on the observation of the parotid gland enlargement, together with the prevalence of glanders at the same time (Jones 2016, p. 664).

Following these reports, and moving into the 1800s, there are increasingly well documented outbreaks of an epizootic disease in cats with well described symptoms and post-mortem results all indicating outbreaks of FIE. The authors of these reports are usually medically qualified. There is one veterinary textbook mention of the disease by Delabere Blaine in his first book, *Canine Pathology* (1817); Blaine was initially trained in medicine and would have been able to use this expertise in his veterinary experience.

The early literature shows that the main cat disease to be observed and recorded was the recurrent epizootics of what was most probably FIE. Many names were used over the years for this disease including cat plague, feline distemper, feline gastro-enteritis, feline agranulocytosis and when the blood picture was recognised, feline panleukopenia, *leucopénie infectieuse du chat* (Fr.), *Leukopenie der Katzen* (Ger.), *leucopenia maligna* (Span.). The isolation of the causal viral entity in France in 1928, and its recognition in Britain (Hindle and Findlay 1932, p. 11) and in the USA (Leasure, Lienhardt and Taberner 1934, p. 30), confirmed its global presence. Vaccine developments by Enders and Hammon (1940, p. 194) and others, followed by the increasing use of immunisation, in developed countries in particular, have brought a large measure of control over the disease.

Two reports of skin disease epizootics in cats in 1671 and 1796 are highly suggestive of *Notoedres cati* infestation (notoedric mange), a highly contagious parasitic skin condition, but one which is now considered to be rare. Recent publications have also identified a pox virus infection of cats with multiple skin ulcerations a feature, sometimes with a fever, inappetence, conjunctivitis and respiratory symptoms – showing some similarity with the early epizootic mentions (Martin et al. 1984, p. 36).

A major part of veterinary practice work, from the 1930s onward, has been in neutering males and females of the species: an essential as otherwise the breeding rate becomes uncontrollable. Feline practice has become a major part of clinical veterinary work. Current estimates in Western Europe (similar to those in North America) show that over 30% of veterinarian working hours are devoted to cat practice, 40% to dogs. Feline nutrition has benefitted from sophisticated research and has enabled food manufacturers to replace the natural all-meat diet of the wild cat.

The welfare and care of cats has varied significantly in quality over the years. From the early 20th century it has steadily improved both in homes and generally because, in many countries, of legislation. However, legislation related to cats is much less restrictive than that for dogs, possibly due to their recognised 'independent' nature, meaning they have less protection.

Finally, another interesting facet of the world of the cat. About 70–80% of cats are affected by plants that produce nepetalactone which is mostly found in *Nepeta cataria*, catmint or catnip, but also in *Actinidia polygama*, the herb Valerian and some other plants. A susceptible cat can detect this chemical at a dilution of one part per million (Sellwood 1964, pp. 259–261). The aromatic chemical binds with the feline olfactory receptors and results in a temporary euphoria. A possible explanation for this behaviour is that the nepetalactone smell mimics a pheromone and stimulates cat social/sexual behaviour. As cats like to play it may just be a simple pleasurable response.

Cats and Public Health

Since cat flesh is not normally consumed by humans the potential public health hazards, seen with other animals, do not exist. In recent years, however, there has been an increasing awareness of the potential hazard existing in the cat as a carrier of *Toxoplasma gondii*. Studies indicate that about 30–40% of cats globally are seropositive to *T. gondii*: the incidence, however, varies widely from 2–3% to 70–80% of cats. It is transmitted through cat faeces, contaminated soil or cat litter. Toxoplasmosis can infect most warm-blooded animals, but felines act as definitive hosts, producing unsporulated oocysts in the intestine which are then excreted in the faeces. The organism was first isolated from a cat by Olafson and Monlux (1942, p. 176). Cats normally acquire the infection through the ingestion of tissue cysts by predation of rodents and birds, the intermediate hosts. It is also possible to contract the disease from sheep or new-born lambs. Toxoplasmosis is known as a global infection in humans, but is usually symptomless. Studies conducted in the United Kingdom (UK) suggest that up to one-third of the population will be infected at some time, but without symptoms.

The human health hazard can occur if women, while pregnant, become infected: this can cause an abortion or stillbirth or it can spread to the unborn foetus and cause congenital toxoplasmosis, a serious condition. Infection can also be dangerous for people with compromised immune systems such as those infected with the Human Immunodeficiency Virus (HIV), patients who have had organ transplants or patients who are undergoing chemotherapy. Lesions in humans usually occur in the eyes, heart, lungs or brain. Human infection in childhood has also been related to later schizophrenia, but this remains unproven. It is advisable to keep children's sandpits covered when not in use.

There is no historical evidence to suggest that cats were recognised as potential sources of human health hazards. Toxoplasmosis, tuberculosis, *Cryptococcosis* and ringworm fungi are now all recognised as feline diseases transmissible to humans. In recent years, the syndrome termed 'cat scratch fever' has been identified as being caused by *Bartonella henselae*, more commonly seen in children following a cat bite or scratch. *Salmonella spp.* infections are now recognised in cats: these can be of zoonotic significance.

References

Enders J.F. and Hammon W.M. (1940) Studies on Vaccines to prevent Feline Panleucopenia. *Proceedings Society Experimental Biology and Medicine* **43**

Hindle, E. and Findlay, G.M. (1932) – Isolation of Feline Panleucopenia Virus. *Journal Comparative Pathology and Therapeutics* **45**

James, P. and Thorpe, N. (1994) *Ancient Inventions.* New York: Ballantine

Jones, B.V. (2016) Glanders and History. *Veterinary Record* **178**

Leasure, E.E., Lienhardt, H.F. and Taberner, F.R. (1934) Studies on Feline Panleucopenia Virus. *North American Veterinarian* **15** No.7

Martin, W.B., Scott, F.M.M., Lauder, I.M. and Nash A. (1984) *Veterinary Record* **115**

Olafson, P. and Monlux, W.S. (1942) Toxoplasmosis in the Cat. *Cornell Veterinarian* **32**

Ottoni, C., Van Neer, W., De Cupere, B., Daligant, J., Guimaraes, S. and others (2017) Domestication of Cats in the Ancient World. *Nature Ecology and Evolution* **1**

Robinson, R. (1984) *Evolution of Domesticated Animals* (Ed. Mason I.L.). New York: Longman

Sellwood, E.H.B. (1964) A Note on Catmint. *Journal of Small Animal Practice* **5**

Spence, L. (1945 reprint 1949) *The Magic Arts in Celtic Britain*. Dover Publications

Strassler, R.B. (2009) *Herodotus: The Histories*. New York: Anchor Books

Verge, J. and Cristoforoni, N.F. (1928) The Virus Origin of a Feline Epizootic Disease. *Compt. Rend. Soc. Biol.* **99**

Walker-Meikle, K. (2011) *Medieval Cats*. London: British Library

Walker-Meikle, K. (2012) *Medieval Pets*. Woodbridge: Boydell Press

Zeuner, F.E. (1963) *A History of Domesticated Animals*. New York: Harper & Row

CHAPTER 24

Avian Species: Poultry, Falcons, Parrots and Others

While certain individual bird species have been extensively selected and bred for human utilisation, the animals, as they are classified in zoological terminology, are best studied as a group. Their basic anatomy, physiology, and susceptibility to many diseases is the same, but there are certain highly significant differences between individual species.

Evolution

Birds are particularly interesting: they are classified as a subgroup of reptiles – the last living examples of the dinosaurs – and are placed in the Superclass Tetrapoda, Class Sauropsida and Subclass Diapsida. Crocodiles are designated as their closest living relatives. Birds are the grouping with the most living species, in excess of 11,000, with almost 70% being passerines or 'perching birds'.

The zoological classification of birds is a contentious issue, with frequent revisions. The names and groupings used here are commonly accepted, but the relationships between a number of species, based on the evolutionary divergence of ancestral species, are frequently adjusted.

Birds made their first appearance in the Jurassic period, over 160 million years ago and, by their DNA evidence, diversified dramatically around the time of the Cretaceous-Palaeogene extinction event about 66 million years ago. They survived the event and spread around the globe. The *Archaeopteryx* fossil found in 1861 gave the first firm evidence that birds were descended from the toothed dinosaurs. While this fossil retained the long bony tail of its ancestor the more advanced avialans lost this and developed the pygostyle bone, and at the same time are reported to have developed an enhanced sense of smell.

The earliest fossil remains of birds, dated to about 160–130 million years ago, have been found in silt rocks from the Tiaojishan Formation in Hebei Province, North-East China. These early Avialans then diversified into a wide variety of forms in the Cretaceous period: the preserved plumage suggests that bird groups were established in this period. Feathers probably evolved as a means of insulation, as temperatures fall towards night-time. The pterosaurs (gliding dinosaurs) are probably not the ancestors of birds; there was a parallel evolution to flight, won by the feathered variant. There is much contention concerning dating of bird evolutionary stages, but most studies agree that the middle to late Cretaceous period was when the common ancestors of modern birds evolved.

The 2014 global DNA study of 45 bird species, by the Avian Phylogenomics Consortium 2014, enabled the reading of the whole genomes of these birds, together with those of three previously sequenced species. The results suggest that the earliest common ancestor of land birds was an apex predator which gave way to the giant 'terror birds' that once dominated the Americas. Many interesting relationships were found – falcons are more closely related to parrots than to eagles or vultures, and the flamingo is more closely related to pigeons than to pelicans.

Birds began to develop in the format that we see today about 65 million years ago. The DNA study reveals much of interest relating to feathers and colouration, and also about the group of some 50 genes that allow birds to sing, a similar grouping to those that give humans the ability to speak. Ultimately such research might produce insights to help improve the health and welfare of wild and domesticated birds. One of the most obvious and defining features of a bird are the wings, evolved from the forelegs. These are more or less developed depending on the species, but are found in all living species. Two extinct species, the moa and the elephant bird, were wingless.

Birds and Humans

Compared to mammals very little is known about the domestication of birds. Being inherently cautious, and with most species being capable of flight, their natural tendency has been to avoid human contact. It has been suggested that such a contact could have evolved as agriculture developed and birds became crop-robbers – of seeds (pigeons, fowl), of grass (geese) or water cultivation in mud (ducks). If so it is unlikely that the keeping of birds would have been earlier than the Neolithic period.

Another important factor for domestication would be the presence of sociability characteristics. Those birds of a more gregarious nature, such as fowl, geese and ducks are much more likely to adapt to be kept in flocks or groups. Pigeons show similar propensities by nesting together. In all cases this sociable behaviour was initially motivated as a defence against predators. Compared with mammals the bird-human relationship developed much later. Initially, but different cultures evolved with differing needs, birds were captured for their feathers as clothing ornamentation, and for use in cockfighting. The consumption of their flesh developed later and their cultivation for egg production much later.

An anthropological view has been expressed that humans first regarded birds as 'protein snacks wrapped in feathers'. Their probable initial human use was in feather art which flourished for thousands of years in both Polynesia and among the indigenous American peoples. The hummingbirds, honey eaters, tanagers, macaws and any bird with beautiful plumage were sacrificed for the feathers to be used in ceremonial wear. The peoples of Papua New Guinea wear elaborate body ornamentation using feathers from the birds of paradise. The Maoris of New Zealand wear cloaks of kiwi feathers. It has been stated that to make a single robe for an Hawaiian royal, thousands of birds would have been killed (Cocker and Tipling, 2013). Some of these objects have survived in museums, most notably the headdress found in the Ethnology Museum, Vienna, which is reputed to have belonged to Moctezuma II (1450–1520). Indigenous North American people still wear feather-ornamented ceremonial headdresses.

The evolution of humans has to be the worst possible happening for birds. They existed long before man and while they would always have had predators, none have been as destructive to them as humans. Since the 17th century some 125 species have become extinct due to humans. Apart from the decimation of the dodo and similar birds, the most tragic occurrence has to be the total slaughter of the passenger pigeon, a remarkably prolific bird species in North America with flocks numbered in millions in the late 1800s, but which became extinct by 1914.

Many other birds were, and are still, treated in similar destructive and cruel ways – cockfighting still exists, in the Philippines in particular; the Yawar Festival in Peru features an Andean Condor tied to the back of a bull; the Arab use of falcon safaris to hunt rare birds; the annual massacre of migrant songbirds as they travel across Cyprus, Malta, Italy and France; and the capture in France of buntings to fatten (often first blinded) and then be drowned in Armagnac for a gourmet's delight.

The economic importance of birds is realised mainly as meat, eggs, feathers and as pets. Of earlier value was the use of guano (bird faeces) as a crop fertiliser, shipped from huge deposits, mostly in the Pacific Ocean region. Birds are also significant symbols in religion and mythology (the phoenix and the roc/rukh), and in culture and folklore.

Natural History and Biology

Birds are members of the Clade Ornithurae, class Aves, which is divided into five main groups, the largest of which are the 27 orders. Of these, six have importance for veterinary intervention and human interaction (Keymer 1962, pp. 29–34).

Birds are vertebrates, characterised by feathers and wings, lack of teeth, clawed feet, horny beaked jaws and the laying of hard-shelled eggs. They have a high meta-bolic rate, a four-chambered heart and a strong but light-weight skeleton. The size differential ranges from the smallest birds about 5 cm to the ostrich at about 2.75 m in height. The wings are the main characteristic, evolved from the forelimb and varying in development, including the presence in some non-flying species. The reproductive and digestive systems are adapted for flying and some seabirds and water birds are uniquely adapted to swim. Most Galliformes (poultry) are essentially terrestrial birds, usually only capable of short periods of flight.

The basic bird skeleton is similar to that of mammals except the bones have air filled cavities and the lower vertebrae are fused to the pelvis to form the synsacrum. Pierre Belon (1517–1564), the French naturalist and author of *L'Histoire de la nature des oyseaux* (*The Story of the Nature of Birds*) 1555, included drawings of a mammalian and avian skeleton identifying homologous bones: this was an early comparative anatomy. Volcher Coiter (1534–1576) established the study of comparative osteology with *De Avium Sceletis et Praecipius Musculis* (*The Skeleton and Muscles of the Bird*) (1576). The book includes detailed anatomical studies with a classification of birds based on their structure and habits.

The alimentary tract of the bird includes a gizzard or ventriculus which aids digestion by grinding the food. The intestines of the goose, largely herbivore, are flaccid; those of the duck, an omnivore, are firmer; and of an eagle, a carnivore, more inflexible. There is no bladder and the urethra opens to the intestines. The complex respiratory system involves an air sac, lungs and bone cavities. The red blood cells retain their nucleus. The brain is well developed, mainly to cope with the complex procedure of flying. The laying of eggs means that a foetus does not have to be carried and with the absence of the bladder also lowering the body weight, flight is aided. The sex of birds is determined by Z and W chromosomes (ZZ male and ZW female), rather than the X and Y chromosomes as in mammals. The incubation of eggs varies by species, from ten days in passerine birds to over 80 days in kiwis (in relation to body size the kiwi lays the largest egg).

Birds are characterised by their great diversity of diet which may include nectar, fruit, seeds, grass, carrion and small mammals or reptiles. They are found in almost every habitat type across all continents, but are most highly developed in the tropical regions.

Social habits are well evolved by species, some being solitary and others being part of groups of all sizes up to flocks. Communication is a major part of bird social life either through visual signals, calls or songs.

Species Domesticated

Within broad categories there are six groupings of birds that are most utilised and largely domesticated by humans:

Order Anseriformes
Family Anatidae – Common duck, Muscovy duck, Goose, Swan
Order Falconiformes
Family Falconidae – Falcons, Hawks
Order Galliformes
Family Phasianidae – Domestic fowl, Pheasants and Partridge, Peafowl, Quail and Grouse
Family Meleagridae – Turkey
Family Numididae – Guinea fowl
Order Columbiformes
Family Columbidae – Pigeons, Doves
Order Psittaciformes
Family Psittacidae – Parrots, African lovebirds, Cockatiels, etc.

Order Passeriformes
Families Fringillidae and Estrildidae – Perching birds including Canary, Bengalese and Zebra finches

In terms of the numbers of birds bred and utilised by humans the Galliformes and Anseriformes dominate, as poultry and game birds for consumption. Columbiformes also are important in some locations for consumption. The Psittaciformes are of interest both as pet birds and zoological specimens, as are certain members of the Passeriformes. In individual value terms the Falconiformes lead, as specialised hunting birds. Three further species which either have, have been or are subjected to domestication are the *ostrich* (order Struthioniformes, family Struthionidae, *Struthio camelus*), the *cormorant* (order Suliformes, family Phalacrocoracidae) and the *pelican* (order Pelecaniformes, family Pelecanidae).

DOMESTICATED BIRDS AND CULTURAL GROUPS

For discussion of the many species that humans have domesticated or utilised it is convenient to group them into three categories – *poultry* (Galliformes, Anseriformes and Columbiformes: all used for consumption of meat and eggs); *falcons* (Falconiformes); *pet birds* (Psittaciformes and Passeriformes). Individual species, as previously identified, are discussed where appropriate.

The domestication of birds is poorly understood. The most important species for humans is the chicken, first domesticated in the Indus Valley region, now Pakistan, about 2000 BC, but possibly as early as 3200 BC (evidence suggests that there was possibly a separate domestication site in China, as early as 6000 BC); the duck was domesticated later, about 2500 BC in the Middle East and the goose much later, about 1500 BC possibly in Germany. Other species were adapted for human use in different global regions at differing times.

English-language names for the bird – chicken, cock, rooster and hen date back to the Middle Ages; chick (newly hatched), cockerel (young male) and pullet (young female) have been adopted in later years. In German, the common name is *küken* and in Dutch *kieken* or *kuiken*. The word poultry is now more generally used for all domestic avian species, but in some countries it specifically refers to chickens (Crawford 1984, pp. 298–310).

The chicken, *Gallus gallus*, is the most widely distributed and utilised of the poultry species. Domesticated from the south-east Asian junglefowl, generally believed to be exclusively from the red junglefowl. It is worth remembering, for the constant debate on the best methods for housing both meat producing and egg laying fowls, that these were originally birds in the Asian rainforest.

The red junglefowl (*Gallus gallus*) is now recognised as the ancestor of the European breeds of domestic chicken, mainly because it most resembles the domestic fowl, although the relationship to some of the heavier Asiatic breeds is less clear-cut (Wood-Gush 1958, pp. 321–326). Delacour (1965) identified five *Gallus* subspecies, of these the Indian type was seen to have been the most likely to have been domesticated.

These birds inhabit south-east Asia, an area ranging approximately from north-west India to southern China and south to Malaysia and Indonesia, and are also found on many Pacific Islands (Zeuner 1963, pp. 443–447, Crawford 1984, pp. 300–302). The hens of all species have drab brownish feathering but the cocks are spectacularly handsome (Lembke 2012, p. 14).

It is known that the initial purpose of domestication was for cockfighting. Birds then gained a religious significance and much later assumed the role of a meat and egg provider. The number of eggs produced by members of the wild species is probably less than 60 in a year, while current domesticated birds produce up to 250 or more a year with a weight of around 60 g or more.

India

Domestication appears to have commenced in the Indus valley during the Harappan culture. Zeuner (1963, pp. 444–445) has described relevant objects (seals and figurines) and bones from Harappa and Mohenjo-daro. Dating of domestication is difficult, it has been suggested that this could have been as early as 3200 BC, but as the peak of the Indus valley civilisation was between 2500–2100 BC it is likely to have advanced more rapidly at that time, as the use of the birds for cockfighting evolved. However, by 1000 BC it had become forbidden to eat fowl in the Indus valley civilisation, indicating that a religious importance had been placed on the bird, and it is assumed also on cockfighting. Birds exerted their fascination in ancient India: the Veda texts (1500–1000 BC) include mention of a member of the cuckoo family – the Asian or Common Koel, *Eudynamys scolopaceus* and its characteristic habit of parasitising crows and other species by laying eggs in their nests, for the host bird to rear.

China

The timing of fowl domestication is unclear. A date of 1400 BC based on translation of an ancient Chinese encyclopaedia published in AD 1609 suggests that these were birds from the west. Another record indicates 1500 BC was the date that Buddhist priests first took the birds to China. However, more recent studies (Lembke 2012, p. 15), along with the excavation of bones and terracotta figurines, suggest that domestication took place in northern China as early as 6000 BC. The Chinese zodiac, which dates from the 5th century BC, includes the rooster as one of its 12 animal symbols. There is also some evidence to suggest that the ancient Chinese raised chickens in large, farmed units.

Persia (Iran)

The arrival of the chicken from India can be traced to a fairly early date. They moved westward to the Middle East and the Mediterranean region – but the exact dates of this are uncertain. The date of the commencement of fowl-keeping in Persia is unclear except that it was in the 1st millennium BC. The chicken was featured on Assyrian coins and seals of the 8th century BC and its existence is recorded in their literature. In the Zoroastrian religion of ancient Persia (Assyria and present-day Iran) in the 6th century BC, the cock played an important role as the guardian of good against evil – the crowing of the cock became known as the 'Herald of the Dawn' and was the symbol of the waking day and thus of the light. One of the symbols of the Zoroastrian religion was a schematic drawing of a priest superimposed on a stylised bird of prey. Translation of the *Avesta*, the sacred text of the religion, indicates that herbal remedies were used in all classes of livestock, birds and humans. The Medes, who were subject to the Assyrians, used the bird in religious rites.

Egypt

The earliest evidence from Egypt is difficult to interpret, the so-called 'chicken hieroglyph' possibly represents a quail or guinea fowl and not a domestic fowl. The first reliable evidence is dated at 1840 BC from graffiti on a Middle Kingdom temple. Later in the reign of Thutmose III (1479–1425 BC) the royal records acknowledge a tribute paid in chickens from an unidentified place east of the Tigris: '. . . four birds of this country. They bear everyday.' Additional archaeological evidence by tomb paintings of poultry at this time exist, and in the tomb of Tutankhamun (r.1333–1323 BC), a painting of a cock on a potsherd was found, dated to about 1350 BC.

Following this event there was a period of steady decline and reduction in trade, with no mention of the chicken. It has been suggested that it was 'removed' when Tutankhamun restored the old religion following Akhenaten's establishment of his new monotheistic religion. The bird was re-established in Egypt in the Ptolemaic period, during 624–525 BC, presumably due to the Greek influence. Reports of the artificial incubation of hen's eggs date from c.400 BC.

Birds were of importance in Egypt, the god Horus (of war, hunting and protection) was depicted as a falcon, as it flew above all and watched. The Sacred Ibis (*Threskiornis aethiopicus*) was much venerated as a symbol of the god Thoth (of writing and knowledge). Many mummified ibis bodies were deposited, in sealed pottery jars as offerings, in the catacombs at Saqqara (dated to between 450–250 BC): some 80,000 mummified birds are estimated to be in the catacombs.

Hellenic World

The chicken reached the Mediterranean from Mesopotamia and was common in the Aegean Sea and Asia Minor region in the 6th century BC, but they may have been present in Greece and Italy before this time. There is evidence of the presence of the fowl in ancient Judea. The absence of any mention of them in the Bible could suggest that they were only used for sport and not for food.

The earliest known European pictorial depictions of poultry – fighting cocks – are found in early Greek pottery from the Corinthian period, dated around 700 BC. In the 6th century BC poultry, both cocks and hens, begin to appear in poetry, and also in Aesop's fables. The fowl is mentioned by the elegiac poet Theognis about 530 BC, and by Pinder (c.522–443 BC) whose odes for athletic contests also included references to gamecocks (fighting birds). By 400 BC the domestic fowl was known throughout the Greek world: Himera (a Greek Sicilian colony) featured cocks on their coinage, as did Selinus, another Sicilian town. These coins show a variety of images, mainly of cocks but also of hens. These can be interpreted as fighters, but there are also strong suggestions of a religious, and a health connection, possibly related to the worship of Aesculapius. That chickens were firmly placed in the Hellenic culture is illustrated by the rather agricultural aphorism of Heraclitus of Ephesus (c.535–475 BC) who wrote 'pigs wash in mud, chickens in dust'.

The gamecock became important to Greek life. It is written that Themistocles, the commander of the Hellenic forces, at the battle of Salamis with the Persians in 480 BC, while addressing the troops before combat, and holding a pair of the birds, said 'These do not fight for country, gods or, for freedom, but because neither would suffer defeat'. It is this characteristic that made cockfighting a popular sport.

By the 5th century BC the chicken had become a widely recognised symbol in the Hellenic world, coins from most of the *coloniae*, even those in the far west, carried the image of the cock in a variety of postures. The Persian origin of the bird was recognised and it was accepted in its role as a divine symbol of light and health. Its primary impact was in cockfighting (even the Athenian government would sometimes organise fighting games). The cock also became an erotic object and was used as a gift to a beloved. Such scenes are depicted on ancient terracotta vases. Before taking poison, Socrates is recorded ordering a cock be sacrificed to Aesculapius for recovery from an illness (399 BC).

The use of the bird as a symbol was widespread. Due to the prolific laying habit of the hen it was associated with fertility: Jews in their marriage ceremony would carry a cock and hen before the bridal couple. This egg producing capacity was almost certainly the factor that triggered the realisation of the economic potential of the chicken. Zeuner (1963) notes the Egyptian Annals of Thutmose III, reigned 1479–1425 BC, which identified birds that laid daily, and the Veneti, an early Indo-European people of north-east Italy, who were reported to have hens that laid two eggs a day. While obviously untrue, these examples suggest that the ancient peoples did have high producing hens and the availability of the eggs initially provided the economic value.

Aristophanes (c.446–c.386 BC), the leading comedy playwright of ancient Athens, observed that every Athenian had a hen, even the poorest. These families would all have a few chickens for the eggs, a bird would only be killed when too old to produce. As the birds were easy to rear, cheap and available, they also become popular as a sacrificial gift to many of the gods. Such intensive poultry keeping, even if in small numbers, must have hastened selection and advanced domestication. There was also a valuable social function, the ancient world had no clocks and the Greeks adopted the Eastern habit of appreciating the cockcrow as an alarm: particularly helpful for the farmer who needed to rise at dawn. They had no taboo against eating the chicken and it gained popularity in their world. The chicken also played a valuable role in the early development of biological science by the studies of Aristotle (384–322 BC), and influenced Greek medical thought.

Roman Empire

Before Rome had established its dominant position chickens were already present on the Apennine peninsula. Coins and artefacts from the Greek *coloniae* in Calabria and Campania illustrate the chicken; the Etruscans also introduced the bird. As Rome developed and expanded, the chicken was absorbed into their culture. The Romans raised farming from a pastoral practice to an agricultural science, and in particular with poultry production. Within a relatively short period of time they developed a poultry industry structure which was adopted throughout the territories of the empire. While they copied the breeding and training of cocks for fighting, they also studied and enhanced the raising of the birds for both meat and eggs. Their recommended practices were labour intensive: this was a different economy, it was slave-based.

Cato (234 –149 BC), in *De Rustica Liber*, wrote a small amount on poultry, and all concerned with fattening birds. For hens it was recommended that when they had laid their first egg they should be 'shut up' and fed cakes of flour or barley meal soaked in water. The feed quantity was to be increased daily and given twice with water, to be also given at noon, but not to be left over one hour. Geese were fattened in a similar way although they could have water earlier and also twice daily. Young pigeons were also fattened: wild birds were caught and a feed of cooked beans and water was to be 'squirted down its throat from one's mouth', this was to be continued for seven days. Then the bird was to be fed with a cooked cake of mashed beans and pine buckwheat, stressing that cooking be thorough and done with cleanliness. When cooked the mixture was kneaded with oiled hands and formed into cakes, these were then soaked in water and fed to the birds until they were replete.

Varro (116–27 BC), in *De Re Rustica*, discusses three types of fowl – barnyard, wild and African. The first is recognised as a chicken, the second has never been satisfactorily explained but may be partridges and the third determined to be a guinea fowl. He recommended the barnyard chicken, and identified five factors for the farmer to consider – careful selection at purchase, breeding, egg production, chick rearing and fattening table birds. Much attention was given to visual characteristics and he warned against buying the 'fighting' breeds (Tanagra, Media or Chalcis). He also recommended and described a caponising method, devised by the Greeks, using a red-hot iron to remove the testicles and smearing potter's clay over the wound. There is no mention of losses so one presumes this brutal procedure was both successful and post-operatively satisfactory.

The Varro treatise survived in translation into the Middle Ages. Much of his counsel was practical and sensible. He advised on henhouse dimensions, perches, nest boxes, windows etc; also suggesting that the poultry man be housed beside the chickens to provide care for the chicks produced. Considerable detail is given on fattening, both through the diet and the use of small cages, with a hole for the bird's head and one for the rear to enable both feeding, and to ensure the birds did not soil themselves. They were force-fed on a nutritious diet for 20–25 days, when they were then said to be 'plump and delectable'. This practice was, however, frowned upon in the early days of the Republic and a law, the *Lex Famia Sumptuaria* of 161 BC, was passed to prevent inordinate expenditure at banquets; among other prohibited items was the eating of fattened fowl. By using caponised birds and cockerels the law could be evaded, but the law was poorly observed and had been dropped by the end of the Republic in 27 BC. The Roman taste for luxury foods was a characteristic of the culture: Horace (65–8 BC) remarked that a fowl drowned in wine and then cooked had a particularly attractive flavour.

Varro's preference was for peacocks and his proposals covered both of these birds as well as pigeons, turtledoves, geese, ducks and thrushes. The Roman taste for diversity was well developed and melded into an organised poultry farming system for supplying the provision dealers and markets. Many wealthy Romans kept aviaries for pleasure, in particular to hold thrushes. The production of fattened thrushes was well organised. The birds were caught by nets in the wild and then kept in large domed houses, either covered with tiles or a net. These were capable of containing, 'several thousand thrushes and blackbirds. Some people like to include other birds, such as ortolans [the bunting *Emberiza hortulana*] and quails, which, when fattened, fetch good prices'.

The construction and water supply were all detailed with an emphasis on cleanliness; special doors are described and few windows, 'as the sight of trees and other birds would make those inside pine with longing and get thin'. Dead birds had to be kept by the custodian for the owner to see. All details are covered including diet, which had to be increased 20 days before they 'are to be taken out'. The act of killing had to be out of sight of those remaining birds.

Harvesting of wild birds was discussed in great detail by Varro who understood the migrating habits of the species and the best time to catch them, including mentioning putting 5000 birds into an aviary and making a good profit if there was a great banquet or triumph to be supplied. Similar detail is given to the production of fattened peacocks, involving the use of a controlled breeding programme adding that when sold 'for fifty denarii each, a price no sheep commands'. Varro was in favour of peacock farming as he stated, 'of all birds it gives the best profit'. Pigeons were also important with pigeon towers being constructed to hold 5000 birds. It was noted that a sick pigeon should receive attention and that if one should die it should be removed, and the other birds prepared for sale. Pigeon farming was obviously popular and Varro states, 'there is no creature more prolific than the pigeon, in the space of forty days it conceives, lays, sits and brings up its young'. In good condition these birds fetched high prices. Turtledoves required similar housing to pigeons, the construction of their houses and feeding routine is described in the treatise. Fattening was recommended at harvest time.

Farming of geese was discussed noting the need for a pool; white birds were recommended, not part-coloured. Each goose was given a separate pen in which to hatch their eggs. The need for green food was stressed, with emphasis on care in feeding and cleanliness. Ducks were also farmed, requiring a pond or tank with running water and fenced enclosure with a netted covering to keep out eagles. A diet of cereals, grapes and occasionally prawns was recommended.

From Varro's lengthy exposition on poultry farming several points are noted: the Romans exploited poultry, taking what were essentially sport and sacrificial creatures, and producing not only a poultry industry, but as they developed a wealthy class of citizen, a desire for gourmet foods which embraced any bird that could be either reared or caught. Varro emphasised good housing, good feed and cleanliness as fundamental to efficient livestock production. Disease was not recorded as a serious constraint to production. All the above is a description of activities in the later years of the 1st century BC – an economy that was well run with an extensive slave force.

Columella (AD 4–70) wrote *De Re Rustica*, which included the most detailed of the Roman poultry texts: it describes the sophistication of the poultry industry in the Graeco-Roman world. In the pragmatic Roman way he identifies the specialised branches of the industry and discusses the marketing procedures and the difficulties in costing these. While Columella was describing what he saw as an ideal industry structure, it is obvious that Roman poultry production was organised well with farmers that had good knowledge of the bird with which they were working. He starts his treatise by observing that rearing chickens could be as profitable as keeping cattle, and that additionally the dung was of great value both on tilled lands and for 'weakly' vines and other plants. The early part of the text follows that of Varro, including describing how to caponise the cocks, using a red-hot iron not to remove their testes but to burn off the spurs, and then as Varro stated, treat the wounds with potters' clay until they heal [this 'operation' is both so ludicrous and yet close to Varro's words that it is suggested that it has arisen by a scribe's error].

The carefully practised breeding methods of the Greeks to produce fighting cocks, using the Tanagra, Rhodes, Chalcis and Median breeds are recognised, but Columella stresses that the objective of Roman farming was to bring in income. He advised that one man should be responsible for 200 hens: to incubate, hatch and rear their progeny and to protect them from snakes, snares laid by man and harmful beasts. White birds were to be avoided as they were both less prolific, weaker and more liable to be taken by eagles; those with five toes and no spurs on their legs should be chosen – a very full description of the ideal hen is given. The chosen cocks should be 'haughty, agile, watchful and crow frequently' as they may have to kill snakes and defend the hens. The use of crossbreeds of the exotic (Greek) cocks and indigenous Roman hens was recommended: these were found to be the most prolific. Instructions for poultry housing construction were detailed, included facing them to where the sun rises in winter, and also to adjoin the bakehouse or kitchen near the smoke, 'which is very good for them'. Details of the three chambers of the hen house are given with openings (to be always closed at night), nest boxes built into the walls and perches for the birds to roost. Sleeping on the floors was to be prevented, as the droppings would accumulate under their feet and cause gout. Emphasis was given to plastering all of the walls inside and outside to prevent cats and snakes from entering, and that the water supply was to be kept pure and clean. Both food and water troughs should have covers with access holes halfway up the sides, for a hen's head only, to prevent the food and water being scratched out or contaminated.

The best foods were recommended as ground barley and chickpeas, or vetch, millet and panic-grass, but only to be purchased at good market prices. If prices were high, farmers were told to use wheat produced in the winnowing process, but never wholegrain; other foods such as bran and flour mix, leaves and seeds of cytisus plants and even grape seeds. Feeding was to be done twice daily, in the early morning and early evening, as this would enable birds to be counted more easily, and also get them ready for the night. For housed birds feeding should be thrice daily, but their yard must be netted to keep out eagles and hawks. An area of dust or cinders should be provided as a wallow. Emphasis was given, as a first essential, to having a conscientious poultry keeper, 'if he is not faithful to his master no poultry farms will make ends meet'.

Before eggs were to be collected for setting, the feed should be improved to encourage laying of larger eggs, the addition of cytisus leaves was believed to aid fertility. Nest boxes had to be kept clean with fresh straw provided regularly to discourage fleas and insects. Those hens which were clucking loudly should be watched and their eggs collected: eggs could be saved for up to ten days before being placed under a broody hen. The older hens were the best to keep as hatchers, the younger were of more value as layers. To cure broodiness in the hens, 'a feather should be passed through their nostrils'.

The instructions were that, on hatching, chicks should be placed with selected hens, up to a maximum of 30. It was also stated that odd numbers of eggs should be set, and not always the same number – setting should always be while the moon was waxing and so the moon would again be waxing when the chicks were hatched. Much detail is given on watching and caring while hatching and early rearing. Columella noted that many people put a little grass, laurel twigs, garlic tops or iron nails under the straw as these were thought to be remedies against thunder 'which addles the eggs and destroys the embryo chicks'. Much detail is given on the care of the sitting hens and placing their food close to their nests. The keeper was instructed to check the nests, turn the eggs and remove any broken ones. When all hatched the chicks were to be placed on a vetch or darnel sieve and then fumigated with sprigs of fleabane, 'for that is calculated to prevent 'pip' [a significant disease problem], from which young birds quickly die'. Great care was stressed for attention to the early rearing of the chicks with the hen, again care against snakes was emphasised.

After 40 days the hen and chicks could be allowed out of the pen, but at all times watched for signs of 'the pip'. As soon as the breeding season was over the farmer is recommended to select and sell the poor specimens to reduce the total flock. Also three-year-old hens, and those which are poor layers or mothers, should be sold. From the middle of November, when the hens cease laying, the costly foods should be withheld and grape fodder substituted until the laying season, which, depending on climate, will start again. The preservation of eggs was of importance. Columella described methods of burying them – in straw in winter or in bran in summer; 'some people cover them first in finely ground salt for six hours, others cover them in beans, natural salt or brine, or harden them in warm brine'. He noted that while salt prevents putrefaction the eggs lose their 'integrity'.

Fattening fowls was said to present no difficulty with a warm house with minimum light, the hens penned in small cages unable to turn around with openings for their heads to feed and for their rump to discharge waste (as described by Varro). Clean straw was essential and it was suggested that 'all feathers be plucked from their heads and under their wings to prevent lice from breeding, and from their rumps to prevent sores'.

Barley meal was the recommended feed with instruction on how not to overfeed and how to feel the crop to ensure the previous meal has been digested. After feeding, birds were let out of their cages for a while so they could use their beaks to remove any insects or irritants. To make birds tender, as well as fat, it was recommended that the feed be mixed with honeyed water, some also used wine and stuffed the birds with soaked wheat bread. Fattening should not exceed 25 days. The biggest birds were reserved for the most sumptuous banquets and 'toil and outlay are substantially repaid'. [In current poultry production a bird aged less than 28 days at slaughter is defined as a 'poussin'.]

Doves and pigeons were fattened in the same way but it was noted that there was less profit in fattening pigeons than in raising them. In country districts, where the birds fly free, they were housed in towers, but in cities they had to be kept in attics – in each case with the walls arranged with small nesting chambers or platforms. All premises should be whitewashed and the outsides plastered. Feed was vetch or pulse, also lentils, millet, darnel and wheat husks. The premises had to be kept clean otherwise 'they often leave their quarters in disgust if they get the chance to escape'. There is much discussion of breeds and types of pigeon, with a stress on not mixing these as the birds do not take well to new partners. When they were growing, to prevent too much exercise and therefore increase weight, it was recommended to pluck the wing feathers and break their legs so that they could not move about, 'the breaking of their legs does not hurt them for more than a day or two, or at the most, three days, and it removes all risk that they will want to escape'.

The rearing of turtledoves was not practised as the birds would neither lay nor rear in captivity. The procedure was to capture them in the wild and fatten indoors. Much less care was required, feed was millet or wheat on the ground and nets to prevent them from flying and losing weight. Platforms around the walls with hemp mats were provided for nesting and it was again stressed that the mats should be kept clean and all droppings carefully kept for use on the fields.

The rearing of thrushes required greater care and expense. For the best results this should take place near where they are caught and 'veteran' birds, kept by the fowlers, should be put among them as they 'will alleviate the grief' of the wild birds and encourage them to take their food and water. Housing needs were the same as pigeons, in sunny quarters, with perches, but not over the feeding area. Recommended feed was chopped dried figs mixed with flour. Columella noted that some prefer to feed figs that have been pre-chewed, he advises against this as chewers cannot be hired for nothing and they are tempted to swallow a certain number of figs – he was always cost conscious! An alternative diet was myrtle and mastic berries, olives and even strawberries. Troughs of millet were to be kept full as a basic feed. Water vessels were the same as those for hens.

In Columella's opinion, 'raising peacocks requires the care of a cultured man rather than of a rough peasant'. He felt they were best raised on little wooded islands off the coast – they cannot fly far, are free of thieves or marauding animals and would largely find their own food. The keeper then just has to give a signal at a fixed time of day, throw down some barley and count the heads. Rearing of chicks had to be on the mainland. A level grassy enclosure with trees was needed, surrounded by a high wall with porticos on three sides for housing the birds and on the fourth a keeper's dwelling. Under the porticos were cage-like enclosures of reeds. The house had to be damp-proof and fitted with low perches (removable for cleaning). One male was allowed for five female birds and aphrodisiac foods (beans roasted over a slow fire) were fed in the early spring. Feeding was in the reed enclosures. The birds had to be watched, and after copulation the females were tended to ensure they only laid eggs in their own quarters. Straw had to be placed under perches as the hens usually lay while perching. Eggs collected from peahens were set under hens, preferably the largest barnyard hens. They should have nine eggs, five peahen's and the rest hen's: on the 10th day the hen's eggs are removed and replaced by fresh ones so that on the 30th day all the eggs should hatch together. The keeper must turn the eggs frequently. On hatching the peafowl chicks were placed in groups of 25 with the hen and treated as ordinary chicks. As they grow, chopped leeks and finely grated cheese were added to the barley meal feed. Locusts, with feet removed, were also recommended as a good food. After six months, feeding was by scattered barley. As the chicks grew they were moved outside, with the hen tethered to a cage that the young peafowl would flutter around. The diseases of chicks were stated to be the same for fowls and peafowl. At seven months the young birds were shut up at night with the rest, and trained to use the perch. Guinea fowl were reared in the same way as peacocks. Columella added, 'they must be given as much food as they can swallow to prepare them for the table at banquets'.

Columella opens his section on geese by quoting Celsus, 'Geese are not easy to rear unless there are both water and grass in plenty. . .'. Geese were recognised as a profitable venture with a low level of work required. They produced both goslings and down, which could be plucked twice a year. Three geese for each gander were suggested. The housing recommended was an isolated yard with separate pens for the geese to sleep and lay eggs. The yard should have a 9 ft wall with porticos including a keeper's dwelling. Under the porticos pens of brick were constructed, each about 3 ft square with strong doors. Water had to be provided by a nearby pond, reservoir or stream, if not possible ponds should be constructed. A grassy field must be sown with vetch, clover, Greek hay and chicory and lettuce. The selected birds should be both large and all white.

Geese lay about three times a year; the eggs should be collected to be placed under hens to hatch; all laying must occur in the enclosure (methods of examining the bird to determine closeness to laying are described). If set under hens there should be five eggs, but not less than three; nettle roots were spread under the eggs for their medicinal properties. Depending on the temperature, hatching takes 25–30 days, the goslings and mother were fed in the pen for the first ten days. When allowed out foods such as lettuce or millet or barley soaked in water were recommended. As they grew, groups of about 20 goslings were penned together overnight, the pens had to be dry with straw or hay and the usual precautions taken against cats, snakes and weasels. At four months the largest birds were selected for fattening, which was considered to be easy: the birds were kept in a warm, dark place and given meal and flour three times a day with ample water available. They were restricted and not allowed to roam, becoming market ready in about two months, or maybe 40 days.

Ducks were treated in a similar manner to geese. Columella also says that 'teal, mallards, coots and suchlike birds' are treated in a similar manner: indicating the diversity of both practices and tastes. Enclosure walls 15 ft high, together with netted covering, were necessary to prevent birds escaping and eagles and hawks entering. Plastered walls were essential to deter cats and ferrets. A central pond in the enclosure must have continually clean water and flagged sides (to prevent erosion) constructed with a gradual slope to the water, as a shelving beach. The pond should be free of weeds but have an island in the middle with water plants, in particular reeds, providing a resting place. The enclosure was of grass with plastered stone cabins about 1 ft square for the birds to use as nests, covered by box or myrtle branches. Food was provided in a water channel with a vegetable diet of seeds, acorns and grape pips and, if available, including crayfish or small water fish. At mating time straw and twigs were strewn in the enclosure for the birds to make nests. It was suggested that if one wished to start a duck preserve it was a good idea to collect eggs from the wild and hatch them under hens: they will then lose their wild instincts, rather than imprisoning wild birds who would pine and not breed.

Palladius (late 4th–early 5th century AD) was the last Roman author of surviving treatises dealing with poultry. Writing his *Opus Agriculturae* (*The Work of Farming*) some 500 years after Columella, it is notable that his text is fundamentally the same. There are a few alterations or additions but nothing of great significance – in other words real practical knowledge of poultry production had made little progress. The most obvious introduction to the new text is the recommendation of the use of certain plants or objects to achieve an effect by some 'mystical' influence. Such beliefs, together with an increasing use of magical spells, was a characteristic of the later Roman Empire.

Palladius recommended that bird housing should be placed along the walls of the farmyard to enable easier collection of the dung, perceived to be of great value as fertiliser, except for that of geese which was seen to be harmful. The dung of the pigeon was most highly rated, in particular when ploughed into salty soils. It was valued for use with vines; after ablaqueation (the 'loosening' of vine roots) the dung was placed on the roots, and also used in cold weather. In a listing of medications the duck is included, in the text it is written that the sight of a swimming duck relieves an animal of internal pain and 'quickly relieves its torment'. This is presumably meant for farm livestock, as it also states that it is even more effective with mules and horses.

The husbandry and rearing of pigeons changed little over the centuries with the use of towers becoming standard for birds feeding in the local countryside. Palladius also suggests that if pieces of esparto rope, 'as used for animal shoes', were scattered on the floor, weasels will be deterred. It was stated that pigeons will not die off or abandon the house if a piece of the strap, belt or rope from a strangled man is hung by the entrances. The hanging of rue twigs 'in many places will deter harmful animals'. Turtle doves were said to be best fattened in a cubicle below the chamber of the pigeon cote. Thrushes, and other birds were recommended to also be fattened in similar cubicles in the tower. Birds fattened out of season would show a good profit, in particular the fieldfare (*Turdus pilaris*) which wintered in Italy in large numbers and was easy to catch. The use of a few prisoner birds was valuable as they 'allayed fear and dejection' in the newly caught: one of Columella's earlier comments.

Poultry farming as described by Palladius is essentially an abridgement of Columella. There is more on the disease – 'pip' (discussed later in this chapter). Goose fattening is discussed based on a barley diet to be taken at will, as well as a special diet, 'if you wish to soften their liver', of mashed figs soaked in water and rolled into little nuggets, to be fed for 20 days [an early liking for foie gras].

The poultry production texts of the significant Roman authors (Cato, Varro, Columella and Palladius) have been made available in a specific publication edited by Ghigi (1939). This is a very useful book with an excellent translation and illustrated by good ancient images of the birds.

Other Birds in Roman Culture

An examination of Roman art, mythology, family life, entertainment and dietary habits show that birds played a significant role in all aspects of their culture. Chickens, geese, ducks, pheasants, peacocks, guinea fowl, pigeons and game birds were an important part of farming and diet for both eggs and meat, as well as an interest in cockfighting (as previously discussed in this chapter). Pliny (AD 23–79) gave good early descriptions of many bird species.

Ostriches

The largest birds, were common in the wild in North Africa and Middle East. They had various names but were usually termed *Struthio camelus* (derived from 'sparrow' and 'long camel-like neck'). The species was valued for its eggs and feathers. There is little evidence that they were farmed or totally domesticated, but there are many descriptions of them being harnessed or ridden and used in ceremonial processions. And, as usual, they were much enjoyed in the amphitheatre either as participants in the *venationes* (staged hunts) or for the amusement afforded by seeing the beheaded birds continue to run and stand. Many birds were also cooked and eaten at banquets. Much of the detail of their capture and use is known from their frequent depiction in pictorial form, in particular in mosaics in North Africa.

Cranes, storks, herons, flamingos and ibises

These birds were well recognised and all eaten at banquets. Some large estates kept flocks of cranes for food, but it is doubtful that they were domesticated. Storks, ibises and flamingos were additionally regarded as being valuable as snake catchers and deterrents. There is also a report of a staged crane-fight, for amusement.

Eagles

Eagles were highly regarded in Roman literature and art as the companion of Jupiter. They were adopted as a symbol by the emperors, and featured as the eagle standard of regiments in the Roman army: the loss of a standard in war was regarded as a great humiliation.

Crows, ravens, pies, starlings, blackbirds and nightingales

All of these birds were popular as pets that could be trained to talk (in both Latin and Greek), but nightingales were particularly favoured as singing birds. This was obviously a very popular pastime and birds would be trained and kept in a cage at the entrance of homes to greet visitors. Parrots were also very popular. There is little evidence that these birds were used for food, except for the parrot which was sometimes used as an ornamental item in banquets. Thrushes, as already described, were consumed in large numbers.

Pelicans

Pelicans are possibly noteworthy in that the Romans did not eat them; they were despised for their voracious appetite and generally disliked. The Egyptians had related the bird to death and funerary texts. Jewish dietary laws forbid the eating of pelican meat, as it is designated 'unclean'. In the Christian religion in Medieval Europe the pelican came to symbolise the Passion of Jesus and the Eucharist, partly replacing the lamb and the flag. This belief was based on the myth that the pelican fed its young with its own blood from its breast. A comprehensive review of the place of birds in Roman life and art is given in Toynbee (2013, pp. 237–282).

Europe – Post-Roman to Enlightenment

Following the Roman imposition of their culture and practices, domestic poultry persisted in farm holdings and households with chickens, and increasingly geese, being found across Europe. Geese had the strongest presence in Germany. Many other birds were also consumed, including waterfowl (mostly ducks) as well as wood-cock, pigeon, blackbirds, finches, rooks, crows, skylarks and swans. Usually nets were used for catching them although bird-lime, a glutinous very sticky product applied to twigs and branches, was widely used in some areas until guns became available.

There is little recorded information on domestic poultry before the 16th century but every smallholding and farm had some chickens, and if grazing was available, geese. The latter were more usually found in wetter regions, in Britain this was usually in the Fenlands of East Anglia. Medieval manuscripts frequently have farm illustrations, including hens tethered by one leg with a group of chicks in her care. Turkeys were introduced to Europe from Mexico in the early 1500s and quickly became established, and on many farms took the place of geese and swan cultivation. They proved to be very suitable for intensive fattening: barley, oats and acorns were favoured.

Fattening of birds for the table became popular as transportation methods improved for farmers to use to get the birds to the markets. Contemporary descriptions of how to make birds 'cram-fat' is found in books such as Gervase Markham's *Cheape and Good Husbandry* 1614, and then much plagiarised in *The Husbandman, Farmer and Grasier's Compleat Instructor* by 'A.S.' in 1697. Much of this content follows the instructions given by Columella: construct a proper house, provide perches and nesting boxes, and special pens for geese and ducks, as well as continuing the strange advice of placing the house near the kitchens so that the smoke blows in.

Caponising was important with emphasis placed on the care to be taken during the operation which was to be 'conducted with delicacy', but little information was given on the actual procedure. William Harrison (1535–1593) in his text *The Description of England*, originally written as part of the introduction to *Holinshed's Chronicles* (1577), gives probably the finest description of English life in the Tudor years, and records that both turkeys and 'Indish' peacocks were caponised 'to improve the quality of the flesh'.

Geese had become a popular bird as they were profitable, not only for the meat, feathers (for quills), down and fat, but also because they were cheap to raise by grazing. Additionally they could be herded, and flocks of up to 2000 birds in wet and marshy areas were not uncommon. The main housing requirement was the inclusion of special wicker pens for sleeping and brooding. Reports of disease in poultry are quite rare, while they occurred they did not appear to be a serious problem for the producers. This possibly underestimates the problem, human and livestock plagues occurring at regular intervals were accepted as a fact of life.

In England, a major market was the Nottingham Goose Fair, this annual gathering was first mentioned in a Charter of King Edward I (1284). This market was originally held for several days, first in September, but after the Gregorian Calendar was introduced, in October. At its peak, when it was held for three weeks in the 1700s, some 20,000 geese would be sold, described at the time by Daniel Defoe in his *A Tour Through the Whole Island of Great Britain* (2nd Ed. London, 1738). Turkey raising developed in England in East Anglia and slowly displaced geese, when it was found that they could be fattened in a similar way to chickens. Defoe recorded droves of 300–1000 turkeys at a time being sent to London. It was said that some drovers coated the feet of geese in tar to give them protection for the long walk to market. As roads improved from the 18th century onwards, special huge wagons pulled by ten to twelve horses were constructed and 'fast carts' of three to four storeys for moving ducks, which could cover up to 100 miles in two days and one night. The horses were harnessed two-abreast to give a smoother ride for the passengers.

While not 'farmed' there was a significant trade in and demand for mallards, plovers, widgeon and sheldrakes which were caught and fed, and then shipped to London poulterers. In fact almost any bird would be eaten. There were vast flocks in the autumn that could be caught by nets. It was estimated in 1824 that over 300,000 skylarks were sold in the London markets. Poulterers would regularly supply blackbirds, rooks, thrushes and other wild fowl as well as domestic poultry.

Quill Production

An important poultry product was the quill, the large hollow feathers of the wing or tail. Quills had many functions including being used as a plectrum or toothpick or being used in fishing floats. However, their major use was as writing instruments, taking the place of the reeds in the Middle Ages. The best were deemed to be from the goose (the largest from each wing), but those from the swan were more durable; turkey and crow quills were also used, but judged to be of a lower quality. Trade grew and quills were imported into Europe from Russia and in the 1800s from Canada. After plucking, the quill had to be dressed, trimmed, hardened and polished before the tip was fashioned by either the end user or sold ready cut. A good quill would be recut several times in its life. Dealers sold them in bundles, graded and priced by quality. In Europe in the early 1800s many millions of quills were used each year, even in the 1890s the British Government Stationery Office still had an annual consumption of some 500,000. As metal pen nibs were introduced the quill pen market died.

Hawks and Falcons

Gervase Markham in his book *Hungers Prevention, or the Whole Art of Fowling*, 1621, classified the birds that were hunted or used in hunting (venery) in three groups:

- 'Fit for foode', listed as 'Pidgeons of all Kinds, Rookes, Pheasants, Partridges, Quailes, Rayles, Blackbyrds, Fellfares, Sparrowes and others'.
- 'Preserved for voice', the singing birds, 'Nightingall, Throstell, Linnet, Larks, Bullfinch, Spynke and others'.
- 'For pleasure only' those used for hunting, 'Hawks of all Kindes, Castrells, Ringtailes, Buzards, Kites' and any bird of prey.

Of these three groupings the latter were by far the most important. They are discussed later in this chapter, together with their management, training and diseases.

Swans

The mute swan, *Cygnus olor*, was a popular food in early medieval Europe and was much favoured at feast and celebration occasions. In Britain, dated from the 12th century the birds were controlled and cared for in an elaborate administration system related to the Crown. The birds were regarded as private property, but living on public rivers, a custom that resulted in the annual marking of birds by clipping or branding the beaks. This procedure appears to have been unique to Britain: a multitude of marks were designed and recorded in registers (many of which survive to this day). The process created many jobs for country people. Much of the law relating to swans and their ownership dealt with beak marks and marking.

The swan owner would pinion his birds, which kept them on certain rivers; each year selected cygnets were removed to fatten for the table, these were kept in hurdled enclosures around a pond. In Britain pinioning of birds was ended in 1978 and beak marking in 1997, being replaced by leg rings. The customs have survived to the present day with the annual ceremony of swan 'upping' conducted on the rivers to mark the Queen's swans. While the bird was popular fare at Royal Feasts and celebrations the complex laws relating to ownership did in fact enable the survival of the species as the killing was controlled. Many other species that were equally valued as food, such as storks and cranes, were hunted to extinction in Britain.

Cormorants

The relationship of the cormorant, *Phalacrocorax carbo*, with humans in Europe is a history full of persecution and extermination by fishermen, to eradicate their very effective competition. In the Asiatic countries, in particular China and Japan, the bird was valued as an aid to fishing. This use was first described to Europe by Odoric of Pordenone (1286–1331), a Franciscan Friar missionary and explorer who visited many Asian countries, spending about three years in China. He described how the fishermen would tie a cord around the neck of the cormorant, just tight enough to prevent swallowing and then would release the bird to dive into the river and catch fish – at which they had great expertise – when a sufficient number had been caught the cord would be loosened for the bird to satisfy its own appetite. The birds required a period of training by the fishermen before they could be 'worked'.

In the Orient, cormorant fishing was not regarded as a sport, it was a method that poorer people used to provide a living. However, when it was introduced to Europe in the early 17th century it first developed in the courtly circles. King James I of England had the birds in 1610 and a colony was established by the Royal court in France about 1619. The practice was well described in *The Ornithology of Francis Willughby* published in London, 1678. The sport had been popular in England under the Stuart regime, collapsed when Oliver Cromwell seized power, but was re-established by Charles II, until interest again declined. In France at Fontainebleau, the sport continued for some time. An effort was made to revive the activity in Britain in the 19th century; birds were purchased from Holland but interest soon declined, influenced by the time and difficulty in training the birds. This proved to be hazardous due to the cormorants accuracy in pecking at the handlers eyes; the revival ended in the late 1800s.

Pigeons – Carrier, Racing and Sport

Pigeons and doves are probably the most common birds in the world, with 42 genera and 310 species. The words 'dove' and 'pigeon' are now interchangeable, but the common domestic or feral pigeon, *Columba livia domestica* is actually known as the rock dove. The homing ability is believed to be a facility termed magnetoreception, but how this actually works is not clearly understood.

The homing instinct in pigeons was recognised in antiquity, the Egyptians and the Assyrians (c.3000 BC) are said to have used them as messenger carriers, and it is believed that they were used to proclaim the names of the winning competitors in the early Greek Olympic Games. Early literature indicates that pigeons were used for regular communication between Baghdad and Damascus in AD 1150 and elsewhere in the Arab and other communities. Use occurred in Europe in the later Middle Ages and was recorded in England in the 1700s. Paul Reuter, the founder of the Press Agency, had a flock of 45 birds to deliver stock market prices to his Brussels Offices. By careful training (with food) birds can be made to make return journeys between two 'homing' places.

Armed forces have all employed the birds. During the Franco-Prussian War (1870–1871) pigeons were used to convey messages and mail to besieged Paris. There was widespread use in the South African (Boer) War (1898–1901). In the Great War (1914–1918) the birds were used both in France and also in naval operations. Some 100,000 birds were donated to the British Army.

Racing pigeons evolved as a sport dating back to the 1700s, well described by John Moore in *Columbarium or the Pigeon House* London, 1753, together with the breeding of pigeons for show – and the evolution of the pigeon-fancier. Pigeon shooting clubs became popular, particularly in Britain from the early 1800s. Initially the guns were rather cumbersome and to aid the shooters the pigeons' feet would be tied together or the wings clipped. Eventually the practice was banned in 1905, but pigeon shooting as a means of bird control continues to be used.

Cockfighting

As described earlier, the first reason for the domestication of the chicken was for fighting, it was widely practised in the East, and in Greek and Roman communities. The sport thrived in Europe from the 11th century in all countries, but is now banned. The practice was first recorded in Britain in London in about 1170 and thrived with Royal Patronage under the Tudor and Stuart monarchies. It was finally banned in Britain in 1849. The breeding and sport had an enormous influence in society for many years. The long story of cockfighting, the breeding, requirements and rules of the sport are well described by Macgregor (2012, pp. 229–235).

Parrots

Fossil study, according to Boehrer (2004, p. IX) indicates that the earliest parrot known to humankind lived in the south of England – some 40 million years ago, in the Middle Eocene period – well before any humans were present. Similar studies have dated the parrot to Australia and Germany also roughly 40 million years ago and in France some 26 million years ago. These birds arrived in Africa and South America much later. A bird said to look like a parrot can be seen in Egyptian hiero-glyphs and wall paintings. But the human interest lies in the ability of the parrot to copy speech.

The first reliable record of the parrot is found in Arrian's biography of Alexander the Great when he mentions that Nearchus (c.327 BC), a friend of Alexander and General in his army, describes, when writing of the Indian campaign, a talking bird. Both the Greeks and the Romans stated that the parrot was of Indian origin. This was believed to be the green bird (there was no mention of the West African grey parrot in the ancient literature), however it is probable that these 'Indian' birds were not parrots but were the, now termed, Indian Hill Mynah (*Acridotheres tristis*). This is a very good clear talker and mimic – the bird is black feathered with a yellow beak. Aristotle also wrote of the Indian bird and noted its power of speech, as well as noting its inclination to be more saucy after drinking wine. Aelian confirmed its Indian origin in his treatise as well as its habit of talking; he also stated that in India the Brahmins thought the ability to imitate human speech made parrots sacred.

Parrots became an important part of Roman life. Pliny (and others) described the green parrot (*psittacus*) with its collar of red and gold neck feathers as well as its reported hard head, adding that it had to be hit with an iron rod to make it talk. Varro recorded that parrots sometimes appeared in public shows. Cages of parrots were carried in Ptolemy II's great pageant. The birds are frequently mentioned in Latin literature, by Ovid among others, not only for their ability to talk but because they were well regarded as pets. A popular use was to have a trained bird in a cage at the entrance of a home to greet visitors. Many images of parrots have survived from the Roman era either in wall or floor mosaics (well shown at Pompeii and at El-Djem in Tunisia), as wall decorations, on silver platters or as figurines. Unfortunately, with the usual Roman tendency to excess, there is a record of a feast for Emperor Elagabalus (AD 218–222) when the dishes were served decorated with parrot heads. According to Boehrer (2004, pp. 20–21) in ancient times parrot was regarded as 'an upper-class delicacy like caviar, the food of only the highest stratum of Roman society'.

With the end of the Roman Empire interest in the parrot in Europe declined, some religious orders and medieval courts did keep them; and many Royal house-holds held collections. The religious interest was much related to the allegorical and evangelical use of different species of birds to discuss moral issues within the

Christian tradition. This was best demonstrated by their inclusion in the bestiary books, of which less than 100 now survive. In the *Liber Bestiarum* MS Bodley 764, written in the mid-13th century, the parrot is included in the species listing, together with an illustration of two green birds with yellow beaks. The text includes the statement that the birds have very 'hard heads' and to teach them heavy blows are necessary to make them learn: an (unfortunate) observation derived from the writings of Pliny.

Parrots featured in many other religious texts, such as the *Holkham Bible* (British Library, Additional MS 47682, folio 10) an illustrated book produced around 1327–1340. The idea had been developed that they were present in the garden of Eden, the earthly paradise. Medieval and later painters liked to include the parrot, and the bird features in the work of many major artists over the years.

The practice of keeping birds as domestic pets had spread across Europe by the 13th century, with the parrot being the most prized of the species. Following the 1492 voyage of Christopher Columbus to the Caribbean region, the US varieties were introduced to Europe. This was followed by a growth in private aviaries, usually associated with large country houses. Later expeditions also found that the native peoples of Central and South America both hunted and ate parrots.

Conrad Gesner (1516–1565) in *Historiae Animalium,* the first work that began to define what became known as zoology, mentions the parrot. The bird continued to have a degree of popularity which increased in the 19th century when the art of taxidermy was perfected. Having a stuffed bird as an ornament or as part of a display cabinet increased the production, and killing, of the birds. However, a sometimes fatal human disease became associated with parrots. Originally termed 'parrot fever', it is now known as ornithosis or psittacosis with its cause elucidated in Europe in 1879 as an infection, by the now termed *Chlamydia psittaci.* As a result, both the interest in, and keeping of, parrots declined. An outbreak in the USA in 1929, created a panic, inflamed by the media, which seriously affected parrot keeping. Now that the disease is understood, controllable and treatable, domestic parrot keeping has retained a place in human affection.

The most popular parrot varieties are macaws, Amazon parrots, cockatiels, parakeets and cockatoos, together with the original green parrot and the African grey. The ability to talk is essentially a feature of parrots kept alone, without other parrots present. The male of this last species is recognised as the best user and learner of speech. Parrots have a reputation of living to a good age: the larger species such as macaws and cockatoos can have lifespans of 80–100 years, the smaller parrots usually live for 15–25 years.

Recognition of Bird Diseases

While the history of birds has the longest timespan of any animal type, it was only in Roman literature that poultry, the primary species utilised by humans, were discussed in any detail. Of the four Latin writers on agricultural matters – Cato, Varro, Columella and Palladius – only Columella deals with disease and its control in any detail. The overall impression is given that to the ancients poultry disease was not a significant problem. There are no mentions of epidemics or enzootic plague-like conditions. An assumption can be made, until other evidence is available, that disease was not a significant limiting problem to production. As most birds were given free access to open air paddocks or pastures this would both have prevented the rapid spread of infection as well as reducing the build-up of infectious micro-organisms. There was, however, also quite extensive use of housing for fattening procedures which could have mitigated against good health.

The Years of Antiquity to AD 400

Varro discusses only one health-related issue for growing chicks, when 'the wings begin to sprout, lice should be constantly picked off their heads and necks, for these are frequently a cause of pining'. The strange advice, to produce capons, is also given: 'burning with a red-hot iron at the lowest part of the leg, until it bursts; and the sore which results is smeared with potters clay'. No adverse consequences of this procedure are noted, nor any comments on its effectiveness. [Note: this translation (Ghigi 1939) differs from that already quoted from an earlier translation, but has some similarity to that quoted from Columella, seen as follows.]

Columella wrote little on disease problems. He advised to keep chicken nests scrupulously clean with fresh straw, 'for the nests get full of fleas and other insects', and newly hatched chicks, should be placed on a 'sieve that has previously been in use and fumigate them with sprigs of fleabane, for that is calculated to prevent Pip, from which young birds quickly die'. Much advice is given on the care of chicks, including, 'they must not be allowed to come into contact with the breath of snakes, for its odour is so foul that they all die'. Snakes must have been a problem, there was advice on preventing their entry and methods to keep snakes away, in particular burning stag's horn or woman's hair.

It was advised that the down on the young chick's rump under the tail should be plucked, to prevent faeces becoming matted. If this happens and creates a blockage, the use of a quill to pierce is recommended. It was stressed that both chicks and mother hen be protected against Pip and 'to avoid it their water must be absolutely fresh'. Emphasis was given to keeping the housing scrupulously clean and to constantly fumigate the premises. If in spite of these measures Pip became a problem then various treatment measures were proposed; for mild cases these included thrusting garlic tops soaked in warm oil down their throats; bathing the beaks, 'in warm human urine then holding them tightly closed till the bitterness compels them to vomit through the nostrils'; and using wild vine grapes mixed with food or squeezed with water as a feed.

In more serious cases, described as 'when the catarrh surrounds the eyes and the bird refuses to eat, an incision should be made and the pus collected under the eyes squeezed out, and then a little salt should be rubbed into the wounds'.

The cause of the disease was attributed to cold and hunger, or drinking stagnant water in the summer, or may arise from allowing the birds to eat figs and unripe grapes. While the causative agent for the disease termed Pip is not known, expert opinion suggests it was probably Infectious Coryza due to *Haemophilus gallinarum* or possibly mycoplasmosis. As disease causation and categorisation was unknown to the ancients it is quite probable that all disease conditions in young birds were termed Pip. This word is still used in some sectors of the poultry industry today.

Fowls for fattening were individually penned preventing the bird from turning round. It was advised that feathers be plucked from their heads and under the wings to prevent lice, and from their rumps to prevent sores. Columella covers in detail the rearing and husbandry of doves, pigeons, thrushes, peacocks and guinea fowl but of chickens only comments, 'Diseases to which chickens are liable also affect these birds and the same remedies should be applied as in the case of hens for Pip. . .'. Geese and ducks are discussed without any mention of disease issues.

It should be noted that Columella recommends a similar procedure as Varro for the caponising of cocks, 'This is not done by removing their genital organs, but by burning their spurs with a red-hot iron . . . and so on'. [It is inconceivable that this procedure would produce a sterilisation effect yet Columella was writing several hundred years later; had nobody noticed, or did it work in some unrecognised manner? It has been suggested that as the spurs are a secondary sex characteristic their removal may have had an effect.]

Palladius in the 4th or 5th century AD wrote the last of the classical Roman agricultural treatises. In the sections on poultry some mention is made of disease. For chickens Pip is again seen as a problem, it 'forms a white film on the tips of their tongues. But this can be easily removed with the nail and by touching the place with ashes and treating the wound with ground garlic. Some people force breadcrumbs soaked in oil down their throats', the wild vine is also recommended (as Columella). This disease could have been Fowl Pox, but the tongue lesion could also have been due to a vitamin A deficiency.

Palladius states that if chickens feed on the bitter lupin, 'a tumour appears on their eyes which can be cured by pricking with a needle and opening up the membrane'.

Cures were also suggested by the application of candytuft juice and mother's milk or ammonia mixed with equal parts of honey and cumin. Lice could be removed by a mixture of ground stavesacre mixed with wine and bitter lupin juice, if applied right under the feathers. No other disease issues are listed for any other poultry species.

The Period of Natural Observation, AD 400–1699

While the work of Palladius, discussed previously, should chronologically be placed in this time period it is best read as the final comment on poultry as developed under the Roman Empire. Following its decline, literature on agriculture generally ceased for some hundreds of years in Europe and when it began again it was with the 'discovery' of the Roman treatises.

From the available literature sources, and using Fleming's works, comment on poultry diseases is seen to be very sparse, it was not until the 1600s that serious observations were recorded. The reports located in this period are identified below.

1111 *England* A 'dreadful' plague visited London, which not only caused a terrible mortality among its citizens but extended itself to cattle, fowls and other domesticated animals. (Holinshed *Saxon Chronicles*, p. 217)

1115 *England* and *Ireland* A very hard winter with snow and frost: 'cattle, birds and people perished'. (Holinshed *Saxon Chronicles*, p. 219, *Annals of the Four Masters* and *Chronic. Scot.*)

1235 *Europe* (Italy?) A pest broke out in quadrupeds '. . . every beast of burden . . . particularly destructive to domestic fowls'. (Tristan Calcho *Misc. Medic. Curios. Col. Agrippa*, 1677, p. 41)

1238 *Europe* A hard winter and 'afterwards a plague broke out among birds, chiefly among fowls'. (Roland *Historia*)
      [The absence of any records in this following period does not indicate a freedom from disease but a lack of surviving records.]

1578 *France* Epizootic disease reported among cats and poultry in Paris region. (Paulet *Recherch. Malad. Epizoöt.*, 1775 Paris)

1609 *England* A hard frost and river Thames frozen from December to April, birds died. (Clark *Examples*)

1614 *Bohemia* (Czechia) A very deadly epizootic disease of fowls reported. 'The fowls collected in groups of six or seven . . . holding their heads close together, would fall to the ground and die'. (Walser *Appenzeller Chronik.*, p. 581)

1694 *Europe* A year of calamities and 'bad air'. Disease and ergotism were widespread many animals, and geese were affected. (Brunner *Ephem. Nat. Curios.*, 1694)

1697 *Germany* 'Fowls, pigeons and geese perished from an epidemic; under their wings were found ulcerated pustules . . . the liver was observed to be dry and parched'. (Stegman *Constat. Mansfeld. Ephem. Nat. Curios.*, p. 384)

1698 *Germany* Outbreak of smallpox in man and also reported in geese and poultry, most perished. (Stegman, p. 108)

The Development of Biological Observations, 1700–1800

An increasing interest was shown in poultry disease by medical and later by early veterinary graduates, geese in Germany provided a particular focus.

1701 *Germany* A long cold winter followed by a dry hot summer and epidemic disease in cattle and other animals, 'and there was a great mortality among young geese in some places'. (Camerarius *Ephem. Nat. Cur.*, pp. 66–67) [most likely Derszy's Disease caused by goose Parvovirus 1, it is serious in goslings]

1712 *Germany* and *Hungary* A 'grievous plague' which killed horses, cattle, pigs and geese and fowls. It was characterised by hard tumours on the breast and groin and was attributed to the stings of hornets who fed from the corpses of animals that had died in the previous year but that had been insufficiently buried. [Later this was attributed to anthrax by John Gamgee]. (Schroekii *Constit. Epid. Eph. Nat. Curios.*, App 27)

1714 *Germany* and *France* Cattle, sheep, pigs, horses and fowls and geese all per- ished, but no details of symptoms given. (Kanold *Jahreshist*, pp. 119–206)

1717 *Hungary* A severe epizootic in turkeys and geese in which large numbers died. The birds sat moping without appetite and, 'then became giddy, stag- gered and died'. Under the feathers were found pustules and scabbed lumps – it was (incorrectly) believed to be smallpox. (Kanold *Breslauer Sammlung*, Vol. I, p. 50)

1718 *Germany* An epidemic in geese and fowls, the most prominent sign was a swelling of the head, they became blinded, emaciated and died. Geese, in particular goslings were most affected. Ducks were little affected. (Kanold *ibid.*, Vol. IV, p. 1175)
Germany Pigeons were seriously affected with 'symptoms of smallpox' (*blat- tern*). (Kanold *ibid.*, Vol. IV, p. 1711)

1719 *Germany* Geese were affected with disease: livers and gall-bladders enlarged and ruptured, body coloured yellow. (Kanold *ibid.*, Vol. X, p. 460)

1726 *Poland* and *Germany* An epizootic in fowls: the birds wasted, would not eat and bodies were covered in lice. In many a growth appeared between the legs near the anus; many died. (Kanold *ibid.*, Vol. XXXVI, p. 556)

1734 *Germany* An, 'epizootic dysentery, accompanied by a swelling of the head, attacked poultry, especially geese . . . they died with their bills open' (Wirth *Lehrbuch der Seuchen und Ansteckenden Krankheiten der Hausthiere* Zurich, 1846, p. 85). [Most likely to have been Avian Influenza, certainly in the fowls, but may have been a concurrent Derszy's Disease in geese]

1737 *Silesia* and *Bohemia* A major outbreak of ergotism had occurred in humans, related to the rye harvest. Experiments on mammals and fowls and dem- onstrated that all the species tested displayed signs of ergot poisoning. (Quotation from Fleming, *Animal Plagues*, 1871)

1741 *Ireland* Reports of deaths in people, horses, cows, sheep, pigs and poultry 'by the plague'. The year was known as *Bliadhain an air* (the year of the slaugh- ter) and was in the worst famine years. (*Famine in Ireland in 1740, 1741*)

1752 *Austria* A 'plague' among fowls was seen in the region of Vienna, an 'immense number were destroyed'. (Plenciz *Opera Med. Phys.*, Vol. I, p. 15) [most likely Avian Influenza]

1754 *Germany* In the winter sheep, pigs and geese and ducks were attacked by 'a disease and died': the flesh was found to be 'black and loosened from the bones'. (*Hannöv. Gen. Anzeig* 1754 and Fischer *Liefladisches Landwirth- schafts- buch*, p. 625)

1757 *France* A 'very peculiar carbuncular epizooty appeared . . . in the province of Brie . . . among horses, cattle, deer, donkeys, pigs, dogs and fowls, and in fish. Humans were also affected'. (A. de Chaignebrun *Relation d'une Maladie Epidemique et Contagieuse*, Paris 1762)

1763 *Europe* This was a year that was noted by medically trained observers and historians as one with many maladies reported in animals, and frequently fatal. These included horses, pigs, sheep, dogs and game birds and poultry. In some regions of France this was diagnosed as 'malignant anthrax' when horses, pigs, dogs and fowls all perished at the same time. [Anthrax is not a recognised disease of poultry.] A specific epizootic which only affected fowls was recorded in Italy and Spain, mortality was almost 100%. Later the same year it was also seen in the South of France. Post-mortem examination of two birds revealed an abnormal liver in the first and a 'corrupted' gizzard surrounded by 'pus globules'. The latter lesions were seen in the second bird. Further reports indicate that this malady was widespread in Spain, France and Italy but not prevalent in northern countries. [Most likely Avian Influenza.] (Webster *A Brief History of Epidemic and Pestilential Diseases*, London 1800, p. 412; Villalba *Epidemiologia Espanola*, Vol. II, p. 219; Richard de Hautesierck *Rec. d'Observations*, Vol. I, p. 169; Tam *Horn-, Schaf-, Pferde-, und Federvieh-Arzneikunst*, p. 543)

1764 *England* 'A mortal pestilence among horses and mules in Provence and among poultry in England'; no details. (*The Repository*)

1767 *Germany* A 'great mortality' reported in geese in Hanover, no details. (*Hannöv. Magazin*, 1767)

1768 *Italy* An 'epizooty among fowls' reported from Genoa; no details. (Franck *Sys. De Med. Poliz.*, Vol. VII, p. 150)

1771 *Germany* A disease outbreak in fowls reported in regions where ergotism (*Kriebel-Krankheit*) was recognised as an important disease – but not seen in ergot-free areas. Housewives complained that hens laid few eggs and they would not hatch. Two fowl were observed by Taube that had shown signs of spasms, would fall on one side, droop their heads and scratch with their feet. They would then get up but appeared cramped. Those observed fed well for 14 days, then refused food and died in the 4th week. [Because of the development of nervous symptoms this was possibly Newcastle Disease.] In Saxony numbers of geese died from 'pityriasis'. On inspection they were found to be covered with lice, but a smaller insect than the recognised goose-louse. [This could have been a mite.] (Taube *Geschichte der Kriebel-Krankheit*; Rohlwes *Die Federviehzucht*, Berlin 1821)

1774 *France* Possibly botulism, 'An epizooty appeared among geese on the banks of the river Meurthe, Lorraine, where in a very short time 600 of these creatures died from diarrhoea and vertigo'. [possibly botulism] (*Gazette de Santé*, February 1774)

1775 *France* Fowls suffered from an epidemic 'that had some analogy with gout', it appeared to be contagious. [Possibly what is now called 'Pullet Disease', of unknown cause.] (Lorry *Mém. de la Societé Royale de Médicine*, Vol. I, p. 1)

1777 *Germany* An epidemic disease in geese. Diarrhoea was the most prevalent symptom. Post-mortem examination showed the stomach and intestines inflamed and gall bladder full of dark green 'stinking' bile. Many 'polypi' in intestines and the rectum held a white excrement with a 'most offensive odour'. [Possibly botulism.] (Rűling *Med. Beschreibung der Stadt Northeim*)

1780 *France* 'Anthracoid maladies' were reported across the country affecting all domestic quadrupeds as well as geese, fowls and turkeys. (Bredin, no reference)

1789 *Italy* A contagious and 'very deadly' disease of fowls was described. The birds were dull, weak with interior of the mouth covered with a 'viscid matter', the anus was red and feathers looked 'soiled and shrivelled'. Followed by a fever, they refused all food and water and death soon followed. Birds had post-mortem examinations: lungs were inflamed, intestines filled with greenish mucus and all those examined had 'great numbers of ascarid worms in gut'. The losses were severe, and continued in 1790. (G. Baroni *Sulla Corrente Epidemia delle Pollastre*, Milan 1789; also Toggia in *Giornale Scientifica et Letterar. di Torino*, 1789 and Brugnone *Descrizione dell' Epizoozia dell Galline Serpeggiante in questa cittá*, Milan 1790)

1796 *USA* A great mortality in both geese and fowls was reported, with a very rapid death. (Webster *op. cit.*, Vol. I, p. 520)

1797 *USA* A disease of 'gallinaceous poultry' was recorded, called 'the gapes' destroying 80% of affected birds in many places. It was most obvious in young turkeys and chickens bred on established farms. A few days after birth the chicks and poults were gasping for breath, sneezing and attempting to swallow. Very few recovered. Post-mortem examination revealed a mass of worms in the trachea. (Wiesenthal, Professor of Anatomy at Baltimore University) [The parasite was named *Sclerostoma Syngamus*, now known as *Syngamus trachea*, the gapeworm. Known to affect a very wide range of both domesticated and wild birds]

Science Evolves with a Developing Veterinary Medicine Discipline, 1800–1900

The establishment of veterinary schools across Europe, together with the growing economic value of domesticated poultry, produces observations and publications with a scientific approach, and a start towards recognition of specific diseases.

1805 *Britain* Gapeworm (*Syngamus trachea*), recognised as a problem in young fowls and turkeys, noting that few recover. (T. Boardman *A Dictionary of the Veterinary Art*, London 1805)

1829 *France* Disease reported in ducks near Toulouse, cause was not ascertained. Examination showed inflammatory changes in the intestines, the colour of bricks, the changes were in several zones which showed a resemblance to the skin disease, shingles; mucous rings formed between the inflamed zones. (Dupuy *Jnl. Pract. Des Sciences Zooatriques*, 1836)

1830 *Poland* Both geese and ducks were attacked by an infection termed 'cholera'; this was currently being diagnosed in many species as an epizootic. The birds had outstretched head and neck which swayed, on land they fell on their sides. Vomiting was frequent, examination showed the lower gut to contain 'a creamy fluid'. In *Germany* a similar malady was seen in geese and also hens, turkeys and ducks. Some birds dropped dead unexpectedly while walking or swimming, vomiting and diarrhoea was frequent. On post-mortem examination the livers were enlarged, gall bladder full and muscles a deep red. Lungs were engorged and intestines contained yellow mucus. (Cohen *Generalbericht d. Med. Colleg. zu Posen*, 1830)

1832 *Germany* 'The disease (cholera) attacked dogs, cats, ducks, hens, and hares . . . it was astonishing how rapidly putrefaction attached anything made of flesh. . .'. (Radius *Mittheilungen*, Vol. IV, p. 68)

France 'An epizooty among fowls was seen in the Upper Garonne'. (*Jnl. de Méd. Vét. Théor. et Pract.*, Vol., VI)

1834 *Germany* A disease observed in the Berlin region affected hens, geese and ducks. A report recorded initial dullness and isolation of affected birds followed by declining appetite, the combs turned blue, feathers soiled and constant diarrhoea of grey, white, green and watery matter, and great thirst. Death was rapid. On examination the intestines looked as if injected with blood but the interior was healthy, as were the other viscera. The pathognomonic feature of the disease was the constant diarrhoea and rapid death. No remedies were of any value. (Halbach *Sanitatsbericht de Provinz Brandenburg*, 1834) [possibly coccidiosis due to *Eimeria maxima*]

1835 *Germany* In Ortelsburg in August and September all fowls, ducks and 300 geese died suddenly 'after suffering for some days from violent diarrhoea'. They often died when eating with a good appetite, 'gave a painful cry, bent their head and neck, threw themselves upon their back and convulsed . . . and died within eight to ten minutes'. Examination revealed enlarged liver and marked inflammation of the intestines and brain. In October 'a mortality appeared among poultry, ducks, and other fowls'.

In Prague, an 'anthracoid disease was seen in poultry', capons and other birds died 'as if struck by lightning'. Examination revealed blood 'as black as coal' and coagulated, the organs were blackened and bodies had a foul smell. In April anthrax broke out in several villages and a considerable number of poultry and geese died.

In Saxony, a 'gangrenous inflammation of the mucous membrane of the intestines' was found in dead poultry. In Eastern Prussia disease occurred in fowls and destroyed many geese. [possibly gangrenous enteritis]

In *France*, many communes in the Alfort region had a 'remarkable mortality among poultry'. The owners reported that the deaths were sudden without any obvious signs.

1836 *France* The disease seen in the previous year recommenced in April and caused widespread poultry losses. Chickens were more affected than ducks or geese, pigeons were also affected but not as seriously. Observers noted that many birds died before showing any signs of illness; almost all affected birds died. Signs were as recorded in 1835 German outbreaks (above) with most deaths occurring at night-time. Post-mortem examination of these birds showed few marked changes other than some inflammation in the intestinal tract and lungs. The opinion was expressed that, 'if, as all are inclined to believe it is due to general causes, the same as other epizooties, some particular circumstances singularly influence its development'.

In May 1836, a disease was observed by Dupuy among geese near Toulouse; the post-mortem appearances included, 'circular patches of variable extent in the rectum . . . the whole intestinal canal was full of purifom mucosities'. (*Recueil de Méd. Vétér.*, Vol. XIII, p. 300; Dupuy *Jnl. de Méd. Vétér. theoret. et pratique*, Vol. VII)

Germany A fatal disease of geese broke out near Munich. Diagnosed as 'cholera' it also affected humans; the geese fell and were unable to rise again, passing a white or greenish fluid from the anus and usually succumbed in about a quarter of an hour. (Kopp *Cholera-Epidemie in Munchen*, p. 169)

1838 *Germany* The 'disease of fowls' called cholera and usually related to human cholera outbreaks occurred, in what was described as a malignant form, in poultry, pheasants, pigeons and other birds. (Gurlt and Hertwig *Magazin.*, Vol. VI, p. 131)

France What was described as the same malady as that seen in Germany but now called 'contagious typhus' caused a great mortality in fowls in 1837 and 1838. (*Recueil de Méd. Vétér.* Vol. XVII, p. 308). In February, a large number of dead ducks were washed ashore on the coast of Landes: the total number was estimated at 20,000, no investigations made. (*Correspondenzbl. d. Wurtemburg, Landw.* Vereins, Vol. XIII)

1842 *England* An outbreak of 'gapes' was described as an epizootic in poultry, partridges and pheasants in several regions but particularly in Somersetshire. The disease is well described noting that the tracheal clumps of worms [*Syngamus trachea*] ranged from five to 14. (*The Veterinarian*, Vol. XIII, p. 648)

Ireland Poultry in Armagh were reported to have died in large numbers. (*The Irish Farmer's and Gardener's Magazine*, August)

A Poultry Industry Emerges

By the middle of the 19th century, poultry (chicken) production was recognised as a possibly significant part of the livestock industry. The main impetus came from the USA, with its rapidly expanding economy and population, also in Britain where additionally a significant hobby had developed based around competitive showing of imported chicken varieties.

During Roman times, as described by Columella, the production of poultry reached a peak that was not excelled until the 20th century. Following the decline of Roman civilisation both organised poultry production, and the careful selection and breeding of well-defined types of birds, vanished. The chicken became a farmyard scavenger, only of real value to the peasant. Rogers (1866), cited by Wood-Gush (1958, pp. 341–342) showed that the number of fowls on 11 English estates varied from seven – 49 over the years 1333–1336: they had an insignificant role in the livestock economy. To the peasant household they were of value; in areas where coins were in short supply fowls were used to pay quit-rents. Marginal images in the *Luttrell Psalter* (1330–1345) show chickens with regularity, including delightful drawings of tethered hens with their chick broods. While poultry as a source of food were not ranked highly by society at large, the breeding of fighting cocks was a sophisticated procedure. There is little or no evidence that these breeding programmes contributed to improving the genetic structure of the then poultry population for food production.

It was only in the beginning of the 19th century that the concept of poultry as a productive species within the farming structure began to develop. The state of poultry production and veterinary knowledge is well illustrated by Boardman (1805) where he writes of 'geese, ducks, turkies and what are called the gallinaceous tribe' and then states, 'the diseases of these creatures are not unworthy of our attention, though their inferior importance may occasion our conferring on them only a small and incidental share of it'.

Poultry were very low on both the livestock and veterinary list. Boardman does give a good, detailed description of the anatomy of the cock, with one veterinary observation – if the crop is over-full it needs to be cut open, emptied and sewn up [known as 'sour crop', due to overeating]. He was also interested in the stones to be found in the gizzard. The section ends with 'Of the diseases of fowls little has been discovered, and less recorded'. He does, later, mention one disease: the finding of the avian bronchial worm (*Syngamus trachea*), but not named. He reported that few birds recover and for chickens and the young turkey, there was no remedy except by taking a bird's feather and stripping it, except for a small end section. This was then passed into the larynx of an affected bird and twisted to catch and remove the worms, but he also recorded that this was of little real help.

Information on domestic poultry in Europe up to the 16th century was mainly published in Greek and Latin, largely based on translations of the ancient texts. In 1600 Ulisse Aldrovani published *Ornithologia,* an encyclopaedic work, the 14th book of Volume II provided a summary of the available poultry knowledge. The first English-language text on the diseases of domestic poultry was the translation of Conrad Heresbach's *Rei Rusticae libri quator,* by Barnaby Googe as *the Fovre Books of Husbandri* (1577). The poultry section deals with chickens, ducks, geese and turkeys, and some other birds. In general, the advice given for both management and disease control is similar to that offered by Aldrovani – as both are based on the writings of Columella.

The first English-luaguage publication dealing solely with domestic poultry was a translation from the French *Discours Economique* by Prudens Choiselat, and published as *A Discourse of Houseboundrie* 1580. The influence of Columella and Varro is obvious, in particular emphasis on ensuring hygiene and cleanliness, and the Roman profitability advice. Other similar works appeared in following years, notably one by Leonard Mascall, *The Husbandlye ordring and Governmente of Poultrie* 1581, again mostly derived from Columella, but with a good description of surgical caponisation. Gervase Markham devoted much space to poultry and their diseases in several of his books in 1614, 1616 and 1631. A valuable publication reviewing the early English printed literature on the diseases of poultry, and other birds was made by Comben (1969, pp. 17–25).

Poultry Diseases and Management in the 19th Century

The expansion of agriculture, as a scientifically based and technologically aided industry, began in the 19th century and was established by the 1850s. Poultry now became of greater interest as an economic source of food. The species had already attracted attention following the importation of Chinese varieties – termed Cochins, Shanghais or Chinas. These started a 'hen craze' in England in the later 19th century and soon specific breeds began to develop, and then were bred with local breeds. The showing of these birds developed rapidly with increasing competition. Gradually more specific production-oriented breeds evolved: in the USA the Plymouth Rock, Wyandotte and Rhode Island Red; in Britain, the Sussex and Orpington, among others (Crawford 1984, pp. 305–307). It was now realised that poultry could be of great value to farming and food production. An anonymous author, writing in *The Complete Farmer or General Dictionary Of Agriculture* 1807, expressed the hope that the farming of poultry would be developed according to scientific principles, and then enunciated husbandry methods that differed little from those advocated by Columella, almost 2000 years before!

A division of interests between the competitive show bird breeders and those who were selecting for meat and egg production occurred. In the late 1800s two significant developments were the introduction of the Leghorn breed, from Italy, and the selection for brown egg colour. In Britain, the Australorp and Cornish strains evolved, and by the early 1900s relatively few breed types had become the root-stocks on which the modern poultry industry has developed. The background and development in the USA has been well described in *American Poultry History 1823–1973* published by the American Poultry Historical Society.

One of the first books of the 19th century to specifically discuss poultry farm-ing was *The Breeding, Rearing and Fattening of all Kinds of Domestic Poultry* by Bonington Moubray, first published in London about 1815. The author discusses the turkey, duck, goose, pea and guinea fowls and the swan; there is also a note on rearing the bustard, 'the flesh is of unrivalled excellence'. As was the custom, the book also includes short sections on pigeons, rabbits, dairy cattle, bees, private brewing and a section on pigs, but the majority of the text is on poultry farming. The name of the author is a pseudonym used by John Lawrence, better known for his numerous works on horses and farriery. The book was successful with eight reprints by 1854. The introduction mentions that poultry have always been regarded as a luxury in Britain, but that in France poultry formed an important part of livestock farming, it also dwells on Egyptian production of chickens and their use of hatching ovens. The available breeds are listed and commented on, some names reveal their identity, and some not: dung-hill fowls, game, Dorking, Poland, Bontharm, Chittagong or Malay, Shackbag, Spanish, 'and their endless sub-varieties'.

Moubray discusses the practice of plucking feathers from living fowls. This was a feature of the farming of geese with the annual stripping of feathers; he also records the selling of plucked live birds in Edinburgh market. He is also strongly critical of the apparently widespread practice, and describes how seabirds were regularly caught, had their down and feathers stripped and then thrown back into the sea to die. He does suggest that much of the cruelty could be prevented by cutting off the feathers with scissors when the bird was in full plumage: he appealed to the clergy to work for reform. This section of his book (pages 35–37) makes uncomfortable reading as he describes a sport practised in Scotland of hanging live birds tied by their legs and men riding at them full speed and catching them by the neck. Another, quoted gourmand speciality, was to roast a goose alive.

The disease section is prefaced by observing that most disease is caused by errors of diet or management and that these should always be controlled to prevent problems. Should disease arise, 'little hope can be derived from medical attempts' and that the greater part of the account of diseases and remedies in books, 'is a farrago of sheer absurdity'. The most common diseases are stated as: 'the Pip' the white skin on the tongue; 'the Roup' an imposthume (abscess or lump) found on the rump of the bird, to be opened and washed out with salty water; 'the Roup' is also a term for 'Catarrh . . . to which gallinaceous fowls are much subject' and the Flux and Constipation. Vermin were said to be a problem unless the chickens were allowed sand and ashes to roll in. The chief disease problem is said to be 'Roupy' when the nostrils run, eyes swollen and the discharge fetid, 'like glanders in horses'. The 'Chip' can affect birds in bad weather and they sit, listless, pining and die. Moubray also writes of the new disease recently reported, Gapes, caused by 'a species of *Fasciola* infecting the trachea of poultry'. Impaction of the crop was obviously common, with incision, evacuation of the contents and stitched, with rapid healing expected. Care was also advised for the cock and to carefully shorten his spurs every three months to prevent them impeding his walk and wounding his legs. Other diseases in geese, pigeons and ducks are noted but with little indication of full symptoms. The book is useful as a guide to poultry practices in the early 19th century, mostly as described by Columella, but sound. The intended readership was the landowner, it was before intensive farming systems had become established, and was intended to aid the commercial farmer in increasing his income.

An interesting comment on poultry diseases is found in *First Aid for Horses, Dogs, Birds and Cattle* published in 1899 by Elliman's, in Slough, England, the manufacturer of a proprietary embrocation. The book is well written but is essentially a vehicle to promote the use of embrocation. Almost 30 diseases of chickens are listed, in most of which the manufacturer has been able to find a use for their product. The list demonstrates that poultry were becoming increasingly of value and not the farmyard scavenger of old, and that the medications for disease were becoming recognised as seldom of use. The list indicates that crop surgery for impaction was common practice, that 'Roup' was a serious infectious condition with respiratory symptoms, 'Pip' is listed again (as Columella), and both round, flat and lungworms are identified as well as lice.

In 1896 Charles Darwin produced a list of the broad groups of chicken types (Darwin 1896). He listed 13 stocks, of these he noted that the Dorking was a five-toed bird with a compact body (this breed, also called Darking, is believed by some to be a descendent of original Roman stock). The listing provided a useful guide for those engaged in the already developed poultry boom, but it does not include the layer and broiler stocks which have come to dominate the poultry industry. The investment in poultry selection and breeding in the 20th century gave the species an evolutionary rate that exceeded all previous development over many centuries.

Poultry Diseases

The rapid development of the poultry industry for meat and egg production has produced one of the most highly intensive animal production systems. This involves lifetime housing, feed control, rigid biosecurity and hygiene. Other poultry fall into two categories – small scale or household flocks usually well controlled, but without rigid biosecurity, and poultry kept by subsistence farmers worldwide.

Disease control in intensive systems forms part of a total management structure aimed at health by using disease prevention programmes based on vaccination or medication as indicated. Small scale flocks are liable for disease outbreaks as climatic and other factors change; subsistence farmed flocks are usually poor producers with a disease burden.

Due to the importance of the poultry industry there is a continuing disease research programme, and an extensive list of viral, bacterial, fungal, parasitic and feed related diseases recognised. Diseases tend to vary by country and management systems but the most serious, considering the total poultry population, are:

Virus Fowl Pox; Infectious Bursal Disease (Gumboro); Newcastle Disease (Ranikhet); Avian Influenza, due to Type A virus H5NI most common; Avian Encephalomyelitis and Infectious Bronchitis

Bacteria Fowl Typhoid (*Salmonella gallinarum*); Infectious Coryza (*Avibacterium paragallinarum*); Pullorum Disease (Salmonellosis) (*Salmonella enteritica*); Chronic Respiratory Disease (Mycoplasmosis) (*Mycoplasma gallisepticum*) and Fowl Cholera (*Pasteurella Multocida*)

Parasites Coccidiosis (*Eimeria spp.*); Ectoparasites: lice, ticks, mites and fleas; Endoparasites: mostly gut nematodes in birds allowed outside housing and gape worms (*Syngamus trachea*)

There are many other disease problems of either an infectious, genetic or nutritional nature that might be found. Usually these are controlled in well-run systems. One particular problem in certain climatic conditions is mycotoxin contamination of feed, most commonly by *Aspergillus flavus*.

Poultry disease control in modern intensive farming is strict biosecurity, good feed supply and controlled management of environment plus a programme for disease recognition, identification and institution of treatment or vaccination as required. In practice this can operate well, but needs investment in buildings, systems and staff.

Wild Birds: Captured and Caged

A particularly interesting book, *The Fowler* by Nicholas Coxe (undated but probably 1780) published in London, deals with all classes of birds that were to be hunted. Apart from the usual land and waterfowl – 'Woodcocks, Felfares, Pigeons, Magpies, Morefoots, Snipes, Gleads, Crows, Rooks, Herons, Partridges, Pheasants, Railes and Quails' – there is an essay on songbirds. This not only details the wide range of birds that were captured to be caged and held in residences, but discusses feeding and diseases. This is a unique commentary on the health problems of 17 species; from the text they appear to be discussed in order of popularity, and possibly of caged populations. The methods of capture and keeping them are discussed in most cases. By far the most detail on capture, feeding and health is devoted to the nightingale, followed by the 'canary bird' indicating their popularity. The information cited here is mostly related to health and disease issues.

Nightingale Would appear to be relatively healthy when caged, but after two to three years are subject to gout, a foot disease with recommended treatment of anointing the feet with butter; also troubled by 'imposthumes' (abscess) and breaking out about their eyes and nib', treatment was with capons-grease (fat).

Canary bird The most diseases are listed for this species: the chief malady is 'surfeit', shown by 'swelling under their bellies . . . sometimes a sinking towards the extreme parts of their bodies', and also with a 'black appearance' [possibly *Trichomas gallinae* infection]. Colds were said to produce similar symptoms, but with a 'red appearance'; treatment was by altering the diet. Moulting was seen as a difficult time when the birds would get 'the Pip', seen as a pimple growing near the tail; it was recommended to take a needle and pierce and then squeeze out the content. Yellow scabs could form about the eyes and head – treat by anointing with oil of sweet almonds or butter and add herbs to the feed. Scouring, is prevented by 'drawing one or two of the tail feathers' and putting saffron in the water. A comprehensive mix of seed types and plants/herbs is given for winter feeding.

Blackbird No diseases mentioned, however the author did not like the song of the bird and stated they could be taught to whistle.

Thrush/Throstle (five types are listed) No diseases mentioned but author stated they were best for 'pot or spit' when they are fat, with frost and snow on the ground.

Robin No diseases mentioned; called 'the little King of the Birds' and very popular because of its song – 'with a Trap-cage and a Meal-worm you may take half a score in a day'.

Wren No diseases mentioned; good songsters and 'easily taught a tune'; as well as feed 'give them a spider or two every three days'.

Woodlark Subject to many diseases: lice 'very common', smoke with tobacco and put fresh gravel and sand on cage floor as they like to bask in the sun; cramp, give fresh gravel to keep the feet clean; giddiness, the result of feeding too much hemp seed, cure by feeding gentles (larvae/maggots of *Calliphora vomitoria*, the bluebottle fly), or hog-lice, (wood louse/weevil) or liquorice in the water. The bird is noted as being an excellent songster.

Sky-Lark Noted to be very hardy. Much instruction on catching the birds plus a note to never feed them salt meat or salt bread.

Linnet Mostly trained to either whistle or copy other birds' songs. Care in feeding, food must always be fresh otherwise will scour and die; food must not be too dry or they will get 'Vent-burnt'.

Goldfinch Stated that they may become 'sick', if so feed a little groundsel; a lump or two of sugar in the cage will help health, as well as a lump of chalk to prevent scouring.

Tit-Lark 'They are easily brought up, being hard; are not subject to cold or cramps as other Birds; and live long if preserved with care.'

Chaffinch 'He is very little subject to Disease; but is inclinable to be very lousy if he be not sprinkled with a little Wine twice or thrice a Month'.

Starling No disease mentioned. 'Bird is kept by all ranks of People, and taught to pipe, whistle or talk'.

Redstart No diseases mentioned. Said to be 'of a very sullen dogged temper in a Cage'.

Bullfinch No diseases mentioned. 'He hath no song of his own, nor whistle, but is very apt to learn anything almost, if taught by the Mouth'.

Greenfinch No disease mentioned. 'This being a hardy heavy Bird, is used for ringing of Bells'. [this is not understood]

Hedge-Sparrow No disease mentioned. Become tame very easily and 'his Song contains very delightful Notes, and he sings early in the Spring with great variety'.

HAWKS AND FALCONS:
HISTORY, MANAGEMENT AND DISEASES

The practice of using birds of prey to catch other birds and small mammals, both for food and also for sport developed in the Eastern countries. Its eventual evolution, however, took two similar, but not identical, courses in Europe and in the East (mainly Arab nations).

Falconry in Europe

Around AD 430 the Huns invaded Eastern Europe and established a significant, but short-lived, foothold. It is believed that this included the introduction of falconry. The earliest European treatises on falconry appear to have been written in the later Byzantine period, the thirteenth century. These two anonymous works, the *Orneosophia* (*The Wisdom of Treating Birds*) and *Ierakosophia* (*The Wisdom of Treating Falcons*), while based in hunting procedures and training, also had a veterinary content. They did not have a significant influence in Medieval Europe and do not appear to have been translated at that time.

The first true European literature was obtained by the translation of an Arabic treatise *Kitab at-mutawakkili*, written by Moamyn: this author's full name is not known but it is suggested to possibly be Hunayn ibn Ishaq (c.AD 809– 873) a physician-translator who also worked on Byzantine and other texts in the Abbasid Caliphate (Viré 1967, pp. 172–176). A copy was obtained by King Frederick II Hohenstaufen (1194–1250) of Swabia (Germany) when he took part in the 6th Crusade in 1228–1229. He had this translated into Latin by Theodore of Antioch, added some comments and issued it in 1241 titled *Scientia Venandi per Aves*. Hohenstaufen had his own aviary and studied falcons, and introduced the Arab custom of placing hoods on the head of the trained birds. He then produced his own book *De Arte Venandi cum Avibus* (*The Art of Hunting with Birds*), published c.1245. This book has been regarded as also making contributions to ornithology and zoology, and enabling progress to be made from Aristotle's initial explanations of nature.

At about the same time Bishop Albert Magnus (c.1200–1280), the theologian and zoologist, published his major work *De Animalibus* (*On Animals*). This was important as he was the first to comment, in text, on Aristotle's writings, and by doing so laid the groundwork for modern zoology. In a previous treatise, *De Falconibus* (*On Falcons*) he discussed the birds and hunting procedures, and prescribed cures for sick and wounded falcons; this was inserted into *De Animalibus* as Book 23, Chapter 40.

There was an active interest in falconry at this time, it became a popular sport for kings and noblemen throughout Medieval Europe. It was confined to the upper and noble classes, mainly due to cost, the time it required and obtaining land suitable for the sport. Additionally, the ownership of these birds conferred status on the individual – as well described in Britain by Dame Juliana Berners in the *Boke of St. Albans* 1486, where mention is also made of the diseases of birds of prey.

The adoption of this method of hunting was appropriated by the courtly classes in Europe from about the 9th century AD and can be recognised pictorially from the 11th century. As seen in the Bayeux Tapestry illustrating events in 1065, showing King Harold Godwinson, with hawk on his wrist meeting William Duke of Normandy. Following their enjoyment by high society in the medieval period for the capture of birds and other game, falconry gradually passed to the yeoman of society. Falconry reached its zenith in the 17th century and then declined, partly due to changes in fashion and also to the introduction of firearms. Gervase Markham, in *Hungers Prevention, or the Whole Art of Fowling* 1621, classified certain birds as, 'for pleasure only' in venery (hunting) as 'Hawks of all kindes, Castrells, Ringtailes, Buzards, Kites', and any bird of prey. The art has survived to the present day, to become once again the occupation of the wealthy.

In Europe two types of birds were involved – the long-winged falcons (Falconidae) and the short-winged hawks (Accipitridae). Falcons were released to fly high, then trained dogs were released to put up the game birds, the falcons then swoop (at speeds estimated to be up to 200 mph). The two most favoured birds were the peregrines (*Falco peregrinus*) and the gyrfalcons (*Falco rusticolus*). These very large birds were initially mainly bred in Scandinavia and Iceland; other falcons used were the sakers, lanners and merlins. Short-winged hawks were trained to fly directly at game when it was put up, the most popular birds being the goshawks and sparrowhawks. The game sought was wide ranging – ducks, pheasants and partridge as well as big birds such as geese, herons, cranes and bustards. All destined for human consumption.

Ownership and use of birds for hunting was based in law in most countries of Europe, this was well established by the start of the 2nd century, as seen in Norman Law. In England, the *Charter of the Forest* issued in 1217, complementary to the *Magna Carta*, gave every free man access to the Royal Forests and eased, but not removed, the hunting restrictions previously imposed by the King.

The management, training and feeding of falcons and hawks was a major occupation in the periods of maximum use (this is well summarised by Macgregor 2012, pp. 175–186). Great expertise was required for the lengthy training process and much specialist equipment was designed (still in use today), in particular the hoods used on the birds and protective arm gloves used by the owners as well as the 'jesses', thongs of soft leather that are knotted around the legs with rings, used to anchor the birds. Special housing was constructed, the mews, often of considerable size. Adult birds were kept here during the annual moult, termed 'mewing'. As a part of training the eyes of the bird would be 'seeled', this involved a thread being passed through the lower eyelids and tied over the head; also used during transport. This procedure was widely practised and no record of it causing harm to the bird appears in the relevant literature. Shipment was handled with great care as the birds were recognised to be prone to stress problems.

There is very limited information available on the diseases and treatments used with hawks and falcons in the Medieval years. Of interest therefore is a manuscript found in the papers of Samuel Pepys, compiled by an anonymous hand at the end of the 15th century. It is a strange collection of charms and recipes, mostly for humans but also including a section on diseases, and cures, of hawks. The text was obviously written for the gentry who were much concerned with social importance and includes the rules for conduct while hawking. Cooking recipes are included for heron, blackbird and cormorant. The manuscript (MS. Pepys 1047) held at Magdalene College, Cambridge has been published (Hodgett, n.d.).

The treatments described are mainly herbal based. The diseases listed are seldom with sufficient symptoms described to allow for any accurate recognition, but an idea can be gained from the problems identified (although some words are difficult to interpret):

- The *rye*, described as a head cold causing swelling.
- The *frounce*, a throat disease described as 'like a scab'; recommended to pick this off with a hazel stick and then medicate (frounce can mean a wrinkle or crease).
- The *peare*, unexplained but appears to be when a bird is unable to moult. The treatment used was an external wash made from a herbal mixture.
- The *cray*, constipation.
- The *cramp*, a disease affecting the wings of hawks.
- The *pies*, described as when the hawk falls, suddenly from the fist or perch. The treatment was to place the bird in herbal smoke. The term is also used for a throat disease and also a 'corn' on the foot.
- The *pip*, a disorder of the tongue of a hawk. [There appears to be some confusion in terminology between this complaint, the frounce and the pies; the pip in poultry usually means a 'scab' on the tongue; also called the frounce.]
- *Casting*, in early English the word meant to vomit, or for a bird of prey to regurgitate. A natural procedure for hawks. The plant-based medication advised is 'to make your hawk break her casting' and its use will 'make her cast'.
- The *polyner*, described as a swelling above the jess (the soft leather thong around the hawk's leg). Treatment advised was to anoint the feet with grease.
- *Enseamed*, a word that was used to describe cleansed or cleared of superfluous fat. The advice to prove this in a hawk was to make it 'cast up' (vomit) and see the colour: yellow indicated the bird is enseamed, if black 'she is bruised within, that is to say she is fat'.
- *Endue*, the heading reads, 'if your bird casts her food and cannot endue'. [Endue meant to digest, or of a hawk to pass the contents of the crop to the stomach.] The interesting cure was, 'take good hot meat while it is alive and if it is a chicken, pluck the skin off the breast and put woman's milk on it and when she casts up her meat give her no more of it'. Other words in the Pepys document that are used in conjunction with diseases of the hawk (some also found in discussing diseases of humans and animals) are: *squat*, to defaecate or to let tail droop or fall; *menson*, dysentery; *boryane*, barren; *feebly*, poor health; *knot*, a hard rounded swelling or growth or mass or lump felt in the stomach or throat; *sere*, a claw or talon, from *serrer*, hold fast, can also mean dried up or withered; *cere*, the soft waxlike covering at the base of the beak through which the nostrils are pierced.

The use of orpiment is recommended for the treatment of 'all manner of vermin on a hawk', to be applied as a powder after washing. Orpiment is a bright yellow naturally occurring mineral, better known as arsenic trisulphide, it was also used as a dye or an artist's pigment. Now known to be extremely toxic.

Falconry in the Middle East

It is believed that falconry began to be practised in the Mesopotamia (Middle Eastern) region about 2000 BC. It is also known that early Mongolian tribes regarded the falcon as a symbol and may also have trained and used the birds. Some early Chinese writings suggest that their emperors about 700 BC participated in the sport; later Saga, the 52nd emperor in AD 818 became interested in falconry, and also banned the eating of meat except that of fish and birds. Early Mesopotamian activity has been described by A H Layard using bas-relief images in ancient Assyrian buildings, these appeared to portray a falconer with a bird on his wrist (*Discoveries in the Ruins of Nineveh and Babylon* 1853). A bas-relief in the palace of the Neo-Assyrian King Sargon II (722–705 BC) at Khorsabad also shows an image of falconry.

The development of falconry reached both a zenith and became a continuing practice in the Middle East. Much of this history has been hidden since it was contained in Arabic language treatises that have been either unavailable or untranslated. A difficulty in translation of ancient texts in a different script is obtaining the correct meaning for specialist words, as well as any nuances that might be present in the original text. A book by Housni Alkhateeb Sheehada, *Mamluks and Animals* (2013), has done much for history and scholarship in examining the veterinary content of the literature produced in the Mamluk period – the mid-13th to the early 16th centuries.

Arabic, or Islamic, falconry literature probably dates from the 8th century AD when it incorporated knowledge from previous Greek, Indian, Persian and other manuscripts. The only important falconry treatise written in the Umayyad period under Caliph Hisham was *Kitab Dawari al-tayr*, *The Book on Birds of Prey*, by Al-Ghatrif, possibly as early as the 8th century. In most Mamluk and other treatises dealing with falcon care and diseases the name of Al-Ghatrif appears, his reputation in the hawking/falconry world was celebrated over many years. Most manuscripts were translated to Arabic during the Umayyad period, and into the early Abbasid. A study by Detlef Möller into the Arabic falconry literature and its evolution from the 8th century to the Mamluk period has been summarised by Sheehada (2013, pp. 115–118). These translations became the basis for the major Arabic writings on falconry. A falconer's manual was issued in the 10th century by Fatamid Caliph al-Aziz Billah and similar books in the 13th century by Abd al-Rahman al-Balal and in the 14th century by Ibn Mangli. By the 15th century there were significantly more authors on the subject. The so-called Golden Age of translation to Arabic of the ancient works was mostly a product of Nestorian Christian monks in the 9th–10th centuries. The heritage of the resulting Arabic literature is essentially Graeco-Byzantine.

It is important also to recognise that when the Arab world was converted to Islam the result was that religious precepts affected many activities, in particular those related to food. Birds of prey (that is, falcons) are considered 'unclean' and therefore followers of the Muslim faith must not have any physical contact with them; the slaughter of animals for human food has to be carried out under the prescribed religious rules, which are obviously impossible in hunting conditions. However, these religious restrictions do not appear to have limited either the enjoyment of falconry, or the eating of the catch, by the Arab elite.

Birds held an esteemed place in Islamic society. Songbirds were caught or purchased in the market, to be released usually on a Friday morning before prayers, in the belief that it was a good deed for which the person would be rewarded on the Day of Judgement. In this environment falconry became recognised as the most sophisticated form of hunting, and a status symbol. The birds employed (in particular the goshawk, sparrow hawk and gyrfalcon) were costly and required much time and great patience to train. Special housing, dietary needs and care resulted in significant cost expenditure. The gyrfalcons were the most highly priced (they had to be transported from northern Europe), and valued in both monetary and status terms.

The early Arabic writings on falconry are much concerned with the Islamic religion and ritual. Discussions on the ritual purity of the prey was a matter of concern since the required ritual for slaughter had not been followed. A book by Hamzah Al-Nashiri on hunting illustrates the influence of the Islamic culture: each chapter discusses a religious topic and its relationship to hunting, with one appendix covering the diseases of hunting birds and another the miracles associated with hunting and the Prophet.

In the 9th century, seen as the beginning of the Golden Age of Islam, Baghdad in the Abbasid reign developed as the centre of Arab thought: a major consequence of this was the great activity in both translation of other works to Arabic as well as the creation of Arabic language texts. One of these was *al-Buzat wa'l-sayd* (*Hawks and Hunting*). During the early 10th century a book by Kushajm titled *Kitab al-Masa'id wa-al-Matarid* appeared, this showed a professional knowledge of falconry and reviewed other Abbasid treatises on hunting. Again, the contents cover the religious aspects of decrees on purity of hunting and the killing of wild animals (discussed by Möller and cited by Shehada, as previously mentioned). Other books appeared on falconry but in general these were compilations of earlier writings; probably the most important of these is *al Jamharah fi al-Bayzarah* by Hasan al-Asadi (c.1230). There are no surviving books on falconry from the Andalusian Caliphate (now Spain) when ruled by the Umayyads, yet the sport was popular there.

Veterinary care of hunting birds was the work of the falconer, the *bazyar*. Particular emphasis was given, in all the treatises, on the care of the birds: there were specialists in the treatment and care of the main species employed – the hawk, peregrine, saker and eagle. Each bird would have its own handler who was responsible for diet, food supply, housing and also selected the hunting grounds. The handlers had assistants, called *hammal*, who were bound by codes of behaviour. The birds had to be trained to work with hunting dogs: this often took time to overcome the natural fear, in both birds and dogs. The most difficult time for handling the birds was in the annual moult (the *qarnasah*) usually a period of some 40 days; they then required careful daily care. Probably with a realisation that few, if any, of the medications and treatments recommended for bird ailments were effective, the emphasis was on preventive medicine, recognising that these birds of prey were not only very delicate, but also highly sensitive to their environment. It required hours of patience to train

them as part of a hunting sport, and the strong message in the Arabic texts was –
preservation of health.

Strict rules were listed for mews cleanliness, care in moulting and control of air
flow, and hours of light and dark depending on the time, before or after a hunting
session. Particular attention was given to the food for each bird – quantities had to
be correct, quality had to be good. The feeding time had to be correct, according
to age and activity. When young birds were moved from their parents to a keeper
also required extra attention to feed and food intake. The food was essentially meat
with the best being from young, healthy sheep. Cattle meat was considered harmful,
camel worse, buffalo even worse and horse the very worst. Meat had to be fresh,
not that which had gone cold after slaughter or killed the previous day. Some meat
of other birds was used (never that of the flamingo or goose) – also bird meat had
to be bled out. When the falcons and hawks were taken on long journeys (always
regarded as a great hazard) the meat supply was a consignment of pigeons also taken
on the journey. Fish were deemed to be an undesirable food. There were some views
expressed which indicate that the rules were not always kept.

During hunting the feeding routine included a carefully mixed dough composed
of various seeds, clay and chalk and lemon juice, called *barud*. Eagles were treated
differently by deprivation of food on some days in hunting training. For all birds
great care was said to be needed in feeding during the moult, after which they were
usually slimmed. A daily physical examination of every bird was a stated routine.
Emphasis was given to examination of the faeces and any regurgitated food – these
were important diagnostic indicators of the health status.

A theory of 'temperaments' in birds was practised, based on being too hot or cold,
or moist. This involved food and it was suggested that different species required
different foods. Temperament was related to foods: pigeon meat was believed to be
dry and therefore suitable for feeding hawks who were said to have a moist temperament. Pigeon meat was thought, for some birds, to help them to rid themselves of
bad 'humours'. The daily excretion of faeces was carefully watched, and measured to
determine the rate of elimination of humours and food. It was important to estimate
the digestion of the food intake to aid judgement on the fitness to hunt. Faeces of a
yellowish tinge were said to be diagnostic of a usually incurable disease called *istarim*,
(but also recorded that if the eyes of the bird were clear and the condition was good
it was probably of little significance).

While the subject of food, feeding and excretion (by faeces or regurgitation) was
obviously important, reading the advice in the 21st century gives an impression of
over-complication to the point of fetish. These were valuable birds, the provision of
much of this 'expert' advice could add to the mystic of owning and caring for such
birds, and also provide prestige to the writers.

Diagnosis of disease in birds was conducted by a process of careful examination,
based on a belief in the Galenic ideas learned from translation of Greek and Latin
treatises. The true condition of the bird was evaluated with particular reference
to the external condition as well as a judgement of the 'balanced condition of the
temperament'. Signs were viewed and judged on the four humours theory and the
main humour being exhibited – the dominant and 'good' humour for a bird was

judged to be yellow bile. Bodily secretions were studied at length – the faeces in particular and also regurgitations, (birds of prey eliminate waste by regurgitation of pellets), to calculate the balance of the humours. It was recognised that urine was eliminated by the alimentary system and therefore there was great concentration on the faeces – consistency, shape and size, colour, smell and also tasting (it is unclear if this was voluntary or obligatory). All to be done every day at dawn for hunting birds. Diagnosis of a problem could also be reached by using different foods and examining the effects on the alimentary tract.

Daily examination included watching the first movements of the bird and use of the oil gland: if used first thing in the morning it was a good sign. An interesting feature of the daily examination was the feeling of the pulse, at the joint of the wing with the body: predictions were made as a result. Attention was given to the recognition of stress, apparently a problem with the frequently volatile and easily excited birds. In such a state they were liable to choke and food would pass to the trachea when they were gasping for breath. Emphasis was placed on the availability of pure, clean water for both drinking and bathing, in desert surroundings water supply was of importance. Much time was devoted to examination and diagnosis – not for disease but as a confirmation of the health status.

Therapeutic procedures were well developed in four categories:

1. Medications, administered orally, in feed or by rectum, ointments for topical use and nasal application for inhalation. Mostly of herbal or mineral origin but additionally urine, animal faeces and blood all feature in the extensive list of substances used. Enemas were used utilising a trimmed bamboo shoot or silver tube, great care was emphasised.

2. Surgical procedures were limited but showed some significant innovations: fracture repair was practised, but it was difficult to restrain the birds to obtain rest. Wing fracture repair invariably failed but leg repair could be successful using resin impregnated bandages with the application of quick-setting coatings such as one composed of Armenian bole (clay), tamarind seeds and gum. Talons were repaired using quick-setting resins, beaks were filed and trimmed if overgrown and foot deformities removed. Eyelids were sewn together as an essential part of taming and training to subdue the bird; it was also recorded that this could result in serious problems.

3. Topical treatments included the use of the cautery, but usually only after other methods had failed, most frequently on the nostrils (for nasal/respiratory conditions) burning each side with a three to four day interval. Control of lice and ticks were stated to have been a major problem for falconry managers. Wounds were a common feature of care, as a result of hunting encounters; woollen sutures were used to close incisions. Skin transplants were advocated when a serious loss had occurred; a donor bird was killed and transplantation and sewing was immediate. The success rate is unclear. Feather implants were also employed when a major loss had occurred.

4. Among other procedures the use of bloodletting was proposed, but the danger of the procedure was emphasised. Taking birds into public baths was not

uncommon and various temperatures were advised for treatments, such as the care of nasal problems or of lice.

This review owes much to the work by Shehada, which provides an excellent starting point for further investigations. It is clear is that the trained bird of prey had become an efficient fighting and killing machine, and was supported in every way.

Avian Welfare and Disease

In overall terms the standards of avian welfare practised by humans over time have been variable and usually poor. While the pragmatic Romans, who developed an effective poultry industry structure, understood that sound management with care produced good results, many of the procedures used in fattening bird species ranged from harmful to cruel, but to the Roman mind were good economic practice. From the 20th century intensive production systems and breeds designed (that is, genetically selected) for these systems evolved to the current state where good welfare practices are in use. Some observers question the humanity of these systems.

Birds kept and trained for sport, both hawks and falcons, and fighting cocks receive good care to ensure that they can be in peak condition to act as the killing machines they have been trained to be. It is difficult to make unbiased comments on the overall welfare management of such situations.

Pleasure or companion birds – parrots, budgerigars, canaries and the multitude of other species employed in this usually confined/caged existence have had dubious standards of welfare throughout history. This is mostly due to a lack of understanding of the habits and nutritional needs of the individual species. For example, Psittacines are gregarious and should not be kept as a solitary bird, but if two or more are kept together, it is unlikely that they will copy the human voice.

Public Health and Poultry Diseases

In past centuries there appears to have been little problem, there is a suggestion that avian influenza was transmitted to humans, but the descriptions are too vague to allow for any conclusions. Poultry meat had a reputation for being a very clean meat and therefore free from possible transmissible diseases.

Research in recent years has shown that there are some transmissible diseases (that is, *Listeria monocytogenes*) to be watched for; these, however, are rare. Disease issues have developed with the increased intensification of poultry production. Problems occur with *Salmonella spp.* and *Campylobacter spp.* contamination of poultry meat during processing, due to the difficulties of effective hygiene in the current mass production systems.

One disease, initially termed 'parrot fever', was found to be sometimes fatal in humans. The cause, *Chlamydia psittaci* infection was elucidated in 1879. Now understood, it is both controllable and treatable. The disease is known as Psittacosis in the psittacine birds (parrots, budgerigars and so on), and Ornithosis in other species (turkeys, pigeons and so on).

References

Boardman, T. (1805) *A Dictionary of the Veterinary Art.* London: George Kearsley

Boehrer, B.T. (2004) *Parrot Culture.* Philadelphia, PA :Pennsylvania University Press

Cocker, M. and Tipling, D. (2013) *Birds and People.* London: Cape

Comben, N. (1969) The Early English Printed Literature on the Diseases of Poultry and Other Birds. *The Veterinarian* **6**

Crawford, R.D. (1984) *Evolution of Domestic Animals* (Ed. Mason I.L.). New York: Longman

Darwin, C. (1896) The Variations of Animals and Plants Under Domestication. New York: Appleton

Delacour, J. (1965) *The Pheasants of the World.* London: Country Life

Ghigi, A. (Ed.) (1939) Poultry Farming as Described by the Writers of Ancient Rome. Milan: Raffaello Bertieri

Hodgett, G.H.J. (n.d.) Stere htt well: Medieval Recipes and Remedies from Samuel Pepys's Library. Adelaide: Mary Martin Books

Keymer, E.F. (1962) Ornithology and the Veterinary Profession, in *Veterinary Annual 1962.* London: Blackwell

Lembke, J. (2012) *Chickens.* New York: Skyhorse

Macgregor, A. (2012) *Animal Encounters.* London: Reaktion Books

Sheehada, H.A. (2013) Mamluks and Animals: Veterinary Medicine in Medieval Islam. Leiden: Brill

Toynbee, J.M.C. (2013) *Animals in Roman Life and Art.* Barnsley: Pen & Sword Archaeology

Viré, F (1967) Sur l'identite de Moamin le Fauconnire. *Comm. l'Academie des Inscriptions et Belles Lettres* April–June

Wood-Gush, D.G.M. (1958) A History of the Domestic Chicken from Antiquity to the 19th Century. *Poultry Science* **38**

Zeuner, F E (1963) *A History of Domesticated Animals.* New York: Harper & Row

CHAPTER 25

Aquatic Species: Fish, Molluscs, Edible Snails and Frogs

Freshwater and Marine Fish

The major civilisations of the Near and Middle East, India and China shared a common characteristic in developing in the proximity of rivers; this ensured a water supply for agriculture and an availability of fish for food. Almost all cultures have used fresh or marine fish as a major food source, in particular those in Asia and the Mediterranean basin, who also took an early interest in confining certain species. Fish cultivation initially developed in coastal Asia and Europe. Peoples in Africa (excepting the North), the Americas and Australia had limited experience with sea-going boats and any fish eaten was river or lake caught. Some aquatic species have attracted a non-food cultivation interest with economic potential in certain colourful, decorative fish and also in molluscs for pearl production; these practices developed in Asia. (The term 'aquaculture' describes the cultivation, or farming, of fish, strictly speaking this refers to freshwater species, with 'mariculture' describing the cultivation of marine fish. Common usage has resulted in aquaculture becoming a generic term for all water-based systems.)

Early paintings and bas-reliefs from Egypt and Mesopotamia show constructed fishponds. Methods of confining fish and feeding them for consumption was practised. Plato (c.427–348 BC) recounting his visit to Egypt recorded that he saw the Royal fishponds and describes the 'taming' of fish (Zeuner 1963, p. 479), which could indicate a cultivation system rather than simply feeding for consumption. Of related interest are early Egyptian paintings (from 1550 BC –1300 BC) in the tombs of high-ranking individuals, which show men fishing in their gardens from channels cut from the Nile. This was a favourite pastime: an early indication of what was to become a popular leisure activity, throughout history.

The first Greek colonisers of Sicily constructed a huge tank for aquaculture at Agrigentum: it was, however, filled in by the 1st century AD, so the system in use was presumably unsuccessful. In his *Bibliotheke* (*Library*) written c.56–30 BC, Diodorus Siculus, a Sicilian, wrote that the waters of rivers and springs were conducted into the tank and 'it supplied fish in great abundance to be used for food . . . swarms of swans settled upon it . . . a delight to look upon'.

Evidence of fishpond cultivation develops as the Roman culture embraced the Mediterranean region, becoming fashionable in Italy in the 1st century BC. The ponds soon attracted a 'snob' value for wealthy people who liked to go fishing at home. Varro (116–27 BC), however, in his writings expressed the view that such behaviour 'had gone too far'. Pliny (AD 23–79), stated that one Licinius Murena invented the first fish farm. Fish were prized by the Romans as food, for leisure fishing and as pets. As a result fish ponds and cultivation/farming in various degrees were widely practised. It is unlikely that the fish were in any way domesticated and there is little evidence of the existence of active breeding programmes. The main economic production of table fish was with the freshwater species in either natural or constructed lakes. These had a controlled water flow, gratings at exit points to confine the fish, and a designated feeding and harvesting plan.

Large fish tanks (*piscinae*) were constructed, usually located near the sea to keep marine fish, ready for the table. Several of these tanks have been found, now under water off the Mediterranean coast located from the South of France to Palestine. Some of the best examples are in Eastern Crete, Cyprus (at Lapithos) and a huge system found in 1964 just off the coast at Caesarea, Israel. This latter is calculated to have been built c.22–9 BC, on the orders of King Herod: the main tank is 115 ft by 58 ft with multiple feeder tanks, holding tanks, and connecting channels together with sluice gates. The Lapithos and Caesarea tanks are cut out of the rock (James and Thorpe 1994, pp. 402–403).

Species Cultivated

Marine

Muraena muraena, Roman eel, moray eel or murena. Found in the Mediterranean and other seas. A popular species in Roman times, unlikely that it was domesticated or bred but mainly fed ready for the table.

Mugil cephalus, grey mullet, *Mullus barbatus* and *Mullus surmuleta*, red mullet or goatfish, also called *Triglia*. Members of the Mugilidae family of about 80 species. Important Mediterranean fish and Roman food, very valued in Roman times. Fish were caught and then kept and fed in ponds or tanks, near the seashore. In Asia the local mullet species, termed milk fish, were cultivated by retention of natural fry in shallow sea lagoons or brackish water ponds.

Labrus mixtus, rainbow wrasse and *Labrus viridis*, green wrasse. Found in the Mediterranean. Popular food with Romans for retention in ponds and tanks for fattening, also enjoyed because of their distinctive colours.

Freshwater

Cyprinus carpio, the common carp. The European and Asian carps are possibly two subspecies. The initial and main area of cultivation was in China where this was recorded in at least 2000 BC. There is evidence that carp were in fishponds in Eastern Europe by AD 200–300 and also in fishponds in the later Roman Empire, but there is no record of their breeding in confinement at this date. In Europe, domestication was advanced by cultivation and breeding in captivity in monastery fishponds between the 7th and 13th centuries. This became a very important activity across Continental Europe until the development of deep sea fishing and salt preservation was able to meet the year-round demand. Carp have continued to be cultivated in Europe in particular in the Eastern countries as food, but in the West more as a sport fish. Indian carps have been cultured for several thousand years but they were not domesticated in the way that the Chinese developed the species.

Tilapia group, classified as *Tilapia* (ten species) and *Sarotherodon* (c.100 species). The Egyptians regarded tilapia as sacred, they appear in bas-reliefs dating from 3000 BC. Scenes depict *S. niloticius* as an important Egyptian fishery species. There is good evidence that they were farmed and bred in specially constructed fishponds from about 2000 BC. Other species of importance have been *S. mossambicus*, *S. spilurus* and *Tilapia zillii*. While essentially freshwater fish, most species will thrive in brackish or even seawater. Some can even tolerate a water temperature up to 42°C. Tilapia species have remained popular as they are a good food source, resistant to disease and will survive in, and tolerate, inadequate environments and poor water quality.

Carassius auratus, goldfish. The wild fish in China is believed to be a variety of *Carassius carassius*, the crucian carp. It is called ji-yu and the domesticated form is jin ji-yu or jin-yu. In Japanese this is kingyo (Zhang Zhong-ge 1984, pp. 381–382). Over the centuries there has been significant breeding work to develop varied colours and forms. Chinese records suggest that the wild form was known as early as AD 249 but serious domestication does not appear to have commenced until the Sung dynasty AD 960–1278. Goldfish were introduced to Japan about AD 1500 and to Europe probably in the early 1600s. They were introduced to England in 1705, Scandinavia by 1740, France 1750 and all Europe during that same century. The first imports from the United States of America (USA) occurred at the beginning of the 19th century (Zhang Zhong-ge 1984, pp. 382–383).

Macropodus chinensis or *Macropodus viridiauratus*, paradise fish. This species, with many variants and subspecies has been bred and cultivated in China for many hundreds of years, it is a small fish with long fins and beautiful colours. Following introduction to Europe and North America, it has become a small but significant part of the economically valuable aquarium market (Axelrod and Vorderwinkler 1962, pp. 432–433).

Salmo salar, Atlantic Salmon and *Oncorhynchus kisutch*, Coho Salmon (one of six Pacific species) the Salmonids, together with the trout also in the Salmo genus: *S. trutta* brown trout, *Oncorhynchus mykiss* (Walbaum) rainbow trout and *S. clarki* cutthroat trout (there are also several other species). These fish have been a significant food source in all areas of the world where they occur naturally. Development of commercial trout and salmon culture began in the period 1850–1870. The first recorded artificial fertilisation, incubation and hatching of eggs is attributed to a German in the late 1700s, with the brown trout.

Bivalve Molluscs

Ostrea edulis, native oyster, *Crassostrea angulate*, cupped oyster. Consumption of wild oysters dates from very early times: they were an easy to harvest and nutritious food. No date is known for the start of cultivation which dates from at least Roman times. Pliny noted that *O. edulis* was first cultivated by Sergius Orata in the 1st century AD when he shipped seed oysters (spats) from near Brindisi to be fattened at Baiae in Lago Lucrino, a seawater lake near Naples.

Napoleon III (1808–1873) directed a French biologist, V Coste, to devise methods to re-establish French oyster beds. He constructed simple methods of collecting oyster spats at sea following spawning in summer, in the following spring these were taken to protected tidal areas or artificial basins. The main objective was to prevent predators – rays, crabs and starfish from reaching the growing oysters. In later years, these basic techniques have been further developed in the coastal regions of many countries (Yonge 1984, p. 429).

China has a history of farming oysters with the objective of producing pearls. Records date from AD 1088, but cultivation had been practised since many years earlier. The insertion was made of not just irritant seed material but also small carvings in specific shapes, that is drops or Buddhas, to produce pearly coated objects of commercial value.

Mytilus edulis, the European mussel. These were also cultivated by the Romans using similar techniques to those of oysters, on suspended ropes in Lago del Fusaro and elsewhere. Since the 13th century mussel cultivation has been practised in the Anse de l'Alguillon near La Rochelle on the Bay of Biscay coast, first on nets but later on 'hedges' of intertwined twigs, branches and stakes: the *bouchet* system.

Suetonius, the Roman writer, stated that one of the reasons that Julius Caesar invaded Britain in 55 BC was the fame of the pearls obtained from British freshwater mussels. Pearls were much prized by Roman women, as they also were by Cleopatra.

Early Domestication and Farming Practices

Egypt

The Nile Valley provides some of the earliest evidence of the importance of fish in the human diet, starting from 7000 BC, the Epipalaeolithic period. Excavations have revealed sophisticated water management systems evolved to handle the Nile and its flooding as early as 5000 BC, fish were probably the basis of the early Nilotic economy. A particular interest was the Nile catfish *(Synodontis batensoda)*, this grows to a large size and is characterised by being an upside-down feeder at the water surface, presumably enabling easier capture. Food remains from this period indicate fish included in the diet comprised 68% *Tilapia*, 30% *Claria*, catfish spp. and the rest *Synodontis*, *Barbus* and *Latus* species. Rock art sites of pre-Neolithic dating south of

Edfu appear to show drawings of sophisticated fish traps (Hendrikx and Vermeersch 2000, pp. 29–31). Fish played a role in the developing culture; images of Nile fish species (tilapia and catfish) appear on bowls (4000–3000 BC) as well as carved ivory fish and later ivory models of fish. Bones from the large catfish were used to engrave pots and the pectoral bones were used as light arrowheads. In the local tongue catfish were called *Nar* (Romer 2012, p. 102, p. 134 and p. 157).

Tilapia became an important part of Egyptian religious belief; they were considered to symbolise the hope of rebirth after death and were designated as sacred. This was probably a recognition of the fish being able to survive the most potentially lethal environments, including partial desiccation. *S. niloticus* is frequently depicted in wall paintings and bas-reliefs from c.3000 BC. There is also evidence from wall paintings (2000 BC) of clearly depicted tilapia cultivation in fishponds. The ponds were well built and drainable: the activity would appear to have been an important part of Egyptian culture (Chimitz 1955, pp. 1–33). There is little clear evidence that catfish were also raised in ponds but such cultivation probably occurred as several varieties of the species are easily adaptable to confinement.

Roman Empire

Romans not only liked to eat seafood, they also found aquatic creatures fascinating – as shown by the images incorporated into mosaic floors, notably in the Pompeii excavations and the Bardo museum in Tunis.

The moray eel was a favourite species, but it was recognised that keeping such a marine fish in restricted spaces needed care. They are known as aggressive creatures yet stories in Roman literature describe how one Marcus Crassus had a favourite moray eel which was adorned with earrings and a jewelled necklace, and would come when called to be fed by hand. Pliny tells of Antonia, daughter of Drusus, who had a favourite lamprey (*Lampetra* spp.) which was adorned with gold earrings on the gills, and much admired at her country house at Baiae, near Naples. [There appears to be some confusion in the translation of ancient texts between morays and lampreys – both eel-like fish.]

The Romans' position as the dominant culture in Europe resulted in a society structured around wealth, and within that, ostentation and 'fashion'. Fish featured strongly in this cultural scene, the red mullets (*Mullus barbatus* and *Mullus surmuleta)* were particular objects of admiration and ostentation, as well as being favoured delicacies. *M. surmuleta* was probably the most valued for both appearance and flavour. There are several stories of the fish being fed and caressed by their owners and single specimens being sold for their weight in silver: behaviour which was much criticised by others. Martial (AD 40–103) in one story satirises a wealthy person who sold a slave for 1200 sesterces, and then bought a 4 lb mullet with the money.

Pliny wrote that the red mullet tasted like an oyster, Galen also commented that the fish was 'prized by men as superior to the rest in tastiness on eating' (*De Alimentorum Facultatibus* III.26). At the height of the red mullet fad, the custom was to bring to the dining table the dying fish in a glass bowl to both assure the diners of its freshness and to admire the changes in colour seen as it perished. Seneca wrote in *Natural Questions* III 18.1.4:

> *There is nothing, you say, more beautiful than a dying surmullet. In the very struggle of its failing breath of life, first a red, then a pale tint suffuses it, and its scales change hue, and between life and death there is a graduation of colour into subtle shades . . . See how the red becomes inflamed, more brilliant than any vermillion! Look at the veins which pulse along its sides. You would think its belly were actual blood. What a bright kind of blue gleamed right under its brow. Now it is stretching out and going pale and is settling into a uniform hue.*

The Greeks named the fish *triglê*, possibly due to a belief that the fish spawned three times a year. Aristotle noted its behaviour in hiding its head in the mud when frightened. The mullet was also dedicated to Hecate, the goddess of crossroads, who looks three ways.

Varro, Columella and Pliny all wrote about fish cultivation. Varro, writing in the 1st century BC, discusses frequently overlooked agriculture revenue sources and identifies fish cultivation citing that 'Marcus Cato sold fish from his farm worth 400,000 sesterces'. Ponds could be of either fresh or saltwater and enclosed, near to the villa; he refers to freshwater ponds and keeping *squali* or *mugiles*, [this is confusing as these are only known as sea fish, Pliny writing in the 1st century AD also refers to them and mentions Aristotle as his source]. Varro is critical of fish snobs but mentions Sergius Orata and Licinius Muraena (also noted by Columella) and lists the famous fishponds, 'of Phillipus, Hortensius and the Lucilli'.

Varro suggests that freshwater ponds are for the common folk, for domestic fish species, but not unprofitable. Seawater ponds were the favourite of the nobility and that they 'appeal more to the eye than the purse', and that they 'exhaust the pouch of the owner, rather than fill it. They are built at great cost, stocked at great cost and are kept at great cost'. He mentions one Hirrus, 'who would take 12,000 sesterces from the buildings around his ponds but then spent all that on fish food'.

Hirrus was recorded as having 'lent Caesar on one occasion 2000 lampreys' [Pliny later said it was 6000, and for a celebration]. There is no mention of how they were transported, or returned, but Hirrus later sold his villa for 4,000,000 sesterces.

Quintus Hortensius had expensive seawater ponds built at Bauli, near Naples, but was said to send to Puteoli (three to four miles away) to buy fish for dinner. His speciality was the barbed mullet which he would feed by hand, and employed fishermen to catch small fish to feed his stock. When the sea was too rough for fishing he would buy salted fish for their food. He was also said to be more concerned over a sick fish than 'an ailing slave' (the only mention of fish disease in his writings). Varro noted that Hortensius was careful that his fish always had clean water, replaced regularly. In discussing the ponds kept by the Lucillus brothers, he was critical of Marcus because his ponds did not have tidal basins, resulting in the water becoming stagnant, whereas his brother Lucius had a channel cut through a mountain to allow a stream of seawater into his ponds so that 'they ebbed and flowed'. He also constructed cooler places for his fish to shelter in hot weather. The ponds Lucius constructed, at great expense, were at Bauli, between Baiae and Misenum; Varro stated, 'the remains can still be seen'. There were many villas in this favoured area of the Italian coast. In his conversational manner Varro was warning that saltwater ponds were an extravagance and more for ostentation than profit, but freshwater ponds could be useful. He stressed the practical point that attention had to be given to water quality and avoidance of stagnant, unshaded ponds. His homely practical advice was widely read and well appreciated for many years.

The most important Roman agricultural author was Columella (AD 4–70). He noted that his ancestors 'even imprisoned saltwater fish in fresh water and fed the grey mullet and parrot wrasse with the same care with which the murry and sea-basse are now reared' and discusses a lake in Umbria, and four to the north-west of Rome, producing basse and gilthead, 'and all fishes that can be found in fresh water'. The lakes are still identifiable.

Later this method of cultivation was abandoned by wealthy patrons and they invested in seawater ponds, which became a symbol of both gluttony and money. Columella mentions two Romans who made fish ponds their particular piscine interest, rejoicing in the names of Sergius Orata (gilthead) and Licinius Muraena (murry).

Discussing the economics of fish farming Columella stated that a fishpond could be a source of profit for a country estate, and very useful if there was poor land available beside the sea. He advised that muddy water was good for flat fish – sole, turbot and flounder (or plaice, translation unsure), also for 'testaceous animals' such as *Murex* spp. molluscs, oysters, small scallops and the sea-acorus or *spondyli* (*Spondylus gaedaropus*, the spring-oyster). Sandy whirlpools were seen to be better for deep sea fish such as gilthead and dentex, but less suitable for shellfish. A rocky seashore was perceived as excellent for rock fish: merle-wrasse, thrush-wrasse and also 'black-tails'. He stated that one must know the qualities of both the sea and shore as well as those of the fish, not all fish will live well in any situation, but cited one exception, the valuable moray, 'which can thrive in strange waters'. Of note in this discussion was the wide knowledge of the fish species, not only naming them but understanding the environments to which they were adapted.

Practical management of ponds was stressed by Columella. Location was a key factor, plus construction, so that incoming tides will expel existing water and replace it with new. Additionally a wind prone site was preferred to enable water to be stirred and moved in the pond. Construction of the pond, either in rock (good, but rare due to cost) or by built and plastered ponds. Emphasis was given to make recesses in the pond floor for fish to shelter, but warning that moray eels should be kept separate as they will eat other fish. Care in construction was stressed, with guarded access points, to keep the fish in and predators out, with all gratings made of brass. Water exit points must be placed opposite entrance points, with it being essential to get incoming water as cold as possible. If the pond's ground level is at sea level then the hole must be excavated to a depth of at least 9 ft and the water channels placed at least 2 ft below the surface. Columella notes the importance of shade and the inclusion of recesses and 'caves' in the walls, for fish to shelter in. It was recommended that rocks with seaweeds or vegetation attached be placed on the bottom of the pond to provide a more natural environment for the fish.

In discussing the choice of fish to be cultivated and fed Columella warned that it did not pay to catch and keep cheap value fish; 'the sluggish grey mullet and greedy basse' do well and are good value. Rocky shore fish were seen as suitable as well as floating morays and rock-dwelling morays (high value). Advice was given that red surmullet is a very delicate fish and intolerant of captivity. Care in feeding was emphasised, noting that flat fish require a softer diet than rock fish, as they lack teeth. It was suggested that decaying shad or pilchard or entrails of several fish (listed) could be used as food, cut-open green figs, ripe crushed arbutus berry or fresh curds from a milk pail can all be fed, but best was the refuse of salted fish; this has a strong odour and flat fish track food by scent. He stressed that fish cultivation should be based on the same principles as terrestrial agriculture – only farm what the land will sustain.

Other fish types such as rock, shore or open sea species could also be fed on salt fish refuse but do best on fresh food – newly caught shad, shrimp, prawn or small goby. If, however, bad weather prevents fishing, a temporary diet could comprise bits of coarse bread or cut up seasonal fruit, as well as dried figs. Columella stresses that fish must be fed every day if they are to be fattened for market: his closing words on fish cultivation reflect the pragmatic Roman approach – if the fish are not fed properly 'a large sum will be knocked off the price'. Columella gave good practical advice. While he made no mention of fish diseases it cannot be presumed they did not exist in these ponds, but it could be assumed that if they were present they did not provide a significant deterrent to the practice. He only described a fattening system, not a breeding cycle and its management.

Pliny (AD 23–79), in *Historia Naturalis* written in the middle years of the 1st century AD, includes the creatures of the sea. It is a jumble of information, some credible and informative, but much incredible and fictional. Pliny tried to collect the information that was known, but was unable to form judgements on topics that he had not experienced. Book IX of *Historia Naturalis* – after discussing tritons, nereids, mermaids and mermen – claims to review all the fish and creatures of the water. The section on oysters mostly discusses the pearls worn by Lollia Paulina, wife of Emperor Caligula, and in particular those owned by Cleopatra. He describes oyster fattening systems, termed *ostriaria*, where they were suspended on ropes in Lago Lucrimo, Naples region, this was a saltwater lake and was rich in organic nutrients and plankton. This continued for many years, also at Lago del Fusaro, near modern Taranto – all in southern Italy. At the end of this book is a short section on 'sea-vermin' and naming what appear to be ectoparasites (*pediculi*) seen on some fish and also on bait laid to catch fish. Book XXXII of *Historia Naturalis* is a collection of stories about fish and claimed remedies for various human diseases, derived from fish or their body parts or organs. Licinius Macer is quoted as stating that lampreys (also translated as morays) are of the female sex only and conceive by coming to the shore and 'engendering with a serpent'. Fishermen were said to entice the lampreys from their lairs by hissing and then catching them (how this is done underwater is not stated). Pliny also wrote that if one hits a lamprey on the head it will not die, but if hit by a fennel stalk they die at once. Finally, a veterinary note: if pigs are bitten by snakes they cure themselves by seeking out and feeding on sea-crabs.

Oppian in the *Halieutica* (*Fishing*), written in verse and dedicated to the Emperor Marcus Aurelius, presents a good overview of the state of fishery knowledge in the 2nd century AD. The text ranges from equipment including boats, sails, ropes, nets, fishing lines, hooks (made of bronze) to an encyclopaedic listing of fish species. Over 150 are named, but with many of these there are difficulties in translation and transliteration, however the majority are recognisable as existing species. There are descriptions of each species, as well as a note on temperament, colours, preferred locale and a review of deep sea, shoreline, freshwater, estuarine, rocky or muddy environment preferences. Behaviours of different species by weather conditions, feeding, mating and breeding characteristics are all listed. Some observations are also made on fish diseases. In the light of later knowledge much of the information on reproduction is now seen as fanciful, these were processes generally not understood at that time. There are sailors' tales quoted, such as the discussion of lampreys bringing a ship to a standstill if they should cling to the ship's hull, even when under full sail. The text, however, indicates a breadth of understanding of aquatic species, demonstrating an interest in nature and natural history, and the ability to collect knowledge.

Palladius, writing *Opus Agriculturae* in the late 5th or early 5th centuries AD, does add an interesting comment on the construction of cisterns for holding river fish and eels. For the final stages of the work, waterproof mortar, made by the incorporation of crushed terracotta, must be used and is then 'polished assiduously to a sheen' with boiled down animal fat, finally a similar layer is used to coat the walls of the cistern.

The *Geoponika,* compiled in 10th century AD, was a distillation of more than a millennium of Greek and Latin writing and consists of many texts now long lost. The content demonstrates the importance of fish in the diets of people in the Roman and Byzantine Empires. Some 58 aquatic species (including crabs, shrimps, octopus) are named: these are not always recognisable. A major section is included on bait for fish (Book 20.7–45) but the text is incomplete and is faulty in parts. Bait mixtures and specific baits are discussed in detail, and some including 'magic' ingredients. The baits are not always attractive, for example, (20.33) 'Knead calf's bile with pearl barley and olive oil and water, make little lumps and use as bait. Chew the same compound, spit it into the water, and they will come to it'.

Various recipes are also given for the production of *garum,* the popular Roman fermented fish sauce. Complex attractant bait recipes are quoted (20.2) from the writings of Oppian: these comprised mixtures of plants, barley, wine, pigs liver, goat fat, garlic and so on. They were to be thrown into the water before the fishermen took their nets to that area and would cause fish to congregate, and be caught. In discussing the keeping of fish, the work of Florentinus (3rd century AD) is cited (20.1) on inland fishponds for freshwater fish and 'those from the sea that will live'. Diets for feeding sea fish and rock fish are advised and a plant, *polysporus,* is suggested for growing on the edge of the ponds and then thrown into the water.

Other Ancient Cultures

Herodotus, travelling between 450–420 BC, makes frequent mention of fish, they formed a significant part of economic activity and diet. He recorded that in Scythia (part of Ukraine bordering the Black Sea) some people catch huge fish called *antakaioi* (a species of sturgeon) in the local rivers, which they then salted for food. He tells of a Babylonian tribe that only eat fish: they dry them, pound them to a powder to make cakes and a type of bread; he writes of a marshland tribe in India who live on raw fish. In Paionia (Macedonia) he sees the people who live over the river in houses on stilts with trap doors in the floor through which they fish to catch *paprakes* and *tilones*, these provide their food and feed for their horses.

In his commentary on Egypt, Herodotus noted that the priests observe scrupulous hygiene but are not allowed to eat fish. One species was determined to be sacred and termed 'scaly' (this was probably a *Tilapia* spp.), the eel was also considered sacred. His descriptions of the Nile and other fisheries in Egypt, contain a mixture of myths, magic and folklore, the beliefs of the time.

Medieval Europe

Fish were an important component of the diet of the medieval church and their institutions. The increasing importance of monasteries demanded a constant supply, as meat (believed to encourage carnal thoughts) was proscribed on Holy days including the Lent period: some orders (Benedictine) totally forbade all meats. As a result, by the 1200s almost half of the days in a year had been designated holy in one way or another. Every monastery had to provide an acceptable diet to their members: the Cellarer was the administrator of food provisions and under him the Keeper of the Fishponds who was responsible for a regular supply (Fagan 2011, p. 314). As fish could only be transported short distances shortages were met by the use of salted fish, but this was always a second choice food. River fishing provided bream, pike and perch but was an unreliable source.

Both monasteries and major secular houses had fishponds, in Britain these were called stewponds (from Medieval English, derived from Old French *estui*, a place of confinement). These could be the size of a small lake with a controlled water flow, in which fish spawned were fed and grew, but it was difficult to produce enough fish for a daily diet and the cultivation became a major enterprise. The first farms developed in the Loire and Rhône valleys in the 11th century based in bream and pike. When carp arrived from the Danube, their farming spread rapidly across Europe from France to the Low Countries, Germany, Bohemia and Poland. The literature indicates that enormous areas and labour were involved, but the enterprises eventually failed, mostly due to neglect of the ponds and their boundaries. Improved methods of sea fishing and salting cod and herring provided a palatable and more economical alternative (Brooker 2006, p. 39 and p. 46).

Carp were never a popular food in Britain, possibly because of the taste, and because they had a reputation for being difficult to catch. This was recorded by Dame Juliana Barnes in her 1468 *Boke of St. Albans*, one of the earliest reports of the British carp. An interesting practice was described by Thomas Pennant (1726–1798). He wrote that a carp was 'very tenacious of life' and could be caught, placed in a net surrounded by wet moss, hung in a cellar or cool place and 'often plunged into water'. If fed frequently, over two weeks, with white bread and milk it would grow fat and superior in taste to those caught from the pond (Pennant 1776, p. 353). Pennant also wrote that such fish produced much roe, which was 'used as a caviar for Jews'. None of the descriptions of monastery fishpond cultivation or freshwater cultivation generally mention any problems with disease.

China

The country has a history of fish cultivation, dating back at least 4000 years. The common carp has been farmed in China for a long time and a system of polyculture ponds developed, with slatted floor pig houses built over the water, ducks swimming on the surface and carp in the pond. The pigs and ducks provide frequent manuring ensuring an adequate food supply; Chinese carp have a better fecundity than the European variety (Wohlforth 1984, pp. 375–377).

Ornamental fish have been pioneered by Chinese fish cultivators. The goldfish was developed from the wild, probably from the 1st century AD, they became objects of wealth in the early dynasties from AD 260–420 and were well domesticated by the time of the Sung dynasty, AD 960–1278. By the 1100s breeding goldfish in ponds became a popular hobby of the wealthy classes. Specialist breeding became established in the Ming dynasty (1368–1644), breeding, cultivation and feeding techniques advanced; the fish were kept in tanks and basins rather than ponds, which developed to fish being kept in bowls in the home. The Qing (Ching) dynasty became the apex of goldfish breeding in China. In the late 1800s, the hobby reached its peak and still remains a major interest in China (Zhang Zhong-ge 1984, pp. 381–383). The goldfish is one of the most highly domesticated of all animals.

China has also been responsible for the development of paradise fish as an ornamental species. The believed original wild ancestor is distributed in China, Korea, Taiwan, India, Ceylon and Malaysia. The fish is much prized by the Chinese for its coloration, mating display, foam nests and male care of the young. There is little background available but the species has been domesticated for many hundreds of years and is now a popular home aquarium species (Zeuner 1963, pp. 482–483, Axelrod and Vorderwinkler 1962, pp. 456–457). Chinese cultivation of oysters for the production of both pearls and pearlised objects also has a history of at least 1000 years.

Hawaiian Islands

In ancient Hawaii, an integrated farming system developed, including massive freshwater and seawater fishponds. The river estuaries and streams were adapted to create fishponds, possibly as early as AD 500. The major ponds studied have been dated back at least 1000 years. The system involved vegetable and plant production in irrigated regions as well as fish cultivation, mainly milkfish and mullet. When Captain Cook reached Hawaii in 1778 at least 360 fishponds existed producing some 900,000 kg of fish per year. By 1985 only seven ponds were in use, the decline followed a decision to allow foreigners to purchase land (Costa-Pierce 1987, pp. 320–331).

Recognition of Fish and Mollusc Diseases

The early literature is fragmented and is frequently difficult to understand: the records were a mixture of observation and belief, which were then the acceptable form of communication (Moulé 1908, pp. 260–262). Fish ailments (usually parasitosis from current recognition) are mentioned in some of the ancient texts (Blancou 2008, p. 86).

The Kahun (el-Lahun) papyrus, the earliest description of animal disease in Egypt, dated from about 1900 BC, has one section that can be interpreted as the treatment of an eye disease in a fish, but the exact meaning is open to debate (Walker 1964, pp. 198–201). An Egyptian wall painting of about 1450 BC depicts a tilapia with a grossly enlarged abdomen, which it is suggested could be due to a neoplasm (Mawdesley-Thomas 1972, pp. 191–284). Other Egyptian papyri have revealed descriptions that have been interpreted as infestations with *Diphyllobothrium* spp (possibly *D. latum*). It has been suggested by Moulé (1911, pp. 543–595) that parasitosis in fish was frequent in antiquity.

The Years of Antiquity to AD 400

The earliest specific observations on fish health appear in Aristotle, *Historia Animalum (History of Animals)*, written some 2350 years ago. He notes (Book VII, 20:21) conditions in which fish either thrive or do not do well and also states,

> *No general plague-like sickness I observed to strike any of the fishes, such as often occurs in humans and attacks horses and cattle . . . . Nevertheless they are thought to have illnesses: the fishermen infer this from the fact that some which are thin and look sickly and have changed colour are caught among many others of the same kind which are fat.*

Aristotle discusses health in differing weather conditions and concludes that 'the fishes, apart from a certain few, are benefited by wet weather' as rainy weather encourages the reeds that grow in the marshes. He also noted that fish migrate to the *Pontus* (Black Sea) because the rivers make the water 'sweeter' and bring down food while some, such as the bonito and grey mullet swim up the rivers. 'They do not thrive in cold places' this statement is followed by a listing of various fish species that are 'blinded' by rain showers and winter storms, many of these have 'white eyes'. Particular note is made of the tunny (tuna) and swordfish who suffer 'oistros-frenzy at the rising of the dog-star' [mid-July the hottest weather/the dog-days]. At this time both species have beside the fins 'a sort of little grub called a gadfly, resembling a scorpion but the size of a spider'; the bite of these parasites, termed *oestros*, created such pain that they were said to cause the swordfish to leap out of the water, sometimes as high as the dolphin. This parasite has not been identified. Moulé (1908, pp. 260–262) has suggested it was probably a copepod.

A similar ectoparasite is described by Oppian in the *Halieutica* (Book II, verses 506–520), again affecting the tuna and swordfish. From the wording Oppian must have been using Aristotle as his source. The verses are quoted in full, translations used the term 'gadfly' for the parasite, as the symptoms described were similar to those recognised in cattle attacked by the gadfly (*Hypoderma bovis*). The clinical descriptions are of interest. The parasites of the fish are now identified as *Brachiella Thynni* in tuna and *Pennatula filosa* in swordfish.

> *The tunny and swordfish are ever attended and companioned by a plague: a fierce gadfly which infests their fins, when the burning Dog-star is newly risen, fixes in them the swift might of its bitter sting, and with sharp assault stirs them to grievous madness, making them drunk with pain. With the lash of frenzy it drives them to dance against their will; maddened by the cruel blow they rush and now here, now there ride over the waves, possessed by pain unending. Often also they leap into well-beaked ships, driven by the stress of their distemper; and often they leap forth from the sea and rush writhing upon the land, and exchange their weary agonies for death, so dire a pain is heavy upon them and abates not. Yea, for oxen also, when the cruel gadfly attacks them and plunges its arrow in their tender flanks, have no more regard for the herdsman nor for the pasture nor for the herd, but leaving the grass and all the folds they rush, whetted by frenzy; no river nor untrodden sea nor ragged ravine nor pathless rocks stays the course of the bulls, when the gadfly hot and sharp impels urging them with keen pains. Everywhere there is bellowing, everywhere range their bounding hoofs: such bitter tempest drives. This pain the fishes suffer even as do the cattle.*

Aristotle (Book VII/VIII) discusses diseases of freshwater fish: the *glanis*, at dog-star time especially swims near the surface and becomes 'star-struck', it is also 'stupefied' by violent thunder, he wrote that this also sometimes happens with carp. Fish described as the *balliros* (possibly bream) and *tilon* are recorded as having an intestinal worm which develops at the time of the dog-star causing them to become weak and appear at the water surface, where they 'are destroyed by heat'. Another fish termed a *chalkis* (this word is also used for other species) can be attacked by a 'violent disease: lice are produced under the gills in large numbers and destroy it'. Aristotle also noted that fishes are killed by mullein (*Verbascum sinuatum*), used by fishers to more easily net fish in rivers either for the table or for transport to lakes (it presumably had an initial stunning or narcotic effect).

Virgil (70–19 BC) wrote *Georgics* (*A Poem of the Land*) and in one place mentions a bovine disease but seemingly implies that this also affects fish (III.540): 'The brood of the unfathomable sea, and all the race of swimmers, wash up along the shoreline like shipwrecked hulls upon the breakers, and the prodigious seals flee up into rivers'.

Blancou (2008, p. 86) cites Paulet who has translated this and interprets the meaning as claiming that bovine pleuro-pneumonia also affected, 'wolves, deer, fallow deer, vipers and fish'. Virgil was a poet and he was only repeating stories that he had been told. Galen (AD 129–210) in *The Aphorisms of Hippocrates* noted worms in the mouth and muscles of a red mullet, but left no further comment.

The Period of Natural Observation, AD 400–1699

After the years of antiquity, which produced a record of practices and observations by the Roman and Greek authors, Europe slowly restructured following the collapse of the Roman Empire. The surviving literature of aquatic interest for this period is found in the ancient annals and chronicles. Those items identified and listed as follows record events concerning fish health. Some of the citations have been sourced from Fleming's *Animal Plagues: Their History, Nature and Prevention* (1871).

444 *England* 'A great mortality among fish'. (*Nicephorus* XV.10)

600 *China* In the 7th century, Sui Dynasty, Chao-Yuan-Fang wrote, 'it is believed that infestation by *Pay-ch'ung* follows the consumption of raw fish'. (*Pay-ch'ung* was translated as designating both *Taenia* sp. and *D. latum*, in Blancou (2008) citing G. Penso (1981) *La conquête du monde invisible. Parasites et microbes à travers les siècles*, Roger Dacosta: Paris p. 37)

916 *Ireland* 'great snow, cold, unusual frost . . . a destruction was brought upon cattle, birds and salmon'. (*Annals of Innisfallen*)

1014 *Bohemia* 'fearful heat and drought . . . rivers were dried up; lakes were corrupted and putrescent . . . especially did immense numbers of fish die'. (Hagek and Liboczan, *Annals Bohemor.* V p. 74)

1046 *England* 'severe winter with frost and snow . . . fishes perished through the great cold and hunger'. (*Anglo-Saxon Chronicles*)

1240 *England* 'Disease attacked the fish on the coast of England . . . There was also a great battle among the fishes on the English coast, by which eleven whales and other monstrous fishes were cast on the shore dead'. (*T. Short* Vol I, p. 143)

1240 *Germany* Albertus Magnus (c.1193–1280) described parasitic worms from horses, dogs, falcons and fishes. Literature searches have failed to reveal any significant records relating to fish disease or health for the almost 300 year period between 1240–1529.

1529 *Germany* The year of 'the sweating in mankind . . . dangerous to eat fish, as it was reported that malignant and contagious disease had been traced to this cause' (Leuthinger *Scriptorum* p. 90).

1554 *Europe* A mention of a parasite designated crustacea, in fish. (H. Salviani, *Aquatilium Animalium Historiae* Vol I (folio) Rome)

1560 *Europe* A mention of parasites in fish in Zurich lake, translation has suggested both a crustacean and also the larvae of *Diphyllobothrium latum*, if so the latter would be the earliest description of the ploceroid larvae. (Conrad Gesner *Historia Animalium – De Aquatilibus*, five vols, Zurich)

1591   *Germany* Mortality of fish in Leipzig region. (Vogels *Annals* p. 268)

1592   *Europe* Thad. Dunus made probably the first recognisable description of '*Diphyllobothrium latum* in *Locarnensis medici epistolae medicinales* . . .' (R. Hoeppli, 1956, 'The Knowledge of Parasites and Parasitic Infections from Ancient Times' *Exp. Parasit* V p. 410)

1592   *Europe* Felix Plater differentiated *Diphyllobothrium latum* from *Taenia* in *Praxeos medicae opus.* (cited by R. Hoeppli, 1956)

1600   *Europe* In *De Alimento*, Francesco Buonamici gives a description of small parasitic creatures on the skin of a fish (regarded as probably copepods by G. Penso (1981) 'La conquête du monde invisible. Parasites et microbes á travers les siècles' Roger Dacosta: Paris p. 134)

1609   *North America* Atlantic coastline. Captain John Smith reported 'crowded, surfacing and dead fish in natural waters of all species'. The live fish had their heads above water and small cod were also seen. (from 'Captain John Smith's America' by J Lankford (1967), Harper and Row)

1634   *England* In one of the earliest entomological compilations, Thomas Muffet (or Moufet) naturalist and physician, had a particular interest in insects in regard to medicine, noted that fish like most other animals could be infested with lice. (*Insectorum Minimorum Animalium Theatrum*)

1655   *Europe* A disease of fish was reported in lakes and ponds, 'people who had eaten them were attacked by a pestilential disease which killed a very great number. Even the dogs which ate the unburied dead were attacked by madness'. (Gothofred, *Chronicles*).

1671   *Europe* A description of a crustacean, probably a *Penella*, found on a swordfish. (S.P. Boccone, 1671, *Recherches et Observations Naturelles*, Paris)

1680   *Europe* Report of the death of many fish in Mansfeldi and Langenbogia lakes, mostly in freshwater and to a lesser degree saltwater lakes. Fish perished in large numbers, 'They had spots of various colours – black, red, yellow and green – dotted here and there over their bodies'. They had a foul odour and a nauseous taste causing vomiting, fever and chest pains in those who consumed them. The fishermen also developed ulcerated faces. The cause was attributed to 'foul nebulae that pervaded the water'. The lake surface was covered in a green scum. The author also wrote, 'Some annals attest that an epidemic disease in fish is a most sure prognostication of a future plague'. (Stegmann *Ephem. Nat. Curios.* Vol II, p. 386 and p. 427)

1691   *England* A discussion of cestodes as parasites of fish. (E. Tyson, 1691 '*Lumbricus hydropicus*, or an essay to prove that hydatids often met with in morbid animal bodies, are a species of worms, or imperfect animals' *Philos. Trans.* London, 17: pp. 506–511.)

1698   *North America* The Council Papers of Virginia for 1698 report that large fish kills resulted from the killing and processing of whales in the Chesapeake river, 'great quantities of fish are poisoned and destroyed and the rivers are made noisesome and offensive'. (S.G. Davidson, 1997, *Chesapeake Waters* Tidewater: Centreville p. 52 and p. 333)

The Development of Biological Observations 1700–1800

1709 *Switzerland* The continent experienced influenza in man, crop diseases and livestock epidemy, 'a pustular epizooty destroyed nearly all the fish in the lake of Zurich'. (*Sendschriben von der Peste in Dantzig*, p. 4)

1711 *Germany* A year of much recorded disease in birds, livestock and in fishes. (Kanold, *Histor. Relationen von der Pestilentz des Hornviehs*. Breslau, 1714)

1714 *Silesia* 'Owing to some local causes the fish died in many lakes in Silesia'. (Kanold, *Jahreshist.*, pp. 119–206)

1717 *Germany* In Silesia, 'there was a great mortality among bees and carp and in Brandenburg . . . the ponds were poisoned by a noxious mist or vapour, so that the surface of the water appeared quite blue, animals which drank from it were killed. Even the fish in the waters died, and were cast upon the banks.'

1722 *Germany* Lake Constance, also bordered by Switzerland and Austria: 'there was a great destruction among the fishes in the lake . . . caused, it is conjectured, by the excessively high temperature in March' then followed by extreme cold, 'When the dead bodies were examined, it was found that the swimming or air-bladders were extremely distended, and that reddish pustules were formed on all the viscera'. (Didier, *Traité de la Peste*, p. 540)

1726 *Germany* An exceedingly dry and hot year, mortality in cattle, deer and the fish perished in ponds and lakes. (*Breslauer Sammlung*, Vol XXXVI p. 690; Vol XXXVII p. 54)

1735 *Europe* In descriptions of fish Carl Linnaeus listed a parasite which he termed *Fasciola intestinalis*, found in the intestinal tract. (first edition of *Systema Naturae*, published in the Netherlands, 1735)

1741 *Ireland* A bad year for both humans and livestock, 'the mortality of the people must have been increased by feeding on the diseased animals. There were . . . shoals of dead fish cast on shore'. (Mr Curry to Dr Petrie in pamphlet, *Famine in Ireland in 1740, 1741*)

1744 *England* Report of parasite 'from eye of sprat, probably a *Lernaeenicus* a crustacean'. (A newly discovered sea-insect called the eye-sucker *Philos. Trans. Roy. Soc. London*. 43 No.472, p. 15)

1746 *Europe* Carl Linnaeus gives a very detailed description of a parasitic crustacean named *Lernea*. (*Fauna Suecica Sistens Animalia Suecica Regni* Ed.1 Stockholm).

1757 *France* 'A peculiar carbuncular epizooty appeared in the province of Brie among horses, cattle, deer, asses, hogs, dogs and fowls, and even in fish'. (A. de Chaignebrun *Relation d'une Maladie Epidemique et Contagieuse* Paris, 1762)

1758 *Europe* Carl Linnaeus reported a crustacean parasite of fish (*Systema Naturae* 10th Edition, Stockholm). In a later edition of *Systema Naturae*, Linnaeus includes a miscellaneous collection of parasites of fish. Volume 1, pages 1069–1327, published in 1766.

1759 *Europe* Report of crustacean, named *Chinensia lagerstromiana*. (J.L. Odhelius *Amoen. Acad. of Linnaeus* 4:257)

1760 *France* In the river Dive, Calvados department, 'an epizootic disease was observed among the fish . . . Two or three kinds of epizootic diseases were seen'. While not producing a general mortality, the majority were seen to be sickly and weak, floating on the surface. Both the gills and cut flesh were pale. Salmon, pike, plaice and other fish were all affected. It was suggested that the cause may be foul water draining to the river after flooding of marshy areas. (Adam, Chabert et al., *Instructions and Observations* 3 p. 331)

1762 *Denmark* Report of crustacean parasite of fish in Norwegian waters. (H. Strom *Physisk og Oeconomisk Beskrivelse over Fogderiet Sondmor* Part 1, Copenhagen)

1763 *North America* The native population of Nantucket 'were attacked by a bilious fever, which killed a large proportion of their number. Immediately after the disease had subsided, a large fish, called blue fish, which had previously been caught in great numbers, suddenly disappeared'. (Webster, Vol I, p. 412)

1763 *England* Report of *Pennella* crustacean parasitism. (J. Ellis, Of the sea pen of *Pennatula phosphorea* of Linnaeus. *Philos. Trans.* 53 p. 419 Pennella)

1767 *Europe* Crustacean parasites of fish described by V. de Bomare. (*De almind-eliga Natur-histoire, Form af et Dictionnaire*, 1767–1770, Copenhagen)

1774 *North America* At Cape Cod a bed of oysters 'perished from disease and at York Island the lobsters mysteriously disappeared'. Dates are confused, could be 1775. (G. Fleming, *Animal Plagues: Their History, Nature and Prevention* 1871, Chapman and Hall p. 465)

1775 *Europe* Report of a crustacean parasite of fish. (J.G. Koelreuter, *Lernaeae* forsan adhuc incognitae *Gadi callarii* L., branchiis firmiter inhaerentis descriptio, *Acad. Theod. Palat.* 3(Phys):57–61)

1775 *Sumatra* 'A remarkable mortality among the finny tribes appears to have been observed at Sumatra; the sea was covered with their dead bodies'. (*Philos. Transac.* Vol IXXI)

1776 *Scandinavia* Reports on miscellaneous fish parasites found in waters off Norway and Denmark (O.F. Muller in *Zoologie Danica* Havniae), also reported in 1777.

1779 *Europe* Mention of two intestinal roundworms in fish, described as belonging to the genera *Cucullanus* and *Caryophilus* by Marcus Elieser Bloch. The latter was later diagnosed as a flatworm by G. Penso (1981, *op. cit.* p. 214).

1779 *Germany* J.F. Blumenbach in *Handbuch der Naturgeschichte*, Gottingen makes general observations on fish parasites.

1779 *Germany* Observations on predation of fish by parasites. (Von Muetzschefahl Nachricht von einigen wasser-insecten an der bartsch. *Oekon. Nachr. d. Cessells. in Schlesien* 6:393–394; 7:2–5)

1780 *Greenland* Report of crustacean fish parasite. (O. Fabricius, *Fauna Groenlandica* 8vo, Hafniae et Lipsiae. Bibliography:ff XI–XVI)

1780 *Denmark* Report of tapeworm (cestode) in fish. (O.F. Muller, Om Baendelorme Nye Saml. of det Kgl. Danske, *Vid-ensk. Selsk. Skrift.* Forste deel, Copenhagen, 1781)

1782 *Germany* Report of helminths in fish. (J.A.E. Goeze, Versuch einer Naturgeschichte der Eingewide wurmer thierischer Korper 471, Blankenburg)

1783 *England* Discussion of crustacean parasites in fish (J. Barbut, Genera Vermium exemplified by various specimens of the animals contained in the Orders of the Intestina et Mollusca Linnaei, (Lernaea) 8 vol. London)

1784 *Germany* Report of crustacean parasite in fish. (J.A.E. Goeze *Von der Fischlernaeen* Leipziger Mag. Naturk. 39–49)

1789 *Atlantic Coasts* Recorded that the codfish did not appear at the Newfoundland Banks at the usual time, nor off British coasts or in Baltic as expected. However, in July great numbers were found dead or dying off the coasts of Norway, Lapland and Archangel (Abbs. *Philosoph. Transac.* 1792). (It had been noted that in 1788 Newfoundland cod were thin and sickly and of no commercial value.)

1790 *Denmark* A notable study by physician/veterinarian P.C. Abildgaard in which he discovered and demonstrated for the first time the life cycle of a parasite and its intermediate host. This was the tapeworm (*Taenia gasterostei*) which has its plerocercoid period in the stickleback and the adult form in several species of seabirds (original paper by P.C. Abildgaard in *Skrivter af Naturhistorie-Selskabet,* 1790 1:1, 26–64). Abildgaard was probably the first worker to introduce experiments into parasitological research to prove his investigation results.

1790 *Europe* Report on crustacean parasite in fish. (J.F. Gmelin, in *Linnaeus Systema Naturae.* Editio decima tertia, aucta, reformata, cura. Lipsiae)

1792 *France* Report on crustacean (*Lerneaus* sp) parasites of fish. (J.G. Brugieres *Dictionaire des Vers. Encyclopedie Methodique* Vol 1, Paris)

1797 *USA* First report of fish parasite in the USA was made by B.H. Latrobe, appointed by Thomas Jefferson as the Surveyor of Public Buildings in charge of the White House and the Capitol. He observed a large crustacean parasite in the mouths of menhaden caught on the York river in Virginia, made careful drawings, naming it *Oniscus praegustator.* (B.H. Latrobe, 1802, A drawing and description of the *Clupea tyrannus* and *Oniscus praegstator Trans. Am. Philos. Soc.* Philadelphia 5:77–81)

1798 *France* Report of crustacea parasitising fish. (G.L. Cuvier, *Tableau elementaire de l'histoire naturelle des animaux* Vol 1, Paris, An 6)

1798 *France* Report of *Pennella* crustacea in fish. (Lamartiniere, *Atlas du Voyage de la Peyrouse,* Paris)

1799 *Germany* Report of nematode in fish. (G.F. Waldheim, Uber einen neu entdeckten Wurm in der Fischblase der Forelle *Cystidicola farionis, Arch. f.d. Physiol.,* Halle, 3(1):95–100)

Science Evolves With a Developing Veterinary Medicine Discipline 1800–1900

The start of the 19th century heralded the progressive organisation of the developing scientific disciplines. Veterinary medicine education was expanding rapidly in Europe, and the realisation was growing that parasites were a significant health problem in all species. Fish health and diseases had not yet featured as a division of veterinary science but some individuals were recognising the problems, in particular Peter Christian Abildgaard (Denmark). In the first half of the century several significant observations were made and, gradually, known clinical symptoms were being connected to causal agents.

1818   *North America* Thomas Say, considered to be the founder of descriptive entomology in the USA, described a crustacean, *Pandarus sinuatus*, from an Atlantic coast dogfish; a common crustacean, *Caligus piscinus*, on codfish and several other crustacea, of *Cymothoa* genus, on marine fishes. (Say's work was published in *J. Acad. Nat. Sci. Phil.* and reviewed by A.J. Mitchell (2001) 'Finfish Health in the United States, 1609–1969' *Aquaculture* 196 pp. 347–438)

1819   *Europe* Encapsulated nematode larvae were found in various species including fish. Rudolphi named these *Ascaris capsularia*; he was followed by von Siebold (1838) who asked whether these immature nematodes have to change their host. He suspected all parasitic nematodes needed an intermediate host, and was the first to recognise muscle *Trichinella* as the larval form. (cited by K. Enigk and H.C. Habil (1989) History of Veterinary Parasitology in Germany and Scandinavia. *Veterinary Parasitology* 33 pp. 65–91)

1823   *England* 'The sea in the vicinity of Exeter emitted noxious effluvia . . . and the fish were nearly dead . . . water was coloured with an oily matter all along the coast.' (Stokes, *Sketch of Epidemic Fever*)

1824   *North America* Charles A. Lesueur, a naturalist attached to the Philadelphia Academy of Natural Sciences, published details of three parasitic crustacea (*Lernaea* genus) found in Lake Erie. (cited by A.J. Mitchell, p. 359)

1825   *Germany* Foot-and-mouth disease in cattle, anthrax in horses, 'many fish in river Wolchow were covered with tumours and foul sores, crabs were found dead on the banks'. (Vieth. *Handbuch der Veterinarkunde* 1831)

1830–1832   *Baltic and East Prussian coast* A heavy mortality in marine fish was reported also fish perished in large numbers in lakes and ponds. 'From Zempelburg lake alone the police have already buried forty tuns full'. The problem was not uncommon, in the autumn large stagnant waters often assumed a green or reddish colour and soon afterwards the fish die. Under the microscope it was seen that the 'slime' was of a vegetable nature of many plants. A further report of occurrence and fish deaths are given for Switzerland and the Leipzig region. (G. Fleming 1882, *Animal Plagues*, Vol II, Balliere, Tindall and Cox, p. 176)

1835–1837   *Ireland* A disease of fish reported (and also in 1836–1837) in Galway at Lough Derg, large numbers of perch, trout and pike, dead on water surface. In 1838 only a few fish died. (G. Fleming 1882, p. 259)

1836   *North America* James Dwight Dana, a naturalist, earth scientist and a professor at Yale College published on a large parasitic copepod of fish called *Argulus catostomi* and also a crustacean parasitising cod called *C. americanus*.

1841   *Europe* Gabriel G. Valentin published the first description of a trypanosome in the blood of a trout (in J. Theordorides, (1980) 'Histoire de la parasitologie' in *Histoire de la médecine, de la pharmacie, de l'art dentaire et de l'art vétérinaire* Vol VII Albin Michel:Laffont pp. 149–175)

1844   *Spain* Two diseases in carp were observed by Casas de Mendoza. Both were described as non-lethal. In one, called *viruela*, the body of the fish was covered in pustules, between the scales, and the second, *musgada*, as excrescences on the back and the head. F. Camarero Rioja has suggested that the former was probably due to a pox virus and the latter to *Flexibacter columnaris* and/or *Saprolegnia* and *Achlya* (the work is cited by J Blancou (2008) 'Early reports on acquatic animal diseases' *Hist. Med. Vet.* 33 pp. 83–99)

At this time, mid-century, there was a developing group of scientists who were beginning to work as specialist fish pathologists in a movement away from the naturalists and systematists. However, fish disease was still very secondary to animal disease as there were no significant fish farming or cultivation activities. Blancou (2008, pp. 93–95) summarised reports by C.G. Ehrenberg (1838) describing a fish skin parasite, *Chilodon spp.* G. Gluge wrote of *Cnidosporidia* 'spores' in fish tissue which J Müller (1841) called *Psorospermia*. Forel and du Plessis (1868) reported high mortality in perch in Swiss and Alpine lakes, thought to be due to colibacillosis infection; various reports indicated that *Strongylus spp.* could be found in the blood vessels of the dolphin and larvae of *Anisakis* could be found in the tissues of certain fish.

More publications began to appear from American authors, J.E. DeKay (1822, 1844) produced work on crustaceans; A.A. Gould a physician, reported on the mollusca, crustacea and annalida (1841) and a leech, *Phylline hippoglossi*, from a marine fish, the first non-crustacean parasite of fish to be recognised in the USA prior to 1850; T.W. Hariss and D.H. Storer also published reports in 1839 of crustacea parasitising fish in North American waters. These papers have all been discussed by Mitchell (2001, pp. 359–360).

By the end of the century the 'naturalist' authors were being replaced with 'scientists' who, having recognised a disease, studied its causation. Such as the report of a mycobacterial infection in fish that was later proven to be transmissible to humans (E. Bataillon et al. (1897) Un nouveau type de tuberculose *Compt. rendus des Séances de la Soc. de Biolog.* **49** 446–449). There was also a report of a skin disease of roach, show-ing yellowish and reddish bruises to the skin, which was diagnosed as a *Proteus* infec-tion (Wyss (1898) in M. Prudhomme (1957) *Inspection sanitaire de poissons, mollusques et crustacés etc* Vigot Frère, Paris, 234). What appears to be the earliest proven report of a bacterial disease, vibriosis, in fish was provided by Canestrini who noted bloody, bruise-like lesions on eels (*Anguilla anguilla*) in the Venetian lagoons (Canestrini G. (1893) La Mallattia Dominate Del Anguille *Atti. Instit. Veneto Serv.* **7** 809–814).

In the 1850s in the USA there were several reports of massive fish kills. At the same time fish culture began to be explored and the health of both cultured and aquarium fish became a subject of serious study. Resulting from this, management practices and early diagnostic technologies were developed, and studies into the pos-sible causes of the diseases were conducted.

The advancement of fish research in the USA was led by J Leidy, who wrote some 600 papers between 1852–1891, and E. Linton who developed the study of entozoan parasites (protozoa, trematodes, cestodes, nematodes and acanthocephala) of fish, writing 63 papers in the later 1800s. This research is reviewed and discussed by Mitchell (2001, pp. 347–438).

One aspect of fish pathology that can be traced from antiquity is the identification of probable neoplasms in fish. The earliest occurs in an Egyptian tomb wall painting depicting probably *Tilapia nilotica*, with an enlarged abdomen, possibly an intra-abdominal tumour. This was reported by Mawdesley-Thomas (1972, pp. 191–284), who reviewed the early literature together with an overview of the topic. Literature search only reveals a few case examples: Olearius (1674) observed exostoses on the vertebral column and spines of a fish; U. Aldrovani in *De Piscibus* (1613) described a 'gibbous' or humped Sea perch, which might have been a tumour and John Hunter (1782) reported on a tumour in the stomach of a cod (*Gadus morhua*). This specimen can be seen in the Hunterian Collection at the Royal College of Surgeons in London. In 1793 W. Bell reported an osteomata in a species of *Chaeton* and in 1843 Rayer described epithelial tumours in trout. Finally Bland-Sutton (1885, pp. 415–475) pro-duced a useful early study of tumours in many species including fish, both marine (cod) and freshwater (pike and goldfish).

By the late 1880s veterinary medicine, human medicine and scientific disciplines were becoming established in their own right. A unique and invaluable source docu-ment is the bibliography of fish parasites, with citations from 330 BC to late AD 1923 (a span of 2253 years), by McGregor (1963). An important overview of fish health publications in the USA, 1609–1969, including a discussion on the leading person-alities in the field is provided by Mitchell (2001, pp. 347–438) and a review of early reports on 'aquatic animal diseases', including a useful bibliography is in Blancou (2008).

More general, but useful, reviews of the animal parasitology field, including fish, are in publications by Hoeppli (1956, pp. 398–419) and from the ancient times Enigk and Habil (1989, pp. 65–91), who deal specifically with German and Scandinavian work from 1200–1950. Much, but general, information involving fish 'problems' from 1490 BC to AD 1850 can be found in *Animal Plagues: Their History, Nature and Prevention* (Fleming, 1871). Jolly and Mawdesley-Thomas (1966, pp. 493–497) review the literature related to diseases of fish, including fish parasites with an extensive bibliography of the Russian literature, and Mawdesley-Thomas and Jolly (1967, pp. 533–541) provide an overview of diseases of the goldfish.

Aquatic Species, Diseases and Welfare

Of all the species of animal life that humankind has attempted to domesticate and cultivate as a food source, fish and other aquatic species (oysters, mussels) present the most diverse selection. They are found in fresh, brackish and saltwater environments, and many species of the finfish in freshwater rivers and lakes have been found to be adaptable to confinement waters.

The diversity available for humankind to exploit was shown by a study (Robins et al., 1991) of fish found in rivers, lakes and along the seaboards of the Atlantic and Pacific Oceans of the USA and Canada (to a depth of 200 m.); the total was just over 2400 species. However, as has become increasingly obvious, these waterborne creatures act as host to a very large number of parasites, bacteria, viruses and fungi as well as being susceptible to a wide selection of toxins, both natural and introduced. Additionally nutritional deficiencies and adverse changes in temperature and water purity are now recognised as important health hazards.

The recognition and understanding of fish diseases has been a slower process than that of other species. This has been due partly to the frequent difficulty in dealing with the aquatic environment, but initially because the first interest in fish was taken by 'naturalists' who were more concerned with systematics and developing a classification of the many varieties and types of aquatic creatures. As a result, taxonomy became the driving influence in fish studies. Fish disease was recognised by Aristotle but there was little study of any diseases until the 19th century.

Fish Culture and Disease

Integrated farming systems that included aquaculture developed in China, South-East Asian countries and the Hawaiian Islands. Various systems were created in places such as on the Mekong River in southwest China and Laos, in many regions of China, and by Chinese immigrants into Thailand, Malaysia and Indonesia. Those that evolved in Hawaii showed a remarkable diversity, development and management. It has been suggested that mariculture (the use of seawater) may have originated in Hawaii (Costa-Pierce 1987, pp. 320–331).

In the Western world, following the end of the Roman Empire, the cultivation of fish became a low priority and only advanced when freshwater carp ponds were attached to monasteries and large secular houses. The religious influence played an important role in the consumption of fish. Before the 17th century there are few records of significant fish disease problems.

The literature review of events associated with fish are dominated by reports of fish kills both in freshwater and marine environments: causes were not known but many of the freshwater ones also record coloured (green or red) contamination of the water. Knowledge today can provide probable answers to the causation of these naturalist descriptions. The main cause of fish kill is due to a low oxygen concentration in the water. This may be created by drought conditions, elevated temperature (prolonged sunshine), overpopulation, algal bloom producing toxicity, as well as certain infectious diseases and parasites. Environmental stress caused by temperatures which are either too cold or too hot, as seen in several of the reports, are significant natural factors.

Algal toxins are a complex disease cause, occurring either when the algal surface scum dies and the decay process uses the available oxygen in the water causing fish death, or when algal bloom such as 'red tide' (*Karenia brevis*) produces a specific toxin. Algal toxins, phytoplankton and bacteria, either alone or acting together, can all result in fish death, as also can some mineral salts leached into the water (such as certain aluminium compounds).

Early recorded recognised symptoms of disease or parasitic conditions included discoloration, open sores, reddening of the skin, bleeding, and black or white spots on the skin. Abnormal shapes, lumps and pop-eyes can all be found often related to parasites. Motility changes such as increases (flashing, whirling, twisting) or decreases (lack of activity, listless, floating), are now all known symptoms.

Identification of Specific Fish Diseases

As observations of disease problems increased, the first specific causal entities recognised were numerous crustacean parasites, usually copepods. From these in the later 1700s, there was the emergence of scientists taking a serious interest in fish pathology and disease. No serious investment in aquaculture was made until effective methods of disease recognition, diagnosis and control were developed, along with technology which provided for effective recycling of water, and an understanding of nutritional requirements. The earliest report of a fish bacterial disease (vibriosis) was made by Canestrini in 1893 and of a viral disease (iridovirus causing lymphocystis) by Weissenberg in 1914. These discoveries began to define the parameters of the problems.

A perspective of how these sectors of fish pathology have developed to the present day, was given in a paper by Snieszko (1975, pp. 446–459). He discusses the parasitism problem, recognising that about 80–90% of both fresh and saltwater fish harbour at least one parasite under natural conditions, but only suffer a disease when the parasite number impairs the functions of the fish. He names early leaders, including B. Hofer who published *Handbuch der Fischkrankheiten*, the first book on fish disease, in German in 1904, and in particular Marianne Plehn (1863–1946), the first veterinarian to become interested in fish pathology.

In its early days fish pathology was a study concentrated in Central and Eastern Europe: Germany, Poland, Czechoslovakia and Russia. Parasitology was concentrated in crustacean studies, but since the 1950s the sporozoan parasites: *Myxosoma cerebralis* (whirling disease of rainbow trout) and others such as *Ceratomyxa shasta* and *Plistophora ovariae* have been recognised, as well as protozoan blood parasites.

The second major disease group to be explored was bacterial, with a major input by Plehn (1911, pp. 609–624) on fish furunculosis in salmonids, caused by *Aeromonas salmonicida*. While initially recognised as a specific condition as early as 1868, it was not until it was observed in Scotland in 1926 that it aroused major concern (due to the threat to the valuable salmon fisheries). The United Kingdom (UK) government appointed a Furunculosis Committee in 1929 to investigate and suggest appropriate courses of action (Mackie et al., 1930, 1933 and 1935). This was a notable event, the disease was seen as the first recognised global epizootic of fishes and, among others, it led to the British Diseases of Fish Act, 1937: believed to be the longest-standing legislative instrument used to control fish disease. Furunculosis is also important as being the first fish disease against which oral immunisation was tried.

Other important recognised bacterial diseases are *Aeromonas liquefacieus* infection, found globally, also called Bacterial Haemorrhagic Septicaemia. Early observers termed the disease Infectious Dropsy. *Myxobacteria* and *Mycobacteria* species are now also recognised as significant agents of fish diseases, as is vibriosis. A particularly interesting disease syndrome, much investigated in Ireland, Scotland and Scandinavia in the 1960s and 1970s, is now termed Ulcerative Dermal Neurosis: a series of papers by Roberts (2015, pp. 404–415) follow the investigative chain. The Roberts papers should be read to give an overall view of major fish bacterial diseases with particular reference to the UK.

Nutritional issues and needs were recognised in Roman times but it has only been since the 20th century that these have been studied scientifically. Iodine deficiency, *Aspergillus flavus* aflatoxin (as a cause of hepatoma in trout), vitamin needs, and fish kills due to a variety of natural toxic incidents, are now all recognised and potentially controllable. Provision and maintenance of health is the product of understanding the fish, the potential disease agents and the all-important environmental factors of the water: temperature, pH, oxygenation, optimum salinity tolerance and cleanliness.

Public Health and Fish Diseases

The human consumption of fish carries several hazards, most of these date back to ancient times, but were not recorded or even recognised. The increasingly strict food hygiene controls introduced during the 20th century has enabled an evaluation of the problems. Most current controls are directed at exogenous factors, primarily water pollution by either municipal or industrial wastes. Specific symptom causing factors in humans are fish poisons such as that found in puffer fish *(fugu)* in Japan and paralytic shellfish poison seen in North America and Japan. Health problems also arise from allergic reactions to certain fish types, food poisoning bacteria, in or on the fish, and spoiled fish toxins. All of these issues would have existed since humans started eating fish.

The most important endogenous disease factors are the parasite intermediate forms to which fish act as secondary hosts. Six of these are now recognised as human health hazards, all of these occur naturally and it can be assumed that they would all have existed in the human food chain from ancient times, in fact there is good archaeological evidence to support this from the first of the six parasites listed below.

1. *Diphyllobothrium latum*, known as the broad or fish tapeworm in humans, can grow up to 10 m in length. It mainly occurs in Scandinavia, West Russia, Baltics and now also in the Pacific Northwest of America. *D. latum* and other members of the species involved, are pseudophyllid cestodes of fish and mammals. It has been found in human remains dating from 4000–10000 years ago excavated on the west coast of South America (which is outside of the believed natural endemic areas). The human is the definitive host and infection is acquired by ingestion of raw or undercooked freshwater fish, including pickled, salted, marinated and smoked forms. Eggs are released into the faeces and pass into freshwater crustacean copepods (first intermediate host) where they develop into procercoid larvae which are eaten by minnows and small fish (second intermediate host) and develop into plerocercoid larvae, which are the infective stage for the definitive host. These fish are eaten by trout, perch and pike which act as the later intermediate hosts to humans. Diphyllobothriasis has been a significant human health problem in the past.

2. *Clonorchis sinensis*, a trematode, the Chinese liver fluke. Said to be the third most prevalent global helminth parasite. Mainly confined to China, Japan and South-East Asia including Eastern Russia. A cause of liver cancer and classified as a group 1 biological carcinogen. A snail (*Parafossarulus* spp. and others) acts as first intermediate host with a second host in freshwater fish, mostly carp spp. (including goldfish). Then to human definitive host where it may live for 20–30 years. Spread by raw, undercooked, salted, pickled and smoked fish.

3. *Opisthorchis viverrini* and *O. felineus*, a trematode, the South-East Asian liver fluke. Mainly found in Thailand and Indo-China. Lifecycle is similar to *Clonorchis sinensis*, and both predispose to cholangiocarcinoma of the gall bladder and ducts of humans. Main definitive hosts are humans, dogs, cats and other mammals.

4. *Heterophyes heterophyes*, a trematode. Main locations are North Africa, Asia Minor, China, Japan and S.E. Asia. The adult form is a minute teardrop shaped fluke in the intestines of fish-eating birds and mammals, including humans. The adult form burrows into the villi of the small intestine. Eggs pass into the water and are ingested by snails and develop to cercaria which burrow into epithelium of fish. The main host fish are *Mugil cephalus* (mullet) and *Tilapia nilotica*. The definitive hosts are humans, cats, dogs and foxes. Infection rates are high in fishermen. Spread by consumption of raw or undercooked or salted or preserved fish.

5. *Paragonimus westermani*, a trematode, the lung fluke of humans, known as the Japanese or Oriental lung fluke. Most frequently found in Eastern Asia and South America. More than 30 species are known in animals, of which ten also infect humans (as well as pigs, dogs and cats). The first intermediate host is a snail and second freshwater crabs or crayfish. When crab meat is eaten raw, undercooked or pickled, the fluke reaches maturity.

6. *Anisakis spp*, this genus of parasitic nematode can produce harmful effects in humans. Most frequently found in herring. Originally recognised in 1845 it is only recently that the complex lifecycle has been understood. There are a number of intermediate hosts, first a crustacean, then fish and squid, and finally whales, seals and dolphins. If the infected fish are eaten by humans they will be infected and act as definitive hosts. Consumption can either result in intestinal infestation and/or serious allergic episodes. The mechanism is complex but the problem is fully controlled by full cooking or blast freezing of fish for seven days at –20°C. This latter process is now compulsory and successful, in the Netherlands, a major consumer of uncooked herring (as a seasonal delicacy, in brine).

A study by Mitchell (2017, pp. 48–58) on human parasites in the Roman Empire shows the health consequences of the Romanisation of their conquered territory. Among other parasites the incidence of *Diphyllobothrium latum* increased (based on archaeological evidence) compared to Bronze and Iron Age Europe. A part of Roman life was the recognition of the value of clean water and the use of this water to develop sanitation – by bath houses, drains, sewers and toilet systems. Cleanliness was not enough, there was little or no knowledge of disease causation, prophylaxis and hygiene.

Archaeological studies have revealed that the Roman population, throughout the empire, was affected with a wide range of endo and ectoparasites. Veterinary, and in particular fish disease related, interests centre on the significant spread of *Diphyllobothriasis*. Studies made, and collated, by Mitchell suggest that the spread was due to the almost universal use of *garum*, a Roman fermented fish sauce that was used for flavouring and also as a medicine. Garum was not cooked, but was a mix fermented in the sun, comprising pieces of fish, herbs, flavouring and salt. It is postulated that this sauce may well have been the vector that enabled the spread of fish tapeworm as it was traded and transported from northern Europe, in terracotta jars across the empire. Mitchell (2015, pp. 389–420) has also recorded that an increase in fish tapeworm infestations appear to have been even more prevalent in medieval Europe. This was possibly related to the widespread adoption of Christianity, with the instruction that fish should be eaten on Fridays and on the many holy feast days during this period.

References

Axelrod, H.R. and Vorderwinkler, W. (1962) *Encyclopedia of Tropical Fishes*. Jersey City, NJ: TFH Publications

Blancou, J. (2008) Early Reports on Aquatic Animal Diseases. *Historia Medicinae Veterinariae* **33** No.3

Bland-Sutton, J. (1885) Tumours in Animals. *Journal Anatomy & Physiology* London **19**

Brooker, C. (2006) The Rise and Fall of the Medieval Monastery. London: Folio

Chimitz, P. (1955) Tilapia and its Culture. A Preliminary Bibliography. *FAO Fisheries Bulletin* **8** No.1

Costa-Pierce, B.A. (1987) Aquaculture in Ancient Hawaii. *Bioscience* **37** No. 5

Enigk, K. and Habil, H.C. (1989) History of Veterinary Parasitology in Germany and Scandinavia. *Veterinary Parasitology* **33**

Fagan, B. (2011) *Elixir: A Human History of Water*. London: Bloomsbury Books

Fleming, G. (1871) Animal Plagues: Their History, Nature and Prevention. London: Chapman and Hall

Hendrikx, S. and Vermeersch, P. (2000) Chapter 2 Prehistory: From the Palaeolithic to the Badarian Culture in *The Oxford History of Ancient Egypt* (Ed. Shaw I.). Oxford: Oxford University Press

Hoeppli, R. (1956) Parasitological Reviews. The Knowledge of Parasites and Parasitic Infections from Ancient Times to the 17th Century. *Experimental Parasitology* **V**

Hofer, B. (1904) *Handbuch der Fischkrankheiten*. Munich: All Fisch-Zeit

James, P. and Thorpe, N. (1994) *Ancient Inventions*. New York: Ballantine

Jolly, D.W. and Mawdesley-Thomas, L.E. (1966) Diseases of Fish: I A Review of the Literature. *Journal Small Animal Practice* **7**

Mackie, T.J., Arkwright, J.A. Pryce-Tannatt, T., Mottram, J.C., Johnston, W.P. and Menzies, W.J.M. (1930, 1933, 1935) *Reports of the Furunculosis Committee*. Edinburgh: HMSO

Mawdesley-Thomas, L.E. (1972) Some Tumours of Fish, *Symposium of the Zoological Society of London* No. 30. London: Academic Press

Mawdesley-Thomas, L.E. and Jolly, D.W. (1967) Diseases of Fish: II The Goldfish *(Carassius auratus)*. *Journal Small Animal Practice* **8**

McGregor, E.A. (1963) *Publications on Fish Parasites and Diseases, 330 BC–AD 1923*, Special Scientific Report – Fisheries No.474. Washington, DC: US Department of the Interior Fish and Wildlife Service

Mitchell, A.J. (2001) Finfish Health in the United States (1609–1969): Historical Perspective. *Aquaculture* **196**

Mitchell, P.D. (2015) Human Parasites in Medieval Europe: Lifestyle, Sanitation and Medical Treatment. *Advances in Parasitology* **90**

Mitchell, P.D. (2017) Human Parasites in the Roman World: Health Consequences of Conquering an Empire. *Parasitology* **144** No.1

Moulé, L. (1908) La parasitologie dans la litterature antique I, L'Oestros des Grecs. *Archive de Parasitologie* **XIII**

Moulé, L. (1911) La parasitologie dans la litterature antique III. Parasites de la peau et des tissus sous-jacents. *Archive de Parasitologie* **XV**

Pennant, T. (1776) *British Zoology*, Vol, III. London: Benjamin White

Plehn, M. (1911) Die Furunkulose der Salmoniden. Zentralblatt Fur Bakteriologie, Parasitenkunde, Infektionskrankheiten und Hygiene **60**

Roberts, R.J. (2015) Veterinarians and Fish Health in the UK: 1890–1990. *Veterinary History* **17**

Robins, C.R., Bailey, R.M., Bond, C.E., Brooker, J.R., Lachner, E.A., Lea, R.N. and Scott, W.B. (1991) *Common and Scientific Names of Fishes from the United States and Canada*, 5th edn. Bethesda, MD: American Fisheries Society (Special Publication 20)

Romer, J. (2012) *A History of Ancient Egypt*. London: Penguin Books

Snieszko, S.F. (1975) History and Present Status of Fish Diseases. *Journal Wildlife Diseases* **11**

Walker, R.E. (1964) The Veterinary Papyrus of Kahun. A Revised Translation and Interpretation. *Veterinary Record* **76**

Wohlforth, G.W. (1984) in *Evolution of Domesticated Animals* (Ed. Mason I.L.). New York: Longman

Yonge, C.M. (1984) in *Evolution of Domesticated Animals* (Ed. Mason I.L.). New York: Longman

Zeuner, F.E. (1963) *A History of Domesticated Animals.* New York: Harper & Row

Zhang Zhong-ge (1984) in *Evolution of Domesticated Animals* (Ed. Mason I.L.). New York: Longman

EDIBLE SNAILS

Snails have formed a part of human diets from prehistoric times, as determined by the presence of shell types of edible snail species from archaeological excavations. While valued as a food source snails are generally regarded as an agricultural pest. From the classical literature it is known that snail consumption was both a recognised part of the Roman diet and that snail cultivation was practised as a part of normal farming.

Species Cultivated and Farmed

Land snails – terrestrial pulmonate gastropod molluscs – belong to a large family of many thousands of species, also found in fresh and seawater. Two families are of importance as a food source.

Helicidae. *Helix pomatia* (aka *H. edulis*), *H. aspersa*, *H. lucorum*, *H. aperta*, *H. vermiculata* (aka *Eobania vermiculata*). All essentially European in origin. *H. pomatia* is the most well-known species. The Helix varieties spread from their original European/Mediterranean habitats with Roman farming development. *H. pomatia* has rather strict environmental needs requiring a calcareous soil, warm nights, dewy mornings and shade. *H. aspersa* has less demanding needs and is more widely spread.

Achatinidae. Both *Achatina achatina* and *Archachatina* spp. are recognised as important sources of animal protein in West Africa, particularly in the coastal regions. Another related species *Achatina fulica* is found in East Africa, this has spread to the East, Pacific and USA in more recent years. Achatina and related species of African land snails can grow up to 38 cm/15 in nose-to-tail in length and weigh up to 1 kg/2¼ lbs.

Edible snails are hermaphrodites: the Helicidae are not self-fertile but the Achatinidae appear to be. *H. pomatia* winters underground closing the shell entrance with a white calcareous operculum. *H. aperta* behaves in a similar matter in the summer. Other species only rarely form an operculum. The operculated species are prized as a food delicacy. Many of the varieties of snails are highly sensitive to their environments and the establishment of a new colony may be difficult (Elmslie 1984, pp. 432–433).

Muricidae. *Murex brandaris* (now *Bolinus brandaris*) the purple dye murex or spiny dye murex. A predatory and edible sea snail. The most important of a large group of related rock snail gastropod species all of whom had a similar dye producing capability. They are mainly located in the Eastern and Central Mediterranean and played an important role in early cultures, in particular the Roman era. The dye was known as Imperial Purple and was used for the fabrics to make the emperor's robes. There is evidence that suggests a similar sea snail was known to, and used by, the early Mexican cultures.

Syrinex aruanus, the Australian trumpet, is the largest sea snail, their meat is both edible and used as bait. The shell can be up to 90 cm/35 in in length and the inshell weight can reach 18 kg/40 lb.

Early Domestication and Farming Practices

Varro (116 BC–27 BC) discusses snails and the work of Quintus Fulvius Lippinus, he also mentions Titus Pompeius in Gaul who had an enclosure for hunting in which he had special places for snails, beehives and for dormice fattening. Varro stated that a place for snails should be selected 'in the open but enclosed by water, they must be shut in by water'. The best situation would be where there was good shade and a little sunshine and where the dew falls. If possible running water should be present and preferably 'by a pipe where it falls on a stone to give a mist'. He suggested little food was needed if there was sufficient natural moist growth. The addition of feeding laurel leaves and bran was advised before killing. In advice on breeding stock Varro identified 'small whites from Reate', a 'larger size from Illyria' and a 'medium size from Africa'. He also mentions very large snails from Africa called *solitannae*, adding that they are 'so large that 80 quadrantes can be put in their shells' (about 2 ½ gallons). Varro noted that snails produce innumerable young and that if you construct large islands the ponds 'will bring you a large haul of money'. He stated that snails may also be fattened by putting them in a large jar lined with must and spelt and with holes for air.

The most informative early literature on edible snails comes from the Roman authors. Pliny, writing in mid-1st century AD, informs us that Quintus Fulvius Lippinus in about 50 BC began farming water snails. He was said to have specialised in giant edible snails from Illyria and Africa and, catering to a very specific market, used both selective breeding and specialised diets, including wine-enriched spelt (*Triticum spelta*, a primitive form of wheat). Pliny added that Fulvius established his 'vivaries' for snails in the vicinity of Tarquinii.

The northern Italian topography was an ideal environment for *H. pomatia*. They would be collected in the spring and placed in selected 'grazing' fields, and in the winter they would be dug up in their operculated form, for sale. In southern Italy and in parts of Sicily, *H. aspersa* would be harvested in a similar manner, but in the summer.

Romans believed snails were of value in medication and for many years were incorporated into skin creams and balms. *H. aspersa* was the principal species used with the suggestion that this would aid skin regeneration and the removal of scar tissue. Snails were also used in divination practices; the Greek poet Hesiod wrote that by watching the activity of snails one could predict the time to harvest: this may have some truth as snail movements are influenced by climatic factors.

The 10th century *Geoponika* compilation noted that to drive ants out of their nests snail shells should be burned with *storax* (Gk. *Styrax*), the resin of *Styrax officinalis*, and then pounded and placed in the ant hills. The flesh of *Helix pomatia* was recommended as a good fish bait in fish traps. Another recipe recommended that, 'ten purple shells be pounded with olive oil and laver (seaweed), then chewed and spat out onto rocks to catch crayfish and morme'.

A recipe to attract octopus and cuttlefish based on sal ammoniac and goats milk butter was suggested; when rubbed on ropes dropped into the water it is claimed to also attract 'purple shells' or *Murex brandaris*. This was important as the dye extracted from these, and related, snails was most expensive.

Archaeological evidence indicates that these sea snails were both harvested, and kept in tanks, dating from the 18th century BC. The early Minoans were said to have 'bred the snails in tanks', but this is unlikely, they probably just used them to store and feed them. The ancients called the dye Tyrian Purple, later this was known as Imperial Purple. It had the claimed attribute of being a powerful long lasting dye, which becoming fixed to the fabric did not fade. The dye was first described by Aristotle and the process of extraction is explained by Pliny, however efforts to reproduce this have only been partially successful. The dye was very expensive, said to have been worth more than its weight in silver and was a much desired luxury item by Roman society. The Murex snail group produce a milky mucous secretion from the hypobranchial glands: when exposed to the air this produces the powerful dye. The extraction process involved lengthy preservation in vats, and the production of a very objectional smell. Chemical analysis shows the active principle to be an organobromine compound.

Recognition and Diseases of Edible Snails

From the only significant ancient writing on snails, by Varro, there are no indications of disease problems. Current literature on snail diseases (not specifically edible snails) suggest that there are three main health issues:

1. Failure to form a complete operculum, this is probably due to a nutritional cause possibly related to over-cleanliness of the vivarium, in confined housing (there are aspects of the process of operculum formation that are not understood).
2. Bacterial infections, in particular with *Pseudomonas* spp. which can rapidly devastate a colony.
3. Infestation with *Riccardoell limacum* and *R. oudemansi*, the slug mite. This can be a particular problem with *H. pomatia* and *H. aspersa*, and also infestation by

Tyrophagus spp. known as a tick or louse. A control method used by current snail farmers is to introduce *Hypoaspis miles,* a predatory mite, which rapidly removes the offending parasites.

Summary

The snail has had a long relationship with humankind. Widely recognised as an agricultural pest it was also found to be an easily harvested source of animal protein, forming a part of human diets dating from very early times. As a dietary constituent it has moved from being a food of the poor to becoming a luxury item. A favourite of Roman meals it is now prized as an example of French cuisine, and is still bred and farmed in private snail gardens (*escargotiéres*) in France and Italy.

Edible terrestrial, freshwater and sea snails are consumed globally and various forms of heliculture have been practised since ancient times. Today *Helix aspersa* is most commonly used in cultivation systems in Europe, but *Achinata* spp are bred in the East for significant export to Europe and the USA. In general, snails are healthy where the environment is well controlled with particular emphasis on moisture, temperature and available food. The sea snail *Murex* was very important in ancient times, there is no evidence that these were 'farmed', but they were kept in a system of tanks before being processed.

While not featuring strongly in folklore and mythology in most societies, the snail did have significance in the Aztec culture: the god Tecciztecatl is always shown with a snail shell on his back, believed to symbolise rebirth.

References – snails

Elmslie, L.J. (1984) in *Evolution of Domesticated Animals* (Ed. Mason I.L.). New York: Longman

EDIBLE FROGS

Frog meat has been recognised as both a high quality protein source as well as a well-flavoured food for many thousands of years. Recognisable frog bones have been found at human sites dating back to the palaeolithic period. The frog (warty species are called toads) is a short-bodied, tailless amphibian of the order *Anura*, there are just under 5000 recorded species (many of which are either extinct or nearly so, due to habitat loss). They represent about 85% of all amphibian species.

Some cultures in the Americas recognised the toxicity of the skin secretions of certain members of the species. Early Mesoamerican societies used the exudates from the cane toad as an hallucinogen, and the early Columbian culture utilised the toxic skin exudate of *Phyllobates terribilis* (golden poison frog) to arm their poisoned darts for hunting. Several other frogs also have toxic skin exudates.

Frogs also feature in the folklore and fairy tales of most societies (to this day, with Kermit in the Muppets). The tradition was particularly strong in American cultures with the Moche people of ancient Peru, who worshipped animals of all types, frequently using the frog image in their pottery. To the present day Panamanian tradition associates the sighting of the Panamanian Golden Frog with good luck.

The main utilisation of frogs by humans has been, and still is, in the consumption of the hind leg meat. In the past there was an ample supply of wild frogs, but now with increased global demand cultivation technologies have evolved.

Species Cultivated and Farmed

A significant number of large edible frogs are known, many of these are eaten and cultivation of several species is undertaken: the degree of success is variable. As far as the literature has revealed, there were no significant cultivation procedures in ancient times. The main edible species currently recognised are identified below, partly derived from Culley (1984, p. 370). In several of these cultivation is practised but the term 'domestication' cannot be truly used.

Europe *Rana ridibunda, R. dalmatina, R. esculenta, R. lessonae, R. temporaria.* Intensive culture is generally poorly developed.

Asia *Rana hexadactyla, R. moodiei, R. tigrina, Glyphoglossus molossus* and some others. Some species under cultivation in India and Philippines with export trade.

North America *Rana catesbeiana, R. pipiens* and other species are found in the wild.

South America *Battachophrynus microphthalmus* is the most commonly consumed species but many other edible varieties are recognised. Very limited cultivation undertaken.

Africa Several edible species are recognised with *Conraua goliath* being probably the most important: also the largest edible frog species, up to 4 kg.

Early Domestication and Farming Practices

It has only been since the 20th century that there has been serious attention to frog farming and cultivation practices. Harvesting from the wild has always provided sufficient supplies; in countries of the East, rice paddies have proved to be a natural environment for frogs and a useful by-product for the farmer. It is believed that now the American bullfrog (*Rana catesbeiana*) is the most widely harvested frog, along with *R. tigrina, R. hexadactyla, R. esculenta* and *R. ridibunda*. Most cultivation is in extensive systems with fenced ponds and flowing water. Intensive systems are also developed with housed frogs but the essential factor is the provision of live food such as small fish and crayfish.

While the ancient literature makes little reference to frogs as a food source the *Geoponika* (10th century AD) makes several references to observations on frogs: Aratus said they were used to determine the onset of bad weather and to predict rain, the tree frog croaking in the morning indicated a pending storm; Africanus wrote that if you rub the pruning knives for vines with goat fat or frog's blood it will help prevent *phtheires*, (literally 'lice', but probably the red spider, *Panonychus ulmi)*. He also said that a lighted candle placed on the riverbank will prevent croaking; Apuleius advised that before land is dug one should take a land frog (toad), place it in an earthenware jar and bury it at night in the middle of the field. When ready to sow, the pot should be dug up and thrown off the land; this will ensure the harvest is not bitter.

Recognition and Diseases of Frogs

No reference to frog disease has been found in the early literature; since the frogs harvested were caught in the wild it can be assumed that only healthy stock was caught. In 1853 the microscopic characters of three parasitic protozoa in frogs were described. At that time there was no association with any specific disease symptoms (Leidy 1854, pp. 241–244). It is noted also, from a report of 1948, that renal adenocarcinoma of the frog is probably the most investigated and documented tumour in the species (Schlumberger and Lucké 1948, pp. 657–754).

Summary

Frogs were one of the hunter/gatherer food sources, but as society has evolved frog meat has become, in certain regions of the world, more of a luxury food item. The classic dish is the French *cuisses de grenouille* (frogs legs) and is mostly eaten in France and Belgium. Other main consumption regions are the southern states of the USA and China, Indo-China and Indonesia. The main production countries are Indonesia, China and the USA.

Apart from use as a human food, the frog has been of great importance to science. Luigi Galvani (1737–1798) pioneered bioelectromagnetics with his use of the isolated frog's leg to discover the link between electricity and the nervous system in 1787: his discovery was termed 'galvanism'. In 1852 H.F. Stannius (1808–1883) used a now termed 'Stannius ligature' on a frog's heart to demonstrate that the ventricles beat independently and at different rates. During the 20th century the frog became a standard animal for student dissection, but this use is now declining. Currently there is a growing study of the chemicals, with frequently strong pharmacological activities, that have been isolated from frog skin.

References frogs

Culley, D.D. (1984) in *Evolution of Domesticated Animals* (Ed. Mason I.L.). New York: Longman

Leidy, J.P. (1854) Some Observations on *Nematoidea imperfecta* and Descriptions of Three Parasitic Infusoriae. *Transactions American Philosophical Society* 1852–1853 **10**

Schlumberger, H.G. and Lucké, B. (1948) Tumours of Fishes, Amphibians and Reptiles. *Cancer Research* **8**

CHAPTER 26

Other Species

Throughout the history of the human race there has been a constant interest in other species, always seeking an advantage that could be seen in utilising the animal; as a food source, for the animal's strength in aiding work or transport, or for its pelt.

Apart from the species discussed in Chapters 17–25, many others have been captured and used, but only a few have been fully tamed and domesticated, most have simply been caged and bred. Eight species (six mammals and two insects), however, have been subjected to varying degrees of domestication and are discussed in the following chapter because they all have a long and interesting relationship with humans. Other species that have attracted human attention are also identified.

CAMELIDS

The subfamily Camelidae belongs to the Order Artiodactyla. They are the only living family of the suborder Tylopoda (pad-footed) named because of the lumps on their feet; the hoofs have been replaced by callous pads ending in claws. They are herbivorous but differ from ruminants. Camelids have slender necks and long legs. There are two tribes: Camelini or Old World camels, and Lamini or New World camels.

Old World Camelids

The distinctive feature of the Camelini is the 'hump', a fatty lump on the back. Three species are recognised: *Camelus dromedaries*, the Dromedary, currently about 93–94% of the old world camels, native of the Middle East, East Africa and South Asia, possesses one hump; *Camelus bactrianus*, the Bactrian Camel, possibly 6% of total, native of Central Asia, possesses two humps; *Camelus ferus*, the Wild Bacterian Camel, now very rare in isolated regions of Mongolia and China, possesses two humps.

The two-humped camel was probably domesticated first and used as a transport animal and a valuable source of hair for tents, clothing and bedding. Camel bones found in Iran and Turkistan have been dated back to 3000–2500 BC. Camel saddles were made in c.1200 BC and the animal was used in warfare and ceremonial duties. Their military use continued up to the 20th century in the British, French and other armies (even the United States of America (USA) had a Camel Corps in the late 1800s).

For the nomadic tribes who first domesticated camels, the animal became their most valuable possession: a means of transport, a source of milk (and yoghurt, essential in a hot climate), of hair and when killed of meat, bones and hide. Camel meat was prized by ancient Greeks and Romans. Camel meat and milk are not Kosher and Jews may not consume them. Muslims can but only with required prayers being spoken. The Romans spread the use of the animal throughout the empire. Small numbers were introduced to Europe but not widely used. The only significant historical disease reference was to a skin disease; this would have been mange, a constant issue with camel care, up to, and including, the present day. A very full and fascinating commentary on the early days and history of the camel in ancient times is in Zeuner (1963, pp. 338–366). Camels were introduced to Australia in the 1860s to aid transport in the arid regions. In the early 20th century, camels were replaced by motor transport, with many of them being released into the wild. This feral population is now estimated as being the world's largest at over 1,000,000.

New World Camelids

There has been much controversy over the relationships between the Lamini camelids found in South America. Four species of the tribe are recognised. Two in the genus *Lama*, the guanaco (*Lama guanicoe*) and the llama (*Lama glama*); and two in the genus *Vicugna*, the vicuna (*Vicugna vicugna*) and the alpaca (*Vicugna pacos*). These four species have a close resemblance and can, at first, be difficult to differentiate. They are all social animals and live in herds. Both the vicuna and the guanaco are wild species mainly living in the high Andes. The llama and alpaca are domesticated. A very full description and history of the New World camelids has been written by Novoa and Wheeler (1984, pp. 116–128).

Llama

The first of the species to be domesticated, from the guanaco, thousands of years ago, probably by the early Moche culture in Peru. The llama was important for meat supply and for its dung as a fertiliser. Later its use as a pack animal was learned, along with the value of its wool; excavations of the many regional cultures all reveal woven fabrics, which are notable in the grave goods. The llama has played an important role in the regional religions, the mythology tells of the Heavenly Llama who drinks water from the oceans and urinates as rain. An essential being for a frequently arid land.

The Inca Empire was very reliant on the llama as a beast of burden (even though the loads were not large), and as a major symbol of Inca ritual and religion. Many were slaughtered at regular sacrifices (see Chapter 9). Very large herds were kept for wool and meat supplies; the *yana*, a llama herder, was an important hereditary post. Following the Spanish conquest huge numbers of llamas were required to provide pack animal transport of silver from the Potosi mines to the coast. Only one disease reference has been found, an enterotoxaemia (possibly clostridial in nature) causing rapid death in corralled animals, probably due to unsanitary conditions.

Alpaca

The other domesticate species which was domesticated from the vicuna several thousands of years ago in one of the early Andean civilisations. There are two alpaca types, the *Suri* and the *Huacaya*. They are herded at a fairly high level in the more temperate mountain areas and are only bred for their wool, which is excellent for clothing. The alpaca is seen in Andean mythology as a gift from *Pachamama* as a provider of meat and fibre.

Guanaco

A wild species widely distributed in South America. While mainly found in the high altitudes it has also adapted to the Patagonian region. It is the main progenitor species of the llama and is prized for its soft warm fibre coat, considered to be second only to that of the vicuna, and also for the pelts from the calves, compared to fox fur. They are hunted, not domesticated.

Vicuna

A wild species with its distribution limited to the *puna* zone of the Andes (4200–4800 m above sea level). They are hunted and caught to be shorn of their very fine wool, this is only produced in small amounts and shearing can only be undertaken every three years. The resultant fabric is both light, silky and costly. In the Inca society it was reserved for royal use. Special local traditional rituals for the vicuna are still held in the mountain regions.

Cervids (Deer)

The Cervidae (reindeer and other deer) belong to the Order Artiodactyla in 23 genera, with 47 species in two main subfamilies. The Capreolinae includes reindeer/caribou, roe deer and moose/elk. The Cervinae includes the muntjac, fallow and chital deer. Of this large family only the reindeer (caribou) has been domesticated to any degree, several of the other deer species have been, and still are, farmed but not domesticated.

As a family, deer are described as hoofed, ruminant, even-toed ungulates. Their particular characteristic is the bearing of antlers, grown and shed annually, always in the male, sometimes in the female. They are notable jumpers and swimmers. Deer have a long history in their relationship with humans; they appear in Palaeolithic cave paintings and in succeeding generations of ornamentation including the Hittites, Celts, Greeks and in Roman mosaics. They feature in Shinto shrines in Japan, in early Mexican sacrifices and were the main animal hunted by the nobility of medieval Europe. Deer also are well recognised in mythology, religions, literature and heraldry.

Deer have been utilised primarily as a source of meat (venison), and for their hides (buckskin) and antlers, first as tools and later for many purposes including ornamentation. Some species have been used to provide milk. Deer have rarely been fully domesticated, but are easily tamed. Deer farming has been practised for many years in China for the production of medicaments used in their traditional system. Deer parks were a feature of medieval Europe (and in Asia), the deer being mainly bred for antler size and hunting.

The word 'deer' and Old English *deor*, Middle English *der*, Old High German *tior*, Old Norse *djur*, *dyr*, Old Frisian *dier* and Old Saxon *diar*. The origin of the 'reindeer' word is not clear. The Norse words *rein* and *ren* are derived from Old Scandinavian, *hreinn* is derived from the Germanic *hran*. The current French for reindeer is *renne* derived from Old French *rangifer*; this is now the generic name used – *Rangifer*.

Disease in farmed (park land) deer was recognised over 500 years ago. Records from English deer parks of the early 1500s identified four ailments: 'garget', 'rotte', 'dooges' and 'wypps'. These vernacular names are no longer in use; however, some comment can be added. 'Garget' was a term used first for ailments of the throat and later for mastitis, as Fletcher (2011, p. 152) noted that necrobacillosis, a form of diphtheria, is a common epidemic in fallow deer this is a likely explanation; 'rotte' was a term used for liver fluke disease (*Fasciola hepatica*) in cattle and sheep, it can be presumed that similar symptoms were observed in deer; 'wypps' is an unknown word, Fletcher (2011, p. 154) has surmised that it might have been lungworm, a common cause of disease in deer; 'dooges' is difficult, but 'dogues' occurs in contemporary animal disease literature referring to the adult flukes found in the livers of infested animals. The relationship of these parasites to 'rotte' was not realised, as 'rotte' was recognised it is possible that 'dooges' were the actual flukes. More recent evidence shows that tuberculosis can be a problem in deer herds and rabies can occur in deer and moose (North America) and liver fluke in many regions. Simulid flies can cause stampedes of reindeer in Russia.

Rangifer tarandus (the reindeer or caribou) is the one cervid species that has been domesticated: found in the northern hemisphere, but only domesticated in Europe, Russia and Siberia. Domestication, in varying degrees, has been undertaken since the Bronze or Iron Ages by the Inuit and other circumpolar peoples; the animals may be kept in large or small herds, or in corralled groups. Aristotle wrote of such an animal (never having seen one), Julius Caesar mentions them, and they are recorded by Conrad Gesner. Domestication varies from use for drawing sledges or riding, or milk production. They are also herded and raised for meat consumption, with their hides and antlers used for tents, clothing and tools (Skjenneneberg 1984, pp. 128–134).

The reindeer, an essential part of the life of the nomadic tribes in northern Scandinavia and Russia, has also become immortalised in Western Christmas customs. An 1823 poem 'A Visit from St. Nicholas', attributed to Clement Moore tells of the flying reindeer and delivery of Christmas presents. St. Nicholas became Santa Claus and the named reindeer had the addition of Rudolph (the red-nosed reindeer) by a 1939 children's book.

Of the many species of deer (apart from reindeer) five have been found to be of particular value:

- *Cervus dama* Fallow deer, the most popular, conserved in parks (first recorded in Scottish deer parks in 1290). Now also farmed in New Zealand, Australia and Germany for meat. Seen as a generally healthy species.
- *Cervus nippon* (Sika deer). Farmed in China and Korea to harvest the growing velvet antlers (*pantil*) and other bodily organs for use in Chinese traditional medicine.
- *Cervus elephas* (Red deer). Mentioned by Columella (AD 65) as a useful parkland species. Farmed in China, and elsewhere, as a source of ingredients for traditional medicine products.
- *Alces alces* (Elk or Moose). Species found in North America and North Europe/Asia. Domesticated in Europe around 200 BC and used for draught, riding, milk and meat. Now limited to herds in Russia for milk production.
- *Moschus spp.* (Musk deer). Grouped with deer but not truly a cervid, more closely related to bovids. Previously believed to be one species, *Moschus moschiferus* is now thought to be seven closely related species. Was hunted, now 'farmed' for the musk, a glandular secretion used as a fixative for perfumes. Males are 'milked' annually to collect about 5 g per session; the animals are productive from about three to twelve years of age (Fletcher 1984, pp. 138–139).

Elephantids

The elephants belong to the order Proboscidea, and family Elephantidae with two genera: *Elephas maximus* the Asian elephant and *Loxodonta africana* the African elephant. The Asian species have attracted humans from very early times, their African cousins have proved to be somewhat intractable. Both species share the common characteristics of being well built, of significant size and possessing a trunk, used for breathing, drinking, conveying food to their mouth and for general investigative purposes. The distinguishing feature is that the African elephant has larger ears and an arched back. African elephants can live for up to 70 years and the Asian up to 50 years.

Elephants are social animals and live in nomadic family groups led by a matriarch. They are highly intelligent and possess a good memory. When trained they are gentle (except the males in the breeding season). Elephants are not truly domesticated as their breeding is not controlled; they are trained after capture at age ten to twenty years. They are valuable for work in logging, being more adaptable than mechanical appliances. They are also used to pull wagons, for tourist rides and ceremonies.

Asian elephants once ranged from Assyria, where the Kings of Babylon hunted them before 800 BC, to Persia, Afghanistan and southern China. Today, in the wild they live in declining numbers in the jungles of South India, Ceylon, Assam, Burma, Thailand and other South-East Asian countries. African elephants are now restricted to the region of the continent below the Sahara desert.

Elephas maximus was found to be tractable over 4000 years ago, the earliest record is in engravings from 2500 BC in the Lower Indus Valley (Olivier 1984, pp. 185–192). Mentions are made in the Sanskrit literature from the 2nd century BC. Elephants became a symbol of power to kings and leaders in Asia. Ancient Sanskrit palm leaf manuscripts include the 4th century BC *Mahabharata* epic, describing elephant warfare and the *Hastyayurveda* of Palakopya, a treatise on elephants, possibly written at least 2000 years ago (see Chapter 8). There were 'veterinary officers' for the elephants in the establishment of the Kings of Ceylon.

Alexander the Great invaded Persia in 331 BC and defeated Darius III who had elephants in his army: the first contact that the West had with these animals. He then invaded India in 335 BC and defeated Porus, King of Taxila at the battle of Hydaspis, capturing the army elephants. He used some in his army and sent some to Aristotle (384–322 BC) his old tutor, who studied them and described their conformation, physiology and diseases with great exactness. He gave us the first, and quite accurate, description of their character 'the tamest and gentlest of all the wild animals is the elephant . . . it both learns and understands . . . it has quick perception and superior understanding'. (*Historia Animalium* Book VIII).

The Greeks valued the elephant as a war weapon. When the Ptolemies had taken control of Egypt, as they could not get any from Asia, they obtained Nubian, African elephants, however when these were used in the battle of Raphia against the Syrians in 217 BC, they were routed by their Asian relatives. The Carthaginians became apprehensive hearing of the new engines of war acquired by the Ptolemies and sourced their own reinforcements from the then Mauritanian race of elephants in the Atlas mountains. They did not have to fight the Ptolemies, but Rome proved to be the aggressor, leading to Hannibal, in the Punic Wars, taking some elephants on his famous (217 BC) trek across the Alps in his last desperate attempt to defeat Rome.

By 280 BC the Romans, finding that elephants were frightened by noise and fire, used them as curiosities in triumphal marches, and as poor victims for slaughter in the Roman arena. They were, however, used in war for many centuries in India, Ceylon, Burma and Thailand. The British in India, in the 18th and 19th centuries, used them as transport animals and then in the teak forests for moving timber.

After the fall of the Roman Empire, elephants are only rarely mentioned in Europe. Emperor Charlemagne received an elephant as a gift from Caliph Haroun-al-Raschid in AD 801. Named Aboul-abbas, the elephant lived for nine years. In 1229 Frederick II returning from the Holy Land brought an elephant to Italy. King Louis of France, in 1254, returning from the Crusades brought one to France and then gave it to Henry III of England – this was the first one ever seen in England and 'created great excitement and interest in London'.

More elephants began to appear in Europe and were known as subjects of great curiosity and fascination. Rembrandt's 1637 drawing (in British Museum) was of

Hansken who had been trained to perform using her trunk, to engage in a sword fight, put a hat on her head or wave a flag. Her skeleton is preserved in the Natural History Museum of Florence.

Loxodonta africana and *Loxodonta cyclotis* the bush and forest elephants are mostly found in the African savannah regions but also in the arid desert of Namibia and forested zone of Central and West Africa. *L. africana* is the largest terrestrial mammal species. Domestication occurred in ancient times, as described with Ptolemy and Hannibal, but their use ceased with the end of the Roman Empire. African tribes have generally praised the elephant as a symbol of wisdom and strength – the tusks being preserved to represent these qualities. An attempt was made in the Congo in the 20th century to revive their training and use for work, but this ceased in the troubles in the 1980s. Diseases of the elephant are discussed in Chapter 8.

The elephant became a part of the Western world, but only as an exhibit in zoos or a curiosity to be trained for the amusement of a circus audience. In Asia, their life is either taking part in parades decked in tassels with people riding on their backs, or labouring moving timber in the teak logging forests. Both of these life situations are very unlike their natural environment of a nomadic life in a small caring family group. The elephant has always fascinated humans who, arguably, have not treated them well. John Donne (1571–1631) summed the animal up perfectly, 'Nature's great masterpiece, an Elephant'.

Leporidae (Rabbits)

Rabbits are mammals of the Leporidae family of the order Lagomorpha. Globally there are some 300 species in eight genera. The common European species is *Oryctolagus cuniculus*, which has been introduced to every continent except North America. It is a prey animal but is domesticated for meat and fur production as well as a pet. There are many specialist breeds of rabbits, some utilised for fur (Angora and Rex) and others for showing.

The Romans used the name *cuniculus*, believed to be derived from an Iberian word. In European languages the rabbit is called *conejo, conelho, coneglio* and *Kaninchen*. The word rabbit is derived from either the Old French *rabotte* or Low Dutch *robbe*. Current Dutch is *robett*. The word cony or coney is derived from the Anglo-Norman word *coning*, from the Old French *conin* which itself is derived from the Latin word *cuniculus*. Cony-wool refers to rabbit fur and a coney-garth was an old term for a rabbit warren. In North America, a jack-rabbit is a hare, and a cotton tail is a rabbit, a different species from the European one.

The European rabbit was first recognised by the Phoenicians in Spain in 1100 BC, later the Romans became interested in rabbits for both food and sport. Early Roman authors such as Varro (116–27 BC) described a *leporia* (enclosures with housing and shelter) in which hares were kept prior to consumption and noted that rabbits would breed under such conditions. They were kept and bred for meat (Romans regarded the unborn rabbit kits as a food delicacy) and sport – hunted with dogs and bows and arrows, also considered suitable for women. The Romans introduced rabbits to many of the countries they conquered.

Later Henry IV of France constructed a 'rabbit garden' at Clichy and Queen Elizabeth I of England housed a colony on a small island. These were not strictly domesticated, but were bred for a purpose; some rabbits escaped and soon there were significant feral populations. More serious rabbit breeding began with the monasteries in the Middle Ages, rabbits were a good food source and monks were allowed to eat the flesh of unborn or newborn rabbits during Lent as it was not considered to be meat. This created serious breeding attempts to get the 'harvest' at the right time. As a result coat-colour mutations appeared and selection began, considered by some people to indicate domestication (Robinson 1984, pp. 234–242). It was soon realised that rabbits had to have human contact from a very early age otherwise they would always be timid.

Global diffusion of the species began with sailors, who would leave some on islands they visited as a future source of food. The rabbit arrived in Australia in 1859 and New Zealand shortly after: it soon became a serious pest. Introduction to North America was unsuccessful probably due to predators. The rabbit has played a role in mythology, religion and folklore in many cultures and countries.

The control of rabbits as a pest in Australia was partially resolved by the introduction of the myxomatosis virus in 1950 as a means of biological control. It reached Europe in 1952 and has enabled a population reduction, but not eradication. Diseases in rabbits were not seen as a significant problem until the species became more seriously bred in the later 20th century. As its place as a pet animal grew, many problems were identified, and several are now controlled by vaccination.

Caviidae (Guinea Pigs)

This small, inoffensive rodent has a very long history of domestication. Its name is confusing, it comes from South America and not Guinea. It is termed *Cavia porcellus*, derived from the original Quecha name of *cuy* or *cui*, still used in South America; in French it is *cobaye*, Spanish *cobayo* and in English usually 'cavy'. It has been used as a 'domesticated' meat animal in the Andes region of Peru, Colombia, Ecuador and Bolivia since around 4000–1000 BC. The animal was previously hunted but as the tribal peoples settled they began to 'farm' the cavy in their homes. It was a situation that suited the animal, it had food, shelter, warmth and protection, and the family had food and pets. The guinea pig has been of importance as a food source in this region for some 4000 years. Disease was not recognised as a problem in the Andean domesticated system.

Following the Spanish conquest it appears that domestication increased, the Inca historian Garcilaso de la Vega wrote in 1591 that the cuy 'makes a tasty meat'. The animal was well received in Europe as a pet, Conrad Gesner wrote the first description in 1554. In the native cultures of the Andean region the cuy features in pottery, paintings and mythology. For many generations they have been used in traditional medicine either by rubbing the animal on the patient, or by sacrifice and examining the organs for a prognosis. As Christianity was introduced the cuy also became a religious symbol – as portrayed in a painting of the Last Supper to be seen in Cuzco cathedral, Jesus is carving a cuy for the meal.

Currently the guinea pig has a major role as a pet in the Western world and is also used as a laboratory animal. Today pet clubs are leading the selection of certain desired characteristics in the species.

Herpestidae (Mongoose)

This agile, active hunting mammal is a member of the Carnivora in the subfamily Herpestinae of 23 species found in Africa, southern Europe and Asia. Three of these have had a long relationship with humans – *Herpestes ichneumon* (ichneumon), *H. edwardsi* (Indian grey mongoose) and *H. auropunctatus* (small Indian or golden spotted mongoose). The name is derived from the Hindi *mungus*, with the plural 'mongooses'. The ichneumon is the largest of the three, but all have similar coarse, long hair and their senses of sight and sound are very acute. They are hunters and eat small mammals, lizards, frogs, worms, insects and in particular, snakes. The mongoose is a fierce animal but is easily tamed, which has to be enacted when they are young.

Early in several civilisations (Egypt, India, Indonesia) the value of a mongoose in the home, as a killer of snakes, rats and mice, was appreciated. Breeding was not controlled. In the New Kingdom in Egypt in the 16th–11th centuries BC, the ich-neumon lived freely in homes as a pet. They were soon regarded as sacred, were kept in temples and mummified when dead. A mongoose cult was centred on Letopolis in the Delta and Herakleopolis, south of Fayoum; as the crocodile was also sacred, the ichneumon's habit of eating crocodile eggs created some local conflicts. Many images can be found in wall paintings, and following the Roman occupation, in mosaic floors, the Romans kept them as pets. Gradually the cat has taken the place of the mongoose, but it is still kept in some houses. In the *Panchatantra* Indian Sanskrit literature of about 100 BC the mongoose is represented as man's friend by protecting him from cobras. Other ancient Indian texts dating back to 1000 BC mention the mongoose. In later stories by the British author Rudyard Kipling a mongoose called Rikki Tikki Tavi is a major character. The mongoose when domesticated will live for up to 20 years, there are no recognised serious disease issues.

Honeybee

Apis mellifera Bees probably appeared by divergence from sphecoid wasps about 100,000,000 years ago (Middle Cretaceous Period), at the same time that angio-sperm vegetation became dominant and increasingly adapted to pollination. The bee evolved as a eusocial insect, socially organised in a system which a single female produces the offspring and non-reproductive individuals care for the young. *Apis mel-lifera* is the domesticated European species that dominates global honey production.

There are several subspecies in Europe, Africa, Middle East and Asia, of these *A. cerana* is the most significant of the domesticated species.

Bees are important, as a provider of honey (and beeswax) but also as a key pollinator of plants. It is estimated that 80% of the crop species cultivated in the EU depend on insect pollination, which is also important for wild flora. Bees have a great genetic diversity; in the 1920s an 'artificial' strain, the Buckfast honeybee, was developed in England to overcome a parasitic infection. Pliny (AD 77) wrote that bees were the 'only insects to have been created for the benefit of man'.

A bee colony, or hive, is an intriguing portrayal of social organisation with three members: the queen, the workers and the drones. The *queen* is pre-selected and specifically fed, when mature she makes a mating flight and will mate with up to 17 drones (which then die) and will store enough sperm to last her life, up to five to six years. She then lays eggs continuously, estimated to be around 200,000 a year. She is fed a highly nutritious diet, named 'royal jelly'. The eggs are of two types: the first to produce male drones and many workers. The drone has only one task, to mate with a queen on her inaugural flight. They complete no work in the colony but just consume food; after summer mating the hive population declines for the winter and the workers will stop feeding the drones or remove them from the hive. The second type, the worker bee, is a non-reproductive female who is trained in a series of tasks to maintain the health of the colony with routine hygienic cleaning and feeding the brood, and collecting nectar and honey. Bees have two dance patterns, one termed the 'round' indicates where good nectar is available and the other, the 'waggle' tells the colony the direction and location of desirable food sources. As workers have a life of about six weeks, the queen has to constantly replenish the stock. In winter, the hive population falls from 50,000–60,000 bees to just the queen and a reduced worker number (Wilson 2004, pp. 10–24).

Bee behaviour is constantly under study and revealing aspects of their practices: in flight they build up a positive charge and when in contact with a plant the negatively charged pollen grains 'fly' to them. Bees can also detect ultraviolet colours and markings on flowers that are invisible to the human eye. Nectar is collected as an energy source and pollen as a protein source. Bees have hygienic behaviour: this is inherited and not all colonies behave in exactly the same manner. Some will rapidly identify and remove dead larvae, or varroa mites.

Humans showed an early interest in honey and its collection from the nests of wild bees. Mesolithic, about 7000 BC, rock paintings found in Spain show honey-collectors with a ladder, indicating that by then it was a common practice. The first images showing domestication and the use of smoke to aid harvesting are found in Egyptian wall paintings c.2500 BC which illustrate long horizontal hives made of baked clay. Aristotle (384–322 BC) mentions the use of smoke and described bees as social creatures – a simile that was taken and used in Greek literature and plays. Moveable combs were developed to enable easier harvesting. The Romans practised bee cultivation and honey collection, with their habits well described by Virgil (70–19 BC). The tubular hive shape was common for many years, Africans used hollow logs hung from tree branches. These were followed by coiled straw cone-shaped baskets. In the Middle Ages, in northern Europe, nests were found in hollow trees, then 'owned' by individuals who created 'doors' so they could harvest the honey.

Honey production became important in Europe based on *A. mellifera*. The first hives crossed the Atlantic in 1621, this led to a development of taller hives using wooden boards, and by 1800 hives were common on the East Coast. They were then introduced in California in 1853 and British Colombia 1858. They had already been taken to Florida by 1763 and then to Cuba and Brazil 1839; Chile and Peru 1857; Australia 1810; New Zealand 1839; Hawaii 1857; and Papua New Guinea in the 1940s. India had developed its own production in Asia with *A. cerana*; interest in China was minimal, honey was not a sought-after taste. The modern hive began with Rev L L Langstroth of Philadelphia who, in 1851, created vertical sided boxes with separate hanging removable wooden frames for the combs. He wrote *The Hive and the Honeybee* in 1853 in which he described his ideas – these were soon accepted and widely used. Now hives could easily hold 50,000 bees and more by adding extra boxes, resulting in more honey production and less swarming, a consequence of crowding (Crane 1984, pp. 403–414).

The bee has played a role in mythology, art and folklore in the Northern hemisphere. A Greek legend tells of Melissa (Bee) a nymph who discovered honey. Medieval bestiaries (and Pliny) told of the knowledge that bees possessed of the weather by always remaining in their hives when it was to rain or became windy – and emphasised the bee as a model for social order and work.

Apart from honey's use as a sweetener it also acquired an early reputation as a medication, in particular for respiratory problems and also as a wound dressing. When used on contaminated wounds honey aids the debridement of dead tissue due to the high sugar content creating osmosis, with some antimicrobial activity due to its low pH. Manuka honey is reputed to have additional activity due to its chemical content.

In recent years much attention has been given to recognition and treatment of bee diseases (such problems were mentioned in the early Roman literature). Aristotle commented on a disease where there was, 'a lassitude of the bees . . . and a malodorousness of the hive'. Now several problems are well identified, in particular European Foulbrood (EFB) due to *Melissococcus plutonius*, which can be treated, and American Foulbrood (AFB) caused by *Paenibacillus larvae* which requires the bee colony to be destroyed. Also important is infestation with *Varroa jacobsoni* mites (originally a parasite of *A. cerana* from Asia), which attack drone cells. Fungal infection with *Nozema ceranae* can be a serious problem as well as deformed wing virus. Another more recent problem, seen mainly in the USA, is termed Colony Collapse Disorder (CCD), the worker bees appear to disappear, the cause has not yet been identified. Bee disease is a complex subject and well described in detail by Vidal-Naquet (2015): now recognised as important it is being increasingly taught in veterinary schools, and also involving government agencies.

Silkworm Moths

Bombyx mori There are many silkworm members of the Lepidoptera with some 14 species recognised for silk production, however, only *Bombyx mori* has been domesticated. It feeds on white mulberry leaves and depends on human intervention to reproduce. The non-mulberry feeding species only contribute less than one tenth total production, they are raised outdoors on appropriate trees and bushes.

Lepidoptera have a complete metamorphosis life cycle of egg, larva, pupa to adult moth. The eggs take around 14 days from hatching to reach the larval stage. The larvae then eat voraciously and constantly until their salivary glands start to produce a silk thread, up to one mile in length, which is wound around the larva to form a cocoon as a protection from predators. When hatching time approaches, the pupa produces an enzyme-containing secretion to dissolve a hole in the cocoon to allow emergence. To prevent this in the silk production process the cocoons are boiled in water to kill the pupa, this also makes it easier to unwind the silk thread. It requires about 2000–3000 cocoons to produce 1 lb (0.4 kg) silk.

The history of silkworm production, sericulture, dates back at least 5000 years to the early Chinese culture. A legend recounted by Shi-Ma-Qian (146–86 BC) tells that Empress Xi-Lung-Shi started the development of sericulture. Silk was loved by Roman aristocrats and shipments were made via the named Silk Road, across Asia to Europe, for many years. China monopolised the practice until moths and cocoons were smuggled out in the 2nd or 3rd centuries AD. Sericulture is recorded in the Indian *Vedas* (1600–1500 BC) demonstrating that they had produced silk cloth independent of China. It is now known that there are many races of silkworm that have been exploited, but none as productive as *B. mori*.

One reason for the high cost of silk is that sericulture requires a high labour input; apart from the unwinding of the cocoon, much time and effort has to be given to aid mating. The domesticated moth has lost the ability to fly any distance and needs human aid to find a mate. These moths have also undergone other changes, it is both significantly larger than its wild ancestor and has lost its colour differentiation. The pupa are eaten in many Eastern cultures. The history of sericulture is well described by Tazima (1984, pp. 416–423): the silk moth is a major figure in Chinese mythology. Several diseases of fungal, viral and parasitic origin are recognised in the larvae and moths. Strict hygiene methods have to be employed. Most natural silk is still produced in China (about 40–45%) and Japan (about 25%).

Many other species have been utilised or farmed by humans. The majority of these have been mammals, but reptiles and snakes have also been included in some places. The more important of these are listed alphabetically, most of these are only semi-domesticated.

Capybara

Hydrochoerus hydrochaeris, the largest living rodent, found in South America (Brazil, Venezuela, Paraguay, Uruguay and Argentina). The name is derived from the Guarani language. The Piaras people of the Orinoco river basin had originally domesticated them to provide a meat source; a Father Anchieta in Brazil in 1565 reported on their breeding for meat. The species was first reported by Alvarez-Nunez in 1541 in Paraguay and first described in 1802 by A Azara, a zoologist. A custom of eating salted capybara in Venezuela at Easter has led to a tradition whereby Catholics are allowed to eat this meat during the Lent and Easter weeks.

Chinchilla

Chinchilla chinchilla and *Chinchilla lanigera*, a small South American rodent originally found in Peru, Bolivia, Argentina and Chile on the slopes of the Andes. Little is known of their history and now they only exist in the wild in Chile. They are the bearers of one of the most exotic furs, possibly they were bred and raised to produce clothing for the Inca royal family. First domesticated in 1855 in Chile, they were taken to the USA in 1918 and then breeding became worldwide. Up to 150 skins are required to make a fur coat. There are no records of disease in the wild animals, but several reports of disease in breeding groups, both infectious and caused by mental stress.

Coypu

Myocastor coypus, also known as nutria. They are large, semi-aquatic, herbivorous rodents found wild in South America (Chile, Argentina, Bolivia). They have been hunted ruthlessly in the wild for meat and fur. Captive breeding began in the Argentine in the late 1800s and then they were also farmed in North America and Europe but this declined in the 1930s. In the 1950s intensive fur-farm breeding began in the USA, Argentina, Poland, Russia and East Europe, this has now declined as a commercial opportunity. Wild coypu seldom live longer than three years, but they can live for up to six years in captivity. The female can become pregnant three times in a year. Coypu escaping from farms cause serious damage to wetlands and are regarded as an invasive species in many countries.

Ferret

Mustela furo, the ferret. Order Carnivora, family Mustelinae. A hunter who follows prey into their burrows. They possess a long lithe body, and have well developed canine teeth to bite and hold. Known in Latin as *viverra* then *furectus* or *furo*. In French *furet*, German *frettchen* and Spanish *huron*, in English usually ferret. Possibly described by Aristotle c.350 BC, later by Strabo (63 BC–AD 24) who recorded their use in Majorca to control a rabbit infestation. Pliny (AD 23–79) mentions the species, and thereafter ferrets are increasingly named in hunting reports and books. Gesner, 1551 described the ferret as the colour of wool dyed in urine. The ferret has remained valuable as a provider of food, controller of rats and a source of sport. Domestication probably began in Iberia many centuries ago.

Fox

Vulpes vulpes, the silver fox (the species usually farmed) is a melanistic form of the red fox. First bred by Charles Dalton in Canada in 1892. From the early 20th century breeding advanced rapidly in Canada, the USA, Scandinavia and Russia. The demand for the fur has declined rapidly in recent years.

Mink

Neovison vison, the American mink. Order Carnivora, family Mustelinae. A hunter with a lithe body, short legs, dense fur and semi-aquatic habits. Probably first bred in captivity in the mid-1800s but this was not initially successful. Later specific fur colour tones were produced and mink farming grew in popularity. Now much decreased due to condemnation of the conditions under which many mink were raised. Mink farming is banned in many countries.

Mongolian gerbil

Meriones unguiculatus, a small rodent whose natural habitat is the semi-desert regions of Mongolia and north China. First captured in 1935 in the Amur river basin and taken to Japan where they were successfully bred. In 1954 they were taken to the USA. Intensive breeding began and they were distributed to Europe. Very attractive pets, also used in laboratory work.

Muskrat

Ondatra zibethicus a medium-sized, semi-aquatic rodent, also named 'musquash'. A native of North America, the genus name comes from the local indigenous language *ondatha*, *zibethicus* means 'musky'. The musk, which is used to mark their territory, was at one time used to fix perfumes. Muskrats have been important providers of fur pelts for the local Native American tribes for centuries. The species was first documented by John Smith in Virginia in 1621. The main value of the species has been in its pelt with thick fur, today sold under the 'Hudson seal fur' name. The meat is also consumed and called 'marsh rabbit'. In some places Catholics are allowed to eat the meat on days when only fish is allowed. In the early 1900s muskrat breeding in captivity commenced, however, the profitability was poor and now only few farms exist. The wild population provides enough for the demand. In many countries, in particular in Europe, where the species has been introduced it is regarded as an invasive pest.

Mouse

Mus musculus domesticus, a small rodent with several subspecies, widely spread in the wild but also closely associated with human habitation. Name is derived from the Latin *mus*, a mouse, but also said to be of Sanskrit origin from *mush*, to steal. The species has a long history, described by Aristotle, known to the Egyptians and the Romans (as a pet, a nuisance or tasty morsel). There has been a constant mouse-human relationship since these early times – either regarding the mouse as an abomination or as an endearing cult creature (Berry 1984, pp. 278–280). Of major importance in laboratory work.

Syrian Hamster

Mesocricetus auratus, also called the Golden Hamster. Their name is said to derive from a vernacular Arabic word. A rodent, now endangered in the wild but extensively studied and bred for use as a pet and laboratory work. First found in Syria, named in 1839 and then captured in 1930; a remarkably prolific species. Of interest are the large flexible cheek pouches, developed to allow the transport of food to their burrows.

Other mammals that have been utilised in some way are – racoon dogs (for fur); civets (for musk); several species of rats (for laboratory studies); and fur bearers such as the beaver, ocelot, racoon, ermine, sable, marten and wolverine (almost all caught from the wild).

References

Berry, R.J. (1984) in *Evolution of Domesticated Animals* (Ed. Mason I.L.). New York: Longman

Crane, E. (1984) in *Evolution of Domesticated Animals* (Ed. Mason I.L.). New York: Longman

Fletcher, J. (1984) in *Evolution of Domesticated Animals* (Ed. Mason I.L.). New York: Longman

Fletcher, J. (2011) Gardens of Earthly Delight: A History of Deer Parks. Oxford: Windgather Press

Novoa, C. and Wheeler, J. (1984) in *Evolution of Domesticated Animals* (Ed. Mason I.L.). New York: Longman

Olivier, R.C.D. (1984) in *Evolution of Domesticated Animals* (Ed. Mason I.L.). New York: Longman

Robinson, R. (1984) in *Evolution of Domesticated Animals* (Ed. Mason I.L.). New York: Longman

Skjenneberg, S. (1984) in *Evolution of Domesticated Animals* (Ed. Mason I.L.). New York: Longman

Tazima, Y. (1984) in *Evolution of Domesticated Animals* (Ed. Mason I.L.). New York: Longman

Vidal-Naquet, N. (2015) *Honeybee Veterinary Medicine*. Sheffield: 5m Publishing

Wilson, B. (2004) The Hive: The Story of the Honeybee and Us. London: John Murray

Zeuner, F. (1963) *A History of Domesticated Animals*. New York: Harper & Row

Animal Self-Medication

Myths, legends and folklore are a feature of the early years of a civilisation. Out of orally transmitted stories, frequently with much fantasy and mystery, a series of procedures and practices developed. In most cultures many of these are related to health and the prevention and treatment of disease. Apart from ritual procedures (always very important), there are also medications, invariably of herbs, plant parts or natural products. Frequently the folklore tells that these treatments were copied from the animals. Traditionally many people hold these beliefs. There are also many stories of animals self-medicating or using natural products to 'heal' themselves.

As science began to develop a base of logical thinking in the 1700s and 1800s attention was given to this subject. In a communication to the Biological Society, Delaunay (1885, p. 290) discusses the subject by noting that some species such as elephants, stags, birds and ants regularly wash and bathe and appear to observe good hygiene rules. Others rid themselves of ectoparasites by using dust, mud or clay, while those who have a fever restrict their diet and seek quiet and dark places. He determined a pattern of health-related behaviours that many animals exhibit, noting that dogs had long been known to eat certain species of grass as an emetic and purgative, and similar behaviour being seen in cats. Delaunay also stated that an animal suffering from 'chronic rheumatism' will avoid the sun. He recounted his observations that chimpanzees will staunch a bleeding wound with leaves or grass, and of those animals who seek water for cooling their bodies. He suggested that veterinary medicine and even human medicine could perhaps profit from a study of the medicine practised by animals.

Study of several aspects of animal self-medication in recent years has helped to build an understanding of some aspects of the subject, now named zoo pharmacognosy, but called by many people 'wild health'. The main topics are now recognised.

Geophagia

Hippocrates (c.460 BC–370 BC) mentions the eating of soil by humans, and the early Egyptians are known to have used clays medicinally. Some indigenous North American tribes were seen to use certain soils to improve the taste of bitter foods. The Tiv tribal people in Nigeria use a craving for soil by women as a sign of pregnancy.

It has been recorded that pregnant women in both Africa and the southern United States of America (USA) will eat soil to alleviate morning sickness, and it has been postulated that it may protect the foetus and mother from food-borne pathogens (Starks and Slabach 2012, pp. 17–18).

Many species of animals and birds have been seen to eat soil – elephants, deer, rabbits, bats, parrots and gorillas, baboons and chimpanzees. The usual explanation is that this is driven by a need for minerals, such as calcium, sodium and iron, to support their essential biological functions. Observations have shown that needs vary with the animal's age, health and season of the year. Sodium rich clays or rock salt deposits are a particular attraction for elephants and gorillas. Elephants have been recorded to regularly travel to rock salt caves to obtain the needed input. In the Himalayas, a similar salt (sodium) craving is seen and is used to capture wild yaks, also the gayal or mithan, a wild bovine in northern East India (see Chapter 18).

Studies have shown that consumption of earth can seldom provide enough mineral supplementation to the diet, but can interfere with the digestion of food. Clay-type soils are the most frequently consumed and it is known that the negatively charged clay molecule will bind easily to a toxin with a positive charge, preventing its absorption and allowing its elimination. Eating may be employed as a preventive measure which would allow the consumption of foods known to contain toxins. A study was organised in the 1990s by J Giraldi, executive director of the World Parrot Trust, to examine the detoxification hypothesis in Macaw parrots on the Manu river, Peru. It was known that the birds avoided mineral rich soils on the riverbank to eat a mineral deficient clay soil, it was assumed that this indicated a need to combat food toxins. A trial was undertaken where birds were fed a food containing quinidine (a toxic alkaloid), with or without an additional offering of the chosen soil. Blood tests showed that those who also ate the clay had their blood toxin (quinidine) level reduced by 60%. Selection of the riverside soil was giving the birds an ecological advantage over other species in allowing them to eat unripe fruits and seeds. Similar studies have been conducted on chimpanzees and baboons. It has also been observed that Amazonian bats visit clay licks; of those captured many were pregnant or lactating, probably indicating that they were consuming large amounts of food. This clay addition would help to detoxify unripe seeds and fruit that they were eating, and prevent harm to their offspring.

Cattle ranchers, by recognised custom, add clay to livestock feeds to inhibit possible pasture/grazing toxins. Many current pig and poultry rations include clay which has been found to be a good supporting matrix in feed, it slows down the transit of food in the gut to allow for better feed digestibility and nutritional uptake, probably by improving the contact between digestive enzymes and nutrients (Gallissot 2017, pp. 38–39). Current pharmacy for animals and humans, utilises a mineral clay, kaolin, to treat alimentary disorders and intestinal ailments.

There are many other observations recorded: some colobus monkeys will eat charcoal; elephants have been seen to pick up either wood or charcoal from forest fires and then exhale 'smoke'. Both cases possibly utilise the detoxifying value of charcoal. It must be noted that geophagia is not always beneficial – pathogenic organisms, parasites, lead or arsenic minerals may all be consumed with lethal effect.

An example of this is the condition seen in range cattle in South Africa termed *Lamziekte*. The cattle were seen to be gnawing on bones and, correctly, it was assumed they had a calcium craving, however, many suffered sudden death afterwards. It was eventually found that the bones were contaminated with botulism-causing bacteria (see Chapter 11).

The eating of soil is practised by both animals and humans, and can be seen to provide the eater with either a vital food ingredient, or an agent that will inactivate toxins or some harmful agents in the food or environment. It should not be considered abnormal; in humans it is termed pica (and regarded by psychiatrists as a mental aberration).

Topical Procedures

Some animals, mammals in particular, use their tongues with great frequency – for grooming, social interaction, sexual behaviour, cleaning their offspring after birth, drinking and aiding the procurement of food, some will also lick mineral rich rocks or salt rocks for the mineral content. Licking is the most common form of wound treatment in animals. Saliva has an antibacterial content and will exert some germicidal effect, and possibly provide a beneficial enzyme content to aid healing. The physical act of licking will also aid the sloughing of dead tissue. Licking as a part of general behaviour must make some contribution to personal hygiene.

Birds will regularly use dust 'baths' which appear to reduce skin mite and insect populations. Some use ants to obtain a similar effect. Chimpanzees can be seen to delouse members of their family and friends. Elephants will roll in mud which leaves a coating of soil, thought to be specifically beneficial to skin health. Buffalo and pigs both seek a wallow or watery mudhole in which to rest in times of high temperature. All of these appear to be instinctive beneficial actions on the part of the animal or bird and frequently can be seen to be enjoyable.

Specific wound treatment has been observed in several of the apes, in particular chimpanzees: they will either hold a hand over the wound or will apply grass and leaves as a dressing to stop blood flow and to protect the site. This positive action may be instinctive or taught by the parents.

Ingestion of Plant and Other Substances

There is a most extensive list of plants which animals and birds are said to select to ingest because of their value in prevention or treatment of various ailments. This is a most contentious topic – the active principle in the plant can be confirmed, but there is little substantive evidence that the ingested material has a specific medicinal effect.

Animals and birds in the wild are generally seen to be healthy, those that are sick are invariably not seen. For the major epizootic diseases, ranging from the cattle virus epidemics to anthrax or other serious bacterial infections it is obvious that self-medication is either not tried or does not work. Apes and other species are seen to eat the leaves of certain plants, some of these are chewed and others swallowed whole, to remove parasites from the gut, either by physical scouring or by anthelmintic effect; it is difficult to quantify the value of this ingestion, or even to know if it is undertaken for a specific reason. Claims for other specific actions, such as pain relief, have been made for certain plants.

One study of chimpanzees in Uganda (Masi 2012, p. 14) showed that when adults ate plants which were believed to be medically useful, the younger chimps tended to copy them, possibly they were learning, but the observers did not see any cases of chimps treating themselves. They noted that as it is very rare to see 'ill' chimpanzees, it was not possible to draw any conclusions. Study of adult gorillas in the Central African Republic eating medicinal plants, showed they were not copied by the younger members of the tribe; again no conclusions were reached.

It would appear that although animals do select certain plants to eat, the reasons for this behaviour is not clearly defined. An interesting and useful overview of these observations has been published in a book by Cindy Engel (2002); the author has drawn her own conclusions, but the text also provides a good starting point for others to continue the study.

Of interest is the fact that some animals will choose certain psychoactive plants or materials to obtain a desired effect. Certain monkeys, birds and elephants are known to enjoy fermented fruits with an alcohol content, this does not appear to be an accidental occurrence. And cats are well known for enjoying the delights of rolling in *Nepeta cataria* (catnip) plants, seemingly just for the mind-bending pleasure (see Chapter 23).

This appendix only provides a summary overview of the subject. It should be remembered that all animals, birds and aquatic creatures are continually fighting a disease onslaught. In the wild we only see the healthy ones, and they are alive perhaps because they have some understanding the need for a healthy diet, exercise and a mental stability (possibly some of these factors could be determined by genetic influences).

References

Delaunay, G. (1885) Medicine as Practised by Animals. *The Veterinary Journal* **20**

Engel, C. (2002) *Wild Health*. London: Weidenfeld & Nicholson

Gallissot, M. (2017) Seaweed and Clay, a New Feed Combination. *Feed Efficiency* June

Masi, S. (2012) Chimps Learn About Nature's Medicine. *New Scientist* 7 January (abstracted from Masi paper in *Physiology & Behaviour* 2011.08.012)

Starks, P.T.B. and Slabach, B.L. (2012) The Scoop on Eating Dirt. *Scientific American* June

Veterinary Journals and Periodicals

The start of formal veterinary education at Lyon, France in 1762 was a defining point in veterinary history, but it was soon realised that this was only the first step in creating an educated profession. The veterinary schools, and others, were making advances by disease observation, keeping records and conducting specific studies. The graduates in the isolation of their practices needed ongoing support. What was needed was the use of the printed word, from an authoritative source, to provide knowledge and to encourage readers to publish their own observations.

The very first periodical veterinary journal appears to have been the German *Archiv für Rossarzte und Pferdeliebhaber* published between 1788–1794, next the *Archiv für Wissenschaftliche ünd Praktische Tierheilkunde*, 1798–1881. By the turn of the century the need for such publications was spreading. In France, the *Recueil de Medicine Vétérinaire* was launched in 1824, in England *The Veterinarian* in 1828 and in Germany *Magazin für die gesamute Tierheilkunde* in 1835. The value of these publications was appreciated, and within the next few years almost every country with a veterinary school produced a journal. Some of these have survived well, in particular the *Rec. de Med. Vét.* Which was published until 1999; at 175 volumes it had one of the longest circulations of any veterinary journal.

As Europe exerted its influence with colonial expansion, the need for veterinary medicine followed, together with the national veterinary periodicals. The major impact was in British involvement in North America, India, Africa, Australia and New Zealand. British journals played a significant role until each country developed their own publications. It is of interest therefore to trace the early growth of these English-language publications.

By strange coincidence the first two British veterinary periodicals appeared on January 1st, 1828. These were *The Veterinarian* and *The Farrier and Naturalist*. They shared a common cause in their criticism of the London Veterinary College and its Professor, Edward Coleman: but there any similarities ended. *The Veterinarian* and its founder editor, William Percivall (1792–1854), had a much broader vision: to collect and spread professional knowledge, and over the next almost 200 years to the present time, there have been a succession of English-language journals and periodicals aimed at the veterinary profession. Mostly these have endeavoured to spread knowledge, a far smaller number have campaigned on a particular issue and generally have been short-lived.

The Veterinarian

The Veterinarian, published monthly between January 1828 and 1902, marked a milestone in the history of the British veterinary profession. It originated with William Percivall, Veterinary Surgeon to the 1st Life Guards. He was aware of the need for improving education for the increasing numbers of veterinary officers but he also perceived the quality of teaching at the London School to be poor. Percivall had not taken on an easy task and he was joined by William Youatt (1778–1847), as joint editor, in November 1828. Youatt's writing approach differed from that of Percivall, he tended to popularise his knowledge whereas Percivall wrote specifically for the profession. The journal had a difficult start, it was poorly patronised and contributors were few: the idea of writing clinical communications was novel. Only in the fourth year of publication did it cover its costs. Percivall dropped out in the early difficult period and the journal probably only survived because Youatt had taken editorial control, he returned in 1847 on Youatt's demise and was sole editor until he died in 1854.

The first issue carried on its title page a quotation from Vegetius, 'Ars veterinaria post medicinam secunda est'; this was Percivall symbolically nailing his message to the masthead. He was recognising the historical context of veterinary medicine as well as its art and science. No editorial names were listed. On page one was an editorial on the concept of veterinary periodical publishing, written in a rather low-key manner. There was no intention to bludgeon a message to the reader.

As the journal grew in readership and acceptance both the content and coverage improved. Of the clinical content a notable contribution was by James Castley in April 1830, when he wrote on laminitis in army horses in the Peninsular campaign: this was the first clinical paper from an army officer and probably the first clinical paper on laminitis. In December 1830, Castley also wrote of the poor quality of regimental veterinary hospitals. In February 1838, the first clinical paper on battle wounds was contributed by J S Beech – *Gunshot, Sabre, Lance and other Wounds*. In later years there were many publications on this most important topic.

An examination of the published communications gives a perspective on the problems of the time, both the diagnostic capabilities as well as the development of therapies and techniques. Not all of the volumes have been examined by the writer but some papers noted include *On Wood-Evil and Moor-evil* by W Cox (Vol 9, 1836, p. 677) the former disease was mastitis and the latter, 'a kind of rheumatism, but clearing on pasture change', both in cattle; *On the Diseases of Cats* (Vol 14, 1841, p. 676), noted as the first paper on the subject, and probably the first clinical communication on the feline topic in the English language; also seen was a paper, *Gasoline as a vermifuge* (Vol 75, 1902, p. 583), this was in the final volume of the journal. At the end of Volume 10 (1837) is a list of the veterinary graduates from the London and Edinburgh Schools, up to October 1837. It shows the origination of students: from the British army (43), India (35) and the USA and Canada (9). At its peak, *The Veterinarian* was almost required reading for those in practice in Britain with a significant readership in English-language countries overseas, in particular in North America.

Percivall wrote his last editorial in the December 1854 issue, he was asking what provision was being made for sick and wounded horses in the army. He refers to the Peninsular and Waterloo campaigns where little was done other than to drag them along at the tail of the regiment. When they could go no further they were destroyed. He was thinking of properly organised veterinary field hospitals: wounded and sick men were, at the time, treated little better. Following Percivall's death *The Veterinarian* was purchased by W J T Morton and J B Simonds and so passed into the hands of the London School. It struggled on for 20 years, entrapped in the inertia of the College. In 1902 it merged into John McFadyean's *The Journal of Comparative Pathology and Therapeutics*. The final issue carried no mention of its closure. The first, trailblazing English-language veterinary journal seemingly vanished without trace.

Farrier and Naturalist

Farrier and Naturalist was issued monthly between January 1828 and December 1829. The first issue was well written and presented, and used the word 'veterinarian' in the Preface. The opening article provides a useful history of the development of veterinary medicine in Britain and an overview of the veterinary schools at Lyons, Alfort, Vienna, Berlin, Copenhagen, Stuttgart, Wurtemburg and Utrecht. A particular mention is made of John Hunter and his interest in studying comparative anatomy.

On page 75, volume 1, there appears an article, strange to today's reader, on *Animal Phrenology*: this also states that plaster casts of the head of Eclipse could be obtained from Deville in the Strand, presumably to study the equine 'bumps'. This is followed by criticism of Coleman's behaviour and lack of 'productivity' at the College. Volume 2 (1829) carried the subtitle '*or Horseman's Chronicle*'.

The Hippiatrist

This journal is the rebadged *Farrier and Naturalist*, now also bearing the subtitle '*and Veterinary Journal*' and was issued monthly between January 1830 and December 1830. In an opening editorial the name change is explained as being a more suitable word to describe the members of the profession, as 'veterinary surgeon' is too cumbersome to include in a title. An interesting difference in the editorial content is the inclusion of material relating to cattle, this represents an important break away from the equine obsession, in spite of the new title. On pages 391–392 there appears an Address, which is in fact another good old go at the Veterinary College, claiming that Coleman still has a lot to learn about the horse. There are no closing words at the end of the last number. It was obviously felt (correctly), by the editors, that their work was done.

The Veterinary Examiner

This short-lived publication, issued monthly between December 1832 and February 1833, was subtitled '*and Monthly Record of Physiology, Pathology and Natural History*' and appeared to have had high minded objectives. No editor name is given but in the third and final issue a piece of editorial material is initialled 'E D S'. Most of the content of the three issues is reprinted from elsewhere. Whoever was behind the publication believed that a knowledge of the history of the veterinary art was an essential to understanding the science.

The first number has a lengthy opening article titled *History of Veterinary Medicine*, in which the author discusses the works of Vegetius (and recognising that most of this was of Greek origin), Columella, Cornelius Celsus, Ruellius (Hippiatrika), Xenophon and then cites significant authors from Britain and Europe up to Bourgelat. An interesting and still valuable overview. On page 24 is an early and perceptive quotation from H W Dewhurst that, 'a knowledge of morbid anatomy is the sheet anchor in ascertaining the symptoms of disease'.

On page 37 there is an article on the British Veterinary Schools. Discussing in turn the Royal Veterinary College, London University (Youatt's lectures); Charles Spooner's Anatomy lectures in his own theatre (Spooner was veterinary surgeon to the Zoological Society); Professor Dick's school in Edinburgh; the Andersonian University, Glasgow where the Professor of Veterinary Surgery was William Cheetham, and the Dublin Veterinary School noting that the Professorship had never been filled.

The second number, January 1833 was mainly composed of a continuation of the article in the previous issue on the *History of Veterinary Medicine*. This concentrates on continental works, mainly French, noting that the *Guide de Marechal* by La Fosse Jnr (1766) was an excellent work that had never been translated into English, and that there were only three copies of La Fosse's *Cours d'Hippiatrique* in the country, one each owned by Moorcroft and Blaine. The third and last number, February 1833, starts at page 81. The subject is again the *History of Veterinary Medicine* discussing the British authors including: Markham, Baret(*sic*), Duke of Newcastle, Snape, Gibson, and John Lawrence. There is a paper by Bracy Clark titled, *The Analogy between Gripes in Horses and Epidemic Cholera*, the author is listed as Fellow Linnaean Society (FLS) and Member Royal Institute of Paris.

Sportsman and Veterinary Recorder

Another short-lived publication, published monthly between January 1835 and June 1836; it is rare. No editor name is given. Much of the comment and editorial content is devoted to attacks on William Youatt, all unsigned. The attacks on Youatt were based on his frequently expressed belief that veterinary medicine and agriculture should be closely related, and that farmers should be educated in veterinary matters. This was an attitude which upset the profession who felt that the 'secrets' of their practice should be kept from the farmer. The veterinarian in practice was having a difficult life due to the large number of quacks and 'cattle and horse doctors'; they needed help to build their professional reputation. *The Sportsman and Veterinary Recorder* made little contribution to the work of the profession. It was intended to boost the image of the College and of Coleman, but it is doubtful that it achieved much. The end of Coleman's career was not far off.

The Centaur

A very rare publication (no copies are now known) with the subtitle '*A Journal of English and Foreign Medical Science and Agriculturalist's, Sportsman's and Naturalist's Register*'. It was published on a weekly basis between December 1836 and January 1837. The first British number ran the masthead line: No.1 London December 3rd 1836. The name of the editor is not given and as far as is known only seven issues appeared. *The Centaur* was the fifth veterinary periodical to appear and was the last of the scandal sheets, later publications all had a more serious veterinary scientific editorial stance.

While no copies of this periodical are available for examination, an outline of the publication was written by Sir Frederick Smith as part of his books on the history of veterinary literature. Smith noted written in ink on the issue, the name 'W Miles' as the editor. Miles, an American, was known as the leader of the student rebellion at the London College in 1836. Miles was also a contributor and wrote a series titled 'Diseases of the Horse' which appeared in each issue: in the judgement of Smith, Miles was a careful clinical observer. It appears that Miles was also the author of another regular column termed, 'Leaves From My Note-Book'. The publication had the primary functions of attacking both the College and William Youatt (then editor of *The Veterinarian*). In several issues there are interesting clinical communications, in one by Charles Clark, *Wounded Abdomen with Protruded Intestine in a half-bred Mare*, the author states that he replaced the gut and the animal survived.

Transactions of the Veterinary Medical Association

The Transactions of the Veterinary Medical Association (VMA) of the Royal Veterinary College appeared in three different formats during 1837–1850. The VMA was formed in 1836 as a successor to the Veterinary Medical Society.

Abstracts of Proceedings of the Veterinary Medical Association

Published as a monthly supplement in *The Veterinarian* from 1837–1841, as an 'exclusive' journal only for members of the profession. Copies contain a wealth of clinical information.

Transactions of the Veterinary Medical Association

Published at the College from 1841–1844 giving fuller reports of the meetings. The Transactions in this form never covered their costs; the policy changed and the series was continued as an 'open' journal.

The Veterinary Record

Subtitled 'and Transactions of the Veterinary Medical Association' published independently from 1845–1850. It was well produced with a strongly clinical, but varied, content including communications from India, translations of Continental publications, proposals and samples of new instruments and some veterinary history contributions. Publication ended suddenly, no reason was disclosed, but the VMA had, for some years been in decline.

Edinburgh Veterinary Review

The *Edinburgh Veterinary Review* was created and edited by John Gamgee, assisted by his father Joseph. It was produced on a monthly basis between July 1858 and 1864. Gamgee was a man of great, but mercurial, talent. His failing was in starting projects that he did not have the support (usually financial) to complete. Gamgee launched his *Review* soon after he had broken with Dick (of the original Edinburgh Veterinary School) and opened his rival Edinburgh 'New Veterinary College' in 1857. Through its columns he endeavoured to educate the country to be aware of the dangers which threatened from cattle plague, and also the need for public health and hygiene measures to be introduced to prevent the sale of diseased meat.

The *Edinburgh Veterinary Review* was well written and provided a vigorous vehicle for Gamgee's papers, as well as allowing him to publish his lectures to public authorities and some of his veterinary lectures and clinical communications. His main contribution was in stressing the danger of the foreign cattle trade introducing cattle plague and the disgrace of the absence of meat inspection controls. Publication ceased at the end of 1864 when Gamgee moved his veterinary school to London and in September 1865 he opened 'The Albert Veterinary College, Limited'.

Veterinary Review and Stockowner's Journal

The *Veterinary Review and Stockowner's Journal* was the continuation of Gamgee's Edinburgh periodical, following his move to London. It was published monthly between January and November 1865. The editors and format remained the same but only eleven numbers appeared. A new section, 'Periscope', was included dealing with farming and agricultural topics including the marketing of 'unsaleable meet' (*sic*). Proceedings of regional Veterinary Society meetings are included as well as a nice historical contribution by Joseph Gamgee, *The Five Epochs of History of Veterinary Science* (pp. 291–299). In the final number Gamgee printed his inaugural address to the first session of The Albert Veterinary College. The Albert College closed in 1868 – and Gamgee departed to the USA.

The Veterinary Journal

The Veterinary Journal was first published in July 1875 and is still published today on a monthly basis.

George Fleming CB, LLD, FRICS was the founder, and editor of *The Veterinary Journal*. He was a man of dynamic energy, rising to be Head of the Army Veterinary Service. He made an outstanding contribution to the profession by starting *The Veterinary Journal* and his prolific authorship of some 13 major books dealing with parasites, obstetrics, rabies, horse shoeing, anatomy and animal plagues as well as numerous contributions to other publications. Fleming started his periodical because he was a forward-looking, modern man and he knew that education was all important to the advancement of the profession. Fleming's army contacts encouraged authors in South Africa, India, Afghanistan and elsewhere. The letter pages were extensive and provide a valuable insight into the affairs of the profession. Fleming had taught himself all the major European languages and would translate papers of interest. Reading it now one can see why he succeeded. His journal was good, he wrote well and was an effective editor. When he retired as Editor in 1894 after 20 years' service, it was recorded that he had held the editorial chair 'with conspicuous zeal and ability'. At the time of writing, the Journal can look back on 145 years of publication.

Quarterly Journal of Veterinary Science in India

The *Quarterly Journal of Veterinary Science in India*, published quarterly between 1882 and 1890, had a subsidiary title *'and Army Animal Management'* and was established by J H Steel MRCVS and Frederick Smith MRCVS when they were both in the army service in India. It was the first veterinary journal in India, and the first English-language publication dealing with tropical diseases. The editorial masthead stated that the Editor was Charles Steel FRCVS, Inspecting Veterinary Surgeon, Bombay Army and Superintendent Army Veterinary School, Poona.

The content had highly topical editorials, good presentation and detailed surveys of health problems, which provided for the first time information that was essential for the control of animal disease in India. Financially the journal never covered its costs and Steel and Smith had to fund the deficit. Production difficulties were significant; the typesetters could not read English but knew the characters, nevertheless considerable time had to be given to corrections. Smith left India in 1885 but remained a co-editor. As Steel Snr. had also returned to the United Kingdom (UK) the whole editorial load fell on J H Steel; he died at the end of 1888 and the journal died with him. Copies are now scarce. It bore on the cover the words *Primus in India*, it was not only first, but it was also of a quality that was not equalled for many years. In volume 1, (page 143) is an editorial headed '*On the Urgent Necessity for an Indian Civil Veterinary Department*': the editors had a strong pioneering streak.

Journal of Comparative Pathology and Therapeutics

The *Journal of Comparative Pathology and Therapeutics* was first published in March 1888 and is still published today on a quarterly basis.

John McFadyean (later Sir John) had considerable success with his first two books. His publishers had confidence in him when he proposed an ambitious venture: he wanted to produce a new type of scientific journal, to be issued quarterly with each number to be about 100 pages, with himself as sole editor. He was determined, as was his publisher, for the periodical to at least cover its costs fairly quickly. It was a huge undertaking but McFadyean wanted an outlet for his own work and also for the rapidly growing disciplines of bacteriology and pathology, as well as a platform for his own opinions.

The first number started with a scientific paper by McFadyean, on *The Pathology of Haemoglobinuria (Azoturia) of Horses*. It was a good and well written paper with colour illustrations. It put the stamp of science and quality on the journal and he had chosen the horse, then the major veterinary interest patient, as his lead subject: he not only discussed the topic expertly, but made his point about honesty in science, careful observation and experimentation, plus caution in reaching conclusions. In the first volume McFadyean wrote 15 editorials: all dealing either with diseases of critical importance or matters of current interest: both tuberculosis and bovine pleuro-pneumonia were discussed.

The journal was successfully launched. Both scientific and literary standards were high: by the time the fourth number was published the financial concerns were forgotten. Recognised teachers sent him good papers, an Abstracts section was included to cover the French and German literature. McFadyean's own contributions were well chosen, well written and well received, but not peer-reviewed (he had confidence). He made the journal, his journal – he was editor, abstractor, translator, reporter and reviewer. He edited the scientific articles that he accepted and only a few items were included in which he was not directly involved. His journal was recognised by the profession as a 'good read', in particular his editorials. In 1902 he absorbed *The Veterinarian*.

The 50th year volume was completed in 1937: it attracted worldwide tributes and included an eight page listing of McFadyean's publications. The 175 page edition was a unique event in British veterinary periodical publishing. McFadyean had to give up his editorial role in 1939, he had completed the first part of volume 53, which was published in 1940. The 100th year was celebrated by volumes 98 and 99. Now in the hands of Elsevier, the *Journal of Comparative Pathology* reached its 132nd year in 2020. The solid groundwork that McFadyean gave it has lasted well.

The Veterinary Record

The Veterinary Record was first published on July 14th, 1888, and is still in publication. The birth of this unique weekly veterinary periodical is due to William Hunting, a student of John Gamgee. He had considered launching a weekly journal for some time, but was always short of funds: his idea was to base it on the valuable clinical presentations given to the increasingly active local veterinary society meetings. In 1888 Thomas Dollar loaned him £50 (it is said he never paid it back) and the *Record* came into being. Issue number one had just 12 pages. Hunting wrote well, followed the latest developments, watched legislation and expressed his opinions with force. Above all he was a practitioner and understood their environment. It was not long before virtually all the British veterinary profession not only read, but eagerly awaited, their weekly copy.

Hunting remained totally in charge for the first 20 years of publication, but in 1905 relinquished his role as lead writer due to his official duties, but remained as editor until his death in 1913. In 1920 the National (now British) Veterinary Association purchased the ownership for £500: a move that saved the Association, membership grew rapidly. In 2021 as the *Record* moved into its 133rd year of publication it has also reduced its frequency to a fortnightly schedule.

The Veterinary News

The Veterinary News was published weekly between 9 January 1904 and 24 September 1920.

A publisher's venture, initially appearing as a supplement to *The Veterinary Journal* it was launched as *The Veterinary News and Bulletin*. The opening editorial was bland, '. . . starts on a new and separate career . . ., week by week', there was no indication of the editor's name, it most probably was Wallis Hoare. The format, layout and general approach was a close copy of *The Veterinary Record*; however, it did not have either the clinical 'punch' or the editorial content to match. When Hoare's health began to fail, about 1918, he passed the editorial role to his friend Henry Gray but there was little he could do. In the post-war years and depression period it was difficult to hold or to generate subscriptions. In the editorial of the last issue, Gray wrote of the difficult times, 'more than half of the profession do not take any publication'.

Tropical Veterinary Bulletin

Published on a quarterly basis starting October 1912 until 1930, this abstracting periodical was issued under the direction of the Hon. Managing Committee of the Tropical Diseases Bureau. The content was devoted to tropical diseases. There were very long, selected, abstracts plus many shorter and some articles simply listed. Quality was good, there was extensive recognition of publications in other languages, in particular German, also some French and some Russian; with comprehensive indexing a reader could get an appreciation of the world publications. In 1930 the publication was absorbed into the *Veterinary Bulletin*. While not in the journal category the *Tropical Veterinary Bulletin* follows the short-lived *Quarterly Journal of Veterinary Science in India* 1882–1890 in recognising the importance of tropical medicine. It was the first English-language publication on the subject.

The Veterinary Review

This periodical, published quarterly between 1917 and 1920, is not to be confused with Gamgee's journal of the same name that closed in 1865. It was a bold initiative by O Charnock Bradley while he was Principal of the Royal (Dick) Veterinary College, Edinburgh. It was the first English-language veterinary periodical solely devoted to review articles. The selection of both authors who, and subjects which, were wide ranging was good. The articles (some on veterinary history) were of a high calibre, in a genre that was not to come into its own for many years, but 1917 was the third year of the first world war. In the first issue Bradley wrote, 'in 1914 there were about 100 periodicals professedly devoted to veterinary science' and in ending the editorial his words were, 'The conditions of the moment are certainly not ideal for the appearance of a periodical'. He was correct, publication ceased with the fourth volume in 1920.

These early publications were major factors in the development and progression of veterinary clinical practice as well as providing trustworthy vehicles for research workers to describe their results. In later years in all countries more specialist veterinary research journals would appear.

British journals were obviously well accepted in all their overseas colonial and dominion countries. In the early days of veterinary medicine in the USA, *The Veterinarian* enjoyed a good readership, encouraged by the editorship of William Youatt who had found a growing market for his books, in particular *The Horse*. British veterinary books were widely circulated in the early years (1700–1800s); in Pennsylvania, with a large German emigrant population German works were widely read.

The important national veterinary periodicals were sponsored and published in almost all cases by the national associations.

United States of America

The first periodical was published by the rather enigmatic George Dadd with the *American Veterinary Journal* 1851–1852 and 1855–1859. Next Alexandre Liautard edited the *American Veterinary Review* in 1877 which, as the national association evolved, became the *Journal of the American Veterinary Association* in 1915 and is still in print together with the *American Journal of Veterinary Research*, launched in 1940.

Australia

The national association in collaboration with their New Zealand colleagues launched the *Australasian Veterinary Journal* in 1882. This ceased when the national association introduced the *Australian Veterinary Journal* in 1925.

New Zealand

Initially a partner in the *Australasian Veterinary Journal* in 1882, then after some years established the *New Zealand Veterinary Journal* in 1952.

India

While still under colonial rule a group of Madras (Chennai) veterinarians launched the *Indian Veterinary Journal* in 1924, still in print. In 1930 the Indian Council of Agricultural Research established the *Indian Journal of Veterinary Science*, now replaced by the *Indian Journal of Veterinary Science and Biotechnology*.

South Africa

In 1927 *The Journal of the South African Veterinary Association* was launched after the national associations unified, still in print. In 1903 the Onderstepoort Veterinary Institute began a publication, in 1933 this was named *Onderstepoort Journal of Veterinary Research and Animal Industry*, to be renamed the *Onderstepoort Journal of Veterinary Research* in 1951.

Canada

Following action by the Canadian Veterinary Medical Association in 1960 the *Canadian Veterinary Journal* commenced publication.

It is fitting to close with the words of William Percivall (1792–1854) who compared the pages of *The Veterinarian* to a safe, 'where records could be placed in custody for future generations'. Veterinary clinical and scientific periodicals, now published worldwide in a profusion of languages and a multiplicity of topics, have become an essential part of the discipline of veterinary medicine, for both clinician and research worker.

Timeline of People and Events

BC dates should be regarded as approximate, and the earliest as presumptive.

BC

c3000–2000   *Huangdi Neijing* Chinese internal medical compendium transmitted orally.

2000–1500   Books of the Veda. *Ayurveda* and *Rigveda*: Sanskrit medical/veterinary texts.

2000–1000   *Zend-Avesta*. Zoroastrian religious texts: instructions on animal healing and care.

2838–2698   **Shen Nang** Probably mythical author of *Pen-tsao Ching* herbal pharmacopoeia.

2700–2600   **Ma Shihuang** Named 'horse doctor' to Emperor Huang di.

2200–2100   **Urlugalidenna** Named on Mesopotamia cylinder seal as 'animal healer'.

1900–1800   El-Lahun Veterinary papyrus, first description of animal diseases.

c1930   Eshnunna Laws nos.55/56 relating to dog control, possibly rabies.

c1800   Hammurabi Legal Code nos. 224/225 refer to 'doctor of animals'.

c1750   **Abil-iliso** Named as 'bovine healer'.

1500–1300   Ugarit tablets. Texts detailing equine ailments and treatments.

c1360   Kikkuli text. Tablets on specialist horse management.

700–600   Assyrian tablets. Fragments suggest an equine almanac.

600–500   **Alcmaeon** Early descriptions of animal dissection and anatomy.

500–400   **Simon of Athens** Wrote early treatise on horse care.

480–420   **Herodotus** Historian, much travelled, discussed animal topics.

470–402   **Democritus** Wrote on anatomy and veterinary topics.

460–375   **Hippocrates** Most famous medical personality of antiquity.

430–354   **Xenophon** Wrote three equine and one dog book: care and management.

428–348   **Plato** Leading Athenian philosopher. Founded Lyceum, first higher learning institute.

400–300 Alexandrian Medical School most productive period.

384–322 **Aristotle** First genuine scientist and contributor to veterinary medicine.

370–287 **Theophrastus** First systemic botanist, identified veterinary medicaments.

c350 Charaka Samahita Hindi medical/veterinary text.

c350 **Mago of Carthage** Notable Carthaginian agricultural author.

335–280 **Herophilus** Anatomist, human dissection and studies at Alexandria.

304–250 **Eristratus** Anatomist, human dissection and studies at Alexandria.

273–232 **King Ashoka** establishes animal sanctuaries and veterinary care (India).

234–149 **Cato** Early agricultural treatise with veterinary advice.

116–26 **Varro** Widely read agricultural treatise with sensible veterinary advice.

70–19 **Virgil** Wrote *Georgics* poem. Recognisable descriptions of animal disease symptoms.

63 BC–AD 14 **Grattius** Wrote about dogs including ailments and management.

AD

25 BC–50 AD **Celsus** Notable medical and veterinary author.

4–70 **Columella** Most complete extant Roman text on agriculture and animal health.

23–79 **Pliny** First encyclopaedia including some animal disease content.

c.100 **Dioscorides** Wrote on medicinal plants, drugs, milks, the dog.

c.100 *Huangdi Neijing* Chinese text transcribed by Han scholars (200 BC–AD 220).

86–160 **Arrian** Writings include work on dogs (style of Xenophon).

170–230 **Aelian** Important author on animals and their characteristics.

100–200 **Oppian** Poet, major work on fish including health and diseases.

129–219 **Galen** Leader of Roman medical world, believed in comparative medicine.

200–300 **Anatolius** Produced farmers' almanac with veterinary content.

200–300 **Martialis** Wrote on cattle cures: doubtful value.

200–300 **Eumelus** Described as 'great horse doctor': only quotations exist.

200–300 **Nemesianus** Poet, wrote on dog training, diseases and breeds.

200–300 Susrata Samahita Hindi medical/veterinary text.

300–400 **Apsyrtus** Most important and original veterinary author of ancient Greece.

300–400 **Hippocrates** (the 'veterinarian') Wrote mainly on equine hoof and digestive tract.

300–400 **Chiron** Anonymous author of *Mulomedicina Chironis*, useful content.

300–400 **Pelagonius** Equine practitioner, wrote *Ars Veterinaria*.

300–400 **Theomnestus** Wrote on the horse, mostly copied from Apsyrtus.

400–450 **Vegetius** Wrote *Artis Veterinariae Sive Mulomedicinae* much sensible content.

400–500 **Palladius** Author of final Roman agricultural treatise, with veterinary chapter.

400–500 **Hierocles** Lawyer, wrote equine text mostly Apsyrtus derived.

526–605 **Alexander of Tralles** Wrote *De Lumbricus* (On worms). First parasitology text.

705–707 *Si mu an jiji* first comprehensive Chinese veterinary text, written by Li-Shi.

720–815 **Geber** Islamic alchemist, laid basis for chemical science.

808–873 **Johannitus** (Hunaya ibn Ishaq). Important Arabic translator of Greek texts.

800–900 Anglo-Saxon *Leech Book*, includes veterinary medicine.

865–932 **Rhazes** Leading Islamic clinician and diagnostician.

980–1037 **Avicenna** Famous Islamic physician, wrote *Canon of Medicine*.

900–1000 *Hippiatrica* Compilation of early veterinary texts ordered by Byzantine Emperor.

900–1000 *Geoponika* Compilation of early agricultural texts ordered by Byzantine Emperor.

1094–1162 **Avenzoar** Andalusian Islamic physician and surgeon (operated on animals).

c1000 *Hastyayurveda* Sanskrit elephant treatise by Muni Palakapya (date questionable).

1098–1179 **Hildegard of Bingen** Abbess, wrote on animal diseases including mange.

1100–1200 *Anatomia Porci* text by Copho on pig anatomy, for medical students.

1135–1204 **Maimonides** Jewish Physician/philosopher, profound thinker on medicine/diet/hygiene.

1200–1280 **Albertus Magnus** Author *De Animalibus* on animals, including disease.

1250? **Jordanus Ruffus** Wrote on hippiatry based on Arabic texts.

1200–1300 **Walter of Henly** Author *Husbandry*, livestock management and disease.

1340–1379 **Jehan de Brie** Treatise on sheep diseases for King of France, described fascioliasis.

1347–1351 The Black Death – 30% to 60% of Europe's population die.

1331–1391 **Gaston Phebus** Author *Livre de Chasse*, hunting text with care of dogs.

1340 **Laurance Rusius** Author *La Marescalia*, complemented Ruffus work.

1350 **Juan Alvares de Salamiella** Spanish treatise on equine diseases.

1355 **Andreas Albrecht** First known German veterinary author.

1480–1533 **Girolamo Frascato** Physician defined animal epidemic diseases and contagion.

1486 *Boke of Seynt Albans* attributed to Juliana Bernes, hunting text, disease mentioned.

1495 **Don Manual Diaz** Printed *Libro de Albeytaria . . .*, based on Ruffus.

1493–1541 **Paracelsus** Brilliant Swiss physician, alchemist, introduced laudanum, defined toxicity.

1516–1590 **Ambrose Paré** French barber-surgeon treated conflict wounds, men and horses.

1522 **Francisco de la Reyna** Author *Libro de Albeytaria* Spanish.

1523 *Boke of Husbandry* by John Fitzherbert, names animal diseases.

1528 *Artis Veterinariae* by Vegetius, printed in Basel in Latin.

1530 *Hippiatrica* compilation translated to Latin by Jean de la Ruellius, printed Paris.

1538 *Geoponika* compilation printed in Venice in Latin.

1566 **Thomas Blundeville** *The Fower Chiefyst Offices . . .* equine management and some diseases.

1599 **Carlo Ruini** *Anatomia Del Cavallo* landmark veterinary medicine text.

1568–1637 **Gervase Markham** Prolific plagiarist author, harmed veterinary progress.

1578–1657 **William Harvey** Described blood circulation, a medical/veterinary breakthrough.

1592–1676 **William Cavendish** Author *Traite d'equitation* magnificent book.

1608 **Yu BenYuan** and **Yu Ben-Heng**, Chinese brothers equine text, many reprints.

1613 **Thomas Spackman** Physician, first English book on rabies.

1626–1697 **Franceso Redi** Italian, described as founder of parasitology.

1646 **Sir Thomas Browne** Physician and polymath first used the word 'veterinarian'.

1664 **Jacques Labessie de Sollysell** Published *Le Parfait Maréchal*, on equine diseases.

1673 **Michael Harward** Innovative veterinary author *The Herdsman's Mate . . .*

1683 **Andrew Snape** Published *The Anatomy of the Horse*.

1698 **Sir John Floyer** Named 'broken wind' in the horse.

1633–1714 **Bernardino Ramazzini** Studied rinderpest, then epidemic control.

1656–1720 **Giovanni Mario Lancisi** Identified rinderpest (1711), proposed controls.

1668–1738 **Herman Boerhaave** Physician, evolved 'clinical' medicine, studied animals.

1680–1750 **William Gibson** Notable author *A New Treatise on Diseases of Horses*.

1708–1777 **Albrecht von Haller** Pupil of Boerhaave, 'founded' physiology.

1714 **Thomas Bates** Described rinderpest in Britain and defined controls.

1679–1729 **Johann Kanold** Early epidemiologist, described rinderpest spread into Europe.

1700–1777 **Gerard von Swieten** Austrian medical leader, saw the need for veterinary medicine.

1726–1808 **Peter Hernquist** Created first Swedish veterinary school.

1729–1799 **Giovanni Battista Morgagni** Credited as founder of pathological anatomy.

1733 **Stephen Hales** (1677–1761) *Essay containing Hemostatics*, explaining blood pressure.

1733–1804 **Joseph Priestley** Isolated 'dephlogisticated air' (oxygen), physiology advanced.

1734–1806 **James Clark** Scottish veterinary practitioner, saw the need for veterinary schools.

1735 **Carl Linnaeus** Formalised binomial nomenclature in *Systema Naturae*.

1737–1789 **Luigi Galvani** Demonstrated animal electricity.

1738–1820 **Johann Gottlieb Wolstein** Opened Vienna Veterinary College.

1739–1795 **Paul Adami** Appointed Professor veterinary medicine at Krakow University.

1740–1801 **Peter Christian Abildgaard** Outstanding veterinarian, created first Danish school.

1743–1794 **Antoine Lavoisier** Named oxygen, founder of modern chemistry.

1746–1846 **William Youatt** Leading British veterinary author of books, and on rabies.

1748 *On the Distemper of Horses* publication of Vegetius AD 450 book in English.

1750–1793 **Charles Vial de Sainbel** Lyon graduate, Heads London School 1791, dies 1793.

1750–1822 **Erik N Viborg** Followed Abilgaard at Danish School. First good book on pigs.

1751–1752 *Encyclopédie* published. Claude Bourgelat wrote several contributions.

1762 **Claude Bourgelat** (1712–1779) Lyon Veterinary School.

1766 **George Stubbs** Publishes *The Anatomy of the Horse*, excellent plates.

1767–1825 **William Moorcroft** Studied at Lyon, first British veterinary graduate.

1770–1845 **Delabere Pritchett Blaine** Gifted author *Canine Pathology*, and clinician.

1780 **Lazzaro Spallanzani** Priest, biological research, first AI in dog.

1793–1866 **William Dick** Opened first Edinburgh veterinary school, many graduates went overseas.

1739–1820 **Philippe-Etienne LaFosse** Author *Cours d'Hippiatrique*, important work.

1803–1873 **Justus von Liebig** Father of organic chemistry and biochemistry.

1816 **R-T-H Laennec** (1781–1826) Invented the stethoscope.

1822–1895 **Louis Pasteur** Established immunology with first bacterial and virus (rabies) vaccines.

1843–1910 **Robert Koch** Established bacteriology, 1881 invented petri dish, 1882 isolated tubercle bacillus.

1850–1903 **Edmond Nocord** Alfort professor, leading bacteriologist.

1853–1933 **Emile Roux** Immunologist, with Pasteur; helped establish Pasteur Institute.

1853–1941 **Sir John McFadyean** Gifted research worker and teacher.

1853 First Mexican veterinary school established, difficult history, University faculty in 1955.

1855 **George Dadd** Opened first veterinary school in the USA, short-lived; competent graduates.

1857 New York College of Veterinary Surgeons, failed, became American Veterinary College to 1899.

1860–1934 **Ferenc Hutyra** Eminent Hungarian researcher and Head Budapest School.

1862 **Andrew Smith** Canada, Created longest viable North American veterinary college in Toronto.

1863 **John Gamgee** (1831–1894) Teacher, author, called first meeting of World Veterinary Association.

1865 **Joseph Lister** (1827–1912) Pioneered antiseptic surgery.

1866 British State Veterinary Service began, as result of rinderpest outbreak.

1866 **Duncan McEachran** (1841–1924) Montreal Veterinary College, excellent course, but short life.

1875 **August Chaveau** (1827–1917) Director Lyon School anatomist and researcher.

1877 **Paul Ehrlich** (1854–1915) Established haematology, important in chemotherapy research.

1880 **Henri Toussaint** (1847–1890) Developed early anthrax vaccine (copied by Pasteur).

1884 **Daniel E Salmon** (1850–1914) First DVM graduate in USA. Headed BAI from 1884–1905.

1888 **Emil von Behring** (1854–1917) Discovered diphtheria antitoxin.

1888 **V Babes** (1854–1926) Discovered piroplasms (*Babesia*).

1889 **Theobald Smith** (1858–1934) Discovered *Babesia bigemina*, cause of Texas Fever.

1889 **Fred Lucius Kilbourne** (1858–1934) Worked with Smith on Texas Fever.

1897 **Hugo Preisz** (1860–1949) Produced first swine fever antiserum.

1898 **Friedrich Loeffler** (1852–1915) Isolated FMD virus, also glanders, swine erysipelas and others.

1898 **Bernhard Bang** (1848–1932) Isolated *Brucella abortus*, cause of bovine abortion.

1902 **Aladár Aujeszky** (1869–1933) Isolated pseudo-rabies virus.

1907 **Jozsef Marek** (1868–1952) Studied poultry virus polyneuritis, named Marek's disease.

1929 **Alexander Fleming** (1881–1955) Discovered penicillin, but could not develop.

1935 **Gerhard Domagk** (1895–1964) Discovered first antibacterial, sulphonamide (*Prontosil*).

1942 **Ernst Chain** (1906–1979) and **Howard Florey** (1898–1968) Purified penicillin, first antibiotic.

2011 Rinderpest. First animal disease to be eradicated globally.

Index